THE FAT COUNTER

High protein diets, low protein diets, good carbs, bad carbs—one thing remains the same: Fat counts. And consumers are increasingly monitoring their fat intake to reduce the risk of heart attacks and other diseases.

If you are among the millions of Americans looking to do just that, you'll want to keep *The Fat Counter* handy. By presenting fat and saturated fat values for thousands of foods, in addition to laying out the difference between good fats and bad ones—*and* demystifying trans fats—this popular nutrition guide is a one-of-a-kind resource.

Now in its sixth edition, *The Fat Counter* presents cutting-edge nutrition news, reliable counts, and helpful tips for healthy eating—all in one convenient, easy-to-use guide.

THE FAT COUNTER

More than one million copies sold!

"An excellent investment."
—*Fitness* magazine

W9-BIX-951

Books by Annette B. Natow and Jo-Ann Heslin

The Antioxidant Vitamin Counter
Calcium Counts
The Calorie Counter (Third Edition)
The Cholesterol Counter (Sixth Edition)
The Complete Food Counter
Count On a Healthy Pregnancy
Eating Out Food Counter
The Fat Attack Plan
The Fat Counter (Sixth Edition)
The Food Shopping Counter (Second Edition)
Get Skinny the Smart Way
The Healthy Heart Food Counter
Megadoses: Vitamins as Drugs
The Most Complete Food Counter
No-Nonsense Nutrition for Kids
The Pocket Encyclopedia of Nutrition
The Pocket Fat Counter (Second Edition)
The Pocket Protein Counter
The Pregnancy Nutrition Counter
The Protein Counter (Second Edition)
The Sodium Counter
The Ultimate Carbohydrate Counter
The Vitamin and Mineral Food Counter

Published by POCKET BOOKS

THE
FAT COUNTER

6th Edition

**Annette B. Natow, Ph.D.
and Jo-Ann Heslin, M.A., R.D.**

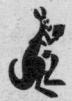

POCKET BOOKS
New York   London   Toronto   Sydney

POCKET BOOKS, a division of Simon & Schuster, Inc.
1230 Avenue of the Americas, New York, NY 10020

Copyright © 1989, 1993, 1995, 1998, 2000, 2005 by
Annette B. Natow and Jo-Ann Heslin

All rights reserved, including the right to reproduce
this book or portions thereof in any form whatsoever.
For information address Pocket Books, 1230 Avenue
of the Americas, New York, NY 10020

ISBN: 0-7434-6440-0

First Pocket Books paperback printing of this revised edition
February 2005

10 9 8 7 6 5 4 3 2 1

POCKET and colophon are registered trademarks of
Simon & Schuster, Inc.

Manufactured in the United States of America

For information regarding special discounts for bulk purchases,
please contact Simon & Schuster Special Sales at 1-800-456-6798 or
business@simonandschuster.com.

To our families, who support us through every project:
Harry, Allen, Irene, Sarah, Meryl, Laura, Marty,
George, Emily, Steven, Rebecca, Joseph, Kristen,
Brian, Karen, and John.

ACKNOWLEDGMENTS

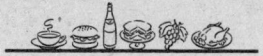

For graciously sharing her knowledge, Karen J. Nolan, Ph.D.

For all her support and help, our agent, Nancy Trichter.

For her suggestions and editing skills, Sara Clemence.

Without the tireless cooperation of Steven Natow, M.D., Stephen Llano, and Sarah Wright, *The Fat Counter, 6th Edition* would never have been completed.

A special thank you to our editor, Micki Nuding.

> *"From hundreds of digestion experiments we have learned . . . that an ounce of pure carbohydrate or pure protein will yield 113 Calories . . . an ounce of fat, 255 Calories . . . the more fat a food contains, the higher its energy value."*

> Mary Swartz Rose, Ph.D.
> *Feeding the Family*
> The Macmillan Company, 1919

CONTENTS

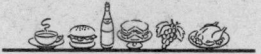

THE EVOLVING FAT STORY

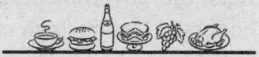

Forget reality TV, the real action is happening on the fat front. In the low fat, high carb corner are true believers, government agencies, and professional organizations who zealously support the "less is best" theory of fat consumption. In the other corner, the high fat, low carb group is led by diet book authors, but following close behind are some respectable researchers and epidemiologists (scientists who study trends in populations).

How did we get to this standoff? If we look at our recent eating history as rounds in a boxing match, Round 1 would be the 1970s. At that point, researchers were examining both sides of the fat issue—moderate to high fat intakes versus low fat intakes. Both sides scored points for their position. Then along came the U.S. Department of Agriculture and the first national dietary guidelines, which convinced many professional groups that low fat was best.

Round 2 was the 1980s, when "all you can eat" low fat eating plans and fat free foods were crowd pleasers. The food industry flooded the market with low fat products and the American public literally ate them up, getting heavier and heavier. The idea that fats make you fat but carbs don't didn't prove true. What was forgotten in this period was the basic premise of low fat eating: eat less fat, but replace the fat with high fiber carbohydrates, fruits, and vegetables. Americans did eat less fat but fiber, fruits, and vegetables never had a chance against low fat cookies, nonfat salad dressings, and plates full of pasta.

Then came Round 3. The low fat group was close to a knockout. Researchers, the government, and many professional groups had endorsed low fat, high carb as the way to go. All that was needed was one last vote by the public to make the decision unanimous. The problem, however, was that the public was having trouble fitting through the revolving doors of the arena. They were heading to the mall to buy this season's wardrobe in the plus size stores.

In the wings, this whole time, was a small but vocal group of unlikely allies—diet book authors touting high fat, low carb eating plans, along with some researchers and epidemiologists. They were seeing something very interesting. People who cut back on carbs and ate more fat didn't get fat. Instead, they were losing weight and their risk for heart disease went down.

So instead of the knockout expected, the high fat group got up off the mat and came back strong. People started shunning carbs, and eating bacon and butter again. The food industry began churning out a whole new selection of low carb, higher fat products.

Stay tuned for Round 4. Researchers are seeing a shift in the basic paradigm of healthy eating. Over the last 35 years (and since the first time *The Fat Counter* was published), we've learned a great deal. We are now redirecting recommendations from a low fat to a moderate fat message. And, more importantly, we realize that not all fats are created equal. Some are good for us, some are bad for us, and some probably should be avoided altogether.

Fast Fat Fact

The simplistic view that all "fats are bad" is no longer accurate.

ALL FATS ARE NOT
CREATED EQUAL

Basic Fat Facts

Fats, or *lipids,* as the scientists would refer to them, is actually an umbrella term for several similar substances. You get fats from the foods you eat, and your body can manufacture some fats. Food fats are made up of strands of *fatty acids.* You can think of these fatty acids as strands of beads that vary in combination and number of beads, depending on their chemical composition.

There are three main types of fatty acids—saturated, monounsaturated, and polyunsaturated. Foods contain a combination of all three, but we label foods as sources of saturated, monounsaturated, or polyunsaturated based on the predominant fat in the food. Recent research suggests that the *type* of fat you eat may be more important than the *amount.*

Good, Bad, and Baddest

Monounsaturated fats fall into the *good* category. Monounsaturated fats—olive oil, nuts, avocados, and olives—are the major fats eaten by people who follow the much-praised Mediterranean diet. But you can't simply dunk Italian bread in

FOOD SOURCES OF DIFFERENT FATS

Type of Fat	Foods	Health Effects
Monounsaturated fats	Olive oil, canola oil, peanut oil, avocados, olives, cashews, peanuts, hazelnuts, macadamia nuts, pine nuts, pistachios, chicken fat	Reduce cholesterol Reduce triglycerides Reduce blood pressure Help control diabetes
Polyunsaturated fats or omega-6 fats	Safflower oil, sesame oil, or soybean oil, corn oil, sunflower oil, nuts, seeds, soybeans, soft margarine	Reduce cholesterol Reduce heart disease risk
Polyunsaturated fats or omega-3 fats	Canola oil, flaxseeds, soybean oil, walnut oil, walnuts, hempseeds, salmon, mackerel, tuna, trout, sardines, herring	Reduce triglycerides Improve immune function Reduce inflammatory diseases Protect against sudden death from heart disease Reduce tumor growth
Saturated fats	Meat, whole milk, cream, ice cream, cheese, butter, lard, poultry, palm oil,	Raise cholesterol Increase heart disease risk Increase stroke

FOOD SOURCES OF DIFFERENT FATS (*continued*)

Type of Fat	Foods	Health Effects
	palm kernel oil, coconut, coconut oil, cocoa butter, bacon, sour cream	risk May increase cancer risk
Trans fats	Cookies, crackers, cakes, candies, shortening, stick margarine, deep-fried foods (french fries, doughnuts), partially hydrogenated oils, hydrogenated vegetable oils	Raise cholesterol Lower HDL "good" cholesterol Raise LDL "bad" cholesterol Increase heart disease risk

olive oil and expect to be healthy. The Mediterranean lifestyle includes not only olive oil, but plenty of fruits and vegetables, less whole milk, cheeses, and meats, and a lot of activity. Research, however, does indicate that when you substitute olive oil and other foods high in monounsaturates for foods high in saturated fat, your risk for heart disease goes down.

Polyunsaturated fats also fall into the *good* category. They not only reduce blood cholesterol but also improve your immune function and protect you against inflammation, another risk factor in the development of heart disease. There are two main groups of polyunsaturated fats: omega-6 and omega-3. Just think of them as two different strands of beads, similar in shape but different in color sequence. Each is important to good health, so eating foods with both is important.

Omega-6 fats are those you usually associate with polyunsaturated fats—most types of vegetable oils. More than 80% of the vegetable oil used in the U.S. is soy oil. Even if you don't use soy oil at home, it's the preferred oil used by food manufacturers and restaurants, so you are probably eating more than you realize. Based on that, it's wise to select another type of vegetable oil for home use. And probably even wiser to vary the type of oil you buy.

Omega-3 fats are in shorter supply in our diets. It's been estimated that the ratio of omega-6 fats to omega-3 fats should range from 5:1 to 10:1 for health benefits. In typical American diets, the ratio is about 20:1. This means you need to make an effort to eat foods higher in omega-3 fats—fish, olive oil, canola oil. Research is showing that this imbalance in the polyunsaturated fats we eat may be contributing to higher risks for cancer, heart disease, and arthritis. The good news is that eating as little as 2 servings of fish a week—a rich source of omega-3 fats—can lower your risks.

Fast Fat Fact

To protect yourself from "sudden cardiac death," which causes half of all heart disease deaths, eat more fish rich in omega-3 fats.

Saturated fats fall into the *bad* category. Saturated fats are those found mainly in animal foods—meats, whole milk, and cheese—and tropical oils, such as palm and coconut. They are twice as potent at raising your blood cholesterol levels as polyunsaturates are at lowering it. You can't eliminate all saturated fats from your diet, and you really don't have to, but it is important to limit them. That's easy when it comes to milk, cream, sour cream, and cheese. Simply choose the nonfat or lower fat versions. When it comes to meat, choose leaner cuts and smaller portions.

Fast Fat Fact

Exercise helps you burn fat. A study showed that your body burns more polyunsaturated fats than saturated fats after exercising. Saturated fats were more likely to be stored; just another reason to eat less of them.

If there was a category called the "baddest" fats, trans fat would fit nicely. Trans fat not only raises total blood cholesterol but also lowers "good" HDL cholesterol. Many feel it's a greater health risk than saturated fats. The good news is that we don't have to eat it.

Almost all the trans fat found in our foods is created artificially by passing hydrogen gas through vegetable oil, a process called *hydrogenation*. Hydrogenated fats or partially hydrogenated fats are more stable for deep-frying and are more solid, so they work well in baking and as the base for stick margarines. It's estimated that we eat 12% to 14% of our daily calories as saturated fat but only 1.5% to 2.5% as trans fat. Cutting down or eliminating foods with trans fats will not eliminate any important nutrients from your diet. In fact, it may help you cut back on less healthy choices like french fries and cakes.

HOW MUCH FAT SHOULD YOU EAT?

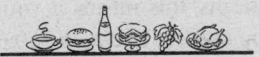

Let's set the record straight. Even though the current research suggests that moderate fat intake may be more healthy, no one is suggesting a *high* fat intake is good for you.

Eating too much fat puts you at risk for:

- Heart disease
- Stroke
- High blood pressure
- High cholesterol
- Cancer
- Obesity
- Diabetes
- Arthritis
- Gout
- Age-related macular degeneration (ARMD), a leading cause of blindness
- Alzheimer's disease, a leading cause of dementia

In 2002, for the first time, the Institute of Medicine of the National Academies of Health gave dietary recommendations for the amount of fat you should eat. The experts recommended a range of fat intake from 20% to 35% of total calories each day. They further recommended that the amount of saturated and trans fat be kept as low as possible, because as the intake of each went up, so did the risk for heart disease.

In practical terms, this means if you regularly eat 1,800 calories a day, somewhere between 360 (20%) and 630 (35%) calories should come from fat. To convert fat calories to grams of fat, all you need to know is that 1 gram of fat = 9 calories. Using the example of 1,800 calories, the grams of fat each day would range between 40 to 70.

The table on page 11 will help you set your own daily target fat intake. First, select the number of calories you eat each day. Next, select the percentage of fat calories you wish to eat, and the chart will give you the grams of fat to aim for daily.

Because no specific recommendation was made for saturated fat, and you were simply advised to keep your intake as low as possible, you may be asking, "How low is low?" The National Cholesterol Education Program has recommended that 7% of daily calories come from saturated fat. Other groups have suggested 10% or less. Using common sense, and knowing that we currently eat between 12% and 14% of our daily calories as saturated fat, anything under 10% would be a significant reduction and provide you with health benefits.

DAILY TARGET FAT INTAKE

Calories per day	Percentage of Fat Calories Each Day in Grams of Fat			
	20%	25%	30%	35%
1,000	22	28	33	39
1,100	24	31	37	43
1,200	27	33	40	47
1,300	29	36	43	51
1,400	31	39	47	54
1,500	33	42	50	58
1,600	36	44	53	62
1,700	38	47	57	66
1,800	40	50	60	70
1,900	42	53	63	74
2,000	44	56	67	78
2,100	47	58	70	82
2,200	49	61	73	86
2,300	51	64	77	89
2,400	53	67	80	93

Fast Fat Fact

When you eat less total fat, you automatically eat less saturated fat and less trans fat.

FINDING FATS IN FOOD

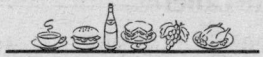

Food surveys show that Americans have heard the message to reduce their intakes of fat, saturated fat, and cholesterol. But hearing and believing a message, and then acting on that information, are two entirely different things. We're hearing but we're not doing.

We may be eating more poultry and fish than red meat, but we still eat 57 pounds a year more of all of them than we did in the 1950s. Meanwhile, our consumption of cheese, high in saturated fat, nearly quadrupled. And the consumption of fats and shortenings has climbed to slightly over 35 pounds per person per year.

Instead of eating less fat, people are trading fats. Less red meat but more poultry and cheese. Less butter but more salad dressing.

These same studies show us that most people are not good at recognizing hidden fats in foods—in pastries, pizza, casseroles, sandwiches, drinks. We need to upgrade our fat-finding skills.

And more importantly, we need to eat less food. Today, we eat 300 more calories every day than we did 20 years ago. By eating more of everything, we also wind up eating more fat. This creates an interesting statistical picture. The percentage of calories we eat as fat each day has gone down, but the actual amount of fat we eat has gone up. Why? Because we are eating more food and we are eating more convenience food that has a lot of hidden fat.

What's On the Label?

Food labels offer a lot of information and are worth reading. There are 3 places to look for information: claims on the front label, the ingredient list, and the nutrition facts panel. Each tells you something different about the food you are buying.

Label claims for fat have been legally defined. If the label says:

Fat Free   In one serving, the food has 0.5 grams of fat or less. Foods in this group can also be called "nonfat."

Low Fat   In one serving, the food has 3 grams of fat or less.

Reduced Fat   In one serving, the food has 25% less fat than the traditional product. Foods in this group can also be call "lower fat."

Light   In one serving, the food has at least 33% fewer calories or 50% less fat than the traditional product. Foods in this group may also be called "lite."

Lean   In one serving, the food has less than 10 grams of total fat, less than 4.5 grams of saturated fat, and less than 95 milligrams of cholesterol.

Extra Lean   In one serving, the food has less than 5 grams of total fat, less than 2 grams of saturated fat, and less than 95 milligrams of cholesterol.

On food labels, ingredients are listed in descending order by amount. The ingredient listed first is found in the largest amount. If fat, butter, or oil is close to the beginning of the list, you can be fairly confident there is a good deal of fat in each serving. The ingredient listing can also help you find "hidden fats." All of the following ingredients add fat to food.

Butter	Oil
Cheese	Partially hydrogenated fat*
Chicken fat	Partially hydrogenated oil*
Cocoa butter	Peanut butter**
Cream	Shortening*
Cream cheese	Sour Cream
Diglycerides	Suet
Fat	Tropical oil*
Hydrogenated fat*	Vegetable fat**
Hydrogenated oil*	Vegetable shortening*
Lard	Whipped cream
Margarine**	Whole milk
Monoglycerides	

* Contains trans fat.   ** May contain trans fat.

The nutrition facts panel tells you the grams of total fat and the grams of saturated fat in a serving of food. Starting in 2006, it will also show the grams of trans fat, though some companies will provide those values sooner. In addition to gram values, "% Daily Value" is also listed.

Daily Values (DV) are standards developed by the Food and Drug Administration (FDA) to represent the needs of a "typical" consumer eating 2,000 calories a day. The Daily Value for total fat is 65 grams. The percentage listed on the individual food label tells you the percent of 65 grams provided by one serving of that food. If the label tells you the food provides 30% of your DV for the day, you know immediately this is a high fat food. The Daily Value for saturated fat is 20 grams. Some labels voluntarily list gram values for monounsaturated and polyunsaturated fats. If they don't, you can subtract the grams of saturated fat from the grams of total fat. The remainder is the approximate sum of monounsaturated and polyunsaturated fats in that food.

No Daily Value will be listed for trans fats when it starts to appear on nutrition labels in 2006. Although a relationship has been shown between eating trans fat and an increased risk for heart disease, the FDA does not feel there is enough information available to set a DV. Foods that are most likely to contain trans fats are:

- foods containing hydrogenated or partially hydrogenated oil
- foods containing shortening
- deep fat-fried foods and snacks
- stick margarines
- cheese foods
- cake and cookie mixes
- crackers

Many food manufacturers are reformulating their products to try to cut down on trans fats. You should be seeing more trans fat-free products as time goes on. And food consumption surveys are already starting to show a small but steady decline in the amount of trans fats we eat yearly.

Nutrition Fact Panel

Nutrition Facts
Serving Size 1 cup
Servings Per Container 2

Amount Per Serving

Calories 280 **Calories from Fat** 120

	% Daily Value*
Total Fat 13 g	20%
Saturated Fat 5 g	25%
Trans Fat 2 g	
Cholesterol 30 mg	10%
Sodium 680 mg	28%
Total Carbohydrate 31 g	10%
Dietary Fiber 0g	0%
Sugar 5 g	
Protein 5g	

← will be added to labels by January 2006

* Percent Daily Values are based on a 2,000 calorie diet.
Your Daily Values may be higher or lower depending
on your calorie needs.

Fast Fat Fact

Total fat is most important. There's little health benefit in choosing a food low in trans fat but high in saturated fat.

What's on Your Plate

Many fats you eat are visible—the fat around a steak, butter, and oil. Others are not that easy to see—fat baked into a muffin or the fat used to fry potato chips may no longer look like fat, but it still adds up. In other cases, it may be tempting to overdo—like pouring dressing on a salad or heaping grated cheese on pasta.

Though a moderate amount of fat adds flavor to foods, helps you feel fuller after a meal, and may have health benefits, all fats are loaded with calories. Snacking on walnuts, rich in omega-3 polyunsaturated fats, is a good idea. But eat a *handful,* not a *canful.* Adding olive oil-rich salad dressing to your greens not only tastes good, but is healthy. Just remember that 2 tablespoons is a serving. Because all fats pack a caloric wallop in a small amount, it's easy to eat too much.

Fast Fat Fact

1 teaspoon of fat = 45 calories
1 teaspoon of carbohydrate (starch and sugar)
= 20 calories
1 teaspoon of protein = 20 calories

When cooking, use nonstick cooking sprays to coat pans. Some brands offer butter or olive oil varieties that can add a punch of flavor to cooked pasta, rice, or potatoes. Measure, don't pour, when adding oil to a frying pan, dressing to your salad, gravy to meat, or sour cream to your potato. A tablespoon or 2 is fine; more starts to pack on calories.

There are now reduced fat versions of old high fat favorites—whipped cream, half & half, sour cream, ice cream, cream cheese, and peanut butter. Switching could save you thousands of calories in a year.

> ### Fast Fat Fact
> *To find out if a food has hidden fat, place it on a napkin or blot the top.*
>
> *· greasy napkin = hidden fat*

Keeping fats moderate:

- Choose lean cuts of meat and poultry
- Eat fried, battered, and breaded foods only occasionally
- Eat lower fat versions of milk, yogurt, cheese, and ice cream
- Measure fats you add on—butter, margarine, sour cream, cream cheese, peanut butter
- Eat nuts and seeds by the handful, not the canful
- Broil, roast, grill, and steam
- Eat tuna and sardines packed in water
- Use tub margarine or whipped butter
- Avoid self-basted turkeys
- Eat small portions of cookies, cakes, candies, and pastries
- Trade pasta in cheese sauce for pasta in tomato sauce

> ### Fast Fat Fact
> *Most nonstick cooking sprays list "0" calories for a ⅓-second spray but it takes 1 second or longer to cover a 10-inch pan.*
>
> *A 1-second spray = 5 to 7 calories, less than 1 tablespoon of oil with 120 calories, but still, seconds count.*

TRACKING FAT

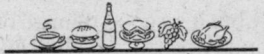

There are many reasons to keep track of the fat you eat. Too much fat puts you at risk for health problems. Too much fat causes you to gain weight. Too much saturated fat increases your risk for heart disease.

Eating the right amount of fat may help you lose weight, control risks for heart disease, and manage diabetes. And, when you make the effort to write down what you eat, you learn a lot about how you eat, why you eat, and when you eat. Many of us eat on the go, substituting meals with a snatch-and-grab lifestyle, giving little thought to what we're eating. If you pay closer attention to what and how much you eat, we guarantee you'll see positive results.

Fast Fat Fact

People cut calories by 10% when they write down what they eat. 30 to 50% of those who keep food records make positive changes in their eating habits.

The Fat Counter, 6th Edition is the best source you can use to count fat. With over 21,000 foods listed, values for everything you eat are at your fingertips. The easiest way to determine how much fat you should be eating each day is to look at the table on page 11 to decide your target daily fat intake.

Use Your Daily Fat·Diary on page 21 to keep track of the fats and calories you eat. You don't have to track your saturated fat intake daily, but it's a good thing to do once in a while to see if you're meeting the recommendations.

Your Daily Fat Diary will tell you a lot about how you eat, why you eat, and what you eat. Research has shown that men are more likely to omit items than women, both sexes are more likely to omit snack items, and meat items are more likely to be underestimated. No one will ever see what you write down, so be honest.

We suggest you note the day and date, because you may eat differently on different days of the week. Some people eat more on weekends or days off; others eat more at work. If you keep track, you may begin to see patterns.

We appreciate that many people eat on a crazy schedule, so the day is broken into 3 periods. That will help you figure out when you do the most eating.

A.M. is from midnight till noon. Many people eat in the middle of the night, so A.M. includes middle-of-the-night noshing, breakfast, and coffee break or morning snack.

Midday is from noon until dinner. It includes lunch and any afternoon or pre-dinner snack, like a drink after work.

P.M. is dinnertime through midnight. It includes your evening meal and after-dinner, TV, and bedtime snacks.

By subtotaling your fats and calories 3 times during the day, you can make adjustments for unexpected situations. For example, if you plan to have a big dinner, you can eat a lighter lunch and skip your afternoon snack to compensate for the extra calories you'll be eating in the evening.

YOUR DAILY FAT DIARY

Your Target Calorie Zone _____
Day _____

Your Daily Fat Grams _____
Date _____

	Food	Portion	Calories	Total Fat	Saturated Fat
AM					
AM Totals					
Midday					
Midday Totals					
PM					
PM Totals					
Daily Totals					

USING YOUR FAT COUNTER

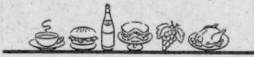

The Fat Counter, 6th Edition lists the portion size, calories, total fat, and saturated fat values for more than 21,000 foods. Now you can compare the values in your favorite foods and, when necessary, choose substitutes before you go out to shop or eat. This will save you time and help you decide what to buy.

The counter section of the book is divided into two parts: Part One: Brand Name, Nonbranded, and Take-Out Foods; and Part Two: Restaurant Chains. Each part lists foods or restaurant chains alphabetically.

In Part One, for each category, you will find nonbranded (generic) foods listed first, in alphabetical order, followed by an alphabetical listing of brand name foods. The nonbranded listings will help you estimate calorie and fat values when you don't see your favorite. They can also help you to evaluate store brands. Large categories are divided into subcategories such as canned, fresh, frozen, and ready-to-eat, to make it easier to find what you're looking for. Some categories have *see* and *see also* footnotes, to help you find related items.

Because we eat out so often, we list more than 500 take-out foods in Part One. These are found in the take-out subcategory in many categories throughout this section. Look there for foods you take out or order in, because these foods are not nutrition labeled.

Most foods are listed alphabetically. But in some cases,

foods are grouped by category. For example, a tuna sandwich is found in the SANDWICH category. Other group categories include:

ASIAN FOOD   Page 36
   includes all types of Asian foods except
   egg rolls and sushi, which are found in
   separate categories

DELI MEATS/COLD CUTS   Page 230
   includes all sandwich meats except
   chicken, ham, and turkey, which are
   found in separate categories

DINNER   Page 233
   includes all by brand name, except
   pasta dinners, which are found in a
   separate category

LIQUOR/LIQUEUR   Page 337
   includes all alcoholic beverages and
   mixed drinks except beer, champagne,
   and wine, which are found in separate
   categories

NUTRITION SUPPLEMENTS   Page 365
   includes all dieting aids, meal
   replacements, and drinks, except
   energy bars and energy drinks, which
   are found in separate categories

SANDWICHES   Page 468
   includes popular sandwich choices

SNACKS   **Page 485**
includes a variety of miscellaneous
snack items such as trail mix, pork
rinds, and cheese puffs

SPANISH FOOD   **Page 519**
includes all types of Spanish and
Mexican foods except salsa and
tortillas, which are found in separate
categories

In Part Two, Restaurant Chains, 97 national and regional restaurants are listed, including candy, coffee, doughnut, ice cream, pizza, burger, seafood, sandwich, and ethnic food chains. Brand name foods are required by law to have nutrition information on labels. Restaurants, however, provide this information voluntarily.

With *The Fat Counter, 6th Edition* as your guide, you will never again wonder how many fats and calories are in the foods you eat.

DEFINITIONS

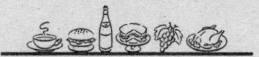

as prep (as prepared): refers to food that has been prepared according to package directions

lean and fat: describes meat with some fat on its edges that is not cut away before cooking, or poultry prepared with skin and fat as purchased

lean only: refers to lean meat that is trimmed of all visible fat, or poultry without skin

shelf stable: refers to prepared products found on the supermarket shelf that are ready-to-eat or ready to be heated and do not require refrigeration

take-out: describes prepared dishes that you purchase ready-to-eat; those included serve as a guide to the calories, fats, and saturated fats in products you may purchase

ABBREVIATIONS

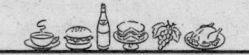

avg	=	average
diam	=	diameter
fl	=	fluid
frzn	=	frozen
g	=	gram
in	=	inch
lb	=	pound
lg	=	large
med	=	medium
mg	=	milligram
oz	=	ounce
pkg	=	package
pt	=	pint
prep	=	prepared
qt	=	quart
reg	=	regular
sec	=	second
serv	=	serving
sm	=	small
sq	=	square
tbsp	=	tablespoon
tr	=	trace
tsp	=	teaspoon
w/	=	with
w/o	=	without
<	=	less than

NOTES

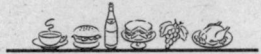

Cals = Calories

Fat = Total fats

Sat Fat = Saturated fats
All fat and saturated fat values are given in grams.

— (dash) indicates that values are not available

tr (trace) = less than 1 gram of fat or saturated fat

0 (zero) indicates there are no calories, fat, or saturated fat in that food

Discrepancies in figures are due to rounding, product reformulation, and reevaluation. Labeling law allows rounding of values. Some the data listed is analysis data obtained directly from manufacturers, not from labels. Therefore, some values may differ from labels because they have not been rounded.

PART ONE

Brand Name, Nonbranded (Generic), and Take-Out Foods

Fast Fat Fact

Some fat in a meal helps you feel fuller longer. A study showed that people who ate fat free muffins ate more calories later on. Those who ate muffins with some fat felt fuller and ate less afterward.

FOOD	PORTION	CALS	FAT	SAT FAT
ABALONE				
fresh fried	3 oz	161	6	1
raw	3 oz	89	1	tr
ACEROLA				
fresh	1	2	tr	—
ACEROLA JUICE				
juice	1 cup	51	1	—
ADZUKI BEANS				
canned sweetened	1 cup	702	tr	—
dried cooked	1 cup	294	tr	—
AKEE				
fresh	3.5 oz	223	20	—
ALCOHOL (see BEER AND ALE, CHAMPAGNE, LIQUOR/LIQUEUR, MALT, WINE)				
ALE (see BEER AND ALE)				
ALFALFA				
sprouts	1 tbsp	1	tr	tr
sprouts	1 cup	40	tr	tr
ALLIGATOR				
cooked	3 oz	126	2	—
ALLSPICE				
ground	1 tsp	5	tr	tr
ALMONDS				
almond butter honey & cinnamon	1 tbsp	96	8	1
almond butter w/ salt	1 tbsp	101	9	1
almond butter w/o salt	1 tbsp	101	10	1
almond meal	1 oz	116	5	tr
almond paste	1 oz	127	8	1
dried unblanched	1 oz	167	15	1
dry roasted unblanched	1 oz	167	15	1
dry roasted unblanched salted	1 oz	167	15	1
dry roasted w/ salt	24 nuts (1 oz)	170	15	1
jordan almonds	10 (1.4 oz)	190	7	1
oil roasted blanched	1 oz	174	16	2
oil roasted blanched salted	1 oz	174	16	2
oil roasted unblanched	1 oz	176	16	2

FOOD	PORTION	CALS	FAT	SAT FAT
praline	17 pieces (1.4 oz)	210	12	1
toasted unblanched	1 oz	167	14	1
Judy's				
Sugar Free Coconut Almond Brittle	¼ piece (1 oz)	90	5	2
Keto				
Chocolatey Covered	1 oz	169	13	6
Lance				
Smoked	1 pkg (0.8 oz)	130	10	1
Low Carb Creations				
Soft Almond Brittle	2 pieces (1 oz)	170	12	2
Mama Mellace's				
Butter Rum	1 oz	150	10	1
Cinnamon Roasted	1 oz	140	9	1
Maranatha				
Almond Butter	2 tbsp	220	18	1
Raw Almond Butter	2 tbsp	190	17	2
Tamari Almonds	¼ cup	160	14	2
Planters				
Almonds	1 oz	170	15	1
Gold Measure Slivered	1 pkg (2 oz)	340	31	3
Honey Roasted	1 oz	160	14	1
Sweet Delights				
Almond Roasters	⅓ pkg (1 oz)	190	14	–
AMARANTH				
leaves cooked	1 cup	28	tr	tr
uncooked	1 cup (6.8 oz)	729	13	3
ANCHOVY				
canned in oil	1 can (1.6 oz)	95	4	1
canned in oil	5	42	2	tr
fresh fillets	3 (0.4 oz)	21	1	–
fresh raw	3 oz	62	4	1
ANGLERFISH				
raw	3.5 oz	72	1	–
ANISE				
seed	1 tsp	7	tr	–
ANTELOPE				
roasted	3 oz	127	2	1

FOOD	PORTION	CALS	FAT	SAT FAT

APPLE
CANNED
| sliced sweetened | 1 cup | 137 | 1 | tr |

Del Monte
| Fruit Pleasures Pie Spiced Apples | ½ cup (4.1 oz) | 70 | 0 | 0 |

Luck's
| Fried Apples | ½ cup (4.7 oz) | 130 | 0 | 0 |

DRIED
cooked w/ sugar	1 cup	232	tr	tr
cooked w/o sugar	1 cup	145	tr	tr
rings	10	155	tr	tr

Sonoma
| Pieces | 10-12 pieces (1.4 oz) | 110 | 0 | 0 |

FRESH
apple	1 lg	125	1	tr
apple	1 sm	63	tr	tr
apple	1 med	81	tr	tr
w/o skin sliced	1 cup	63	tr	tr
w/o skin sliced & cooked	1 cup	91	tr	tr
w/o skin sliced & microwaved	1 cup	95	tr	tr

Chiquita
| Apple | 1 med (5.4 oz) | 80 | 0 | 0 |

Cool Cut
| Apples & Caramel Dip | 1 pkg (4.25 oz) | 180 | 5 | 2 |

Tastee
| Candy Apple | 1 (3 oz) | 160 | 5 | 2 |
| Caramel Apple | 1 (3 oz) | 160 | 5 | 2 |

FROZEN
| sliced w/o sugar | 1 cup | 83 | 1 | tr |

Stouffer's
| Escalloped | 1 cup (6 oz) | 180 | 3 | 0 |

TAKE-OUT
| baked | 1 (5.3 oz) | 126 | tr | tr |
| baked no sugar | 1 (5.9 oz) | 82 | 1 | tr |

APPLE JUICE
frzn as prep	1 cup	111	tr	tr
frzn not prep	1 can (6 oz)	350	1	tr
juice + vitamin C	1 cup	117	tr	tr

FOOD	PORTION	CALS	FAT	SAT FAT
mulled cider	1 serv	265	1	tr
After The Fall				
Organic	1 bottle (10 oz)	110	0	0
Vermont Apple	1 bottle (8 oz)	90	0	0
Vermont Apple	1 bottle (10 oz)	110	0	0
Apple & Eve				
100% Juice	8 fl oz	110	0	0
Cider	8 fl oz	110	0	0
Eden				
Organic Juice	8 oz	80	0	0
Everfresh				
Apple Juice	1 can (8 oz)	110	0	0
Hansen's				
Junior Juice 100%	1 box (4.23 oz)	60	0	0
Langers				
100% Cider	8 oz	120	0	0
100% Juice	8 oz	120	0	0
Diet Cocktail	8 oz	60	0	0
Mott's				
100% Juice	1 box (8 oz)	120	0	0
100% Juice	8 fl oz	120	0	0
100% Natural	8 fl oz	120	0	0
Nantucket Nectars				
100% Pressed	8 oz	100	0	0
NutraBalance				
Plus Fibre	1 pkg (8 oz)	120	0	0
Ocean Spray				
100% Juice	8 oz	110	0	0
Odwalla				
Spiced Harvest Cider	8 fl oz	130	0	0
Snapple				
Snapple Apple	8 fl oz	120	0	0
Squeezit				
Green Apple	1 bottle (7 oz)	110	0	0
Swiss Miss				
Hot Apple Cider Mix	1 serv	84	tr	0
Hot Apple Cider Mix Low Calorie	1 serv	14	0	0
Tropicana				
Season's Best	8 oz	110	0	0

FOOD	PORTION	CALS	FAT	SAT FAT
Turkey Hill				
Herbal Cider w/ Chamomile & Lemongrass	1 cup	100	0	0
Veryfine				
100% Juice	1 bottle (10 oz)	150	0	0
Juice-Ups	8 fl oz	120	0	0
White House				
Juice	8 oz	120	0	0
APPLESAUCE				
sweetened	½ cup	97	tr	tr
unsweetened	½ cup	52	tr	tr
Eden				
Organic	½ cup	50	0	0
Organic Sweet Cinnamon	½ cup	50	0	0
Jok'n'Al				
Low Carb	1 tbsp	10	0	0
Mott's				
Single-Serve Cinnamon	1 pkg (4 oz)	100	0	0
Single-Serve Natural	1 pkg (4 oz)	50	0	0
Single-Serve Original	1 pkg (4 oz)	100	0	0
White House				
Applesauce	½ cup (4.4 oz)	90	0	0
Chunky	½ cup (4.4 oz)	90	0	0
Cinnamon	½ cup (4.5 oz)	100	0	0
Natural Plus	½ cup (4.4 oz)	70	0	0
APRICOT JUICE				
nectar	1 cup	141	tr	tr
APRICOTS				
CANNED				
halves heavy syrup pack w/ skin	1 cup (9.1 oz)	214	tr	tr
halves water pack w/ skin	1 cup (8.5 oz)	65	tr	tr
halves water pack w/o skin	1 cup (8 oz)	51	tr	tr
heavy syrup	3 halves	99	tr	tr
juice pack	3 halves	51	tr	tr
puree from heavy syrup pack w/ skin	¾ cup (9.1 oz)	214	tr	tr
puree from light pack w/ skin	¾ cup (8.9 oz)	160	tr	tr
puree from water pack w/ skin	¾ cup (8.5 oz)	65	tr	tr

FOOD	PORTION	CALS	FAT	SAT FAT
puree juice pack w/ skin	1 cup (8.7 oz)	119	tr	tr
water pack	3 halves	30	tr	tr
Del Monte				
Halves Unpeeled Lite	½ cup (4.3 oz)	60	0	0
Orchard Select Halves Unpeeled	½ cup (4.4 oz)	80	0	0
DRIED				
halves	4	32	tr	tr
halves cooked w/o sugar	½ cup	153	tr	tr
Del Monte				
Sun Dried	⅓ cup (1.4 oz)	80	0	0
Sonoma				
Dried	10 pieces (1.4 oz)	120	0	0
FRESH				
apricots	1	17	tr	tr
Chiquita				
Apricots	3 med (4 oz)	60	1	0
FROZEN				
sweetened	½ cup	119	tr	tr
ARROWHEAD				
corm boiled	1 med	9	tr	—
flour	1 cup	457	tr	tr
ARTICHOKE				
CANNED				
Progresso				
Hearts	2 pieces (2.9 oz)	30	0	0
Hearts Marinated	2 pieces (1.1 oz)	170	5	1
S&W				
Marinated Hearts	2 pieces (1 oz)	20	2	0
FRESH				
cooked	1 med	60	tr	tr
hearts cooked	½ cup	42	tr	tr
FROZEN				
cooked	1 pkg (9 oz)	108	1	tr
Birds Eye				
Hearts	½ cup	40	0	0
ARUGULA				
fresh	½ cup	3	tr	tr

FOOD	PORTION	CALS	FAT	SAT FAT
ASIAN FOOD (*see also* DINNER, EGG ROLLS, SUSHI)				
CANNED				
chow mein chicken	1 cup	95	tr	tr
Chun King				
Beef Pepper Oriental BiPack	1 cup (8.8 oz)	98	2	1
Chow Mein Beef BiPack	1 cup (8.6 oz)	78	1	tr
Chow Mein BiPack Chicken	1 cup (8.8 oz)	98	3	1
Chow Mein Pork BiPack	1 cup (8.6 oz)	78	2	1
Hot & Spicy Chicken BiPack	1 cup (8.6 oz)	98	3	1
Sweet & Sour Chicken BiPack	1 cup (8.9 oz)	161	2	1
La Choy				
Beef Pepper Oriental BiPack	1 cup (8.8 oz)	98	2	1
Chow Mein Beef BiPack	1 cup (8.6 oz)	78	1	tr
Chow Mein Chicken BiPack	1 cup (8.9 oz)	98	3	1
Chow Mein Shrimp BiPack	1 cup (8.6 oz)	52	1	tr
Main Entree Chow Mein Chicken	1 cup (9.3 oz)	80	4	1
Oriental Beef w/ Noodles BiPack	1 cup (8.8 oz)	156	3	1
Oriental Chicken w/ Noodles BiPack	1 cup (8.7 oz)	154	4	1
Sweet & Sour Chicken BiPack	1 cup (8.9 oz)	161	2	1
Teriyaki Chicken BiPack	1 cup (8.6 oz)	109	3	1
FRESH				
wonton wrappers	1	23	tr	tr
Azumaya				
Round Wraps	10	160	1	0
Square Wraps	6	160	1	0
Wrappers Large Square	3	170	1	0
Nasoya				
Egg Roll Wrappers	3	170	1	0
Won Ton Wrappers	8	160	1	0
FROZEN				
Amy's				
Bowls Teriyaki	1 pkg (10 oz)	300	2	0
Skillet Meals Teriyaki Stir Fry	1 cup	320	3	0
Stir Fry Asian Noodle	1 pkg (10 oz)	240	5	1
Stir Fry Thai	1 pkg (9.5 oz)	270	11	7
Banquet				
Fried Rice w/ Chicken & Egg Rolls	1 meal (8.5 oz)	330	9	3
Birds Eye				
Easy Recipe Creations Oriental Lo Mein	2¼ cups	230	4	1

FOOD	PORTION	CALS	FAT	SAT FAT
Easy Recipe Creations Sesame Ginger Teriyaki	2¼ cups	140	2	0
Easy Recipe Creations Spicy Szechuan Cashews	2¼ cups	180	5	1
Green Giant				
Create A Meal LoMein Stir Fry as prep	1¼ cups (10 oz)	320	70	2
Create A Meal Sweet & Sour Stir Fry as prep	1¼ cups (10 oz)	290	7	1
Create A Meal Szechuan Stir Fry as prep	1¼ cups (10 oz)	340	15	4
Create A Meal Teriyaki Stir Fry as prep	1¼ cups (10 oz)	240	6	1
La Choy				
Beef Pepper Oriental	1 cup (7.1 oz)	151	1	tr
Chow Mein Vegetable	1 cup (8.9 oz)	108	2	tr
Lean Cuisine				
Everyday Favorites Oriental Style Dumplings	1 pkg (9 oz)	300	6	2
Everyday Favorites Teriyaki Stir Fry	1 pkg (10 oz)	290	4	1
Rice Gourmet				
Chicken Teriyaki Rice Bowl	1 bowl (10.9 oz)	430	6	1
Stouffer's				
Chicken Chow Mein w/ Rice	1 pkg (10.6 oz)	260	5	1
Tyson				
Chicken Fried Rice Kit w/ Sauce	1 pkg (14 oz)	440	6	2
Weight Watchers				
Smart Ones Chicken Chow Mein	1 pkg (9 oz)	200	2	1
Smart Ones Hunan Style Rice & Vegetables	1 pkg (10.34 oz)	280	0	2
Smart Ones King Pao Noodles & Vegetables	1 pkg (10 oz)	250	8	1
Smart Ones Spicy Szechaun Style Vegetables & Chicken	1 pkg (9 oz)	220	2	1
MIX				
Annie Chun's				
Meal Kit Garlic Scallion	1 serv	230	5	1
TAKE-OUT				
buddha's delight w/ cellophane noodles fat choi jai	1 serv (7.6 oz)	211	4	1
cashew chicken	1 serv	406	29	5

FOOD	PORTION	CALS	FAT	SAT FAT
cha siu bao steamed buns w/ chicken filling	1 (2.3 oz)	160	3	1
chop suey cantonese chicken	1 serv	570	17	3
chop suey w/ beef & pork	1 cup	300	17	4
chop suey w/ pork	1 cup	375	29	8
chow mein chicken	1 cup	255	10	4
chow mein pork	1 cup	425	24	8
chow mein shrimp	1 cup	221	10	1
chow mein vegetable	1 serv (8 oz)	90	3	0
filipino chicken adobo	1 serv (15 oz)	555	26	7
fried rice chicken	1 serv	314	89	1
fried rice vegetable	1 cup	210	9	1
fried rice w/ egg	6.7 oz	395	20	–
general tsao's chicken	1 serv	723	35	5
kung pao chicken	1 cup	409	29	5
lo mein pork	1 serv	323	40	1
moo goo gai pan chicken	1 cup	272	35	4
phad thai	1 serv (9.2 oz)	232	9	1
sesame seed paste bun	1 (2.5 oz)	220	6	1
shrimp & snow peas	1 cup	220	148	2
shrimp chips	1¼ cups (1 oz)	140	6	3
shu mai chicken & vegetable dumplings	6 (3.6 oz)	160	5	1
soba noodles w/ vegetables	1 serv	276	39	2
spring roll	1 (3.5 oz)	112	2	–
stir fry beef & broccoli	2 cup	512	202	10
stir fry garlic green beans	1 serv	68	0	0
stir fry vegetable	1 serv	235	70	2
sweet & sour chicken w/o rice	1 serv	416	95	1
sweet & sour pork	1 serv (8 oz)	250	8	3
sweet red bean bun	1 (2.5 oz)	130	1	0
szechuan chicken w/ lo mein	1 cup (5.3 oz)	190	1	0
szechuan cold noodles	1 serv	334	0	1
tempura seafood & vegetable	1 serv	590	185	6
tempura vegetables	5 pieces (4 oz)	270	15	3
teriyaki beef w/ sticky rice	1 serv	664	105	–
teriyaki chicken plain	¾ cup	399	27	6
teriyaki chicken w/ rice	1 serv (11 oz)	430	6	1
wonton fried	½ cup (1 oz)	111	8	1

FOOD	PORTION	CALS	FAT	SAT FAT
ASPARAGUS				
CANNED				
spears	½ cup	23	1	tr
Del Monte				
Cuts & Tips	½ cup (4.4 oz)	20	0	0
Spears Extra Long	½ cup (4.4 oz)	20	0	0
Spears Tender Young	½ cup (4.4 oz)	20	0	0
Tips Hand Selected	½ cup (4.4 oz)	20	0	0
Green Giant				
Cut Spears	½ cup (4.2 oz)	20	0	0
Cut Spears 50% Less Sodium	½ cup (4.2 oz)	20	0	0
Extra Long Spears	4.5 oz	20	0	0
Spears	4.5 oz	20	0	0
LeSueur				
Spears Extra Large	4.5 oz	20	0	0
S&W				
Green	6 pieces (4.5 oz)	15	0	0
FRESH				
cooked	½ cup	22	tr	tr
cooked	4 spears	14	tr	tr
raw	½ cup	16	tr	tr
raw	4 spears	15	tr	tr
FROZEN				
cooked	4 spears	17	tr	tr
cooked	1 pkg (10 oz)	82	1	tr
Birds Eye				
Cuts	½ cup	25	0	0
Jumbo Spears	3 oz	20	0	0
Green Giant				
Harvest Fresh Cuts	⅔ cup (3 oz)	25	0	0
ATEMOYA				
fresh	½ cup	94	1	—
AVOCADO				
fresh mashed	1 cup	407	40	6
fresh peeled california	1	306	30	4
fresh peeled florida	1	340	27	5
Chiquita				
Fresh	⅓ med (1 oz)	55	5	1

FOOD	PORTION	CALS	FAT	SAT FAT
TAKE-OUT				
guacamole	1 serv (2.2 oz)	105	10	1
BACON				
breakfast strips cooked	3 strips	156	12	4
gammon lean & fat grilled	4.2 oz	274	15	–
pan fried	3 strips	109	9	3
Armour				
Star cooked	1 strip	38	3	–
Black Label				
Center Cut cooked	3 slices (0.5 oz)	70	6	2
Cooked	2 slices (0.5 oz)	80	7	3
Low Salt cooked	2 slices (0.5 oz)	80	7	3
Health Is Wealth				
Uncured Sliced	2 slices (0.5 oz)	70	7	3
Hormel				
Bacon Bits	1 tbsp (7 g)	30	2	1
Bacon Pieces	1 tbsp (7 g)	25	2	1
Microwave cooked	2 slices (0.5 oz)	70	5	2
Old Smokehouse				
Cooked	2 slices (0.5 oz)	80	7	3
Oscar Mayer				
Bacon Bits	1 tbsp (0.2 oz)	25	2	1
Bacon Pieces	1 tbsp (0.2 oz)	25	2	1
Center Cut cooked	2 slices (0.4 oz)	70	5	2
Cooked	2 slices (0.5 oz)	70	6	2
Lower Sodium cooked	2 slices (0.5 oz)	70	5	2
Thick Cut cooked	1 slice (0.4 oz)	60	5	2
Range Brand				
Cooked	2 slices (0.7 oz)	100	9	4
Ready Crisp				
Fully Cooked	3 slices (0.5 oz)	70	6	3
Red Label				
Cooked	2 slices (0.5 oz)	80	7	3
Shannon				
Irish	1 oz	70	5	2
BACON SUBSTITUTES				
meatless	1 strip	16	1	tr
Bac-Os				
Chips or Bits	1½ tbsp (7 g)	30	2	0

FOOD	PORTION	CALS	FAT	SAT FAT
Lightlife				
Fakin' Bacon Bits	1 tsp	45	1	0
Smart Bacon	2 strips (0.8 oz)	45	2	0
Louis Rich				
Turkey Bacon	1 slice (0.5 oz)	35	3	1
Morningstar Farms				
Breakfast Strips	2 (0.5 oz)	60	5	1
Worthington				
Stripples	2 strips (0.5 oz)	60	5	1
BAGEL				
cinnamon raisin	1 lg	359	2	tr
cinnamon raisin toasted	1 lg	363	2	tr
egg	1 mini	72	1	tr
egg	1 lg	364	3	1
mini onion	1 (1.4 oz)	100	0	0
oat bran	1 lg	334	2	tr
onion	1 lg	363	2	tr
plain	1 lg	360	2	tr
plain	1 mini	72	tr	tr
poppy seed	1 lg	360	2	tr
Atkins				
Cinnamon Raisin	1	200	4	1
Onion	1	190	5	1
Plain	1	190	5	1
Otis Spunkmeyer				
Barnstormin' Blueberry	1 (3.6 oz)	250	3	0
Barnstormin' Cinnamon Raisin	1 (3.6 oz)	230	2	0
Barnstormin' Onion	1 (3.6 oz)	230	2	0
Barnstormin' Plain	1 (3.6 oz)	240	3	0
Pepperidge Farm				
Mini	1 (1.4 oz)	120	0	0
Plain	1 (3.5 oz)	290	1	0
Sara Lee				
Blueberry	1 (2.8 oz)	210	1	0
Cinnamon Raisin	1 (2.8 oz)	220	1	0
Egg	1 (2.8 oz)	210	1	1
Oat Bran	1 (2.8 oz)	210	1	0
Onion	1 (2.8 oz)	210	0	0
Plain	1 (2.8 oz)	210	1	1

FOOD	PORTION	CALS	FAT	SAT FAT
Poppy Seed	1 (2.8 oz)	210	1	0
Sesame Seed	1 (2.8 oz)	210	2	1
Thomas'				
Everything	1 (3.6 oz)	300	4	1
Multi-Grain	1 (3.6 oz)	280	2	1
Plain	1 (3.6 oz)	280	2	1
Uncle B's				
Plain	1 (2.8 oz)	210	1	0
Wonder				
Blueberry	1 (3 oz)	210	1	1
Cinnamon Raisin	1 (3 oz)	210	1	0
Onion	1 (3 oz)	210	1	0
Plain	1 (3 oz)	210	1	0
Rye	1 (3 oz)	220	1	0
Wheat	1 (3 oz)	210	1	0
BAKING POWDER				
baking powder	1 tsp	2	0	0
low sodium	1 tsp	5	0	0
Calumet				
Baking Powder	¼ tsp (1 g)	0	0	0
Clabber Girl				
Baking Powder	1 tsp	0	0	0
Davis				
Baking Powder	1 tsp	0	0	0
Rumford				
Aluminum Free	⅛ tsp	0	0	0
BAKING SODA				
baking soda	1 tsp	0	0	0
BALSAM PEAR (BITTER GOURD)				
leafy tips cooked	½ cup	10	tr	–
leafy tips raw	½ cup	7	tr	–
pods cooked	½ cup	12	tr	–
BAMBOO SHOOTS				
canned sliced	1 cup	25	1	tr
fresh	½ cup	21	tr	tr
fresh cooked	½ cup	12	tr	tr
Chun King				
Bamboo Shoots	2 tbsp (0.8 oz)	3	tr	0

FOOD	PORTION	CALS	FAT	SAT FAT
La Choy				
Bamboo Shoots	2 tbsp (0.8 oz)	3	tr	0
BANANA				
banana chips	1 oz	147	10	8
fresh	1 med	109	tr	tr
fresh mashed	1 cup	207	1	tr
fresh sliced	1 cup	138	1	tr
powder	1 tbsp	21	tr	tr
whole dried	1 piece (1.2 oz)	130	1	0
Chiquita				
Fresh	1 med (4.4 oz)	110	0	0
Rainforest Farms				
Slices Dried	5 slices (1.3 oz)	60	0	0
BARBECUE SAUCE				
barbecue	1 cup	188	5	1
Atkins				
Barbecue Sauce	1 tbsp	15	1	0
Bull's Eye				
Original	2 tbsp	50	0	–
Carb Options				
Original	2 tbsp	10	0	0
Healthy Choice				
Hickory	2 tbsp (1.1 oz)	26	0	0
Hot & Spicy	2 tbsp (1.1 oz)	25	0	0
Original	2 tbsp (1.1 oz)	25	0	0
House Of Tsang				
Hong Kong	1 tbsp (0.6 oz)	10	0	0
Hunt's				
Bold Hickory	2 tbsp (1.2 oz)	47	tr	0
Bold Original	2 tbsp (1.2 oz)	46	tr	0
Hickory & Brown Sugar	2 tbsp (1.3 oz)	75	tr	0
Honey Hickory	2 tbsp (1.2 oz)	54	tr	0
Honey Mustard	2 tbsp (1.2 oz)	48	tr	0
Hot & Spicy	2 tbsp (1.2 oz)	48	tr	0
Light Original	2 tbsp (1.2 oz)	23	tr	0
Mesquite	2 tbsp (1.2 oz)	40	tr	0
Mild	2 tbsp (1.2 oz)	41	tr	0
Mild Dijon	2 tbsp (1.2 oz)	39	tr	0
Open Range Original	2 tbsp (1.2 oz)	39	tr	0

FOOD	PORTION	CALS	FAT	SAT FAT
Open Range Premier	2 tbsp (1.3 oz)	56	tr	0
Open Range Smokey	2 tbsp (1.2 oz)	37	tr	0
Original	2 tbsp (1.2 oz)	40	tr	0
Teriyaki	2 tbsp (1.2 oz)	46	tr	0
Kraft				
Char-Grill	2 tbsp (1.3 oz)	60	0	0
Extra Rich Original	2 tbsp (1.2 oz)	50	0	0
Hickory Smoke	2 tbsp (1.2 oz)	40	0	0
Hickory Smoke Onion Bits	2 tbsp (1.2 oz)	45	0	0
Honey	2 tbsp (1.3 oz)	50	0	0
Honey Hickory	2 tbsp (1.3 oz)	60	0	0
Honey Mustard	2 tbsp (1.3 oz)	60	0	0
Hot	2 tbsp (1.2 oz)	40	0	0
Hot Hickory Smoke	2 tbsp (1.2 oz)	40	0	0
Kansas City Style	2 tbsp (1.2 oz)	50	0	0
Mesquite Smoke	2 tbsp (1.2 oz)	40	0	0
Molasses	2 tbsp (1.3 oz)	70	0	0
Onion Bits	2 tbsp (1.2 oz)	45	0	0
Original	2 tbsp (1.2 oz)	40	0	0
Roasted Garlic	2 tbsp (1.2 oz)	50	0	0
Spicy Honey	2 tbsp (1.3 oz)	60	0	0
Teriyaki	2 tbsp (1.3 oz)	60	1	0
Thick'N Spicy Brown Sugar	2 tbsp (1.2 oz)	60	0	0
Thick'N Spicy Hickory Bacon	2 tbsp (1.2 oz)	60	1	0
Thick'N Spicy Hickory Smoke	2 tbsp (1.2 oz)	50	0	0
Thick'N Spicy Honey	2 tbsp (1.3 oz)	60	0	0
Thick'N Spicy Honey Mustard	2 tbsp (1.3 oz)	60	0	0
Thick'N Spicy Kansas City Style	2 tbsp (1.3 oz)	60	0	0
Thick'N Spicy Mesquite Smoke	2 tbsp (1.2 oz)	50	0	0
McIlhenny				
Sauce	2 tbsp (1.1 oz)	70	5	1
Muir Glen				
Garlic Mesquite	2 tbsp (1.3 oz)	40	0	0
Hot & Smoky	2 tbsp (1.2 oz)	40	0	0
Original	2 tbsp (1.2 oz)	40	0	0
Steel's				
Sugar Free	2 tbsp	15	0	0
BARLEY				
flour	1 cup	511	2	tr

FOOD	PORTION	CALS	FAT	SAT FAT
malt flour	1 cup	585	3	1
pearled cooked	1 cup (5.5 oz)	193	1	tr
pearled uncooked	1 cup	704	2	tr

BARRACUDA
fresh	3 oz	122	8	—

BASIL
fresh chopped	2 tbsp	1	tr	tr
ground	1 tsp	4	tr	—
leaves fresh	5	1	tr	tr

BASS
freshwater raw	3 oz	97	3	1
sea cooked	3 oz	105	2	1
sea raw	3 oz	82	2	tr
striped baked	3 oz	105	3	1
striped bass farm raised	4 oz	110	3	1

BAY LEAF
crumbled	1 tsp	2	tr	tr

BEAN SPROUTS (see ALFALFA, SPROUTS)

BEANS (see also individual names)
CANNED
baked beans plain	½ cup	118	1	tr
baked beans vegetarian	½ cup	118	1	tr
baked beans w/ beef	½ cup	161	5	2
baked beans w/ franks	½ cup	184	9	3
baked beans w/ pork	½ cup	134	2	1
baked beans w/ pork & sweet sauce	½ cup	140	2	1
baked beans w/ pork & tomato sauce	½ cup	124	1	tr
refried beans	½ cup	134	1	1

Amy's
Vegetarian Baked	½ cup	120	5	1

B&M
99% Fat Free Baked Beans	½ cup (4.6 oz)	160	1	0
Barbeque Baked Beans	½ cup (4.6 oz)	210	1	0
Brick Oven Baked	½ cup (4.6 oz)	180	2	1
Extra Hearty Baked	½ cup (4.6 oz)	190	2	1
Maple Baked	½ cup	150	1	0
Vegetarian 99% Fat Free	½ cup	150	1	0

FOOD	PORTION	CALS	FAT	SAT FAT
Bush's				
Barbecue	½ cup (4.6 oz)	160	1	0
Maple Cured Bacon	½ cup	150	1	1
Original	½ cup	150	1	0
Vegetarian	½ cup (4.6 oz)	130	0	0
Chi-Chi's				
Refried	½ cup (4.2 oz)	100	1	0
Refried Beans Fat Free	½ cup (4.2 oz)	120	0	0
Refried Beans Vegetarian	½ cup (4.2 oz)	100	1	0
Eden				
Organic Baked w/ Sorghum & Mustard	½ cup (4.6 oz)	150	0	0
Friend's				
Original Baked	½ cup (4.6 oz)	170	1	0
Gebhardt				
Chili	½ cup (4.6 oz)	134	1	tr
Refried Jalapeno	½ cup (4.5 oz)	105	3	1
Refried No Fat	½ cup (4.5 oz)	92	tr	0
Refried Traditional	½ cup (4.5 oz)	109	3	1
Refried Vegetarian	½ cup (4.5 oz)	118	2	tr
Green Giant				
Pork And Beans w/ Tomato Sauce	½ cup (4.5 oz)	120	1	0
Spicy Chili	½ cup (4.5 oz)	110	1	0
Three Bean Salad	½ cup (4.2 oz)	90	0	0
Health Valley				
Honey Baked	½ cup	110	0	0
Honey Baked No Salt	½ cup	110	0	0
Heartland				
Iron Kettle Baked	½ cup (4.6 oz)	150	1	0
Hormel				
Beans & Wieners	1 can (7.5 oz)	290	12	4
Hunt's				
Big John's Beans & Fixin's	½ cup (4.7 oz)	127	4	1
Homestyle Country Kettle	½ cup (4.6 oz)	152	2	1
Homestyle Special Recipe	½ cup (4.7 oz)	185	3	1
Mix & Serve	½ cup (4.7 oz)	125	3	1
Pork & Beans	½ cup (4.6 oz)	157	5	2
Pork & Beans	½ cup (4.5 oz)	130	1	tr
Kid's Kitchen				
Microwave Meals Beans & Weiners	1 cup (7.5 oz)	310	13	5

FOOD	PORTION	CALS	FAT	SAT FAT
Old El Paso				
Mexe-Beans	½ cup (4.6 oz)	110	1	0
Refried	½ cup (4.2 oz)	110	2	1
Refried Fat Free	½ cup	100	0	0
Refried Spicy	½ cup (4.3 oz)	140	3	2
Refried Vegetarian	½ cup (4.1 oz)	100	1	0
Refried With Cheese	½ cup (4.2 oz)	130	4	2
Refried With Green Chilies	½ cup (4.3 oz)	110	1	0
Refried With Sausage	½ cup (4.1 oz)	200	13	5
Open Range				
Ranch	½ cup (4.4 oz)	124	3	1
Pringles				
Vegetarian	1 cup (7.9 oz)	250	1	0
Rosarita				
3 Bean Recipe Bacon & Jalapeno	½ cup (4.6 oz)	117	2	0
3 Bean Recipe Chiles & Chicken	½ cup (4.6 oz)	115	1	0
3 Bean Recipe Chilies & Chorizo	½ cup (4.6 oz)	111	2	0
3 Bean Recipe Onions & Peppers	½ cup (4.6 oz)	104	1	0
Fiesta Beans Bacon & Jalapenos	½ cup (4.6 oz)	117	2	0
Fiesta Beans Chicken & Chilies	½ cup (4.6 oz)	115	1	0
Fiesta Beans Chilies & Chorizo	½ cup (4.6 oz)	110	2	0
Fiesta Beans Onions & Peppers	½ cup (4.6 oz)	104	1	0
Refried Bacon	½ cup (4.5 oz)	116	3	1
Refried Green Chile	½ cup (4.5 oz)	110	3	2
Refried Low Fat Black	½ cup (4.5 oz)	107	1	0
Refried Nacho Cheese	½ cup (4.5 oz)	108	2	1
Refried No Fat	½ cup (4.5 oz)	120	0	0
Refried No Fat Green Chiles & Lime	½ cup (4.5 oz)	101	tr	0
Refried No Fat w/ Zesty Salsa	½ cup (4.5 oz)	105	tr	0
Refried Onion	½ cup (4.5 oz)	114	3	1
Refried Spicy	½ cup (4.5 oz)	118	3	1
Refried Traditional	½ cup (4.5 oz)	108	1	1
Refried Vegetarian	½ cup (4.5 oz)	237	5	1
S&W				
Barbecue Beans Ranch Recipe	½ cup (4.5 oz)	100	2	1
Taco Bell				
Home Originals Fat Free Refried Beans	½ cup (4.6 oz)	110	0	0
Home Originals Fat Free Refried Beans w/ Mild Chilies	½ cup (4.5 oz)	110	0	0

FOOD	PORTION	CALS	FAT	SAT FAT
Home Originals Refried Beans	½ cup (4.7 oz)	140	3	1
Van Camp				
Baked Fat Free	½ cup (4.6 oz)	132	tr	tr
Baked Original	½ cup (4.7 oz)	143	1	tr
Baked Southern Style Sauteed Onion	½ cup (4.8 oz)	145	1	tr
Baked Sweet Hickory & Bacon	1 can (4.8 oz)	143	1	tr
Beanee Weenee BBQ	1 cup (7.7 oz)	290	12	3
Beanee Weenee Baked	1 cup (9.1 oz)	410	14	4
Beanee Weenee Microwave	1 cup (7.5 oz)	260	11	3
Beanee Weenee Original	1 cup (9.1 oz)	320	14	4
Beanee Weenee Zestful	1 cup (7.7 oz)	300	12	3
Brown Sugar	½ cup (4.6 oz)	170	3	1
Pork And Beans	½ cup (4.6 oz)	110	2	1
Vegetarian	½ cup (4.6 oz)	110	1	0
FROZEN				
Natural Touch				
Nine Bean Loaf	1 in slice (3 oz)	160	8	2
MIX				
Melting Pot				
Terrazza Napoli Mixed Beans	1 cup	200	2	0
TAKE-OUT				
baked beans	½ cup	161	5	2
barbecue beans	3.5 oz	120	tr	tr
four bean salad	3.5 oz	100	tr	tr
frijoles w/ cheese	1 cup	225	8	4
refried beans	½ cup	43	2	1
three bean salad	¾ cup	230	11	1
BEAR				
simmered	3 oz	220	11	—
BEAVER				
roasted	3 oz	140	6	—
simmered	3 oz	141	5	—
BEECHNUTS				
dried	1 oz	164	14	2
BEEF (see also BEEF DISHES, VEAL)				
CANNED				
corned beef	3 oz	85	5	4
corned beef	1 oz	71	4	—

FOOD	PORTION	CALS	FAT	SAT FAT
Armour				
Chopped Beef	2 oz	170	15	7
Corned Beef	2 oz	120	7	3
Potted Meat	1 can (3 oz)	120	7	3
Tripe	3 oz	90	2	1
Hormel				
Corned Beef	2 oz	120	7	3
Cubed Beef	½ cup (4.9 oz)	130	3	1
Potted Meat	4 tbsp (2 oz)	100	8	4
Treet				
Luncheon Loaf	2 oz	130	11	4
Luncheon Loaf 50% Less Fat	2 oz	110	8	3
DRIED				
Armour				
Sliced	7 slices (1 oz)	60	2	1
Hormel				
Pillow Pack	10 slices (1 oz)	45	1	tr
FRESH				
bottom round lean & fat trim 0 in Choice roasted	3 oz	172	8	3
bottom round lean & fat trim 0 in Select braised	3 oz	171	6	2
bottom round lean & fat trim 0 in Select roasted	3 oz	150	24	2
bottom round lean & fat trim 0 in braised	3 oz	193	26	3
bottom round lean & fat trim ¼ in Choice braised	3 oz	241	15	6
bottom round lean & fat trim ¼ in Choice roasted	3 oz	221	14	5
bottom round lean & fat trim ¼ in Select braised	3 oz	220	13	5
bottom round lean & fat trim ¼ in Select roasted	3 oz	199	11	4
brisket flat half lean & fat trim 0 in braised	3 oz	183	8	3
brisket flat half lean & fat trim ¼ in braised	3 oz	309	24	9
brisket point half lean & fat trim 0 in braised	3 oz	304	24	10

FOOD	PORTION	CALS	FAT	SAT FAT
brisket point half lean & fat trim ¼ in braised	3 oz	343	29	12
brisket whole lean & fat trim 0 in braised	3 oz	247	17	6
brisket whole lean & fat trim ¼ in braised	3 oz	327	27	11
chuck arm pot roast lean & fat trim 0 in braised	3 oz	238	14	6
chuck arm pot roast lean & fat trim ¼ in braised	3 oz	282	20	8
chuck blade roast lean & fat trim 0 in braised	3 oz	284	21	8
chuck blade roast lean & fat trim ¼ in braised	3 oz	293	22	9
corned beef brisket cooked	3 oz	213	16	5
eye of round lean & fat trim 0 in Choice roasted	3 oz	153	5	8
eye of round lean & fat trim 0 in Select roasted	3 oz	137	4	1
eye of round lean & fat trim ¼ in Choice roasted	3 oz	205	12	5
eye of round lean & fat trim ¼ in Select roasted	3 oz	184	10	4
flank lean & fat trim 0 in braised	3 oz	224	14	6
flank lean & fat trim 0 in broiled	3 oz	192	11	5
ground extra lean broiled medium	3 oz	217	14	5
ground extra lean broiled well done	3 oz	225	14	5
ground extra lean fried medium	3 oz	216	14	5
ground extra lean fried well done	3 oz	224	14	5
ground extra lean raw	4 oz	265	19	8
ground lean broiled medium	3 oz	231	16	6
ground lean broiled well done	3 oz	238	15	6
ground regular broiled medium	3 oz	246	18	7
ground regular broiled well done	3 oz	248	17	7
ground 97% fat free irradiated	4 oz	160	8	3
ground low-fat w/ carrageenan raw	4 oz	160	7	4
porterhouse steak lean & fat trim ¼ in Choice broiled	3 oz	260	19	8
porterhouse steak lean only trim ¼ in Prime broiled	3 oz	185	9	4

FOOD	PORTION	CALS	FAT	SAT FAT
rib eye small end lean & fat trim 0 in Choice broiled	3 oz	261	19	8
rib large end lean & fat trim 0 in roasted	3 oz	300	24	10
rib large end lean & fat trim ¼ in broiled	3 oz	295	24	10
rib large end lean & fat trim ¼ in roasted	3 oz	310	25	10
rib small end lean & fat trim 0 in broiled	3 oz	252	18	7
rib small end lean & fat trim ¼ in broiled	3 oz	285	22	9
rib small end lean & fat trim ¼ in roasted	3 oz	295	24	10
rib whole lean & fat trim ¼ in Choice broiled	3 oz	306	25	10
rib whole lean & fat trim ¼ in Choice roasted	3 oz	320	27	11
rib whole lean & fat trim ¼ in Prime roasted	3 oz	348	30	12
rib whole lean & fat trim ¼ in Select broiled	3 oz	274	21	9
rib whole lean & fat trim ¼ in Select roasted	3 oz	286	23	9
shank crosscut lean & fat trim ¼ in Choice simmered	3 oz	224	12	5
short loin top loin lean & fat trim 0 in Choice broiled	3 oz	193	10	4
short loin top loin lean & fat trim 0 in Choice broiled	1 steak (5.4 oz)	353	19	7
short loin top loin lean & fat trim 0 in Select broiled	1 steak (5.4 oz)	309	14	5
short loin top loin lean & fat trim ¼ in Choice braised	3 oz	253	18	7
short loin top loin lean & fat trim ¼ in Choice broiled	1 steak (6.3 oz)	536	38	15
short loin top loin lean & fat trim ¼ in Prime broiled	1 steak (6.3 oz)	582	43	17
short loin top loin lean & fat trim ¼ in Select broiled	1 steak (6.3 oz)	473	31	12

FOOD	PORTION	CALS	FAT	SAT FAT
short loin top loin lean only trim 0 in Choice broiled	1 steak (5.2 oz)	311	14	5
short loin top loin lean only trim ¼ in Choice broiled	1 steak (5.2 oz)	314	15	6
shortribs lean & fat Choice braised	3 oz	400	36	15
t-bone steak lean & fat trim ¼ in Choice broiled	3 oz	253	18	7
t-bone steak lean only trim ¼ in Choice broiled	3 oz	182	9	4
tenderloin lean & fat trim 0 in Select broiled	3 oz	194	11	4
tenderloin lean & fat trim ¼ in Choice broiled	3 oz	259	19	7
tenderloin lean & fat trim ¼ in Choice roasted	3 oz	288	22	9
tenderloin lean & fat trim ¼ in Choice broiled	3 oz	208	12	5
tenderloin lean & fat trim ¼ in Prime broiled	3 oz	270	20	8
tenderloin lean & fat trim ¼ in Select roasted	3 oz	275	21	8
tenderloin lean only trim 0 in Select broiled	3 oz	170	7	3
tenderloin lean only trim ¼ in Choice broiled	3 oz	188	10	4
tenderloin lean only trim ¼ in Select broiled	3 oz	169	7	3
tip round lean & fat trim 0 in Choice roasted	3 oz	170	8	3
tip round lean & fat trim 0 in Select roasted	3 oz	158	6	2
tip round lean & fat trim ¼ in Choice roasted	3 oz	210	13	5
tip round lean & fat trim ¼ in Prime roasted	3 oz	233	15	6
tip round lean & fat trim ¼ in Select roasted	3 oz	191	10	4
top round lean & fat trim 0 in Choice braised	3 oz	184	6	2

FOOD	PORTION	CALS	FAT	SAT FAT
top round lean & fat trim 0 in Select braised	3 oz	170	5	2
top round lean & fat trim ¼ in Choice braised	3 oz	221	11	4
top round lean & fat trim ¼ in Choice broiled	3 oz	190	9	3
top round lean & fat trim ¼ in Choice fried	3 oz	235	13	5
top round lean & fat trim ¼ in Prime broiled	3 oz	195	9	3
top round lean & fat trim ¼ in Select braised	3 oz	175	7	3
top round lean & fat trim ¼ in Select braised	3 oz	199	8	3
top sirloin lean & fat trim 0 in Choice broiled	3 oz	194	10	4
top sirloin lean & fat trim 0 in Select broiled	3 oz	166	6	3
top sirloin lean & fat trim ¼ in Choice broiled	3 oz	228	14	6
top sirloin lean & fat trim ¼ in Choice fried	3 oz	277	19	8
top sirloin lean & fat trim ¼ in Select broiled	3 oz	208	12	5
tripe raw	4 oz	111	4	2
Healthy Choice				
Ground Extra Lean	4 oz	130	4	2
Laura's Lean				
Eye Of Round Steak Or Roast	4 oz	140	4	2
Flank Steak	4 oz	140	5	2
Ground 92% Lean	4 oz	160	9	4
Ground Round 96% Lean	4 oz	140	5	2
Ribeye Steak	4 oz	145	5	2
Sirloin Steak	4 oz	140	5	2
Sirloin Tip Steak Or Roast	4 oz	120	3	2
Strip Steak	4 oz	140	4	2
Tenderloin Filet	4 oz	140	5	2
Top Round Steak Or Roast	4 oz	130	3	1
Maverick Ranch				
Filet Mignon	4 oz	120	4	2

FOOD	PORTION	CALS	FAT	SAT FAT
Ground	4 oz	130	5	2
Ground Round	4 oz	130	4	2
Ground Sirloin & Chuck	4 oz	130	5	2
NY Strip Steak	4 oz	150	7	3
Rib Eye Steak	4 oz	170	10	4
Top Round Steak & Roast	4 oz	110	4	2
Top Sirloin	4 oz	160	8	3
Organic Valley				
Extra Lean Ground	3 oz	130	6	3
Extra Lean Patties	1 (3.2 oz)	130	6	3
FROZEN				
patties broiled medium	3 oz	240	17	7
READY-TO-EAT				
dried beef	5 slices (21 g)	35	tr	—
smoked beef cooked	1 sausage (1.4 oz)	134	12	—
Alpine Lace				
Roast Beef 97% Fat Free	2 oz	70	2	1
Boar's Head				
Corned Beef Brisket	2 oz	80	4	2
Eye Round Pepper Seasoned	2 oz	90	3	2
Italian Style Oven Roasted Top Round	2 oz	80	2	1
Roast Beef Cajun	2 oz	80	3	2
Top Round Deluxe	2 oz	90	3	2
Top Round Oven Roasted No Salt Added	2 oz	90	3	2
Healthy Choice				
Deli-Thin Roast Beef	6 slices (2 oz)	60	2	1
Fresh-Trak Roast Beef	1 slice (1 oz)	30	1	0
Jordan's				
Healthy Trim 97% Fat Free Roast Beef Medium	1 slice (1 oz)	30	1	1
Healthy Trim 97% Fat Free Roast Beef Rare	1 slice (1 oz)	30	1	1
Tyson				
Beef Strips Seasoned	1 serv (3 oz)	140	6	2
TAKE-OUT				
roast beef medium	2 oz	70	2	1
roast beef rare	2 oz	70	2	1

FOOD	PORTION	CALS	FAT	SAT FAT
BEEF DISHES				
CANNED				
corned beef hash	3 oz	155	10	5
Armour				
Corned Beef Hash	1 cup (8.3 oz)	440	30	14
Corned Beef Hash w/ Peppers & Onions	1 cup (8.3 oz)	270	30	14
Roast Beef Hash	1 cup (8.4 oz)	400	25	12
Roast Beef In Gravy	½ cup (4.6 oz)	150	4	2
Stew	1 cup (8.6 oz)	220	12	5
Dinty Moore				
Meatball Stew	1 cup (8.4 oz)	250	15	7
Sliced Potatoes & Beef	1 can (7.5 oz)	230	9	4
Stew	1 cup (8.2 oz)	230	14	7
Stew	1 cup (8.3 oz)	230	14	7
Hormel				
Beef Goulash	1 can (7.5 oz)	230	11	5
Roast Beef With Gravy	2 oz	60	2	1
Mary Kitchen				
Corned Beef Hash	1 cup (8.3 oz)	410	27	10
Corned Beef Hash 50% Reduced Fat	1 cup	280	12	5
Roast Beef Hash	1 cup (8.3 oz)	390	24	10
Sausage Hash	1 cup (8.3 oz)	410	27	9
FROZEN				
Banquet				
Sandwich Toppers Creamed Chipped Beef	1 pkg (4 oz)	120	6	3
Sandwich Toppers Gravy & Salisbury Steak	1 pkg (5 oz)	210	16	7
Sandwich Toppers Gravy & Sliced Beef	1 pkg (4 oz)	70	2	1
MIX				
Hamburger Helper				
BBQ Beef as prep	1 cup	320	10	4
Beef Pasta as prep	1 cup	270	10	4
Beef Romanoff as prep	1 cup	280	10	4
Beef Stew as prep	1 cup	260	10	4
Beef Taco as prep	1 cup	280	10	4
Beef Teriyaki as prep	1 cup	290	10	4
Cheddar & Broccoli as prep	1 cup	350	15	6

FOOD	PORTION	CALS	FAT	SAT FAT
Cheddar Melt as prep	1 cup	310	12	5
Cheddar'n Bacon as prep	1 cup	330	15	6
Cheeseburger Macaroni as prep	1 cup	360	16	6
Cheesy Hashbrowns as prep	1 cup	400	19	6
Cheesy Italian as prep	1 cup	320	14	6
Cheesy Shells as prep	1 cup	330	15	6
Chili Macaroni as prep	1 cup	290	10	4
Fettuccine Alfredo as prep	1 cup	300	13	5
Four Cheese Lasagne as prep	1 cup	330	14	5
Italian Parmesan w/ Rigatoni as prep	1 cup	300	11	4
Lasagne as prep	1 cup	270	10	4
Meat Loaf as prep	⅙ loaf	270	14	6
Meaty Spaghetti & Cheese as prep	1 cup	290	10	4
Mushroom & Wild Rice as prep	1 cup	310	12	5
Nacho Cheese as prep	1 cup	320	13	5
Pizza Pasta w/ Cheese Topping as prep	1 cup	280	10	4
Pizzabake as prep	⅙ pie	270	10	4
Potatoes Au Gratin as prep	1 cup	280	13	5
Potatoes Stroganoff as prep	1 cup	250	11	5
Reduced Sodium Cheddar Spirals as prep	1 cup	300	13	5
Reduced Sodium Italian Herby as prep	1 cup	270	10	4
Reduced Sodium Southwestern Beef as prep	1 cup	300	10	4
Rice Oriental as prep	1 cup	280	10	4
Salisbury as prep	1 cup	270	10	4
Spaghetti as prep	1 cup	270	10	4
Stroganoff as prep	1 cup	320	13	5
Swedish Meatballs as prep	1 cup	290	14	5
Three Cheeses as prep	1 cup	340	15	5
Zesty Italian as prep	1 cup	300	10	4
Zesty Mexican as prep	1 cup	280	10	4
REFRIGERATED				
Hormel				
Beef Roast Au Jus	1 serv (5 oz)	200	9	4
Morton's Of Omaha				
Beef Pot Roast w/ Gravy	1 serv (3 oz)	160	5	2
Smithfield				
Beef Tips w/ Gravy	½ cup	170	5	2

FOOD	PORTION	CALS	FAT	SAT FAT
Tyson				
Roast Beef In Brown Gravy	1 serv + gravy (3.5 oz)	160	6	3
SHELF-STABLE				
Dinty Moore				
Microwave Cup Corned Beef Hash	1 pkg (7.5 oz)	350	22	9
Microwave Cup Hearty Burger Stew	1 pkg (7.5 oz)	240	13	5
Microwave Cup Stew	1 pkg (7.5 oz)	190	10	5
Hormel				
Microcup Meals Stew	1 cup (7.5 oz)	190	10	4
Lunch Bucket				
Beef Stew	1 pkg (7.5 oz)	170	9	4
TastyBite				
Beef Roganjosh	1 pkg (9.5 oz)	270	15	2
Meatballs Vindaloo	1 pkg (9.5 oz)	270	18	5
TAKE-OUT				
beef bourguignon	1 serv (7 oz)	254	16	7
bubble & squeak	5 oz	186	13	–
bulgoghi korean grilled beef	1 serv (5.2 oz)	256	15	5
cornish pasty	1 (8 oz)	847	52	–
greek moussaka	1 serv (8.5 oz)	450	33	14
irish stew	1 cup (7 oz)	280	16	9
kebab indian	1 (5.4 oz)	553	40	–
kheena	6.7 oz	781	71	–
koftas	5	280	22	–
peppered steak	1 cup	331	73	4
pot roast w/ gravy	1 serv (6 oz)	320	10	4
samosa	2 (4 oz)	652	62	–
shepherds pie	1 serv (7 oz)	282	16	6
steak & kidney pie w/ top crust	1 slice (5 oz)	400	26	–
stew	6 oz	208	13	–
stew w/ vegetables	1 cup	220	11	4
stroganoff	¾ cup	260	19	11
swiss steak	4.6 oz	214	9	3
toad in the hole	1 (4.7 oz)	383	29	–
BEEFALO				
roasted	3 oz	160	5	2
BEER AND ALE				
alcohol free beer	7 fl oz	50	tr	–

FOOD	PORTION	CALS	FAT	SAT FAT
ale brown	10 oz	77	0	0
ale pale	10 oz	88	0	0
beer light	12 oz can	100	0	0
beer regular	12 oz can	146	0	0
black & tan	1 serv (12 oz)	146	0	0
boilermaker	1 serv	216	0	0
lager	10 oz	80	0	0
mead	1 serv	250	0	0
pilsener lager beer	7 fl oz	85	tr	—
shandy	1 serv	125	0	0
stout	10 oz	102	0	0
Amstel				
Light	1 bottle (12 oz)	95	0	0
Anchor				
Liberty Ale	1 bottle (12 oz)	188	0	0
Porter	1 bottle (12 oz)	205	0	0
Steam	12 oz	152	0	0
Beck's				
Beer	1 bottle (12 oz)	143	0	0
Blue Moon				
White	1 bottle (12 oz)	171	0	0
Bud				
Ice Light	1 bottle (12 oz)	110	0	0
Budweiser				
Beer	1 bottle (12 oz)	143	0	0
Ice	1 bottle (12 oz)	148	0	0
Light	1 bottle (12 oz)	110	0	0
Busch				
Beer	1 bottle (12 oz)	133	0	0
Ice	1 bottle (12 oz)	173	0	0
Light	1 bottle (12 oz)	110	0	0
Clausthaler				
Beer	1 bottle (12 oz)	96	0	0
Colt 45				
Malt Liquor	1 bottle (12 oz)	172	0	0
Coors				
Extra Gold	1 bottle (12 oz)	147	0	0
Light	1 bottle (12 oz)	102	0	0
Nonalcoholic	1 bottle (12 oz)	73	0	0
Nonalcoholic	1 bottle (12 oz)	73	0	0

FOOD	PORTION	CALS	FAT	SAT FAT
Original	1 bottle (12 oz)	148	0	0
Corona				
Extra	1 bottle (12 oz)	148	0	0
Light	1 bottle (12 oz)	109	0	0
Deschutes				
Bachelor ESB	1 bottle (12 oz)	180	0	0
Black Butt Porter	1 bottle (12 oz)	185	0	0
Cascade Ale	1 bottle (12 oz)	140	0	0
Mirror Pond Pale	1 bottle (12 oz)	175	0	0
Edison				
Light	1 bottle	109	0	0
Genesee				
12 Horse	1 bottle (12 oz)	152	0	0
Genny Light	1 bottle (12 oz)	96	0	0
Guinness				
Draught	1 bottle (12 oz)	125	0	0
Foreign Extra Stout	1 bottle (12 oz)	176	0	0
Hamm's				
Beer	1 bottle (12 oz)	144	0	0
Light	1 bottle (12 oz)	110	0	0
Heineken				
Beer	1 bottle (12 oz)	166	0	0
I.C.				
Light	1 bottle (12 oz)	96	0	0
Icehouse				
5.0	1 bottle (12 oz)	132	0	0
5.5	1 bottle (12 oz)	149	0	0
J.W. Dundee				
Honey Brown	1 bottle (12 oz)	150	0	0
Keystone				
Light	1 bottle (12 oz)	100	0	0
Kilarney's				
Red Lager	1 bottle (12 oz)	197	0	0
Killian's				
Beer	1 bottle (12 oz)	163	0	0
Lowenbrau				
Beer	1 bottle (12 oz)	160	0	0
Michelob				
Ultra Low Carbohydrate	1 bottle (12 oz)	95	0	0

FOOD	PORTION	CALS	FAT	SAT FAT
Weinhard's				
Ale	1 bottle (12 oz)	147	0	0
Amber Ale	1 bottle (12 oz)	169	0	0
Dark	1 bottle (12 oz)	150	0	0
Hefeweizen	1 bottle (12 oz)	128	0	0
BEET JUICE				
juice	7 oz	72	0	0
BEETS				
CANNED				
harvard	½ cup	89	tr	tr
pickled	½ cup	75	tr	tr
sliced	½ cup	27	tr	tr
Del Monte				
Pickled Crinkle Style Sliced	½ cup (4.5 oz)	80	0	0
Sliced	½ cup (4.3 oz)	35	0	0
Whole	½ cup (4.3 oz)	35	0	0
Green Giant				
Harvard	⅓ cup (3.1 oz)	60	0	0
Sliced	½ cup (4.2 oz)	35	0	0
Sliced No Salt Added	½ cup (4.2 oz)	35	0	0
Whole	½ cup (4.2 oz)	35	0	0
Greenwood				
Harvard	1 serv (4.4 oz)	100	0	0
Pickled	1 oz	25	0	0
LeSueur				
Baby Whole	½ cup (4.3 oz)	35	0	0
S&W				
Julienne	½ cup (4.3 oz)	30	0	0
Pickled Sliced	1 oz	15	0	0
Pickled Whole	1 oz	15	0	0
Sliced	½ cup (4.3 oz)	30	0	0
Whole Small	½ cup (4.3 oz)	30	0	0
Veg-All				
Small Sliced	½ cup	40	0	0
FRESH				
greens cooked	½ cup	20	tr	tr
greens raw	½ cup	4	tr	tr
greens raw chopped	½ cup	4	tr	tr
raw sliced	½ cup (2.4 oz)	29	tr	tr

FOOD	PORTION	CALS	FAT	SAT FAT
sliced cooked	½ cup (3 oz)	38	tr	tr
whole cooked	2 (3.5 oz)	44	tr	tr
whole raw	2 (5.7 oz)	70	tr	tr

BEVERAGES *(see* BEER AND ALE, CHAMPAGNE, COFFEE, DRINK MIXERS, ENERGY DRINKS, FRUIT DRINKS, ICED TEA, LIQUOR/LIQUEUR, MALT, MILKSHAKE, SODA, TEA/HERBAL TEA, WATER, WINE*)*

BISCUIT
MIX

FOOD	PORTION	CALS	FAT	SAT FAT
buttermilk	1 (2 oz)	191	7	2
plain	1 (2 oz)	191	7	2
Bisquick				
Buttermilk	½ cup	150	6	3
Cheese Garlic	½ cup	160	7	2
Cinnamon Swirl	½ cup	150	4	1
Mix	⅓ cup (1.4 oz)	160	6	2
Reduced Fat	⅓ cup	140	3	1
Kentucky Kernel				
Biscuit	¼ cup (1 oz)	171	5	1
MiniCarb				
Buttery as prep	1	255	21	12
REFRIGERATED				
buttermilk	1 (1 oz)	98	4	1
plain	1 (1 oz)	98	4	1
1869 Brand				
Buttermilk	1 (1.1 oz)	100	5	2
Hungry Jack				
Butter Tastin' Flaky	1 (1.2 oz)	100	5	1
Cinnamon & Sugar	1 (1.2 oz)	110	4	1
Flaky	1 (1.2 oz)	100	5	1
Flaky Buttermilk	1 (1.2 oz)	100	5	1
Pillsbury				
Big Country Butter Tastin'	1 (1.2 oz)	100	4	1
Big Country Buttermilk	1 (1.2 oz)	100	4	1
Big Country Southern Style	1 (1.2 oz)	100	4	1
Buttermilk	1 (2.2 oz)	150	2	0
Country	1 (2.2 oz)	150	2	0
Grands Blueberry	1 (2.1 oz)	210	9	3
Grands Butter Tastin'	1 (2.1 oz)	200	10	3
Grands Buttermilk	1 (2.1 oz)	200	10	3

FOOD	PORTION	CALS	FAT	SAT FAT
Grands Buttermilk Reduced Fat	1 (2.1 oz)	190	7	2
Grands Extra Rich	1 (2.1 oz)	220	12	3
Grands Flaky	1 (2.1 oz)	200	9	2
Grands Golden Corn	1 (1.2 oz)	210	10	3
Grands HomeStyle	1 (2.1 oz)	210	10	3
Grands Southern Style	1 (2.1 oz)	200	10	3
Southern Style Flakey	1 (1.2 oz)	100	5	1
Tender Layer Buttermilk	1 (2.2 oz)	160	5	1
TAKE-OUT				
buttermilk	1 (2 oz)	212	10	3
oatcakes	2 (4 oz)	115	5	—
plain	1 (35 g)	276	34	9
tea biscuit	1 (3 oz)	210	3	2
w/ egg	1 (4.8 oz)	316	20	6
w/ egg & bacon	1 (5.2 oz)	458	31	8
w/ egg & ham	1 (6.7 oz)	442	27	6
w/ egg & sausage	1 (6.3 oz)	581	39	15
w/ egg & steak	1 (5.2 oz)	410	28	9
w/ egg cheese & bacon	1 (5.1 oz)	477	31	11
w/ ham	1 (4 oz)	386	18	11
w/ sausage	1 (4.4 oz)	485	32	14
w/ steak	1 (4.9 oz)	455	26	7
BISON				
roasted	3 oz	122	2	1
BLACK BEANS				
dried cooked	1 cup	227	1	tr
Bean Cuisine				
Pasta & Beans Mediterranean Black Beans & Fusilli	1 serv	210	1	0
Eden				
Organic	½ cup (4.6 oz)	100	0	0
Green Giant				
Black Beans	½ cup (4.5 oz)	50	0	0
Old El Paso				
Black Beans	½ cup (4.6 oz)	100	1	0
Refried	½ cup (4.2 oz)	120	2	0
Progresso				
Black Beans	½ cup (4.6 oz)	110	1	0

FOOD	PORTION	CALS	FAT	SAT FAT
BLACKBERRIES				
canned in heavy syrup	½ cup	118	tr	—
fresh	½ cup	37	tr	—
unsweetened frzn	1 cup	97	1	—
BLACKBERRY JUICE				
Clear Fruit				
Blackberry Rush	8 oz	90	0	0
Everfresh				
Clear Fruit Blackberry Rush	8 oz	90	0	0
Kool-Aid				
Scary Blackberry Ghoul-Aid Drink as prep w/ sugar	1 serv (8 oz)	100	0	0
BLACKEYE PEAS				
CANNED				
w/pork	½ cup	199	4	1
Eden				
Organic	½ cup (4.6 oz)	90	1	0
Green Giant				
Blackeye Peas	½ cup (4.4 oz)	90	0	0
DRIED				
cooked	1 cup	198	1	tr
Hurst				
HamBeens California w/ Ham	1 serv	120	1	0
FROZEN				
Birds Eye				
Blackeye Peas	½ cup	110	1	0
BLINTZE				
Cohen's & Wilton				
Cheese	1	80	3	1
Golden				
Cheese	1 (2.1 oz)	80	2	1
Potato	1	90	4	1
Ratner's				
Cheese	1 (2.2 oz)	90	2	1
TAKE-OUT				
cheese	1 (2.7 oz)	160	9	4
BLUEBERRIES				
canned in heavy syrup	1 cup	225	1	—

FOOD	PORTION	CALS	FAT	SAT FAT
fresh	1 cup	82	1	–
unsweetened frzn	1 cup	78	1	–
Sonoma				
Dried	¼ cup (1.3 oz)	140	0	0
Tree Of Life				
Organic	1 cup (5 oz)	80	0	0

BLUEBERRY JUICE
After The Fall

Maine Coast	1 cup (8 oz)	90	0	0

BLUEFIN

fillet baked	4.1 oz	186	6	1

BLUEFISH

fresh baked	3 oz	135	5	1

BOAR

wild roasted	3 oz	136	4	1

BOK CHOY (see CABBAGE)

BONITO

fresh	3 oz	117	4	–

BORAGE

fresh chopped	½ cup	9	tr	–
fresh chopped cooked	3½ oz	25	1	–

BOTTLED WATER (see WATER)

BOYSENBERRIES

in heavy syrup	1 cup	226	tr	–
unsweetened frzn	1 cup	66	tr	–

BRAINS

beef pan-fried	3 oz	167	13	3
beef simmered	3 oz	136	11	2
lamb braised	3 oz	124	9	2
lamb fried	3 oz	232	19	5
pork braised	3 oz	117	8	2
veal braised	3 oz	115	8	–
veal fried	3 oz	181	14	–
Armour				
Pork Brains In Milk Gravy	⅔ cup (5.5 oz)	150	5	3

FOOD	PORTION	CALS	FAT	SAT FAT
BRAN				
corn	1 cup (2.7 oz)	170	1	tr
oat	½ cup (1.6 oz)	116	3	1
oat cooked	½ cup (3.8 oz)	44	1	tr
rice	½ cup (2.1 oz)	187	12	2
wheat	½ cup (2 oz)	63	1	tr
Hodgson Mill				
Oat	¼ cup	120	3	1
Wheat Unprocessed	¼ cup	30	0	0
Quaker				
Oat Bran	½ cup (1.4 oz)	150	3	1
BRAZIL NUTS				
dried unblanched	1 oz	186	19	5
BREAD				
CANNED				
boston brown	1 slice (1.6 oz)	88	1	tr
B&M				
Brown Bread	½ in slice (2 oz)	130	1	0
Brown Bread Raisins	½ in slice (2 oz)	130	1	0
FROZEN				
Kineret				
Challah	⅛ loaf (2 oz)	150	4	1
Marie Callender's				
Cornbread & Honey Butter	1 piece + butter	210	11	5
Original Garlic	1 piece	190	8	6
Parmesan & Romano Garlic	1 piece	200	10	3
New York				
Garlic	1 slice (2 oz)	190	8	2
Garlic Reduced Fat	1 slice (2 oz)	160	4	1
Texas Garlic Toast	1 in slice (1.4 oz)	160	9	2
Pepperidge Farm				
Garlic	1 slice (1.8 oz)	170	10	3
Garlic Sourdough 30% Reduced Fat	1 slice (1.8 oz)	170	7	1
Mozzarella Garlic Cheese	1 slice (2 oz)	201	10	5
MIX				
cornbread	1 piece (2 oz)	189	6	2
Atkins				
Caraway Rye as prep	1 slice	150	0	0
Country White as prep	1 slice	70	0	0

FOOD	PORTION	CALS	FAT	SAT FAT
Sourdough as prep	1 slice	70	0	0
Buitoni				
Focaccia Rosemary & Garlic	1 piece (1 oz)	110	1	0
Carbolite				
Bread Mix as prep	1 slice	45	5	1
Hodgson Mill				
European Cheese & Herb	¼ cup (1.2 oz)	130	1	0
Honey Whole Wheat	¼ cup (1.2 oz)	120	1	0
Keto				
Quick Bread All Flavors as prep	1 slice	55	0	0
MiniCarb				
Country White as prep	1 slice	80	3	0
Zia Foods				
Cornbread Blue Cornmeal	1 piece (1.2 oz)	110	6	–
READY-TO-EAT				
baguette parisian	2 oz	120	0	0
baguette whole wheat	2 oz	140	0	0
challah	1 slice (2 oz)	160	3	1
cracked wheat	1 slice	65	1	tr
egg	1 slice (1.4 oz)	115	2	1
french	1 slice (1 oz)	78	1	tr
french	1 loaf (1 lb)	1270	18	4
gluten	1 slice	47	tr	tr
italian	1 slice (1 oz)	81	1	tr
italian	1 loaf (1 lb)	1255	4	1
navajo fry	1 (5 in diam)	296	9	2
navajo fry	1 (10.5 in diam)	527	15	3
oat bran	1 slice	71	1	tr
oat bran reduced calorie	1 slice	46	1	tr
oatmeal	1 slice	73	1	tr
oatmeal reduced calorie	1 slice	48	1	tr
pita	1 reg (2 oz)	165	1	tr
pita	1 sm (1 oz)	78	tr	tr
pita whole wheat	1 reg (2 oz)	170	2	tr
pita whole wheat	1 sm (1 oz)	76	1	tr
protein	1 slice	47	tr	tr
pumpernickel	1 slice	80	1	tr
raisin	1 slice	71	1	tr
rice bran	1 slice	66	1	tr
rye	1 slice	83	1	tr

FOOD	PORTION	CALS	FAT	SAT FAT
rye reduced calorie	1 slice	47	1	tr
seven grain	1 slice	65	1	tr
sourdough	1 slice (1 oz)	78	1	tr
vienna	1 slice (1 oz)	78	1	tr
wheat reduced calorie	1 slice	46	1	tr
wheat berry	1 slice	65	1	tr
wheat bran	1 slice	89	1	tr
wheat germ	1 slice	74	1	tr
white	1 slice	67	1	tr
white reduced calorie	1 slice	48	1	tr
white toasted	1 slice	67	1	tr
white cubed	1 cup	80	1	tr
whole wheat	1 slice	70	1	tr
Arnold				
Bran'nola Country Oat	1 slice (1.3 oz)	110	2	0
Country Buttermilk	1 slice (1.3 oz)	110	2	0
Country Wheat	1 slice (1.3 oz)	100	2	0
Country White	1 slice (1.3 oz)	110	2	0
Natural 100% Whole Wheat	1 slice (1.3 oz)	90	1	0
Raisin Cinnamon	1 slice (1 oz)	80	2	0
Atkins				
Rye	1 slice	60	1	1
White	1 slice	60	1	1
Bread Du Jour				
French	3 in slice (2 oz)	140	1	0
Damascus				
Mountain Shepard Lahvash	⅓ loaf (2 oz)	135	0	0
Pita	1 (2 oz)	130	0	0
Pita Whole Wheat	1 (2 oz)	160	0	0
Wraps Honey Wheat	½ wrap (2 oz)	130	0	0
Wraps Plain	½ wrap (2 oz)	130	0	0
Wraps Spinach	1 (4 oz)	280	0	0
Wraps Tomato	1 12-inch (4 oz)	240	0	0
Ecce Panis				
Country Wheat	1 slice (2 oz)	150	0	0
Freihofer's				
Country Potato	1 slice (1.3 oz)	100	1	0
Country White	1 slice (1.3 oz)	100	1	0
Whole Wheat 100%	1 slice (1.3 oz)	90	2	0
Whole Wheat Light	2 slices	80	1	0

FOOD	PORTION	CALS	FAT	SAT FAT
Gold Medal				
100% Whole Wheat	1 slice	70	2	0
Home Pride				
Wheat	1 slice (1 oz)	80	1	0
La Mexicana				
Wraps Chocolate	1 (1.3 oz)	120	3	1
Wraps Southwestern Mild Chili	1 (1.3 oz)	120	4	1
Wraps Spinach	1 (1.3 oz)	120	4	1
Wraps Tomato Basil	1 (1.3 oz)	120	4	1
Mediterranean Magic				
Focaccia	⅓ loaf (1.8 oz)	140	2	0
Milton's				
Healthy Multi-Grain	1 slice (1.4 oz)	110	1	0
Pepperidge Farm				
Apple Cinammon	1 slice (1 oz)	80	2	0
Deli Swirl Rye & Pump·	1 slice	80	1	0
Farmhouse Butter Topped Wheat	1 slice	110	2	1
Farmhouse Country Wheat	1 slice	110	2	0
Farmhouse Hearty White	1 slice (1.5 oz)	110	2	0
Farmhouse Sesame Wheat	1 slice	110	2	0
Farmhouse Sourdough	1 slice (1.5 oz)	110	2	1
Jewish Rye	1 slice	80	1	0
Natural Whole Grain Whole Wheat	1 slice (1.2 oz)	90	1	0
Natural Whole Grain Honey Oat	1 slice (1.2 oz)	90	2	0
Sandwich Pocket Wheat	1 (2 oz)	160	1	1
Sandwich Pocket White	1 (2 oz)	150	1	0
Swirl Cinnamon	1 slice (1 oz)	90	3	1
Swirl Raisin Cinnamon	1 slice (1 oz)	80	2	0
Stroehmann				
100% Whole Wheat	1 slice (1.3 oz)	90	1	0
D'Italiano Italian No Seeds	1 slice (1 oz)	80	1	0
D'Italiano Italian Seeded	1 slice (1 oz)	80	1	0
Family White	1 slice (0.8 oz)	65	1	0
Homestyle Split Top Wheat	1 slices (0.8 oz)	60	0	0
Homestyle Split Top White	1 slice (0.8 oz)	65	1	0
Honey Cracked Wheat	1 slice (1.2 oz)	80	1	0
King White	1 slice (0.8 oz)	65	1	0
New York Rye	1 slice (1 oz)	80	1	0
Potato	1 slice (1.2 oz)	100	2	0
Ranch White	1 slice (0.8 oz)	65	1	0

FOOD	PORTION	CALS	FAT	SAT FAT
Rye	1 slice (1.1 oz)	80	1	0
Twelve Grain	1 slice (1.2 oz)	90	1	0
TastyBite				
Nan Kontos Massala	½ loaf (1.4 oz)	120	3	1
Nan Kontos Onion	½ loaf (1.4 oz)	120	4	1
Nan Kontos Roghani	½ loaf (1.4 oz)	125	3	2
Nan Kontos Tandoori	½ loaf (1.4 oz)	120	3	2
Roti Kontos Missy	½ loaf (1.4 oz)	125	4	2
Toufayan				
Wraps Sundried Tomato Basil	1 (2 oz)	183	5	1
Wraps Wheat	1 (2 oz)	183	5	1
Valley Lahvosh				
Valley Wraps	1 (1 oz)	100	1	0
ZA				
Pit-Za Hearty Multi-Grain	⅓ bread (2 oz)	130	2	0
Pit-Za Salt-Free Garlic Whole Wheat	⅓ bread (2 oz)	150	1	0
REFRIGERATED				
Pillsbury				
Crusty French Loaf	⅕ loaf (2.2 oz)	150	2	1
Grands Wheat	1 (2.1 oz)	200	8	2
TAKE-OUT				
chapatis as prep w/ fat	1 bread (1.6 oz)	95	2	1
chapatis as prep w/o fat	1 (2½ oz)	141	1	–
cornbread	2 in x 2 in (1.4 oz)	107	2	1
cornstick	1 (1.3 oz)	101	4	1
focaccia	1 piece (2 oz)	130	3	0
focaccia onion	1 piece (4.6 oz)	282	10	1
focaccia rosemary	1 piece (3.5 oz)	251	7	1
focaccia tomato olive	1 piece (4.7 oz)	270	8	1
garlic bread	2 slices (2 oz)	190	8	2
irish soda bread	1 slice (2 oz)	174	3	1
naan	1 bread (3.5 oz)	286	9	5
papadums fried	2 (1.5 oz)	81	4	–
paratha	1 bread (2.1 oz)	201	10	7
BREAD COATING				
Don's Chuck Wagon				
Chicken Baking Mix	¼ cup (1 oz)	95	0	0
Fish & Chips Mix	¼ cup (1 oz)	100	0	0
Fish Mix	¼ cup (1 oz)	95	0	0

FOOD	PORTION	CALS	FAT	SAT FAT
Mushroom Batter Mix	¼ cup (1 oz)	95	0	0
Onion Ring Mix	¼ cup (1 oz)	100	0	0
Seafood Bake & Fry Mix	¼ cup (1 oz)	95	0	0
Luzianne				
Cajun Chicken Coating Mix	2 tbsp (1 oz)	100	1	0
Oven Fry				
Extra Crispy For Chicken	⅛ pkg (0.5 oz)	60	1	0
Extra Crispy For Pork	⅛ pkg (0.5 oz)	60	2	0
Shake 'N Bake				
Buffalo Wings	1/10 pkg (0.4 oz)	40	1	0
Classic Italian Chicken or Pork	⅛ pkg (0.4 oz)	40	1	0
Country Mild Recipe	⅛ pkg (0.3 oz)	35	2	1
Glazes Barbecue Chicken Or Pork	⅛ pkg (0.4 oz)	45	1	0
Glazes Honey Mustard Chicken Or Pork	⅛ pkg (0.4 oz)	45	1	0
Glazes Tangy Honey Chicken Or Pork	⅛ pkg (0.4 oz)	45	1	0
Home Style Flour Recipe For Chicken	⅛ pkg (0.4 oz)	40	1	0
Hot & Spicy Chicken Or Pork	⅛ pkg (0.4 oz)	40	1	0
Original For Chicken	⅛ pkg (0.4 oz)	40	1	0
Original For Fish	¼ pkg (0.7 oz)	80	2	0
Original For Pork	⅛ pkg (0.4 oz)	45	1	0
BREAD MACHINE MIX				
Betty Crocker				
Harvest Wheat	1/11 loaf	140	3	1
Home-Style White	1/11 loaf	130	2	0
Carbsense				
Harvest Wheat as prep	1 slice	60	0	0
Fleischmann's				
Apple Cinnamon	⅛ loaf	160	1	0
Cinnamon Raisin	⅛ loaf	160	1	0
Country White	⅛ loaf (1.6 oz)	170	3	1
Cranberry Orange	⅛ loaf	150	2	0
Honey Oatmeal	⅛ loaf	160	1	0
Italian Herb	⅛ loaf	160	2	1
Sourdough	⅛ loaf	150	2	1
Stoneground Wheat	⅛ loaf	160	1	0
Keto				
Cinnamon Raisin as prep	1 slice	79	0	0
French Loaf as prep	1 slice	79	0	0

FOOD	PORTION	CALS	FAT	SAT FAT
Sourdough Rye as prep	1 slice	79	1	–
Ketogenics				
Low Carb Honey Wheat as prep	1 slice	80	1	1
Low Carb Original White as prep	1 slice	62	0	0
Low Carb Pumpernickel Rye as prep	1 slice	80	2	1
Sassafras				
Apricot Oatmeal	1 slice (1.4 oz)	140	1	0

BREADCRUMBS

FOOD	PORTION	CALS	FAT	SAT FAT
dry	1 cup	426	6	1
dry seasoned	1 cup (4 oz)	441	3	1
fresh	⅔ cup	76	1	tr
Keto				
Low Carb Cajun	½ cup	185	1	–
Low Carb Italian	½ cup	185	1	–
Low Carb Original	½ cup	185	1	–
Progresso				
Garlic & Herb	¼ cup (1 oz)	100	2	0
Italian Style	¼ cup (1 oz)	110	2	0
Parmesan	¼ cup (1 oz)	100	2	0
Plain	¼ cup (1 oz)	110	2	0
Ronzoni				
Italian Flavored	¼ cup	120	2	1

BREADFRUIT

FOOD	PORTION	CALS	FAT	SAT FAT
fresh	¼ small	99	tr	–
seeds cooked	1 oz	48	1	tr
seeds raw	1 oz	54	2	tr
seeds roasted	1 oz	59	tr	tr

BREADNUTTREE SEEDS

FOOD	PORTION	CALS	FAT	SAT FAT
dried	1 oz	104	tr	tr

BREADSTICKS

FOOD	PORTION	CALS	FAT	SAT FAT
onion poppyseed	1	64	1	–
plain	1	41	1	tr
plain	1 sm	25	1	tr
Bread Du Jour				
Original	1 (1.9 oz)	130	1	0
Sourdough	1 (1.9 oz)	130	1	0

FOOD	PORTION	CALS	FAT	SAT FAT
New York				
Garlic Soft	1 (1.5 oz)	140	4	1
Pepperidge Farm				
Snack Sticks Wheat	9 (1 oz)	130	4	1
Pillsbury				
Soft	1 (1.4 oz)	110	2	0
Soft Garlic & Herb	1 (2.1 oz)	180	7	2
Stella D'Oro				
Grissini Style Fat Free	3 (0.5 oz)	60	0	0
Original	1 (0.4 oz)	45	1	0
Potato 'N Onion	1 (0.4 oz)	45	1	0
Roasted Garlic	1 (0.4 oz)	45	1	0
Roasted Garlic	1 (0.4 oz)	45	1	0
Sesame	1 (0.4 oz)	50	3	0
Snack Stix Cracked Pepper	4 (0.5 oz)	70	2	0
Snack Stix Salted	4 (0.5 oz)	70	2	0
Sodium Free	1 (0.4 oz)	45	1	0
Wheat	1 (0.3 oz)	40	1	0

BREAKFAST BARS (see CEREAL BARS, ENERGY BARS)

BREAKFAST DRINKS

FOOD	PORTION	CALS	FAT	SAT FAT
orange drink powder	3 rounded tsp	93	0	0
orange drink powder as prep w/water	6 oz	86	0	0
Carnation				
Instant Breakfast French Vanilla as prep w/ 2% milk	1 serv	250	5	—
Instant Breakfast French Vanilla as prep w/ fat free milk	1 serv	220	1	—
Instant Breakfast French Vanilla as prep w/ whole milk	1 serv	280	8	—

BROAD BEANS

FOOD	PORTION	CALS	FAT	SAT FAT
canned	1 cup	183	1	tr
dried cooked	1 cup	186	1	tr
fresh cooked	3½ oz	56	tr	tr

BROCCOFLOWER

FOOD	PORTION	CALS	FAT	SAT FAT
fresh raw	½ cup (1.8 oz)	16	tr	tr

FOOD	PORTION	CALS	FAT	SAT FAT
BROCCOLI				
FRESH				
chinese broccoli (gai lan) cooked	1 cup (3.1 oz)	19	1	tr
chopped cooked	½ cup	22	tr	tr
raw chopped	½ cup	12	tr	tr
FROZEN				
chopped cooked	½ cup	25	tr	tr
spears cooked	10 oz pkg	69	tr	tr
spears cooked	½ cup	25	tr	tr
Birds Eye				
Chopped	⅓ cup	25	0	0
Cuts	½ cup	25	0	0
Florets	1 cup	25	0	0
In Cheese Sauce	½ cup	70	4	2
Fresh Like				
Spear	3.5 oz	26	tr	–
Green Giant				
Butter Sauce	4 oz	50	2	1
Cheese Sauce	⅔ cup (3.9 oz)	70	3	1
Chopped	¾ cup (2.8 oz)	25	0	0
Cuts	1 cup (2.9 oz)	25	0	0
Harvest Fresh Cut	⅔ cup (3.2 oz)	25	0	0
Harvest Fresh Spears	3.5 oz	25	0	0
Select Florets	1⅓ cups (2.9 oz)	25	0	0
Select Spears	3 oz	25	0	0
Health Is Wealth				
Broccoli Munchees	2 (1 oz)	60	2	0
Stouffer's				
Au Gratin	1 serv (4 oz)	100	4	2
Tree Of Life				
Cuts	1 cup (3.1 oz)	25	0	0
BROWNIE				
FROZEN				
Greenfield				
Fat Free Homestyle	1 (1.3 oz)	110	0	0
Otis Spunkmeyer				
Blue Yonder w/ Walnuts	1 (2 oz)	230	10	3
Weight Watchers				
Brownie A La Mode	1 (3.14 oz)	190	4	2

FOOD	PORTION	CALS	FAT	SAT FAT
Double Fudge Brownie Parfait	1 (5.3 oz)	190	3	2
MIX				
plain	1 (1.2 oz)	139	7	1
plain low calorie	1 (0.8 oz)	84	2	1
Atkins				
Kitchen Fudge as prep	1 (2 inch)	60	0	0
Aunt Paula's				
Low Carb Chef Fudge Brownie as prep	1 (2.5 inch)	89	5	2
Betty Crocker				
Chocolate Chunk as prep	1	180	9	2
Dark Chocolate Fudge as prep	1	170	7	1
Dark Chocolate w/ Syrup as prep	1	170	7	1
Fudge as prep	1	170	7	1
German Chocolate Coconut Pecan Filling as prep	1	200	8	2
Hot Fudge as prep	1	170	8	2
Original as prep	1	180	6	1
Peanut Butter as prep	1	180	8	3
Stir'n Bake w/ Mini Kisses as prep	1 serv	220	7	3
Turtle w/ Caramel & Pecans as prep	1	170	8	1
Walnut as prep	1	180	9	1
Estee				
Brownie Mix as prep	2	100	4	2
Keto				
Chocolate Fudge as prep	1	59	3	–
MiniCarb				
Chocolate Brownie as prep	1	220	17	4
No Pudge!				
All Flavors	1	100	0	0
Sweet Rewards				
Low Fat Fudge as prep	1	130	3	1
Reduced Fat Supreme as prep	1	140	3	1
READY-TO-EAT				
plain	1 lg (2 oz)	227	9	2
plain	1 sm (1 oz)	115	5	1
w/ nuts	1 (1 oz)	100	4	2
Dolly Madison				
Fudge	1 (3 oz)	330	11	4

FOOD	PORTION	CALS	FAT	SAT FAT
Entenmann's				
Little Bites	3 (2.2 oz)	290	16	3
Ultimate Fudge	1 (1.6 oz)	220	13	4
Greenfield				
Blondie Fat Free Apple Spice	1 (1.3 oz)	110	0	0
Health Valley				
Bar w/ Fudge Filling	1 bar	110	0	0
Hostess				
Brownie Bites	3 (1.3 oz)	170	9	2
Fudge	1 (3 oz)	330	11	4
Light	1 (1.4 oz)	140	3	1
Lance				
Fudge Nut	1 (2.25 oz)	340	13	3
Little Debbie				
Brownie Lights	1 (2 oz)	190	3	0
Brownie Loaves	1 (2.1 oz)	260	15	3
Fudge	1 pkg (2.1 oz)	270	13	3
Tastykake				
Fudge Walnut	1 (3 oz)	370	17	4
Tom's				
Fudge Nut	1 pkg (2.5 oz)	300	13	3
REFRIGERATED				
Toll House				
Brownie Dough	½₂ pkg (1.5 oz)	180	7	3
TAKE-OUT				
plain	1 2 in sq (2.1 oz)	243	10	3
BRUSSELS SPROUTS				
FRESH				
cooked	½ cup	30	tr	tr
cooked	1 sprout	8	tr	tr
raw	½ cup	19	tr	tr
raw	1 sprout	8	tr	tr
FROZEN				
cooked	½ cup	33	tr	tr
Birds Eye				
Brussels Sprouts	11 sprouts	35	0	0
Green Giant				
Butter Sauce	⅔ cup (3.6 oz)	60	2	2

FOOD	PORTION	CALS	FAT	SAT FAT
BUCKWHEAT				
groats roasted cooked	1 cup (5.9 oz)	647	1	tr
groats roasted uncooked	1 cup (5.7 oz)	567	4	1
BUFFALO				
burger	4 oz	150	5	3
water buffalo roasted	3 oz	111	2	1
BULGUR				
cooked	1 cup (6.3 oz)	151	tr	tr
uncooked	1 cup (4.9 oz)	479	2	tr
TAKE-OUT				
tabbouleh	½ cup	120	4	0
BURBOT (FISH)				
fresh baked	3 oz	98	1	tr
BURDOCK ROOT				
cooked	1 cup	110	tr	–
fresh	1 cup	85	tr	–
BUTTER				
clarified butter	3½ oz	876	99	62
ghee cow's milk	1 tbsp	126	14	–
ghee vegetable oil	1 tbsp	126	14	–
stick	1 stick (4 oz)	813	92	57
stick	1 pat (5 g)	36	4	3
whipped	4 oz	542	61	38
whipped	1 pat (4 g)	27	3	2
whipped	1 tbsp	70	7	5
Breakstone's				
Salted	1 tbsp (0.5 oz)	100	11	7
Cabot				
Butter	1 tbsp	100	11	7
Corman				
Light	1 tbsp	55	6	3
Hotel Bar				
Stick	1 tbsp (0.5 oz)	100	11	7
Keller's				
European	1 tbsp (0.5 oz)	100	11	7
Land O Lakes				
Salted	1 tbsp (0.5 oz)	100	11	8

FOOD	PORTION	CALS	FAT	SAT FAT
Ultra Creamy Salted	1 tbsp (0.5 oz)	110	12	8
Organic Valley				
Butter	1 tbsp (0.5 oz)	100	11	8
Unsalted	1 tbsp (0.5 oz)	110	12	8
BUTTER BEANS				
CANNED				
Green Giant				
Butter Beans	½ cup (4.5 oz)	90	0	0
Van Camp				
Butter Beans	½ cup (4.6 oz)	110	1	0
FROZEN				
Birds Eye				
Speckled	½ cup	100	0	0
BUTTER SUBSTITUTES				
stick	1 stick	811	91	32
Keto				
Butta	1 tsp	43	5	5
Molly McButter				
Natural Butter	1 tsp	5	0	0
Natural Cheese	1 tsp	5	0	0
Roasted Garlic	1 tsp	5	0	0
Mrs. Bateman's				
Butterlike Baking Butter	1 tbsp (0.5 oz)	36	1	tr
Butterlike Saute Butter	1 tbsp (0.5 oz)	40	2	1
Olivio				
Spread	1 tbsp	80	8	1
BUTTERBUR				
canned fuki chopped	1 cup	3	tr	–
fresh fuki	1 cup	13	tr	–
BUTTERFISH				
baked	3 oz	159	9	–
fillet baked	1 oz	47	3	–
BUTTERNUTS				
dried	1 oz	174	16	tr
BUTTERSCOTCH (see also CANDY)				
Hershey				
Chips	1 tbsp (0.5 oz)	80	4	4

FOOD	PORTION	CALS	FAT	SAT FAT
Nestle				
Morsels	1 tbsp	80	4	4
CABBAGE *(see also COLESLAW)*				
chinese bok choy shredded cooked	½ cup	10	tr	tr
chinese pak-choi raw shredded	½ cup	5	tr	tr
chinese pe-tsai raw shredded	1 cup	12	tr	tr
chinese pe-tsai shredded cooked	1 cup	16	tr	tr
danish raw	1 head (2 lbs)	228	2	tr
danish raw shredded	½ cup (1.2 oz)	9	tr	tr
danish shredded cooked	½ cup (2.6 oz)	17	tr	tr
green raw	1 head (2 lbs)	228	2	tr
green raw shredded	½ cup (1.2 oz)	9	tr	tr
green shredded cooked	½ cup (2.6 oz)	17	tr	tr
napa cooked	1 cup (3.8 oz)	13	tr	0
red raw shredded	½ cup	10	tr	tr
red shredded cooked	½ cup	16	tr	tr
savoy raw shredded	½ cup	10	tr	tr
savoy shredded cooked	½ cup	18	tr	tr
Greenwood				
Sweet & Sour Red	½ cup	100	0	0
Lohmann				
Red Cabbage Sweet & Sour	¼ cup	40	0	0
TAKE-OUT				
korean kimchee	½ cup	22	tr	–
northern white kimchi	½ cup	79	1	–
stuffed cabbage	1 (6 oz)	373	22	12
sweet & sour red cabbage	4 oz	61	3	–
CACTUS				
napoles fresh sliced	½ cup (1.5 oz)	7	tr	–
pricklypear fresh	1 cup (5.3 oz)	56	1	–
CAKE *(see also CAKE MIX)*				
angelfood	1 cake (11.9 oz)	876	3	tr
battenburg cake	1 slice (2 oz)	204	10	–
boston cream pie frzn	⅙ cake (3.2 oz)	232	8	2
carrot w/ cream cheese icing home recipe	1 cake 10 in diam	6175	328	66
cheesecake	1 cake 9 in diam	3350	213	120

FOOD	PORTION	CALS	FAT	SAT FAT
cheesecake	1/6 cake (2.8 oz)	256	18	9
cherry fudge w/ chocolate frosting	1/8 cake (2.5 oz)	187	9	3
coffeecake fruit	1/8 cake (1.8 oz)	156	5	1
cream puff shell	1 (2.3 oz)	239	17	4
crumpet	1 (2.3 oz)	131	1	–
devil's food cupcake w/ chocolate frosting	1	120	4	4
devil's food w/ creme filling	1 (1 oz)	105	4	2
eccles cake	1 slice (2 oz)	285	16	–
eclair	1 (1.4 oz)	149	10	–
fruitcake	1 piece (1.5 oz)	139	4	tr
fruitcake dark home recipe	1 cake 7½ in x 2¼ in	5185	228	48
jelly roll lemon filled	1 slice (3 oz)	210	2	1
madeira cake	1 slice (1 oz)	98	4	–
pound	1 cake 8½ x 3½ x 3 in	1935	94	52
pound	1/10 cake (1 oz)	117	6	3
pound fat free	1 cake (12 oz)	961	4	1
pound cake home recipe	1 loaf 8½ in x 3½ in	1935	94	21
sheet cake w/ white frosting home recipe	1 cake 9 in sq	4020	129	42
sheet cake w/o frosting home recipe	1 cake 9 in sq	2830	108	30
sheet cake w/o frosting home recipe	1/9 cake	315	12	3
sour cream pound	1/10 cake (1 oz)	117	5	1
sponge	1/12 cake (1.3 oz)	110	1	tr
sponge cake dessert shell	1 (0.8 oz)	70	2	1
sponge w/ creme filling	1 (1.5 oz)	155	5	1
tiramisu	1 cake (4.4 lbs)	5732	421	217
toaster pastry apple	1 (1¾ oz)	204	5	1
toaster pastry blueberry	1 (1¾ oz)	204	5	1
toaster pastry brown sugar cinnamon	1 (1¾ oz)	206	7	2
toaster pastry cherry	1 (1¾ oz)	204	5	1
toaster pastry strawberry	1 (1¾ oz)	204	5	1
treacle tart	1 slice (2.5 oz)	258	10	–
vanilla slice	1 slice (2½ oz)	248	13	–
white w/ white frosting	1/16 cake	260	9	2
white w/ white frosting	1 cake 9 in diam	4170	148	33

FOOD	PORTION	CALS	FAT	SAT FAT
yellow w/ chocolate frosting	⅛ cake (2.2 oz)	242	11	3
yellow w/ chocolate frosting	1 cake 9 diam	3895	175	92
Amy's				
Toaster Pops Apple	1	140	3	0
Toaster Pops Strawberry	1	140	3	0
Baby Watson				
Cheesecake	1 slice (3 oz)	260	18	11
Carousel				
New York Cheese Cake	1 cake (3 oz)	250	19	11
Dolly Madison				
Angel Food	1 slice (2.1 oz)	160	2	0
Apple Crumb	1 (1.6 oz)	160	5	2
Banana Dream Flip	1 (3.5 oz)	390	16	3
Bear Claw	1 (2.75 oz)	270	10	4
Carrot	1 (4 oz)	360	8	3
Chocolate Snack Squares	1 (1.6 oz)	210	10	6
Cinnamon Buttercrumb	1 (1.6 oz)	170	6	2
Cinnamon Buttercrumb Low Fat	1 (1.5 oz)	140	2	0
Cinnamon Stix	1 (1.3 oz)	170	9	4
Creme Cakes	2 (1.9 oz)	210	8	4
Cupcakes Chocolate	1 (2 oz)	210	7	3
Cupcakes Spice	1 (2 oz)	230	10	4
Dunkin' Stix	1 (1.3 oz)	170	9	4
Frosty Angel	1 (3.5 oz)	330	6	4
Holiday Cupcakes	1 (1.9 oz)	180	3	1
Honey Bun	1 (3.7 oz)	440	25	11
Koo Koos	1 (1.8 oz)	200	9	6
Mini Coconut Loaf	1 (3.5 oz)	350	10	2
Mini Pound Cake	1 (3.2 oz)	310	11	5
Raspberry Square	1 (1.8 oz)	190	8	4
Sweet Roll Apple	1 (2.2 oz)	200	6	2
Sweet Roll Cherry	1 (2.2 oz)	210	6	3
Sweet Roll Cinnamon	1 (2.2 oz)	230	7	3
Texas Cinnamon Bun	1 (4.2 oz)	440	15	6
Zingers Devil's Food	2 (2.6 oz)	270	8	4
Zingers Lemon	1 (1.4 oz)	150	6	3
Zingers Raspberry	1 (1.4 oz)	150	6	3
Zingers Yellow	2 (2.5 oz)	280	8	3
Drake's				
Coffee Cake Low Fat	1 (1.1 oz)	110	2	1

FOOD	PORTION	CALS	FAT	SAT FAT
Mini Coffee Cakes	4 (1.83 oz)	220	9	2
Yodel's	1 (1 oz)	150	9	–
Dutch Mill				
Dessert Shells Chocolate Covered	1 (0.5 oz)	80	5	2
Entenmann's				
Apple Puffs	1 (3 oz)	270	13	4
Coffee Cake Cheese Filled Crumb	1 serv (1.9 oz)	200	10	3
Coffee Cake Crumb	1 serv (2 oz)	250	12	3
Cupcakes Light Chocolate Creme Filled	1 (2 oz)	160	0	0
Hot Cross Buns	1 (2.3 oz)	230	7	2
Stollen Fruit	⅛ cake (2 oz)	210	7	2
Ultimate Crumb Cake	⅒ cake	250	13	3
Fillo Factory				
Apple Turnovers Vegan	5 (5 oz)	270	5	0
Goody Man				
Happy Birthday Cupcake Chocolate	1 (1.75 oz)	200	6	3
Happy Birthday Cupcake White	1 (1.75 oz)	190	5	2
Greenfield				
Blondie Fat Free Chocolate Chip	1 (1.3 oz)	110	0	0
Hostess				
Angel Food	⅛ cake (2 oz)	160	2	0
Chocodiles	1 (1.6 oz)	240	11	8
Chocolicious	1 (1.6 oz)	190	7	3
Coffee Crumb	1 (1.1 oz)	130	5	2
Crumb Cake Light	1 (1 oz)	100	2	0
Cupcakes Chocolate	1 (1.8 oz)	180	6	3
Cupcakes Orange	1 (1.5 oz)	160	5	2
Cupcakes Light Chocolate	1 (1.6 oz)	140	2	1
Ding Dongs	2 (2.7 oz)	360	19	12
Ho Ho's	2 (2 oz)	250	12	8
Honey Bun Glazed	1 (2.7 oz)	320	19	9
Honey Bun Iced	1 (3.4 oz)	410	24	11
Shortcake Dessert Cups	1 (1 oz)	100	2	1
Sno Balls	1 (1.8 oz)	180	5	3
Suzy Q's	1 (2 oz)	230	9	4
Sweet Roll Cherry	1 (2.2 oz)	210	6	3
Sweet Roll Cinnamon	1 (2.2 oz)	230	7	3
Twinkies	1 (1.5 oz)	150	5	2
Twinkies Light	1 (1.5 oz)	130	2	1

FOOD	PORTION	CALS	FAT	SAT FAT
Jell-O				
Dessert Delights Cheesecake	1 bar (1.4 oz)	160	7	3
Dessert Delights Chocolate Fudge Pudding	1 bar (1.4 oz)	150	6	3
Kellogg's				
Pop-Tarts Apple Cinnamon	1 (1.8 oz)	210	6	1
Pop-Tarts Blueberry	1 (1.8 oz)	210	5	1
Pop-Tarts Brown Sugar Cinnamon	1 (1.8 oz)	210	6	1
Pop-Tarts Cherry	1 (1.8 oz)	200	5	1
Pop-Tarts Chocolate Graham	1 (1.8 oz)	210	6	2
Pop-Tarts Frosted Apple Cinnamon	1 (1.8 oz)	190	3	1
Pop-Tarts Frosted Blueberry	1 (1.8 oz)	200	5	1
Pop-Tarts Frosted Brown Sugar Cinnamon	1 (1.8 oz)	210	7	2
Pop-Tarts Frosted Cherry	1 (1.8 oz)	200	5	1
Pop-Tarts Frosted Chocolate Vanilla Creme	1 (1.8 oz)	200	5	1
Pop-Tarts Frosted Chocolate Fudge	1 (1.8 oz)	200	5	1
Pop-Tarts Frosted Grape	1 (1.8 oz)	200	5	1
Pop-Tarts Frosted Raspberry	1 (1.8 oz)	210	5	1
Pop-Tarts Frosted S'mores	1 (1.8 oz)	200	6	1
Pop-Tarts Frosted Strawberry	1 (1.8 oz)	200	5	1
Pop-Tarts Frosted Wild Berry	1 (2 oz)	210	5	1
Pop-Tarts Frosted Wild Watermelon	1 (2 oz)	210	5	1
Pop-Tarts Low Fat Blueberry	1 (1.8 oz)	190	3	1
Pop-Tarts Low Fat Cherry	1 (1.8 oz)	190	3	1
Pop-Tarts Low Fat Frosted Brown Sugar Cinnamon	1 (1.8 oz)	190	3	1
Pop-Tarts Low Fat Frosted Chocolate Fudge	1 (1.8 oz)	190	3	1
Pop-Tarts Low Fat Frosted Strawberry	1 (1.8 oz)	190	3	1
Pop-Tarts Low Fat Strawberry	1 (1.8 oz)	190	3	1
Pop-Tarts Strawberry	1 (1.8 oz)	200	5	1
Lance				
Dunking Sticks	1 (2.75 oz)	180	10	3
Fig Cake	½ piece (2.1 oz)	110	2	5
Fig Cake Fat Free	½ piece (2.1 oz)	100	0	0
Honey Bun	1 (3 oz)	330	13	5
Pecan Twirls	1 pkg (2 oz)	220	9	4
Swiss Rolls	1 (2.5 oz)	170	9	5

FOOD	PORTION	CALS	FAT	SAT FAT
Little Debbie				
Angel Cakes Lemon	1 (1.6 oz)	130	1	0
Angel Cakes Raspberry	1 (1.6 oz)	130	1	0
Banana Nut Loaves	1 (1.9 oz)	220	10	2
Banana Twins	1 (2.2 oz)	250	10	3
Be My Valentine Chocolate	1 (2.2 oz)	280	13	3
Be My Valentine Vanilla	1 (2.2 oz)	290	14	3
Blueberry Loaves	1 (2 oz)	220	10	2
Chocolate Chip	1 (2.4 oz)	310	15	4
Christmas Tree Cake	1 pkg (1.5 oz)	190	10	2
Coconut Creme	1 (1.7 oz)	210	10	3
Coffee Cake Apple	1 (2.1 oz)	230	7	2
Cupcake Creme Filled Chocolate	1 (1.6 oz)	180	9	2
Cupcake Creme Filled Orange	1 (1.7 oz)	210	10	3
Cupcake Creme Filled Strawberry	1 (1.7 oz)	210	10	3
Devil Cremes	1 (1.6 oz)	190	8	2
Devil Squares	1 (2.2 oz)	270	13	3
Easter Basket Cake Chocolate	1 (2.4 oz)	300	14	4
Easter Basket Cake Vanilla	1 (2.5 oz)	320	10	4
Fall Party Cake Chocolate	1 (2.4 oz)	290	14	3
Fall Party Cake Vanilla	1 (2.5 oz)	310	15	4
Fancy Cakes	1 (2.4 oz)	300	15	4
Frosted Fudge	1 (1.5 oz)	200	10	3
Golden Cremes	1 (1.5 oz)	150	5	2
Holiday Cake Roll Cherry Creme	1 (2.1 oz)	260	12	3
Holiday Snack Cake Chocolate	1 (2.4 oz)	300	14	3
Holiday Snack Cake Vanilla	1 (2.5 oz)	320	15	4
Honey Bun	1 (1.8 oz)	220	13	4
Pecan Spinwheels	1 (1 oz)	110	4	1
Snack Cake Chocolate	1 (2.5 oz)	310	15	4
Strawberry Shortcake Roll	1 (2.1 oz)	230	8	2
Swiss Rolls	1 (2.1 oz)	270	12	3
Zebra Cakes	1 (2.6 oz)	330	16	4
Marie Callender's				
Cobbler Apple	1 serv (4.25 oz)	370	20	9
Cobbler Berry	1 serv (4.25 oz)	370	21	5
Cobbler Cherry	1 serv (4.25 oz)	380	19	8
Cobbler Peach	1 serv (4.25 oz)	380	18	6
Natural Touch				
Toaster Square Blueberry	1 (2.8 oz)	180	2	1

FOOD	PORTION	CALS	FAT	SAT FAT
Toaster Squares Date Walnut	1 (2.8 oz)	200	3	1
Pepperidge Farm				
Apple Turnover	1 (3.1 oz)	330	14	3
Blueberry Turnover	1 (3.1 oz)	340	16	3
Cherry Turnover	1 (3.1 oz)	320	13	3
Large Layer Chocolate Fudge	⅛ cake (2.4 oz)	260	11	3
Large Layer Coconut	⅛ cake (2.4 oz)	260	11	3
Large Layer Vanilla	⅛ cake (2.4 oz)	250	11	3
Mini Turnover Apple	1 (1.4 oz)	140	8	2
Mini Turnover Cherry	1 (1.4 oz)	140	8	2
Mini Turnover Strawberry	1 (1.4 oz)	140	7	2
Peach Turnover	1 (3.1 oz)	340	15	3
Raspberry Turnover	1 (3.1 oz)	330	14	3
Philadelphia				
Snack Bars Classic Cheesecake	1 (1.5 oz)	200	13	6
Pillsbury				
Apple Turnovers	1 (2 oz)	170	8	2
Cherry Turnovers	1 (2 oz)	180	8	2
Sara Lee				
Cheesecake 25% Reduced Fat	¼ cake (4.2 oz)	310	13	8
Cheesecake Cherry Cream	¼ cake (4.7 oz)	350	12	5
Cheesecake Chocolate Chip	¼ cake (4.2 oz)	410	21	14
Cheesecake French	⅙ cake (3.9 oz)	350	21	13
Cheesecake French Strawberry	⅙ cake (4.3 oz)	320	14	9
Cheesecake Strawberry Cream	¼ cake (4.7 oz)	330	12	5
Coffee Cake Butter Streusel	⅙ cake (1.9 oz)	220	12	6
Coffee Cake Crumb	⅛ cake (2 oz)	220	9	2
Coffee Cake Pecan	⅙ cake (1.9 oz)	230	12	5
Coffee Cake Raspberry	⅙ cake (1.9 oz)	220	8	3
Coffee Cake Reduced Fat Cheese	⅙ cake (1.9 oz)	180	6	2
Layer Cake Coconut	⅛ cake (2.8 oz)	260	14	10
Layer Cake Double Chocolate	⅛ cake (2.8 oz)	260	13	9
Layer Cake Fudge Golden	⅛ cake (2.8 oz)	260	13	10
Layer Cake German Chocolate	⅛ cake (2.9 oz)	280	14	9
Layer Cake Vanilla	⅛ cake (2.8 oz)	260	14	10
Original Cheesecake	¼ cake (4.2 oz)	350	18	9
Pound Cake All Butter	¼ cake (2.7 oz)	320	16	9
Pound Cake Chocolate Swirl	¼ cake (2.9 oz)	330	16	8
Pound Cake Family Size	⅙ cake (2.7 oz)	310	17	9
Pound Cake Reduced Fat	¼ cake (2.7 oz)	280	11	3

FOOD	PORTION	CALS	FAT	SAT FAT
Pound Cake Strawberry Swirl	¼ cake (2.9 oz)	290	11	3
Strawberry Shortcake	⅛ cake (2.5 oz)	180	7	5
Sinbad				
Baklava	1 piece (2 oz)	337	20	4
Snack & Smile				
Mini Loaf Apple Cinnamon	1 loaf (2 oz)	190	8	2
Mini Loaf Banana	1 loaf (2 oz)	200	8	2
Mini Loaf Blueberry	1 loaf (2 oz)	190	8	2
Mini Loaf Carrot	1 loaf (2 oz)	200	8	2
SnackWell's				
Streusel Squares Apple Cinnamon	1 (1.5 oz)	150	3	0
Streusel Squares Cherry	1 (1.5 oz)	150	3	0
Super				
Bun	1 (2.5 oz)	270	16	4
Tastykake				
Banana Creamie	1 (1.5 oz)	170	7	1
Bear Claw Apple	1 (3 oz)	280	7	2
Bear Claw Cinnamon	1 (3 oz)	300	8	2
Big Texas	1 (3 oz)	300	9	2
Breakfast Bun Chocolate Raisin	1 (3.2 oz)	330	8	2
Bunny Trail Treats	1 (1.3 oz)	150	6	1
Chocolate Creamie	1 (1.5 oz)	180	8	1
Chocolate Krimpies	2 (2.2 oz)	240	10	2
Coffee Roll Glazed	1 (3 oz)	300	9	2
Coffee Roll Vanilla	1 (3.2 oz)	320	9	2
Cupcakes	2 (2.1 oz)	200	5	1
Cupcakes Butter Cream Cream Filled Iced	2 (2.2 oz)	240	8	2
Cupcakes Chocolate Cream Filled Iced	2 (2.2 oz)	230	8	1
Cupcakes Low Fat Vanilla Cream Filled	2 (2.2 oz)	190	2	0
Cupid Kake	1 (1.3 oz)	150	6	1
Honey Bun Glazed	1 (3.2 oz)	350	17	4
Honey Bun Iced	1 (3.2 oz)	350	17	4
Junior Chocolate	1 (3.3 oz)	330	12	2
Junior Coconut	1 (3.3 oz)	310	8	4
Junior Koffee Kake	1 (2.5 oz)	270	9	2
Junior Pound Kake	1 (3 oz)	320	13	5
Kandy Kakes Chocolate	3 (2 oz)	250	13	8

FOOD	PORTION	CALS	FAT	SAT FAT
Kandy Kakes Coconut	2 (2.7 oz)	330	18	13
Kandy Kakes Peanut Butter	2 (1.3 oz)	190	9	5
Koffee Kake Cream Filled	2 (2 oz)	240	10	2
Koffee Kake Low Fat Apple	2 (2 oz)	170	2	0
Koffee Kake Low Fat Lemon	2 (2 oz)	180	3	0
Koffee Kake Low Fat Raspberry	2 (2 oz)	170	2	0
Koffee Kakes	1 (2 oz)	210	7	1
Kreepy Kakes	2 (2.2 oz)	240	8	2
Kreme Krimpies	2 (2 oz)	230	9	1
Krimpets Butterscotch Iced	2 (2 oz)	210	5	1
Krimpets Jelly Fillled	2 (2 oz)	190	3	1
Krimpets Strawberry	2 (2 oz)	210	5	1
Kringle Kake	1 (1.3 oz)	150	6	1
Santa Snacks	2 (2.2 oz)	240	8	2
Sparkle Kake	1 (1.3 oz)	150	6	1
Tasty Tweets	2 (2.2 oz)	240	8	2
Tropical Delight Coconut	2 (2 oz)	190	9	5
Tropical Delight Guava	2 (2 oz)	190	7	4
Tropical Delight Papaya	2 (2 oz)	200	7	4
Tropical Delight Pineapple	2 (2 oz)	200	7	4
Vanilla Creamie	1 (1.5 oz)	190	9	1
Witchy Treat	1 (1.3 oz)	150	6	1
Tom's				
Honey Bun	1 pkg (3 oz)	360	20	—
Honey Bun Jelly Filled	1 pkg (4 oz)	490	29	10
Marble Pound	1 pkg (2.5 oz)	300	16	4
Texas Cinnamon Roll	1 pkg (4 oz)	360	6	2
Tortuga				
Cayman Island Rum Cake	1 piece (2 oz)	194	9	2
Weight Watchers				
Chocolate Raspberry Royale	1 (3.5 oz)	190	3	1
Chocolate Eclair	1 (2.1 oz)	150	4	1
Danish Coffee Cake Apple Cinnamon	1 piece (1.9 oz)	160	3	1
Danish Coffee Cake Cheese	1 piece (1.9 oz)	160	3	1
Danish Coffee Cake Raspberry	1 piece (1.9 oz)	160	3	1
Double Fudge	1 piece (2.75 oz)	190	4	2
French Style Cheesecake	1 piece (3.9 oz)	170	4	2
New York Style Cheesecake	1 piece (2.5 oz)	150	5	3
Strawberry Parfait Royale	1 (5.24 oz)	180	2	1
Triple Chocolate Eclair	1 (2.14 oz)	160	5	1

FOOD	PORTION	CALS	FAT	SAT FAT
TAKE-OUT				
angelfood	1/12 cake (1 oz)	73	tr	tr
apple crisp	½ cup (5 oz)	230	5	1
baklava	1 oz	126	9	4
basbousa namoura	1 piece (1 oz)	60	3	0
boston cream pie	1/6 cake (3.3 oz)	293	12	4
cannoli w/ cannoli cream	1	369	21	–
carrot w/ cream cheese icing	1/12 cake (3.9 oz)	484	29	5
cheesecake w/ cherry topping	1/12 cake (5 oz)	359	23	13
chocolate w/ chocolate frosting	1/8 cake (2.2 oz)	235	11	3
coffeecake cheese	1/6 cake (2.7 oz)	258	12	4
coffeecake crumb topped cheese	1/6 cake (2.7 oz)	258	12	4
coffeecake crumb topped cinnamon	1/9 cake (2.2 oz)	263	15	4
cream puff w/ custard filling	1 (4.6 oz)	336	20	5
dutch honey cake	1 slice (0.8 oz)	70	0	0
eclair w/ chocolate icing & custard filling	1	205	10	–
french apple tart	1 (3.5 oz)	302	15	9
fruitcake	1/3 cake (2.9 oz)	302	10	1
gingerbread	1/9 cake (2.6 oz)	264	12	3
panettone	1/12 cake (2.9 oz)	300	12	9
petit fours	2 (0.9 oz)	120	7	3
pineapple upside down	1/9 cake (4 oz)	367	14	3
pound fat free	1 oz	80	tr	tr
pound cake	1 slice (1 oz)	120	5	1
sacher torte	1 slice (2.2 oz)	240	11	5
sheet cake w/ white frosting	1/9 cake	445	14	5
strudel apple	1 piece (2½ oz)	195	8	2
tiramisu	1 piece (5.1 oz)	409	30	15
trifle w/ cream	6 oz	291	16	–
yellow w/ vanilla frosting	1/8 cake (2.2 oz)	239	9	2
CAKE ICING				
chocolate ready-to-use	1/12 pkg (1.3 oz)	151	7	2
glaze home recipe	1/12 recipe (1 oz)	97	2	tr
vanilla ready-to-use	1/12 pkg (1.3 oz)	159	6	2
Betty Crocker				
HomeStyle Mix Coconut Pecan as prep	2 tbsp	160	2	3
HomeStyle Mix White Fluffy as prep	6 tbsp	100	0	0

FOOD	PORTION	CALS	FAT	SAT FAT
Party Frosting Chocolate w/ Stars	2 tbsp (1.2 oz)	140	5	2
Rich & Creamy Butter Cream	2 tbsp (1.3 oz)	140	5	2
Rich & Creamy Cherry	2 tbsp (1.2 oz)	140	5	2
Rich & Creamy Chocolate	2 tbsp (1.2 oz)	130	5	2
Rich & Creamy Cream Cheese	2 tbsp (1.2 oz)	140	5	2
Rich & Creamy Dark Chocolate	2 tbsp (1.3 oz)	130	6	2
Rich & Creamy French Vanilla	2 tbsp (1.2 oz)	140	5	2
Rich & Creamy Milk Chocolate	2 tbsp (1.3 oz)	130	5	2
Rich & Creamy Rainbow Chip	2 tbsp (1.2 oz)	140	5	2
Rich & Creamy Vanilla	2 tbsp (1.2 oz)	140	5	2
Toppers Milk Chocolate	2 tbsp (1.2 oz)	130	5	2
Toppers Vanilla	2 tbsp (1.2 oz)	140	5	2
Duncan Hines				
Chocolate Creamy Homestyle	2 tbsp	130	5	2
Milk Chocolate Creamy Homestyle	2 tbsp	130	5	2
Vanilla Creamy Homestyle	2 tbsp	140	5	2
Estee				
Frosting as prep	⅕ pkg	100	0	0
Sweet Rewards				
Ready-To-Spread Reduced Fat Chocolate	2 tbsp (1.2 oz)	120	2	1
Ready-To-Spread Reduced Fat Vanilla	2 tbsp (1.2 oz)	130	2	1
CAKE MIX				
angelfood	½ cake (1.8 oz)	129	tr	tr
angelfood	10 in cake (20.9 oz)	1535	2	tr
carrot w/o frosting	2 layers (29.6 oz)	2886	133	22
carrot w/o frosting	½ cake (2.5 oz)	239	11	2
chocolate pudding type w/o frosting	½ cake (2.7 oz)	270	14	3
chocolate pudding type w/o frosting	2 layers (32.4 oz)	3234	172	35
chocolate w/o frosting	½ cake (2.3 oz)	198	8	2
chocolate w/o frosting	2 layers (26.8 oz)	2393	92	21
coffeecake crumb topped cinnamon	⅛ cake (2 oz)	178	5	1
devil's food w/o frosting	½ cake (2.3 oz)	198	8	2
devil's food w/ chocolate frosting	1 cake 9 in diam	3755	136	56

FOOD	PORTION	CALS	FAT	SAT FAT
devil's food w/ chocolate frosting	1/16 cake	235	8	4
fudge w/o frosting	1/12 cake (2.3 oz)	198	8	2
gingerbread	1 cake 8 in sq	1575	39	10
gingerbread	1/9 cake (2.4 oz)	207	7	2
white w/o frosting	1/12 cake (2.2 oz)	190	5	1
white w/o frosting	2 layer cake (26 oz)	2265	57	9
yellow w/ chocolate frosting	1/16 cake	235	8	3
yellow w/o frosting	1/12 cake (2.2 oz)	202	6	1
yellow w/o frosting	2 layers (26.5 oz)	2415	71	12
yellow w/ chocolate frosting	1 cake 9 in diam	3895	175	92
Betty Crocker				
Angel Food Fat Free	1/12 cake	140	0	0
Angel Food Fat Free Confetti as prep	1/12 cake	150	0	0
Cheesecake Chocolate Chip as prep	1/8 cake	410	28	13
Cheesecake Original as prep	1/8 cake	400	27	12
Cheesecake Strawberry Swirl as prep	1/8 cake	380	25	11
Pineapple Upside Down as prep	1/6 cake	420	14	3
Quick Bread Banana	1/12 cake	170	7	1
Quick Bread Cinnamon Streusel as prep	1/14 cake	180	7	2
Quick Bread Cranberry Orange as prep	1/12 cake	170	6	2
Quick Bread Lemon Poppy Seed as prep	1/12 cake	170	7	1
Stir'n Bake Carrot Cake w/ Cream Cheese Frosting as prep	1/6 cake	260	7	2
Stir'n Bake Coffee Cake w/ Cinnamon Streusel as prep	1/6 cake	230	2	1
Stir'n Bake Devils Food w/ Chocolate Frosting as prep	1/6 cake	240	7	2
Stir'n Bake Yellow w/ Chocolate Frosting as prep	1/6 cake	240	7	2
SuperMoist Butter Pecan as prep	1/12 cake	240	10	2
SuperMoist Butter Yellow as prep	1/12 cake	260	11	6
SuperMoist Carrot as prep	1/10 cake	320	15	3
SuperMoist Cherry Chip	1/10 cake	300	13	3
SuperMoist Chocolate Fudge as prep	1/12 cake	270	12	3

FOOD	PORTION	CALS	FAT	SAT FAT
SuperMoist Golden Vanilla as prep	1/12 cake	240	10	2
SuperMoist Lemon as prep	1/12 cake	240	10	2
SuperMoist Milk Chocolate as prep	1/12 cake	240	10	2
SuperMoist Pineapple as prep	1/12 cake	250	7	2
SuperMoist Spice as prep	1/12 cake	240	10	2
SuperMoist Strawberry as prep	1/12 cake	250	10	2
SuperMoist White as prep	1/12 cake	230	14	2
SuperMoist White Light as prep	1/10 cake	210	3	1
Bisquick				
Mix	1/3 cup (1.4 oz)	160	6	2
Reduced Fat	1/3 cup (1.4 oz)	140	3	1
Carbolite				
Cheesecake Chocolate as prep	1/8 cake	260	25	–
Carbsense				
Zero Carb Baking Mix	1 oz	110	1	1
Dromedary				
Date Bread	1/11 cake (2 oz)	190	7	2
Date Nut Roll	1/2 in slice	80	2	–
Gingerbread	1 piece (2 in x 2 in)	100	2	–
Pound	1/2 in slice	150	6	–
Duncan Hines				
Angel Food as prep	1/12 pkg (1.3 oz)	140	0	0
Butter Recipe Golden as prep	1/12 cake	320	16	7
Cupcake Yellow as prep	1	180	0	2
Dark Chocolate Fudge as prep	1/12 cake	290	15	3
Devil's Food Moist Deluxe as prep	1/12 cake (1.5 oz)	290	15	3
French Vanilla	1/12 cake (1.5 oz)	250	11	2
Fudge Marble Moist Deluxe as prep	1/12 cake (1.5 oz)	250	17	2
Lemon Supreme Moist Deluxe	1/12 cake (1.5 oz)	250	17	2
White Moist Deluxe as prep	1/12 cake	190	6	1
Yellow Moist Deluxe as prep	1/12 cake (1.5 oz)	250	17	11
Yellow Moist Deluxe as prep	1/12 cake	250	11	2
Estee				
Chocolate as prep	1/8 cake	190	4	2
White as prep	1/8 cake	200	4	2
Hodgson Mill				
Gingerbread Whole Wheat	1/4 cup (1 oz)	110	0	0
Jell-O				
No Bake Cherry Cheesecake as prep	1/6 cake (4.8 oz)	340	12	5

FOOD	PORTION	CALS	FAT	SAT FAT
No Bake Double Layer Chocolate as prep	⅛ cake (4.4 oz)	260	12	5
No Bake Double Layer Cookies And Creme as prep	⅛ cake (4.5 oz)	390	19	7
No Bake Double Layer Lemon as prep	⅛ cake (4.4 oz)	260	12	4
No Bake Homestyle Cheesecake as prep	⅙ cake (4.6 oz)	360	15	4
No Bake Peanut Butter Cup as prep	⅛ cake (3.8 oz)	380	23	10
No Bake Reduced Fat Strawberry Swirl Cheesecake as prep	⅛ cake (4 oz)	250	6	2
No Bake Strawberry Cheesecake as prep	⅛ cake (4.8 oz)	340	12	5
Real Cheesecake as prep	⅛ cake (4.6 oz)	360	16	6
MiniCarb				
Carrot as prep	1 slice	280	20	3
Chocolate as prep	1 slice	230	18	4
Zero Carb Baking Mix not prep	½ cup	55	1	0
Sweet Rewards				
Reduced Fat White as prep	1/12 cake	180	3	1
Reduced Fat Yellow as prep	1/12 cake	200	5	1
CALABAZA				
fresh	½ cup	32	tr	—
CALZONE				
TAKE-OUT				
beef and cheese	1	330	35	5
cheese	1 (12 oz)	1020	54	24
pepperoni	1	450	19	9
CANADIAN BACON				
grilled	1 pkg (6 oz)	257	12	4
Boar's Head				
Canadian Bacon	2 oz	70	3	1
Hormel				
Sandwich Style	3 slices (2 oz)	70	3	2
Jones				
Slices	3	70	3	1
Oscar Mayer				
Canadian Bacon	2 slices (1.6 oz)	50	2	1

FOOD	PORTION	CALS	FAT	SAT FAT
Yorkshire Farms				
Uncured	3 oz	100	4	2

CANADIAN BACON SUBSTITUTES
Yves

FOOD	PORTION	CALS	FAT	SAT FAT
Canadian Veggie Bacon	1 serv (2 oz)	80	1	0

CANDY

FOOD	PORTION	CALS	FAT	SAT FAT
boiled sweets	¼ lb	327	0	–
butterscotch	1 oz	112	1	tr
butterscotch	1 piece (6 g)	24	tr	tr
candied cherries	1 (4 g)	12	tr	tr
candied citron	1 oz	89	tr	–
candied lemon peel	1 oz	90	tr	–
candied orange peel	1 oz	90	tr	–
candied pineapple slice	1 slice (2 oz)	179	tr	tr
candy corn	1 oz	105	0	0
caramels	1 piece (8 g)	31	1	1
caramels	1 pkg (2.5 oz)	271	6	5
caramels chocolate	1 piece (6 g)	22	tr	tr
caramels chocolate	1 bar (2.3 oz)	231	2	tr
carob bar	1 (3.1 oz)	453	28	7
crisped rice bar almond	1 bar (1 oz)	130	6	1
crisped rice bar chocolate chip	1 bar (1 oz)	115	4	1
dark chocolate	1 oz	150	10	6
fondant chocolate coated	1 lg (1.2 oz)	128	3	2
fondant chocolate coated	1 sm (0.4 oz)	40	1	1
fondant mint	1 oz	105	0	0
fruit pastilles	1 tube (1.4 oz)	101	0	–
gumdrops	10 sm (0.4 oz)	135	0	0
gumdrops	10 lg (3.8 oz)	420	0	0
hard candy	1 oz	106	0	0
jelly beans	10 sm (0.4 oz)	40	tr	–
jelly beans	10 lg (1 oz)	104	tr	–
lollipop	1 (6 g)	22	0	0
marzipan	1 oz	128	7	1
milk chocolate	1 bar (1.55 oz)	226	14	8
milk chocolate crisp	1 bar (1.45 oz)	203	11	7
milk chocolate w/ almonds	1 bar (1.45 oz)	215	14	7
nougat nut cream	0.5 oz	49	4	–
peanut bar	1 (1.4 oz)	209	14	2

FOOD	PORTION	CALS	FAT	SAT FAT
peanuts chocolate covered	10 (1.4 oz)	208	13	6
peanuts chocolate covered	1 cup (5.2 oz)	773	50	22
pretzels chocolate covered	1 (0.4 oz)	50	2	1
pretzels chocolate covered	1 oz	130	5	2
sesame crunch	20 pieces (1.2 oz)	181	12	2
sesame crunch	1 oz	146	9	1
sweet chocolate	1 bar (1.45 oz)	201	14	8
sweet chocolate	1 oz	143	10	6
truffles	4 pieces (1.1 oz)	190	14	13
100 Grand				
Bar	1 bar (1.5 oz)	200	8	5
3 Musketeers				
Bar	2 fun size (1.2 oz)	140	4	3
Bar	1 (2.1 oz)	260	8	4
5th Avenue				
Snack Size	1 bar (0.58 oz)	80	4	2
Almond Joy				
Snack Size	1 (0.6 oz)	90	5	4
Altoids				
All Flavors	3 pieces	10	0	0
Andes				
Chocolate Covered Mint Patties	1 (0.5 oz)	60	1	1
At Last!				
Chocolate Almond	1 bar	120	10	6
Chocolate Crisp	1 bar	110	9	6
Chocolate Mint	1 bar	110	10	6
Chocolate Peanut Butter	1 bar	100	8	5
Chocolate Peanut Butter	1 bar	120	11	7
Atkins				
Endulge Caramel Nut Chew	1 bar (1.23 oz)	140	9	4
Endulge Chocolate Bar	1 bar (1.1 oz)	150	12	7
Endulge Chocolate Crunch	1 bar (1 oz)	150	12	7
Endulge Peanut Butter Cups	3 pieces	160	13	6
Baby Ruth				
Bar	1 bar (2.1 oz)	270	13	7
Fun Size	1 bar (1 oz)	130	6	4
Barricini				
Dark Chocolate Raspberry Creme Shells	1 piece (0.3 oz)	47	3	1

FOOD	PORTION	CALS	FAT	SAT FAT
Bittyfinger				
Bars	2	170	7	4
Body Smarts				
Chocolate Peanut Crunch	2 bars (1.8 oz)	210	6	4
Breath Savers				
Sugar Free Mint Cinnamon	1 piece (2 g)	10	0	0
Sugar Free Peppermint	1 piece (2 g)	10	0	0
Sugar Free Spearmint	1 piece (2 g)	10	0	—
Sugar Free Wintergreen	1 piece (2 g)	10	0	—
Butterfinger				
BB's	1 pkg (1.7 oz)	230	9	6
Bar	1 (2.1 oz)	270	11	5
Fun Size	1 bar	100	4	2
Cadbury				
Milk Chocolate Roast Almond	10 blocks (1.4 oz)	220	13	7
Cape Cod Provisions				
Cranberry Bog Frogs	3 pieces (1.9 oz)	250	12	10
CarbSlim				
Crunch Bites Chocolate Caramel	1 pkg	122	14	12
Crunch Bites Peanut Butter	1 pkg	171	14	12
Carbolite				
Caramel	1 bar	100	5	3
CarbAway	1 bar	100	5	3
CarboSnack	1 bar	110	6	3
Chocolate Truffle	1 bar (1 oz)	122	8	5
Chocolate Almond	1 bar (1.75 oz)	298	21	11
Chocolate Crisp	1 bar (1.75 oz)	256	14	11
Chocolate Peanut Butter	1 bar (1.75 oz)	256	21	7
Crispy Caramel	1 bar (1 oz)	130	9	5
Milk Chocolate	1 bar (1.75 oz)	263	18	11
Peanut Butter Cup	1	170	14	7
Pecan Cluster	1 bar	120	8	3
Carmello				
Snack Size	1 (0.66 oz)	90	4	3
Cary's Of Oregon				
English Toffee Milk Chocolate Almond	1 piece (0.75 oz)	110	8	4
Charleston Chew				
Chocolate	½ bar	120	3	—
Strawberry	½ bar	120	3	—

FOOD	PORTION	CALS	FAT	SAT FAT
Vanilla	½ bar	120	3	—
Charms				
Blow Pop	1 (0.6 oz)	70	0	0
Lollipop Sour	1 (0.6 oz)	70	0	0
Lollipop Sweet	1 (0.6 oz)	70	0	0
Chunky				
Bar	1 (1.4 oz)	210	11	6
Cloud Nine				
Australian Orange Peel	½ bar (1.5 oz)	220	13	7
Butter Nut Toffee	½ bar (1.5 oz)	230	14	8
Cool Mint Crisp	½ bar (⅓ oz)	220	13	7
Espresso Bean Crunch	½ bar (1.5 oz)	220	14	8
Malted Milk Crunch	½ bar (1.5 oz)	230	14	8
Milk Chocolate	½ bar (1.5 oz)	230	15	8
Oregan Red Raspberry	½ bar (1.5 oz)	230	15	8
Peanut Butter Brittle	½ bar (1.5 oz)	230	15	8
Sundried Cherry	½ bar (1.5 oz)	230	13	8
Toasted Coconut Crisp	½ bar (1.5 oz)	230	14	9
Vanilla Dark	½ bar (1.5 oz)	230	15	8
Crunch				
Fun Size	4 bars	210	11	7
Daboga				
Organic Milk Chocolate	1 bar (2 oz)	318	20	14
Del Monte				
Radical Raizins Cinnamon	1 pkg (0.7 oz)	70	0	0
Radical Raizins Rainbow	1 pkg (0.7 oz)	70	0	0
Doctor's CarbRite				
Sugar Free Dark Chocolate	1 oz	124	8	—
Sugar Free Dark Chocolate With Almonds	4 sq (1 oz)	132	10	4
Sugar Free Milk Chocolate	1 oz	128	9	—
Sugar Free Milk Chocolate With Peanuts	4 sq (1 oz)	132	10	4
Sugar Free Milk Chocolate With Soy Crisps	4 sq (1 oz)	120	8	4
Sugar Free Mint Chocolate	1 oz	128	9	—
Dove				
Dark Chocolate	¼ bar (1.5 oz)	230	14	8
Dark Chocolate	1 bar (1.3 oz)	200	12	7
Dark Chocolate Minatures	7 (1.5 oz)	220	14	8

FOOD	PORTION	CALS	FAT	SAT FAT
Milk Chocolate	¼ bar (1.5 oz)	230	13	8
Milk Chocolate	1 bar (1.3 oz)	200	12	7
Milk Chocolate Miniatures	7 (1.5 oz)	230	13	8
Dream				
Caramel & Nougat In Milk Chocolate	1 bar (1 oz)	90	3	2
Estee				
Caramels Vanilla & Chocolate	5	115	5	1
Dark Chocolate	½ bar (1.4 oz)	200	14	8
Milk Chocolate	½ bar (1.4 oz)	230	17	10
Milk Chocolate w/ Almonds	½ bar (1.4 oz)	230	17	9
Milk Chocolate w/ Crisp Rice	½ bar (1.2 oz)	370	26	15
Milk Chocolate w/ Fruit & Nuts	½ bar (1.4 oz)	220	16	9
Mint Chocolate	½ bar (1.4 oz)	200	14	8
Peanut Brittle	⅓ box (1.3 oz)	160	9	2
Peanut Butter Cups	5	200	12	7
Sugar Free Assorted Fruit	5	30	0	0
Sugar Free Assorted Mint	5	30	0	0
Sugar Free Butterscotch	2	25	0	0
Sugar Free Fruit Gum Drops	23	80	0	0
Sugar Free Gourmet Jelly Beans	26	70	0	0
Sugar Free Gummy Apple Rings	5	70	0	0
Sugar Free Gummy Bears Assorted Fruit	17	100	0	0
Sugar Free Licorice Gum Drops	11	90	0	0
Sugar Free Peppermint Swirl	3	30	0	0
Sugar Free Sour Citrus Slices	9	60	0	0
Sugar Free Toffee	5	30	0	0
Sugar Free Tropical Fruit	5	30	0	0
Fauchon				
Assorted	3 pieces (1.1 oz)	170	11	8
Favorite Brands				
Candy Corn	24 pieces (1.4 oz)	150	0	0
Cinnamon Imperials	52 (0.5 oz)	80	0	0
Circus Peanuts	5 pieces (1.6 oz)	160	0	0
Gummallo Apple Ring	5 pieces (1.4 oz)	120	0	0
Gummallo Peach Ring	5 pieces (1.4 oz)	120	0	0
Gummi Bears	18 pieces (1.4 oz)	130	0	0
Gummi Dinos	7 pieces (1.3 oz)	120	0	0
Gummi Worms	4 pieces (1.4 oz)	130	0	0
Jelly Beans	13 (1.4 oz)	150	0	0

FOOD	PORTION	CALS	FAT	SAT FAT
Marshmallow Eggs	3 (1.3 oz)	140	0	0
Neon Worms	4 pieces (1.4 oz)	120	0	0
Sour Gummi Bears	16 pieces (1.4 oz)	110	0	0
Sour Gummi Worms	4 pieces (1.6 oz)	130	0	0
Ferrero Rocher				
Candy	1 piece (0.4 oz)	73	5	2
Godiva				
Chocolatier Dark Chocolate w/ Raspberry	1 bar (1.5 oz)	220	11	4
Chocolatier Milk Chocolate	1 bar (1.5 oz)	230	13	5
Milk Chocolate w/ Whole Almonds	1 bar (⅓ oz)	230	15	4
Mochaccino Mousse	2 pieces (1.25 oz)	210	15	4
Truffles Assorted	2 pieces (1.5 oz)	220	13	6
Goetze's				
Cow Tales	1 pkg (1 oz)	110	3	1
Gol D Lite				
Milk Chocolate Crisp	1 bar	125	9	6
Seashell Truffle	1 piece	54	3	0
Goldenberg's				
Peanut Chews	3 pieces (1.3 oz)	180	9	2
Goo Goo Supreme				
With Pecans	1 pkg (1.5 oz)	188	5	2
Goobers				
Peanuts	1 pkg (1.38 oz)	210	13	5
Haviland				
Chocolate Covered Thin Mints	6 (1.5 oz)	170	5	3
Hershey				
Amazin' Fruit Gummy Candy	1 snack pkg (0.7 oz)	60	0	0
Bar	1 (0.6 oz)	100	6	3
Candy-Coated Milk Chocolate Eggs	4 pieces	90	5	3
Cookies 'n' Mint	1 bar (0.6 oz)	90	5	2
Hugs	1 piece	25	2	1
Hugs w/ Almonds	1 piece	25	2	1
Kisses	1	25	2	1
Kisses w/ Almond	1	25	2	1
Milk Chocolate	1 bar (0.6 oz)	90	5	4
Milk Chocolate w/ Almonds	1 bar (0.6 oz)	100	6	3
Miniature Milk Chocolate	1 (0.3 oz)	45	3	2
Nuggets Cookies 'n' Creme	1 (0.35 oz)	50	3	2

FOOD	PORTION	CALS	FAT	SAT FAT
Nuggets Cookies 'n' Mint	1 (0.35 oz)	50	3	2
Nuggets Milk Chocolate	1 (0.35 oz)	50	3	2
Nuggets Milk Chocolate w/ Almonds	1 (0.35 oz)	50	3	2
PayDay Snack Size	1 (0.66 oz)	90	5	1
Pot Of Gold Solitaires	5 pieces	90	6	3
ReeseSticks Snack Size	2 pieces (1.2 oz)	190	11	5
S'mores	1 bar	240	11	6
Special Dark Miniature	1 (0.3 oz)	45	2	0
Sweet Escapes Chocolate Toffee Crisp	1 bar (0.66 oz)	80	4	2
Sweet Escapes Peanut Butter Crispy	1 bar (0.7 oz)	70	3	1
Sweet Escapes Triple Chocolate Wafer	1 bar (0.7 oz)	80	3	2
Tastetations Butterscotch	3 pieces (0.6 oz)	60	2	1
Tastetations Caramel	3 pieces (0.6 oz)	60	2	1
Tastetations Chocolate	3 pieces (0.6 oz)	60	1	1
Tastetations Chocolate Mint	3 pieces (0.6 oz)	60	2	1
Tastetations Peppermint	3 pieces (0.6 oz)	60	0	0
Hint Mint				
All Flavors	2 pieces	10	0	0
Jolly Rancher				
Lollipops All Flavors	1 (0.6 oz)	60	0	0
Joyva				
Halvah Chocolate Covered	1 serv (2 oz)	380	25	5
Halvah Marble	1 serv (2 oz)	390	25	4
Judy's				
Sugar Free Almond Caramel Cluster	1 piece (1.5 oz)	200	15	4
Sugar Free Cashew Caramel Cluster	1 piece (1.5 oz)	190	14	5
Sugar Free English Toffee	1 piece (1.5 oz)	220	17	5
Sugar Free Macadamia Caramel Cluster	1 piece (1.5 oz)	220	20	5
Sugar Free Peanut Brittle	¾ cup	100	6	1
Sugar Free Pecan Almond Cluster	1 piece (1.5 oz)	220	19	4
Junior Mints				
Snack Size	1 box (0.7 oz)	75	1	1
Just Born				
Hot Tamales	1 pkg (2.1 oz)	220	0	0
Mike and Ike Berry Fruits	1 pkg (2.1 oz)	220	0	0
Mike and Ike Cherry & Bubble Gum	1 pkg (2.1 oz)	220	0	0
Mike and Ike Chewy Grape	1 pkg (2.1 oz)	220	0	0
Mike and Ike Lemon Watermelon	1 pkg (2.1 oz)	220	0	0
Mike and Ike Original	1 pkg (1.2 oz)	220	0	0

FOOD	PORTION	CALS	FAT	SAT FAT
Mike and Ike Strawberry & Banana	1 pkg (2.1 oz)	220	0	0
Mike and Ike Tropical Fruits	1 pkg (2.1 oz)	220	0	0
Super Hot Tamales	1 pkg (2.1 oz)	220	0	0
Teenee Beanee Assorted Fruits	36 pieces (1.4 oz)	150	0	0
Teenee Beanee Berry Berry	36 pieces (1.4 oz)	150	0	0
Teenee Beanee Tropical Mix	36 pieces (1.4 oz)	150	0	0
Kit Kat				
Bar	1 (0.5 oz)	80	4	3
Klein				
Sugar Free Hard Candy All Flavors	3 pieces	12	0	0
Krackel				
Bar	1 (0.6 oz)	90	5	3
Miniature	1 (0.3 oz)	45	3	2
Lambertz				
Petits Soleils Chocolate Coated Gingerbread	1 piece (0.4 oz)	47	2	1
Lance				
Chocolaty Peanut Bar	1 (2 oz)	290	15	4
Cinnamon Chews	1 pkg (1.06 oz)	120	1	0
Fruit Chews	1 pkg (1.06 oz)	120	1	0
Gum Ball Pops	1 (0.45 oz)	45	0	0
K-Nuts	4 pieces (1.5 oz)	240	15	5
Mint Chews	1 pkg (1.06 oz)	120	1	0
Peanut Bar	1 (1.75 oz)	270	15	3
Pop-A-Lance	1 piece (0.42 oz)	45	0	0
Popcorn'n'Carmel	1 bar (0.75 oz)	90	0	0
Starlight Mints	3 pieces (1 oz)	60	0	0
Strawberry Chews	1 pkg (1.06 oz)	120	1	0
Suckers	3 pieces (0.5 oz)	50	0	0
Whistle Pop	1 (0.67 oz)	70	0	0
Landies Candies				
Sugar Free Almond Clusters	2 pieces (1.5 oz)	240	17	7
Sugar Free Bon Bons Peanut Butter	2 (1.5 oz)	240	17	7
Sugar Free Coconut Clusters	2 pieces (1.5 oz)	250	18	12
Sugar Free Cookies & Cream	2 pieces (1.5 oz)	240	15	8
Sugar Free Dark Almond Bark	1 piece (1.5 oz)	230	15	7
Sugar Free Dark Miniature Bars	7 pieces (1.5 oz)	230	14	8
Sugar Free Milk Miniature Bars	7 pieces (1.5 oz)	240	15	9
Sugar Free Mint Discs	7 pieces (1.5 oz)	240	15	9
Sugar Free Peanut Clusters	2 (1.5 oz)	240	17	7

FOOD	PORTION	CALS	FAT	SAT FAT
Sugar Free White Almond Bark	1 piece (1.5 oz)	230	15	10
Sugar Free White Caps	6 pieces (1.5 oz)	230	15	8
Lean Protein Bites				
Milk Chocolate	1 pkg (1 oz)	120	6	3
Peanut Butter	1 pkg (1 oz)	120	5	4
White Chocolate	1 pkg (1 oz)	120	4	2
Lifesavers				
Big Tablet Candy Cane	4 pieces (0.5 oz)	60	0	0
Cards 'N Candy	4 pieces (0.4 oz)	40	0	0
Christmas Tin	4 pieces (0.5 oz)	60	0	0
Egg-Sortment	1 roll (0.4 oz)	40	0	0
Gummi Bunnies	3 pkg (1.6 oz)	140	0	0
Gummi Savers Five Flavor	1 roll (1.5 oz)	130	0	0
Gummi Savers Five Flavor	1 pkg (1.8 oz)	160	0	0
Gummi Savers Mixed Berry	1 roll (1.5 oz)	130	0	0
Gummi Savers Mixed Berry	1 pkg (1.8 oz)	160	0	0
Gummi Savers Tangy Fruits	1 roll (1.5 oz)	130	0	0
Gummi Savers Tangy Fruits	1 pkg (1.8 oz)	160	0	0
Gummi Savers Variety	2 pkg (1.3 oz)	120	0	0
Gummi Savers Wacky Frootz	1 roll (1.5 oz)	130	0	0
Gummi Savers Wacky Frootz	1 pkg (1.8 oz)	160	0	0
Gummi Shapes Barnum's Animals	1 pkg (0.8 oz)	70	0	0
Holes Five Flavor	20 pieces (5 g)	20	0	0
Holes Island Fruit	20 pieces (5 g)	20	0	0
Holes Sour 'N Sweet	16 pieces (5 g)	20	0	0
Holes Sunshine Fruits	20 pieces (0.2 oz)	20	0	0
Holes Super Tart	20 pieces (5 g)	20	0	0
Holes Wild Fruits	20 pieces (5 g)	20	0	—
Lollipops Candy Cane	1 (0.4 oz)	40	0	0
Lollipops Christmas	1 (0.4 oz)	40	0	0
Lollipops Easter	1 (0.4 oz)	40	0	0
Lollipops Fruit Flavors	1 (0.4 oz)	45	0	0
Lollipops Swirled Flavors	1 (0.4 oz)	40	0	0
Lollipops Valentine	1 (0.4 oz)	40	0	0
Roll Butter Rum	2 pieces (5 g)	20	0	0
Roll Candy Cane	4 pieces (0.4 oz)	40	0	0
Roll Cryst-O-Mint	2 pieces (5 g)	20	0	0
Roll Five Flavor	2 pieces (5 g)	20	0	0
Roll Fruits On Fire	2 pieces (5 g)	20	0	0
Roll Pep-O-Mint	3 pieces (5 g)	20	0	0

FOOD	PORTION	CALS	FAT	SAT FAT
Roll Spear-O-Mint	3 pieces (5 g)	20	0	0
Roll Sunshine Fruits	2 pieces (5 g)	20	0	0
Roll Tangy Fruit Swirl	2 pieces (5 g)	20	0	0
Roll Tangy Fruit Watermelon	1 piece (5 g)	20	0	0
Roll Tangy Fruits	2 pieces (5 g)	20	0	0
Roll Tropical Fruits	2 pieces (5 g)	20	0	0
Roll Wild Cherry	1 piece (5 g)	20	0	0
Roll Wild Flavors	2 pieces (5 g)	20	0	0
Roll Wild Sour Berries	2 pieces (5 g)	20	0	0
Roll Wint-O-Green	3 pieces (5 g)	20	0	0
Sack'it Butter Rum	4 pieces (0.5 oz)	60	0	0
Sack'it Five Flavor	4 pieces (0.5 oz)	60	0	0
Sack'it Holiday Tin	4 pieces (0.5 oz)	60	0	0
Sack'it Pep-O-Mint	4 pieces (0.5 oz)	60	0	0
Sack'it Tangy Fruits	4 pieces (0.5 oz)	60	0	0
Sack'it Wild Cherry	4 pieces (0.5 oz)	60	0	0
Sack'it Wint-O-Green	4 pieces (0.5 oz)	60	0	0
Sugar Free Iced Mint	1 piece (2 g)	10	0	0
Sugar Free Vanilla Mint	1 piece (2 g)	10	0	0
Valentine Book	2 pieces (5 g)	20	0	0
Lindt				
Dark Chocolate 70% Cocoa	4 blocks (1.4 oz)	220	17	10
Lindor Truffles Dark Chocolate	3 pieces	220	18	13
Low Carb Chef				
Gummi Bears	14 pieces	138	0	0
Jelly Beans	37 pieces	120	0	0
Sugar Free Caramel Marshmallow Treats	3 pieces	140	7	5
Sugar Free Cherry Cordials	3 pieces	250	8	5
Sugar Free Coconut Clusters	4 pieces	210	18	13
Sugar Free Milk Chocolate Covered Vanilla Caramels	3 pieces	160	8	5
Sugar Free Peanut Butter Cups	1 piece	200	16	8
Sugar Free Peanut Butter Truffles	2 pieces	200	16	8
Sugar Free Peanut Clusters	4 pieces	210	17	5
Sugar Free Pecan Turtles	1 piece	120	13	6
Sugar Free Peppermint Patties	3 pieces	150	9	5
M&M's				
Almond	1.5 oz	220	12	4
Almond	1 pkg (1.3 oz)	200	11	4

FOOD	PORTION	CALS	FAT	SAT FAT
Mint	1 pkg (1.7 oz)	230	10	6
Mint	1.5 oz	200	9	5
Peanut	½ bag king size (1.6 oz)	240	12	5
Peanut	1 fun size (0.7 oz)	110	5	2
Peanut	1 pkg (1.7 oz)	250	13	5
Peanut	1.5 oz	220	11	5
Peanut Butter	1 fun size (0.7 oz)	110	6	4
Peanut Butter	1 pkg (1.6 oz)	240	13	8
Peanut Butter	1.5 oz	220	12	8
Plain	1 pkg fun size (0.7 oz)	100	4	3
Plain	1.5 oz	200	9	5
Plain	½ pkg king size (1.6 oz)	220	9	6
Plain	1 pkg (1.7 oz)	240	10	6
Mars				
Almond Bar	2 fun size (1.3 oz)	190	10	3
Almond Bar	1 bar (1.8 oz)	240	13	4
Milk Duds				
Snack Size	4 boxes (1.3 oz)	160	6	2
Milky Way				
Bar	2 fun size (1.4 oz)	180	7	4
Bar	⅓ king size (1.2 oz)	160	6	3
Bar	1 (2.1 oz)	280	11	5
Dark	1 bar (1.8 oz)	220	8	5
Dark	1 fun size (0.7 oz)	90	3	2
Miniature	5 (1.5 oz)	190	7	4
Mon Cheri				
With Hazelnuts	2 pieces	120	9	5
Mounds				
Bar	1 (0.68 oz)	90	5	4
Mr. Goodbar				
Miniature	1 (0.3 oz)	45	3	1
Necco				
Bridge Mix	¼ cup (1.5 oz)	180	9	5
Chocolate Covered Raisins	30 pieces (1.5 oz)	170	7	5
Malted Milk Balls	11 pieces (1.5 oz)	180	6	6

FOOD	PORTION	CALS	FAT	SAT FAT
Mint	1 piece	12	tr	–
SkyBar	1 bar (1.5 oz)	190	9	5
Nestle				
Buncha Crunch	1 pkg (1.4 oz)	90	10	6
Crunch	1 bar (1.55 oz)	230	12	7
Crunch Disk	1 (1.2 oz)	180	9	6
Crunchkins	5 pieces	190	10	6
Jingles Milk Chocolate Butterfinger	5 pieces	180	8	4
Jingles Milk Chocolate Crunch	7 pieces	220	11	7
Jingles White Crunch	7 pieces	230	14	8
Milk Chocolate	1 bar (1.45 oz)	220	13	8
Nesteggs Milk Chocolate Butterfinger	5 pieces	210	10	5
Nesteggs Milk Chocolate Crunch	5 pieces	190	10	6
Nesteggs White Crunch	7 pieces	230	14	8
Pearson's Egg Nog	2 pieces	60	2	1
Toll House Brownie Bar	2 pieces (2 oz)	250	12	5
Toll House Cookie Bar	1 piece (1 oz)	130	6	3
Treasures Butterfinger	3 pieces	180	9	5
Treasures Crunch	4 pieces (1.4 oz)	210	11	7
Treasures Peanut Butter	4 pieces	250	17	7
Turtles Bite Size	4 pieces	210	12	4
Turtles Bite Size	1 piece (0.4 oz)	50	2	1
White Crunch	1 bar (1.4 oz)	220	13	8
Newman's Own				
Organic Peanut Butter Cups Dark Chocolate	3 pieces (1.2 oz)	180	12	6
Organic Peanut Butter Cups Milk Chocolate	3 pieces (1.2 oz)	180	12	6
Organic Peppermint Cups	3 pieces (1.2 oz)	180	12	6
Organics Espresso Sweet Dark Chocolate	1 bar (1.2 oz)	190	12	7
Nibs				
Cherry	1 pkg (0.49 oz)	45	0	0
Licorice	1 pkg (0.49 oz)	40	0	0
Nips				
Butter Rum	2 pieces	60	2	1
Caramel	2 pieces	60	2	1
Chocolate	2 pieces	60	2	1
Chocolate Parfait	2 pieces	60	2	1
Coffee	2 pieces	50	2	2

FOOD	PORTION	CALS	FAT	SAT FAT
Vanilla Almond Cafe	2 pieces	50	1	1
Oh Henry!				
Bar	1 (1.8 oz)	120	5	3
Palmer				
Milk Chocolate Lollipop	1 (0.9 oz)	130	7	4
Pearson's				
Irish Cream Parfait	2 pieces	60	2	2
Mint Patties	1	30	1	tr
Perlege				
Sugar Free Belgium Chocolate All Flavors	1 bar (3.5 oz)	532	42	–
Sugar Free Cream Filled Belgian Chocolate All Flavors	1 bar (1.5 oz)	226	16	10
Pez				
Candy	1 roll (0.3 oz)	35	0	0
Candy Sugar Free	1 roll (0.3 oz)	30	0	0
Planters				
Original Peanut Bar	1 pkg (1.6 oz)	230	14	2
Pure De-Lite				
Caramel	1 bar	120	5	4
Caramel Crisp	1 bar	120	6	4
Caramel Nougat	1 bar	110	5	3
Caramel Peanut Butter	1 bar	120	6	3
Caramel Pecan	1 bar	130	7	4
Sugar Free Dark Chocolate	1 bar	173	14	8
Sugar Free Milk Chocolate w/ Mint	1 bar	187	14	9
Sugar Free Milk Chocolate	1 bar	187	14	9
Sugar Free Milk Chocolate w/ Almonds	1 bar	190	14	9
Sugar Free Milk Chocolate w/ Coconut	1 bar	190	14	9
Sugar Free Milk Chocolate w/ Orange	1 bar	187	14	9
Sugar Free Milk Chocolate w/ Peanuts	1 bar	190	14	9
Sugar Free White Chocolate	1 bar	187	14	9
Truffle Bar Caramel	1 bar	140	8	5
Truffle Bar Dark Mint	1 bar	160	12	8
Truffle Bar Hazelnut	1 bar	160	12	7
Truffle Bar Peanut Butter	1 bar	160	11	7
Raisinets				
Candy	1 pkg (1.58 oz)	200	8	5
Fun Size	3 pkg	200	8	5

FOOD	PORTION	CALS	FAT	SAT FAT
Reese's				
FastBreak	1 bar (2 oz)	270	13	5
Nutrageous	1 bar (0.6 oz)	95	6	2
Peanut Butter Cups	1 (0.28 oz)	40	3	1
Peanut Butter Cups Miniature	1 (0.3 oz)	42	2	1
Pieces	25 (0.7 oz)	100	4	4
ReeseSticks Peanut Butter	2 pieces (1.2 oz)	190	11	5
Ritter Sport				
Dark Chocolate Whole Hazelnuts	6 pieces (1.3 oz)	210	15	8
Rokeach				
Cotton Candy	2 cups (1 oz)	110	0	0
Rolo				
Caramels In Milk Chocolate	3 pieces (0.64 oz)	90	4	2
Russell Stover				
Assorted Creams	3 pieces (1.4 oz)	180	7	4
Looney Tunes Peanut Butter Nougat w/ Peanuts in Milk Chocolate	1 snack size (0.7 oz)	90	5	2
Low Carb Pecan Delights	1 pkg (1 oz)	130	9	5
Peanut Butter & Grape Jelly	1 piece (0.8 oz)	100	6	2
Peanut Butter & Red Raspberry Cups	2 (1.2 oz)	140	9	3
Pecan Delights	1 pkg (2 oz)	280	18	5
Pecan Roll	1 (1.75 oz)	260	18	2
S'mores	3 (1.4 oz)	210	12	7
Sugar Free Peanut Butter Cups	4 pieces (1.3 oz)	200	13	6
Sugar Free Pecans & Caramel	2 pieces (1.2 oz)	170	12	3
Simply Lite				
Sugar Free Lil'l Bits Chocolatey	36 pieces (1.4 oz)	130	5	5
Sugar Free Lil'l Bits Peanut Buttery	36 pieces (1.4 oz)	140	5	5
Sugar Free Patteez	5 pieces (1.3 oz)	110	3	2
Skittles				
Original	2 pkg fun size (1.6 oz)	180	2	0
Original	½ king size (1.3 oz)	150	2	0
Original	1.5 oz	170	2	0
Original	1 pkg (2.8 oz)	250	3	1
Tropical	1 bag (2.2 oz)	250	3	1
Tropical	1.5 oz	170	2	0
Tropical	2 bags fun size (1.4 oz)	160	2	0

FOOD	PORTION	CALS	FAT	SAT FAT
Wild Berry	1 bag (2.2 oz)	250	3	1
Wild Berry	1.5 oz	170	2	0
Wild Berry	2 bags fun size (1.4 oz)	160	2	0
Smucker's				
Fruit Fillers Strawberry	1 pkg (0.9 oz)	80	0	0
Jelly Beans	1 pkg (0.7 oz)	70	0	0
Snickers				
Bar	1 bar (2.1 oz)	280	14	5
Bar	2 bars fun size (1.4 oz)	190	9	4
Bar	⅓ king size (1.2 oz)	170	8	3
Cruncher	3 fun size (1.4 oz)	230	13	5
Miniatures	4 (1.3 oz)	170	8	3
Munch Bar	1 (1.4 oz)	230	15	4
Peanut Butter	1 bar (2 oz)	310	20	7
Sno Caps				
Candies	1 pkg (2.3 oz)	300	13	8
Speakeasy				
Organic Mints All Flavors	4 pieces (2 g)	10	0	0
Starburst				
California Fruits	8 pieces (1.4 oz)	160	3	1
California Fruits	1 stick (2.1 oz)	240	5	1
Original Fruits	⅓ king size (1.2 oz)	140	3	1
Original Fruits	8 pieces (1.4 oz)	160	3	1
Original Fruits	1 stick (2.1 oz)	240	5	1
Strawberry Fruits	1 stick (2.1 oz)	240	5	1
Strawberry Fruits	8 pieces (1.4 oz)	160	3	1
Tropical Fruits	8 pieces (1.4 oz)	160	3	1
Tropical Fruits	1 stick (2.1 oz)	240	5	1
Steel's				
Salt Water Taffy Assorted	3 pieces (1 oz)	90	1	0
Sugar Babies				
Tidbits	1 pkg	180	2	–
Swedish Fish				
Original	19 pieces (1.4 oz)	160	0	0

FOOD	PORTION	CALS	FAT	SAT FAT
Sweet'N Low				
Sugar Free Butter Toffee	4 pieces (0.5 oz)	30	1	1
Sugar Free Butterscotch	1 piece	7	0	0
Sugar Free Cinnamon	1 piece	7	0	0
Sugar Free Fancy Fruit	1 piece	7	0	0
Sugar Free Fruit Flavors	1 piece	7	0	0
Sugar Free Hard Candy Coffee	4 pieces (0.5 oz)	30	0	0
Sugar Free Peppermint	1 piece	7	0	0
Sugar Free Soft Candy Fruitie Flavors	1 piece	11	tr	—
Sugar Free Soft Candy Tropical Flavors	1 piece	11	tr	—
Sugar Free Watermelon	1 piece	7	0	0
Sugar Free Wild Cherry	1 piece	7	0	0
Symphony				
Bar	1 (0.6 oz)	100	6	4
W/ Almonds & Chocolate Chips	1 bar (0.6 oz)	90	6	4
Tobler				
Orange Dark Chocolate	5 pieces (1.5 oz)	240	13	8
Toblerone				
Milk Chocolate w/ Honey & Almond Nougat	½ bar (1.76 oz)	170	9	5
Tom's				
Cherry Sours	1 pkg (2.25 oz)	210	0	0
Jelly Beans	1 pkg (2.25 oz)	230	0	0
Tootsie				
Pop	1	60	0	0
Torras				
Sugar Free Dark Chocolate	1 oz	136	10	6
Sugar Free Milk Chocolate	1 oz	140	10	6
Sugar Free Milk Chocolate w/ Almonds	1 oz	146	10	5
Sugar Free Milk Chocolate w/ Hazelnuts	1 oz	148	11	6
Sugar Free White Chocolate	1 oz	138	10	6
Tropical Source				
Butterscotch Dream	4 pieces (0.5 oz)	60	0	0
Chocolate Dairy Free California Raisin & Currant	½ bar (1.5 oz)	230	13	8
Chocolate Dairy Free Hazelnut Espresso Crunch	½ bar (1.5 oz)	250	17	8

FOOD	PORTION	CALS	FAT	SAT FAT
Chocolate Dairy Free Maple Almond Granola	½ bar (1.5 oz)	230	15	9
Chocolate Dairy Free Mint Candy Crunch	½ bar (1.5 oz)	220	13	8
Chocolate Dairy Free Red Raspberry Crush	½ bar (1.5 oz)	230	15	9
Chocolate Dairy Free Sundried Jungle Banana	½ bar (1.5 oz)	230	13	8
Chocolate Dairy Free Toasted Almond	½ bar (1.5 oz)	250	17	8
Chocolate Dairy Free Wild Rice Crisp	½ bar (1.5 oz)	230	14	8
Cool Peppermint	4 pieces (0.5 oz)	60	0	0
Lollipops All Flavors	1	24	0	0
Mango Papaya	4 pieces (0.5 oz)	60	0	0
Twix				
Caramel	1 fun size (0.5 oz)	80	4	2
Caramel	1 pkg (2 oz)	280	14	5
Caramel	1 (1 oz)	140	7	3
Caramel	1 king size (0.8 oz)	120	6	2
Peanut Butter	1 (0.9 oz)	130	8	3
Twizzlers				
Cherry	1 piece	35	0	0
Chocolate	1 piece	30	0	0
Licorice	1 piece	35	0	0
Pull'n'Peel Cherry	1 piece (1 oz)	90	0	0
Strawberry	1 piece	35	0	0
Unique Origin				
Guaranda Dark Chocolate	1 piece (0.3 oz)	54	4	3
Very Special				
Chocolate Bottles Liquor Filled	3 pieces (1 oz)	150	6	4
Werther's				
Original	3 pieces (0.5 oz)	60	1	1
Whatchamacallit				
Bar	1 (0.58 oz)	80	4	2
Whitman's				
Pecan Roll	1 bar (2 oz)	300	20	3
Snoopy Treats Caramel Peanuts Milk Chocolate	1 snack size (1.4 oz)	80	5	3
Whoppers				
Malted Milk Balls	1 pkg (0.7 oz)	100	4	3

FOOD	PORTION	CALS	FAT	SAT FAT
York				
Chocolate Covered Peppermint Bites	15 pieces (1 oz)	150	3	2
Peppermint Patty	1 (0.49 oz)	50	1	1
HOME RECIPE				
fondant	1 piece (0.6 oz)	57	0	–
fudge brown sugar w/ nuts	1 piece (0.5 oz)	56	1	tr
fudge brown sugar w/ nuts	1 recipe 60 pieces (30.7 oz)	3453	88	15
fudge chocolate	1 recipe 48 pieces (29 oz)	3161	70	43
fudge chocolate marshmallow	1 recipe (43.1 oz)	5182	207	125
fudge chocolate marshmallow	1 piece (0.7 oz)	84	3	2
fudge chocolate marshmallow w/ nuts	1 recipe 60 pieces (43.1 oz)	5182	207	125
fudge chocolate marshmallow w/ nuts	1 recipe 60 pieces (46.1 oz)	5742	258	127
fudge chocolate marshmallow w/ nuts	1 piece (0.8 oz)	96	4	2
fudge chocolate w/ nuts	1 piece (0.7 oz)	81	3	1
fudge chocolate w/ nuts	1 recipe 48 pieces (32.7 oz)	3967	150	52
fudge peanut butter	1 recipe 36 pieces (20.4 oz)	2161	38	9
fudge peanut butter	1 piece (0.6 oz)	59	1	tr
fudge vanilla	1 recipe 48 pieces (27.5 oz)	2893	42	26
fudge vanilla w/ nuts	1 recipe 60 pieces (31 oz)	3666	117	33
fudge vanilla w/ nuts	1 piece (0.5 oz)	62	2	1
peanut brittle	1 recipe (17.6 oz)	2288	95	25
peanut brittle	1 oz	128	5	1
praline	1 piece (1.4 oz)	177	10	1
praline	1 recipe 23 pieces (31.8 oz)	4116	220	17
taffy	1 piece (0.5 oz)	56	1	tr
taffy	1 recipe 48 pieces (25 oz)	2677	24	15
toffee	1 recipe 48 pieces (19.4 oz)	2997	182	113
toffee	1 piece (0.4 oz)	65	4	2

FOOD	PORTION	CALS	FAT	SAT FAT
truffles	1 piece (0.4 oz)	59	4	3
truffles	1 recipe 49 pieces (21.5 oz)	2985	210	132
CANTALOUPE				
dried	3.5 pieces (1.4 oz)	140	0	0
fresh cubed	1 cup	57	tr	–
fresh half	½	94	1	–
Chiquita				
Wedge	¼ med (4.7 oz)	50	0	0
CARAWAY				
seed	1 tsp	7	tr	tr
CARDAMOM				
ground	1 tsp	6	tr	tr
CARDOON				
fresh cooked	3½ oz	22	tr	tr
fresh shredded	½ cup	36	tr	tr
CARIBOU				
roasted	3 oz	142	4	1
CARISSA				
fresh	1	12	tr	–
CAROB				
carob mix	3 tsp	45	0	0
carob mix as prep w/ whole milk	9 oz	195	8	5
flour	1 tbsp	14	tr	tr
flour	1 cup	185	1	tr
Sunspire				
Carob Chips Unsweetened	13 pieces (0.5 oz)	70	3	3
Carob Chips Vegan	13 pieces (0.5 oz)	70	3	3
CARP				
fresh	3 oz	108	5	1
fresh cooked	1 fillet (6 oz)	276	12	2
fresh cooked	3 oz	138	6	1
roe raw	1 oz	37	tr	–

FOOD	PORTION	CALS	FAT	SAT FAT
CARROT JUICE				
canned	6 oz	73	tr	tr
CARROTS				
CANNED				
slices	½ cup	17	tr	tr
slices low sodium	½ cup	17	tr	tr
Del Monte				
Sliced	½ cup (4.3 oz)	35	0	0
Green Giant				
Sliced	½ cup (4.2 oz)	25	0	0
LeSueur				
Baby Whole	½ cup (4.2 oz)	35	0	0
S&W				
Julienne	½ cup (4.3 oz)	30	0	0
Sliced	½ cup (4.3 oz)	30	0	0
Whole Small	½ cup (4.3 oz)	30	0	0
FRESH				
baby raw	1 (½ oz)	6	tr	tr
raw	1 (2.5 oz)	31	tr	tr
raw shredded	½ cup	24	tr	tr
slices cooked	½ cup	35	tr	tr
Dole				
Shredded	1 cup (3 oz)	40	0	0
Earthbound Farms				
Organic Mini Peeled	½ cup	30	0	0
FROZEN				
slices cooked	½ cup	26	tr	tr
Birds Eye				
Baby Whole	½ cup	40	0	0
Sliced	½ cup	35	0	0
Fresh Like				
Carrots Slice	3.5 oz	42	tr	–
Green Giant				
Harvest Fresh Baby	⅔ cup (3 oz)	20	0	0
Select Baby Cut	¾ cup (2.8 oz)	30	0	0
CASABA				
cubed	1 cup	45	tr	–
fresh	⅒	43	tr	–

FOOD	PORTION	CALS	FAT	SAT FAT
CASHEWS				
cashew butter w/o salt	1 tbsp	94	8	2
dry roasted salted	1 oz	163	13	3
dry roasted w/ salt	18 nuts (1 oz)	160	13	3
oil roasted	1 oz	163	14	3
oil roasted salted	1 oz	163	14	3
Bowlby's				
Bits Cashew	½ cup	200	19	3
Frito Lay				
Salted	1 oz	180	15	3
Lance				
Cashews	1 pkg (1⅛ oz)	200	16	3
Maranatha				
Cashew Butter	2 tbsp	190	15	3
Tamari Cashews	¼ cup	160	13	3
Planters				
Fancy Oil Roasted	1 oz	170	14	3
Fancy Oil Roasted	1 pkg (2 oz)	340	29	6
Halves Lightly Salted Oil Roasted	1 oz	160	13	3
Halves Oil Roasted	1 oz	170	14	3
Honey Roasted	1 oz	150	12	2
Honey Roasted	1 pkg (2 oz)	310	24	4
Munch'N Go Honey Roasted	1 pkg (2 oz)	310	24	4
Munch'N Go Singles Oil Roasted	1 pkg (2 oz)	330	28	6
Oil Roasted	1 pkg (1 oz)	160	14	3
Oil Roasted	1 pkg (1.5 oz)	250	21	4
Sweet Delights				
Cashew Roasters	⅓ pkg (1 oz)	170	14	—
CASSAVA				
fresh	3½ oz	120	tr	tr
CATFISH				
channel breaded & fried	3 oz	194	11	3
channel raw	3 oz	99	4	1
CAULIFLOWER				
FRESH				
cooked	½ cup (2.2 oz)	14	tr	tr
flowerets cooked	3 (2 oz)	12	tr	tr
flowerets raw	3 (2 oz)	14	tr	tr

FOOD	PORTION	CALS	FAT	SAT FAT
green cooked	1½ cups (3.2 oz)	29	tr	tr
green raw	1 head 7 in diam (18 oz)	158	2	tr
green raw	1 (2.2 oz)	20	tr	tr
green raw floweret	1 (0.9 oz)	8	tr	tr
raw	½ cup (1.8 oz)	13	tr	tr
FROZEN				
cooked	½ cup	17	tr	tr
Birds Eye				
Cauliflower	½ cup	20	0	0
Fresh Like				
Florets	3.5 oz	26	tr	—
Green Giant				
Cheese Sauce	½ cup (3.5 oz)	60	3	1
Florets	1 cup (2.8 oz)	25	0	0
CAVIAR				
black	1 tbsp	40	3	—
red	1 tbsp	40	3	—
CELERIAC				
fresh cooked	3½ oz	25	tr	—
raw	½ cup	31	tr	—
CELERY				
diced cooked	½ cup	13	tr	tr
fresh	1 stalk (1.3 oz)	6	tr	tr
raw diced	½ cup	10	tr	tr
seed	1 tsp	8	tr	tr
Dole				
Stalks	2 med (3 oz)	15	0	0
McCormick				
Celery Salt	¼ tsp	0	0	0
CELTUCE				
raw	3½ oz	22	tr	—
CEREAL				
bran flakes	¾ cup (1 oz)	90	1	tr
corn flakes	1¼ cups (1 oz)	110	tr	tr
corn flakes low sodium	1 cup (0.9 oz)	100	tr	tr

FOOD	PORTION	CALS	FAT	SAT FAT
corn grits white regular & quick as prep w/ water & salt	¾ cup (6.4 oz)	109	tr	tr
corn grits white regular or quick as prep	¾ cup (6.4 oz)	109	tr	tr
corn grits yellow regular & quick as prep w/ water & salt	¾ cup (6.4 oz)	109	tr	tr
corn grits yellow regular & quick not prep	1 cup (5.5 oz)	579	2	tr
crispy rice	1 cup (1 oz)	111	tr	tr
crispy rice low sodium	1 cup (0.9 oz)	105	tr	tr
farina as prep w/ water	¾ cup (6.1 oz)	88	tr	tr
farina not prep	1 tbsp (0.4 oz)	40	tr	0
granola	½ cup (2.1 oz)	285	15	3
oatmeal instant w/ cinnamon & spice as prep w/ water	1 pkg (5.6 oz)	177	2	tr
oatmeal instant w/ raisins & spice as prep w/ water	1 cup (5.5 oz)	161	2	tr
oatmeal instant w/ bran & raisins as prep w/ water	1 pkg (6.8 oz)	158	2	tr
oatmeal instant as prep w/ water	1 cup (8.2 oz)	138	2	tr
oatmeal regular & quick as prep w/ water	¾ cup (6.1 oz)	149	2	tr
oatmeal regular & quick not prep	⅓ cup (0.9 oz)	104	2	tr
oatmeal instant cooked w/o salt	1 cup	145	2	tr
oatmeal quick cooked w/o salt	1 cup	145	2	tr
oatmeal regular cooked w/o salt	1 cup	145	2	tr
puffed rice	1 cup (0.5 oz)	56	tr	tr
puffed wheat	1 cup (0.4 oz)	44	tr	tr
shredded mini wheats	1 cup (1.1 oz)	107	1	tr
shredded wheat rectangular	1 biscuit (0.8 oz)	85	tr	tr
shredded wheat round	2 biscuits (1.3 oz)	136	1	tr
sugar-coated corn flakes	¾ cup (1 oz)	110	1	tr
whole wheat hot natural as prep w/ water	¾ cup (6.4 oz)	113	1	tr
Albers				
Hominy Quick Grits uncooked	¼ cup	140	1	0
Alpen				
Corn Flakes	1 serv (1 oz)	110	tr	—
No Salt No Sugar	1 serv (2 oz)	200	3	—
Regular	1 serv (2 oz)	200	3	—

FOOD	PORTION	CALS	FAT	SAT FAT
Atkins				
Banana Nut Harvest	⅔ cup	100	3	0
Blueberry Bounty w/ Almonds	⅔ cup	100	2	0
Crunchy Almond Crisp	⅔ cup	100	2	0
Aunt Paula's				
Hot Flax Cereal	1 serv (1½ oz)	100	5	5
Back To Nature				
Hi-Protein	⅔ cup	140	1	0
Muesli	½ cup	160	3	1
Puff Wheat	½ cup	160	3	1
Ultra Flax	¾ cup	150	2	1
Barbara's Bakery				
Apple Cinnamon O's	¾ cup	110	1	0
Bite Size Shredded Oats	1¼ cups (2 oz)	220	3	1
Cinnamon Puffins	1¼ cups (2 oz)	100	1	0
Cocoa Crunch Stars	1 cup (1 oz)	110	1	0
Frosted Corn Flakes	1 cup (1 oz)	110	1	0
Fruit Juice Sweetened Breakfast O's	1 cup (1 oz)	120	2	0
Fruit Juice Sweetened Brown Rice Crisps	1 cup (1 oz)	120	1	0
Fruit Juice Sweetened Corn Flakes	1 cup (1 oz)	110	0	0
GrainShop	⅔ cup (1 oz)	90	1	0
Honey Crunch Stars	1 cup (1 oz)	110	0	0
Honey Nut Toasted O's	¾ cup	120	2	1
Organic Fruity Punch	1 cup (1 oz)	110	1	0
Organic Soy Essence	¾ cup (1 oz)	100	1	0
Puffins	¾ cup (0.9 oz)	90	1	0
Shredded Spoonfuls	¾ cup (1.1 oz)	110	2	0
Shredded Wheat	2 biscuits (1.4 oz)	140	1	0
Carbsense				
Hot Cereal Country Spice not prep	½ cup	130	6	1
Hot Cereal Roasted Hazelnut not prep	½ cup	140	9	1
Deliciously Slim				
Granola Cranberry Cashew	¾ cup	230	13	1
Granola Strawberry Almond	¾ cup	230	13	1
Erewhon				
Apple Stroodles	¾ cup	110	1	0
Aztec	1 cup	110	0	0
Banana O's	¾ cup	110	0	0

FOOD	PORTION	CALS	FAT	SAT FAT
Brown Rice Cream	¼ cup	170	1	0
Corn Flakes	1¼ cups	210	3	0
Crispy Brown Rice	1 cup	110	0	0
Crispy Brown Rice No Salt Added	1 cup	110	0	0
Fruit'n Wheat	¾ cup	170	2	0
Kamut Flakes	⅔ cup	110	0	0
Raisin Bran	1 cup	170	1	0
Rice Twice	¾ cup	120	0	0
Whole Wheat Flakes	1 cup	180	1	0
Expert Foods				
Low Carb Hot Cereal Sub	½ cup	24	0	0
General Mills				
Basic 4	1 cup (1.9 oz)	200	2	0
Boo Berry	1 cup (1 oz)	120	1	0
Cheerios	1 cup (1 oz)	110	2	0
Cheerios Apple Cinnamon	¾ cup (1 oz)	120	2	0
Cheerios Frosted	1 cup (1 oz)	120	1	0
Cheerios Honey Nut	1 cup (1 oz)	120	2	0
Cheerios Multi Grain	1 cup (1 oz)	110	1	0
Cheerios Team	1 cup (1 oz)	120	1	0
Chex Corn	1 cup (1 oz)	110	0	0
Chex Honey Nut	¾ cup	120	1	0
Chex Morning Mix Cinnamon	1 pkg (1.1 oz)	130	4	1
Chex Morning Mix Fruit & Nut	1 pkg (1.1 oz)	180	4	1
Chex Morning Mix Honey Nut	1 pkg (1.1 oz)	130	4	1
Chex Multi-Bran	1 cup (2 oz)	200	2	0
Chex Rice	1¼ cups (1.1 oz)	120	0	0
Cinnamon Grahams	¾ cup (1 oz)	120	1	0
Cinnamon Toast Crunch	¾ cup (1 oz)	130	4	1
Cocoa Puffs	1 cup (1 oz)	120	1	0
Cookie Crisp	1 cup (1 oz)	120	1	0
Count Chocula	1 cup (1 oz)	120	1	0
Country Corn Flakes	1 cup (1 oz)	120	0	0
Fiber One	½ cup (1 oz)	60	1	0
Franken Berry	1 cup (1 oz)	120	1	0
French Toast Crunch	¾ cup (1 oz)	120	1	0
Gold Medal Raisin Bran	1⅓ cups (1.9 oz)	170	2	0
Golden Grahams	¾ cup (1 oz)	120	1	0
Harmony	1¼ cups (1.9 oz)	200	4	0
Honey Nut Clusters	1 cup (1.9 oz)	210	3	0

FOOD	PORTION	CALS	FAT	SAT FAT
Kaboom	1¼ cups (1 oz)	120	1	0
Kix	1⅓ cups (1 oz)	120	1	0
Kix Berry Berry	¾ cup (1 oz)	120	2	0
Lucky Charms	1 cup (1 oz)	120	1	0
Nature Valley Low Fat Fruit Granola	⅔ cup (1.9 oz)	210	3	0
Newquick	¾ cup (1 oz)	120	2	0
Oatmeal Crisp Almond	1 cup (1.9 oz)	220	5	1
Oatmeal Crisp Apple Cinnamon	1 cup (1.9 oz)	210	2	0
Oatmeal Crisp Raisin	1 cup (1.9 oz)	210	2	0
Para Su Familia Cinnamon Stars	1 cup (1 oz)	120	1	0
Para Su Familia Fruitis	1 cup (1 oz)	120	1	0
Para Su Familia Raisin Bran	1¼ cups (2 oz)	170	2	0
Raisin Nut Bran	¾ cup (1.9 oz)	200	4	1
Reese's Puffs	¾ cup	130	3	1
Snack'N Dash Cinnamon Toast Crunch	1 pkg (1.2 oz)	140	4	1
Snack'N Dash Honey Nut Cheerios	1 pkg (1 oz)	110	1	0
Snack'N Dash Lucky Charms	1 pkg (1 oz)	110	1	0
Sunrise Organic	¾ cup (1 oz)	110	1	0
Total Brown Sugar & Oat	¾ cup (1 oz)	110	1	0
Total Corn Flakes	1⅓ cups (1 oz)	110	0	0
Total Raisin Bran	1 cup (1.9 oz)	170	1	0
Total Whole Grain	¾ cup (1 oz)	110	1	0
Trix	1 cup (1 oz)	120	1	0
Wheat Hearts	¼ cup (1.3 oz)	130	1	0
Wheaties	1 cup (1 oz)	110	1	0
Wheaties Energy Crunch	1 cup (1.9 oz)	210	3	0
Wheaties Frosted	¾ cup (1 oz)	110	1	0
Wheaties Raisin Bran	1 cup (1.9 oz)	180	1	0
Grainfield's				
Brown Rice	1 serv (1 oz)	110	1	—
Crisp Rice	1 serv (1 oz)	112	tr	—
Raisin Bran	1 serv (1 oz)	90	2	—
Wheat Flakes	1 serv (1 oz)	100	1	—
Gram's Gourmet				
Cream Of Flax not prep	½ cup	142	5	1
Crunch Granolas All Flavors	½ cup	349	30	6
Hansen's				
Orange & Chocolate	½ cup	230	14	4
Strawberry & Yogurt	½ cup	230	9	4

FOOD	PORTION	CALS	FAT	SAT FAT
Toasted Nut Crunch	½ cup	230	6	1
Tropical Cluster	½ cup	210	5	3
Health Valley				
10 Bran O's Apple Cinnamon	¾ cup	100	0	0
Bran w/ Apples & Cinnamon	¾ cup	160	0	0
Golden Flax	½ cup	190	3	—
Granola 98% Fat Free Date Almond	⅔ cup	180	1	—
Healthy Crunches & Flakes Almond	¾ cup	130	0	0
Healthy Crunches & Flakes Apple Cinnamon	¾ cup	130	0	0
Healthy Crunches & Flakes Honey Crunch	¾ cup	130	0	0
Hot Cereal Cups Amazing Apple!	1 pkg	220	2	—
Hot Cereal Cups Banana Gone Nuts!	1 pkg	240	3	—
Hot Cereal Cups Maple Madness!	1 pkg	240	2	—
Hot Cereal Cups Terrific 10 Grain!	1 pkg	220	3	—
Oat Bran O'S	¾ cup	100	0	0
Organic Amaranth Flakes	¾ cup	100	0	0
Organic Blue Corn Bran Flakes	¾ cup	100	0	0
Organic Bran w/ Raisin	¾ cup	160	0	0
Organic Fiber 7 Flakes	¾ cup	100	0	0
Organic Healthy Fiber Flakes	¾ cup	100	0	0
Organic Oat Bran Flakes	¾ cup	100	0	0
Organic Oat Bran Flakes w/ Raisins	¾ cup	110	0	0
Puffed Honey Sweetened Corn	1 cup	110	0	0
Puffed Honey Sweetened Crisp Brown Rice	1 cup	110	0	0
Raisin Bran Flakes	1¼ cup	190	0	0
Real Oat Bran	½ cup	200	3	—
Healthy Choice				
Almond Crunch With Raisins	1 cup (2 oz)	210	3	0
Golden Multi-Grain Flakes	¾ cup (1.1 oz)	110	0	0
Toasted Brown Sugar Squares	1 cup (2 oz)	190	1	0
Hi-Lo				
Low Carb Cereal	½ cup	90	2	0
Hodgson Mill				
Bulgur Wheat w/ Soy Grits	¼ cup	116	1	0
Cracked Wheat	¼ cup	110	1	0
Multi Grain w/ Flaxseed & Soy	⅓ cup	160	3	1

FOOD	PORTION	CALS	FAT	SAT FAT
Kashi				
Breakfast Pilaf as prep	½ cup (4.9 oz)	170	3	—
Go Apple Spice	½ cup (4.9 oz)	270	3	—
Go Banana Almond	½ cup (4.9 oz)	280	4	—
Go Berry Tart	½ cup (4.9 oz)	260	3	0
Go Blueberry Bliss	½ cup (4.9 oz)	260	3	—
Go Cherry Vanilla	½ cup (4.9 oz)	260	3	—
Go Just Peachy	½ cup (4.9 oz)	260	3	—
GoLean	¾ cup (1.4 oz)	120	1	—
Good Friends	¾ cup (1 oz)	90	1	—
Honey Puffed	1 cup (1 oz)	120	1	—
Medley	½ cup (1 oz)	100	1	—
Pillows Apple	¾ cup (1.9 oz)	200	1	—
Pillows Chocolate	¾ cup (1.9 oz)	200	1	—
Pillows Strawberry Crisp	¾ cup (1.9 oz)	200	1	—
Puffed	1 cup (0.9 oz)	70	tr	—
Kellogg's				
All-Bran	½ cup (1.1 oz)	80	1	0
All-Bran Bran Buds	⅓ cup (1 oz)	80	1	0
All-Bran Extra Fiber	½ cup (0.9 oz)	50	1	0
Apple Jacks	1 cup (1.2 oz)	120	0	0
Cocoa Frosted Flakes	¾ cup (1.1 oz)	120	0	0
Cocoa Krispies	¾ cup (1.1 oz)	120	1	1
Complete Oat Bran Flakes	¾ cup (1 oz)	110	1	0
Complete Wheat Bran Flakes	¾ cup (1 oz)	90	1	0
Corn Flakes	1 cup (1 oz)	100	0	0
Corn Pops K-Sentials	1 oz	100	0	0
Cracklin' Oat Bran	¾ cup (1.7 oz)	190	7	2
Crispix	1 cup (1 oz)	110	0	0
Froot Loops K-Sentials	1 oz	100	1	0
Frosted Flakes	¾ cup (1.1 oz)	120	0	0
Granola Low Fat	½ cup (1.7 oz)	190	3	1
Honey Crunch Corn Flakes	¾ cup (1.1 oz)	120	1	0
Just Right Crunchy Nuggets	1 cup (2 oz)	210	2	0
Just Right Fruit & Nut	1 cup (2.1 oz)	220	2	0
Low Fat With Raisins	⅔ cup (2.1 oz)	220	3	1
Mini-Wheats Frosted	1 cup (1.8 oz)	180	1	0
Mini-Wheats Strawberry Squares	¾ cup (1.8 oz)	170	1	0
Mini-Wheats Apple Cinnamon Squares	¾ cup (1.9 oz)	180	1	0

FOOD	PORTION	CALS	FAT	SAT FAT
Mini-Wheats Blueberry Squares	¾ cup (1.9 oz)	180	1	0
Mini-Wheats Frosted Bite Size	24 pieces (2.1 oz)	200	1	0
Mini-Wheats Raisin Squares	¾ cup (1.9 oz)	180	1	0
Mueslix Apple & Almond Crunch	¾ cups (1.9 oz)	200	5	1
Mueslix Raisin & Almond	⅔ cup (1.9 oz)	200	3	0
Nutri-Grain Almond Raisin	1¼ cups (1.7 oz)	180	3	0
Nutri-Grain Golden Wheat	¾ cup (1 oz)	100	1	0
Product 19	1 cup (1 oz)	100	0	0
Raisin Bran	1 cup (2.1 oz)	200	2	0
Rice Krispies	1¼ cups (1.2 oz)	120	0	0
Rice Krispies Razzle Dazzle	¾ cup (1 oz)	110	0	0
Rice Krispies Treats	¾ cup (1 oz)	120	2	0
Smacks	¾ cup (1 oz)	100	1	0
Smart Start	1 cup (1.8 oz)	180	1	0
Special K	1 cup (1.1 oz)	110	0	0
Keto				
Cocoa Crisp	½ cup	110	2	0
Frosted Flakes All Flavors	¾ cup	110	1	0
Hot Cereal Apple Cinnamon	2 scoops	150	4	1
Hot Cereal Strawberry & Creme	2 scoops	150	4	1
Low Carb Crispy Soy	¾ cup	110	2	–
Oatmeal Old Fashioned	2 scoops	150	4	1
Kolln				
Crispy Oats	1 cup (1.8 oz)	190	3	1
Oat Bran Crunch	⅔ cup (2.1 oz)	220	5	1
Oat Muesli Fruit	¾ cup (2 oz)	200	5	1
Lundberg				
Purely Organic Hot'n Creamy Rice	⅓ cup	190	2	0
McCann's				
Irish Oatmeal	1 oz	110	2	–
Irish Oatmeal Instant Apples & Cinnamon	1 pkg (1 oz)	130	2	0
Irish Oatmeal Instant Maple & Brown Sugar	1 pkg (1 oz)	160	2	0
Irish Oatmeal Instant Regular	1 pkg (1 oz)	100	2	0
MiniCarb				
Milk Chocolate Hot Cereal not prep	½ cup	140	6	1
Morning Traditions				
Banana Nut Crunch	1 cup (2 oz)	250	6	1

FOOD	PORTION	CALS	FAT	SAT FAT
Blueberry Morning	1¼ cups (1.9 oz)	220	3	1
Cranberry Almond Crunch	1 cup (1.9 oz)	220	3	0
Great Grains Crunchy Pecan	⅔ cup (1.9 oz)	220	6	1
Great Grains Raisins Dates & Pecans	⅔ cup (1.9 oz)	210	5	1
Nabisco				
100% Bran	⅓ cup (1 oz)	80	1	0
Cream Of Wheat Instant as prep	1 cup	120	0	—
Cream Of Wheat Quick as prep	1 cup	120	0	—
Cream Of Wheat Regular as prep	1 cup	120	0	—
Frosted Shredded Wheat Bite Size	1 cup (1.8 oz)	190	1	0
Honey Nut Shredded Wheat Bite Size	1 cup (1.8 oz)	200	2	0
Original Shredded Wheat	2 biscuits (1.6 oz)	160	1	0
Original Shredded Wheat 'N Bran	1¼ cups (2.1 oz)	200	1	0
Original Shredded Wheat Spoon Size	1 cup (1.7 oz)	170	1	0
Post				
Alpha-Bits	1 cup (1 oz)	130	2	0
Alpha-Bits Marshmallow	1 cup (1 oz)	120	1	0
Bran Flakes	¾ cup (1 oz)	100	1	0
Cocoa Pebbles	¾ cup (1 oz)	120	1	1
Fruit & Fibre Dates Raisins & Walnuts	1 cup (1.9 oz)	210	3	1
Fruit & Fibre Peaches Raisins & Almonds	1 cup (1.9 oz)	210	3	1
Fruity Pebbles	¾ cup (1 oz)	110	1	0
Golden Crisp	¾ cup (1 oz)	110	0	0
Grape-Nuts	¾ cup (1 oz)	100	1	0
Grape-Nuts Flakes	¾ cup (1 oz)	100	1	0
Honey Bunches Of Oats	¾ cup (1 oz)	120	2	1
Honey Bunches Of Oats With Almonds	¾ cup (1.1 oz)	130	3	1
Honeycomb	1⅓ cups (1 oz)	110	1	0
Post Toasties	1 cup (1 oz)	100	0	0
Raisin Bran	1 cup (2 oz)	190	1	0
Selects Blueberry Morning	¾ cup (1.3 oz)	140	2	0
Waffle Crisp	1 cup (1 oz)	130	3	0
Quaker				
Instant Grits Original	1 pkg (1 oz)	100	0	0
Multigrain	½ cup (1.4 oz)	130	2	0
Oatmeal Instant	1 pkg (1 oz)	100	2	0
Oatmeal Instant Apples & Cinnamon	1 pkg (1.2 oz)	130	2	1
Oatmeal Instant Bananas & Cream	1 pkg (1.2 oz)	130	3	1

FOOD	PORTION	CALS	FAT	SAT FAT
Oatmeal Instant Blueberries & Cream	1 pkg (1.2 oz)	130	3	1
Oatmeal Instant Cinnamon & Spice	1 pkg (1.6 oz)	170	2	1
Oatmeal Instant Kid's Choice Chocolate Chip Cookie	1 pkg (1.5 oz)	160	3	1
Oatmeal Instant Kid's Choice Cookie'n Cream	1 pkg (1.5 oz)	160	3	1
Oatmeal Instant Kid's Choice Fruity Marshmallow	1 pkg (1.4 oz)	150	2	1
Oatmeal Instant Kid's Choice Oatmeal Raisin Cookie	1 pkg (1.5 oz)	160	2	1
Oatmeal Instant Kid's Choice Radical Raspberry	1 pkg (1.4 oz)	150	3	1
Oatmeal Instant Kid's Choice S'mores	1 pkg (1.5 oz)	160	3	1
Oatmeal Instant Kid's Choice Strawberries'n Stuff	1 pkg (1.4 oz)	150	2	1
Oatmeal Instant Kid's Choice Twisted Strawberry Banana	1 pkg (1.4 oz)	150	2	1
Oatmeal Instant Maple & Brown Sugar	1 pkg (1.5 oz)	160	2	0
Oatmeal Instant Peaches & Cream	1 pkg (1.2 oz)	140	3	1
Oatmeal Instant Raisin & Spice	1 pkg (1.5 oz)	150	2	1
Oatmeal Instant Raisin Date & Walnut	1 pkg (1.3 oz)	140	3	1
Oatmeal Instant Strawberries & Cream	1 pkg (1.2 oz)	140	3	1
Oatmeal Nutrition for Women Golden Brown Sugar	1 pkg (1.6 oz)	170	2	1
Oatmeal Quick'n Hearty Microwave	1 pkg (1 oz)	110	2	1
Oatmeal Quick'n Hearty Microwave Apple Spice	1 pkg (1.6 oz)	170	2	1
Oatmeal Quick'n Hearty Microwave Brown Sugar Cinnamon	1 pkg (1.5 oz)	150	2	1
Oatmeal Quick'n Hearty Microwave Cinnamon Double Raisin	1 pkg (1.6 oz)	170	2	1
Oatmeal Quick'n Hearty Microwave Honey Bran	1 pkg (1.4 oz)	150	2	1
Oats Old Fashion	½ cup (1.4 oz)	150	3	1
Oats Quick	½ cup (1.4 oz)	150	3	1
Oats Steel Cut	½ cup (1.4 oz)	150	3	1
Whole Wheat Hot Natural	½ cup (1.4 oz)	130	1	0
Sunbelt				
Berry Basic	½ cup (1.9 oz)	220	6	2
Granola Banana Nut	½ cup (1.9 oz)	250	9	4

FOOD	PORTION	CALS	FAT	SAT FAT
Granola Cinnamon Raisins	½ cup (1.9 oz)	200	3	1
Granola Fruit & Nut	½ cup (1.9 oz)	240	7	2
Muesli 5 Whole Grains	½ cup (1.9 oz)	210	2	1
Uncle Sam				
Cereal	1 cup (1.9 oz)	190	1	0
Weetabix				
Cereal	2 biscuits (1.2 oz)	100	1	–
Wheatena				
Cereal	⅓ cup (1.4 oz)	150	1	0
CEREAL BARS (see also ENERGY BARS)				
granola	1 (1 oz)	134	7	1
Barbara's Bakery				
Nature's Choice Apple Cinnamon	1 (1.3 oz)	120	2	0
Nature's Choice Blueberry	1 (1.3 oz)	120	2	0
Nature's Choice Cherry	1 (1.3 oz)	120	2	0
Nature's Choice Granola Carob Chip	1 (0.7 oz)	80	2	0
Nature's Choice Granola Cinnamon & Raisin	1 (0.7 oz)	80	2	0
Nature's Choice Granola Oats 'N Honey	1 (0.7 oz)	80	2	0
Nature's Choice Granola Peanut Butter	1 (0.7 oz)	80	3	0
Nature's Choice Raspberry	1 (1.3 oz)	120	2	0
Nature's Choice Strawberry	1 (1.3 oz)	120	2	0
Nature's Choice Triple Berry	1 (1.3 oz)	120	2	0
Cap'n Crunch				
Bar	1 (0.8 oz)	90	2	1
Berries Bar	1 (0.8 oz)	90	2	–
Dolly Madison				
Apple	1 (1.3 oz)	120	2	0
Blueberry	1 (1.3 oz)	120	2	0
Raspberry	1 (1.3 oz)	120	2	0
Strawberry	1 (1.3 oz)	120	2	0
Entenmann's				
Apple Cinnamon	1 (1.3 oz)	140	3	1
Blueberry	1 (1.3 oz)	140	3	1
Multi-Grain Chocolate Chip	1	140	3	1
Multi-Grain Rainbow Chip	1	180	8	3
Multi-Grain Real Raspberry	1	140	3	1

FOOD	PORTION	CALS	FAT	SAT FAT
Oatmeal Apple Cinnamon	1 (1.3 oz)	140	3	1
Oatmeal Apple Raisin	1 (1.3 oz)	140	3	0
Raspberry	1 (1.3 oz)	140	3	0
Strawberry	1 (1.3 oz)	140	3	1
Estee				
Rice Crunchie Chocolate	1 (0.7 oz)	50	0	0
Rice Crunchie Chocolate Chip	1 (0.7 oz)	50	0	0
Rice Crunchie Peanut Butter	1 (0.7 oz)	60	1	0
Rice Crunchie Vanilla	1 (0.7 oz)	60	0	0
General Mills				
Milk 'N Cereal Bars Chex	1 bar (1.6 oz)	160	4	2
Milk 'N Cereal Bars Cinnamon Toast Crunch	1 bar (1.6 oz)	180	4	2
Oatmeal Crisp Apple	1 bar (1.4 oz)	150	2	0
Oatmeal Crisp Strawberry	1 bar (1.4 oz)	140	2	0
Glenny's				
Chocolate Crunch Creamy Low Fat	1 bar (1.75 oz)	190	3	1
Chocolate Crunch Roasted Peanut	1 bar (1.75 oz)	200	4	1
Chocolate Crunch Toasted Almond	1 bar (1.75 oz)	200	4	0
Health Valley				
98% Fat Free Raisin Cinnamon	⅔ cup	180	1	—
98% Fat Free Tropical	⅔ cup	180	1	—
Blueberry	1	140	0	0
Breakfast Bakes Apple Cinnamon	1 bar	110	0	0
Breakfast Bakes California Strawberry	1 bar	110	0	0
Breakfast Bakes Mountain Blueberry	1 bar	110	0	0
Breakfast Bakes Red Raspberry	1 bar	110	0	0
Chocolate Chip	1	140	0	0
Crisp Rice Bars Apple Cinnamon	1	110	0	0
Crisp Rice Bars Orange Date	1	110	0	0
Crisp Rice Bars Tropical Fruit	1	110	0	0
Date Almond	1	140	0	0
Fiber 7 Flakes w/ Strawberry	1 bar	110	0	0
O's Almond	¾ cup	120	0	0
O's Apple Cinnamon	¾ cup	120	0	0
O's Honey Crunch	¾ cup	120	0	0
Oat Bran Flakes w/ Blueberry	1 bar	110	0	0
Raisin	1	140	0	0
Raisin Bran Flakes w/ Apple Raisin	1 bar	110	0	0
Raspberry	1	140	0	0

FOOD	PORTION	CALS	FAT	SAT FAT
Strawberry	1	140	0	0
Hershey's				
Crispy Rice Snacks Peanut Butter	1 bar (0.5 oz)	60	2	tr
Hostess				
Apple	1 (1.3 oz)	120	2	0
Banana Nut	1 (1.3 oz)	120	2	0
Blueberry	1 (1.3 oz)	120	2	0
Raspberry	1 (1.3 oz)	120	2	0
Strawberry	1 (1.3 oz)	120	2	0
Kudos				
Chocolate Coated Chocolate Chip	1	120	5	3
Chocolate Coated Peanut Butter	1	90	3	1
Low Fat Blueberry	1 (0.7 oz)	90	2	0
Snickers	1	100	4	2
With M&M's	1	90	3	1
Little Debbie				
Raspberry	1 (1.3 oz)	130	3	0
S'mores Granola Treats	1 (1 oz)	130	5	2
Strawberry	1 (1.3 oz)	130	3	0
Nabisco				
Nutter Butter Granola Bar	1 (1 oz)	120	8	1
Oreo Granola Bar	1 (1 oz)	120	4	1
Nature Valley				
Low Fat Chewy Orchard Blend	1 bar (1 oz)	110	2	0
Nutri-Grain				
Apple Cinnamon	1 (1.3 oz)	140	3	1
Blueberry	1 (1.3 oz)	140	3	1
Cherry	1 (1.3 oz)	140	3	1
Fruit-full Squares Apple	1 (1.7 oz)	180	4	1
Fruit-full Squares Banana	1 (1.7 oz)	190	5	1
Fruit-full Squares Cinnamon Raisin	1 (1.7 oz)	180	4	1
Minis Strawberry	1 pkg (1.5 oz)	160	3	1
Mixed Berry	1 (1.3 oz)	140	3	1
Twists Low Fat Apple Cinnamon	1 (1.3 oz)	140	3	1
Twists Low Fat Banana Strawberry	1 (1.3 oz)	140	3	1
Twists Low Fat Strawberry Blueberry	1 (1.3 oz)	140	3	1
Quaker				
Chewy Chocolate Chip	1 (1 oz)	120	4	2
Chewy Cookies 'n Cream	1 (1 oz)	110	3	1
Chewy Peanut Butter Chocolate Chunk	1 (1 oz)	120	3	1

FOOD	PORTION	CALS	FAT	SAT FAT
Chewy Graham Slam Chocolate Chip	1 (1 oz)	110	2	—
Chewy Graham Slam Peanut Butter	1 (1 oz)	110	2	—
Chewy Low Fat Chocolate Chunk	1 (1 oz)	110	2	—
Chewy Low Fat Oatmeal Raisin	1 (1 oz)	110	2	1
Chewy Low Fat S'mores	1 (1 oz)	110	2	1
Fruit & Oatmeal Apple Cinnamon	1 (1.3 oz)	130	3	—
Fruit & Oatmeal Bites Apple Crisp	1 pkg	140	3	0
Fruit & Oatmeal Bites Strawberry	1 pkg	140	3	0
Fruit & Oatmeal Bites Very Berry	1 pkg	140	3	0
Fruit & Oatmeal Low Fat Cherry Cobbler	1 (1.3 oz)	140	3	—
Fruit & Oatmeal Low Fat Strawberry	1 (1.3 oz)	140	3	—
Fruit & Oatmeal Low Fat Strawberry Banana	1 (1.3 oz)	130	3	—
Fruit & Oatmeal Low Fat Strawberry Cheesecake	1 (1.3 oz)	130	3	1
Rice Krispies				
Treats	1 (0.8 oz)	90	2	1
Treats Peanut Butter Chocolate	1 (0.8 oz)	110	4	1
Treats Cocoa	1 (0.8 oz)	100	4	1
SnackWell's				
Country Fruit Medley	1 (1.3 oz)	130	3	0
Fat Free Apple Cinnamon	1 (1.3 oz)	120	0	0
Fat Free Blueberry	1 (1.3 oz)	120	0	0
Fat Free Strawberry	1 (1.3 oz)	120	0	0
Hearty Fruit'n Grain Crisp Autumn Apple	1 (1.3 oz)	130	3	0
Hearty Fruit'n Grain Mixed Berry	1 (1.3 oz)	120	3	0
Hearty Fruit'n Grain Orchard Cherry	1 (1.3 oz)	130	5	1
Sunbelt				
Apple	1 (1.3 oz)	130	3	0
Blueberry	1 (1.3 oz)	130	3	0
Chewy Granola Almond	1 (1 oz)	130	7	2
Chewy Granola Apple Cinnamon	1 (1.2 oz)	140	3	0
Chewy Granola Chocolate Chip	1 (1.2 oz)	160	7	3
Chewy Granola Oatmeal Raisin	1 (1.2 oz)	130	3	0
Chewy Granola Oats & Honey	1 (1 oz)	120	5	2
Granola Fudge Dipped Chocolate Chip	1 (1.5 oz)	200	10	4
Granola Fudge Dipped Macaroon	1 (1.4 oz)	190	10	4

FOOD	PORTION	CALS	FAT	SAT FAT
Weight Watchers				
Apple Cinnamon	1 (1 oz)	100	2	1
Blueberry	1 (1 oz)	100	2	1
Raspberry	1 (1 oz)	100	2	1
CHAMPAGNE				
mimosa	1 serv	117	tr	tr
punch	1 serv	113	0	0
sekt german champagne	3.5 fl oz	84	0	0
Andre				
Blush	4 fl oz	88	0	0
Brut	4 fl oz	84	0	0
Cold Duck	4 fl oz	100	0	0
Extra Dry	4 fl oz	92	0	0
Ballatore				
Spumante	4 fl oz	92	0	0
Eden Roc				
Brut	4 fl oz	92	0	0
Brut Rose'	4 fl oz	99	0	0
Extra Dry	4 fl oz	84	0	0
Tott's				
Blanc de Noir	4 fl oz	88	0	0
Brut	4 fl oz	80	0	0
Extra Dry	4 fl oz	84	0	0
CHAYOTE				
fresh cooked	1 cup	38	1	—
raw	1 (7 oz)	49	1	—
raw cut up	1 cup	32	tr	—
CHEESE (see also CHEESE DISHES, CHEESE SUBSTITUTES, COTTAGE CHEESE, CREAM CHEESE, NEUFCHATEL)				
american	1 oz	93	7	4
american cheese food	1 pkg (8 oz)	745	56	35
american cheese spread	1 jar (5 oz)	412	30	19
american cold pack	1 pkg (8 oz)	752	56	35
american cheese spread	1 oz	82	6	4
beaufort	1 oz	115	9	6
bel paese	1 oz	112	9	—
blue	1 oz	100	8	6
blue crumbled	1 cup (4.7 oz)	477	39	25

FOOD	PORTION	CALS	FAT	SAT FAT
brick	1 oz	105	8	5
brie	1 oz	95	8	–
cacio di roma sheep's milk cheese	1 oz	130	10	6
caerphilly	1.4 oz	150	13	–
camembert	1 oz	85	7	4
camembert	1 wedge (1⅓ oz)	114	9	6
cantal	1 oz	105	9	6
caraway	1 oz	107	8	–
chabichou	1 oz	95	8	5
chaource	1 oz	83	7	4
cheddar	1 oz	114	9	6
cheddar low fat	1 oz	49	2	1
cheddar low sodium	1 oz	113	9	6
cheddar reduced fat	1.4 oz	104	6	–
cheddar shredded	1 cup	455	37	24
cheshire	1 oz	110	9	–
cheshire reduced fat	1.4 oz	108	6	–
colby	1 oz	112	9	6
colby low fat	1 oz	49	2	1
colby low sodium	1 oz	113	9	6
comte	1 oz	114	9	5
coulommiers	1 oz	88	7	5
crottin	1 oz	105	9	6
derby	1.4 oz	161	14	–
edam	1 oz	101	8	5
edam reduced fat	1.4 oz	92	4	–
emmentaler	1 oz	115	9	–
feta	1 oz	75	6	4
fontina	1 oz	110	9	5
frais	1.6 oz	51	3	–
gjetost	1 oz	132	8	5
gloucester double	1.4 oz	162	14	–
goat fresh	1 oz	23	2	1
goat hard	1 oz	128	10	7
goat semisoft	1 oz	103	8	6
goat soft	1 oz	76	6	4
gorgonzola	1 oz	107	9	–
gouda	1 oz	101	8	5
gruyere	1 oz	117	9	5
lancashire	1.4 oz	149	12	–

FOOD	PORTION	CALS	FAT	SAT FAT
leicester	1.4 oz	160	14	–
limburger	1 oz	93	8	5
lymeswold	1.4 oz	170	16	–
maroilles	1 oz	97	8	5
monterey	1 oz	106	9	–
morbier	1 oz	99	8	5
mozzarella	1 oz	80	6	4
mozzarella	1 lb	1276	98	60
mozzarella fresh	1 oz	80	6	4
mozzarella low moisture	1 oz	90	7	4
mozzarella part skim	1 oz	72	5	3
muenster	1 oz	104	9	5
parmesan grated	1 oz	129	9	5
parmesan grated	1 tbsp (5 g)	23	2	1
parmesan hard	1 oz	111	7	5
picodon	1 oz	99	8	5
pimento	1 oz	106	9	6
pont l'eveque	1 oz	86	7	4
port du salut	1 oz	100	8	5
provolone	1 oz	100	8	5
pyrenees	1 oz	101	8	5
quark 20% fat	1 oz	33	1	–
quark 40% fat	1 oz	48	3	–
quark made w/ skim milk	1 oz	22	tr	–
queso anego	1 oz	106	9	5
queso asadero	1 oz	101	8	5
queso chichuahua	1 oz	106	8	5
queso fresco	1 oz	41	2	–
queso manchego	1 oz	107	8	–
queso panela	1 oz	74	5	–
raclette	1 oz	102	8	5
reblochon	1 oz	88	7	5
ricotta part skim	½ cup (4.4 oz)	171	10	6
ricotta part skim	1 cup (8.6 oz)	340	19	12
ricotta whole milk	1 cup (8.6 oz)	428	32	20
ricotta whole milk	½ cup (4.4 oz)	216	16	10
romadur 40% fat	1 oz	83	6	–
romano	1 oz	110	8	–
roquefort	1 oz	105	9	5
rouy	1 oz	95	8	5

FOOD	PORTION	CALS	FAT	SAT FAT
saint marcellin	1 oz	94	8	5
saint nectaire	1 oz	97	8	5
saint paulin	1 oz	85	6	4
sainte maure	1 oz	99	8	5
selles sur cher	1 oz	93	8	5
stilton blue	1.4 oz	164	14	–
stilton white	1.4 oz	145	13	–
swiss	1 oz	107	8	5
swiss cheese food	1 pkg (8 oz)	734	55	–
swiss processed	1 oz	95	7	5
tilsit	1 oz	96	7	5
tome	1 oz	92	7	5
triple creme	1 oz	113	11	7
vacherin	1 oz	92	8	5
wensleydale	1.4 oz	151	13	–
whey cheese	1 oz	126	8	5
yogurt cheese	1 oz	80	7	3
Alouette				
Garlic & Herbs	2 tbsp (0.8 oz)	70	7	5
Alpine Lace				
American Jalapeno Peppers	1 slice (1 oz)	80	6	4
American Less Fat Less Sodium White	1 slice (1 oz)	50	6	4
American Less Fat Less Sodium Yellow	1 slice (1 oz)	80	6	4
Cheddar Reduced Fat	1 slice (1 oz)	70	5	3
Colby Reduced Fat	1 slice (1 oz)	80	5	3
Fat Free Parmesan	2 tsp (5 g)	10	0	0
Feta Reduced Fat	1 oz	50	3	2
Feta Reduced Fat Sun Dried Tomato & Basil	1 oz	50	3	2
Goat Reduced Fat	1 oz	40	3	2
Mozzarella Reduced Fat	1 oz	70	3	2
Muenster Reduced Sodium	1 slice (1 oz)	100	9	5
Provolone Smoked Reduced Fat	1 slice (1 oz)	70	5	3
Swiss Reduced Fat	1 slice (1 oz)	90	6	4
Athenos				
Feta	1 oz	80	6	4
Boar's Head				
American	1 oz	100	9	6
Baby Swiss	1 oz	110	9	6
Canadian Cheddar	1 oz	110	10	6

FOOD	PORTION	CALS	FAT	SAT FAT
Double Glouster Yellow	1 oz	110	10	6
Feta	1 oz	60	4	3
Havarti	1 oz	110	10	7
Havarti w/ Dill	1 oz	110	10	7
Havarti w/ Jalapeno	1 oz	110	10	7
Lacey Swiss	1 oz	90	6	4
Longhorn Colby	1 oz	110	9	5
Monterey Jack	1 oz	100	9	6
Monterey Jack w/ Jalapeno	1 oz	100	9	6
Mozzarella	1 oz	90	7	4
Muenster	1 oz	100	8	5
Muenster Low Sodium	1 oz	100	8	5
Provolone Picante Sharp	1 oz	100	8	5
Swiss	1 oz	110	8	5
Swiss No Salt Added	1 oz	110	8	5
Bonbel				
Mini Babybel	1 piece (0.7 oz)	70	6	4
Borden				
Lite Line Sharp Cheddar	1 oz	50	2	–
Lite Line Swiss	1 oz	50	2	–
Boursin				
Garlic & Fine Herbs	2 tbsp	120	13	9
Breakstone's				
Ricotta	¼ cup (2.2 oz)	110	8	5
Cabot				
American	1 slice (0.7 oz)	80	7	4
Cheddar	1 oz	110	9	5
Cheddar Smoked	1 oz	110	9	5
Cheddar Light 50% Reduced Fat	1 oz	70	5	3
Cheddar Light 50% Reduced Fat Jalapeno	1 oz	70	5	3
Cheddar Light 75% Reduced Fat	1 oz	60	3	2
Colby Jack	1 oz	110	9	5
Fancy Blend Shredded	¼ cup	100	7	4
Monterey Jack	1 oz	110	9	5
Mozzarella Shredded	¼ cup	80	6	4
Pepper Jack	1 oz	110	9	5
Swiss Slices	1 slice (1 oz)	110	8	5
Cedar Grove				
Marble Colby	1 oz	110	9	6

FOOD	PORTION	CALS	FAT	SAT FAT
Organic Tomato Basil Cheddar	1 oz	110	9	6
Chavrie				
Goat's Milk	2 tbsp	50	4	3
Cheez Whiz				
Light	2 tbsp (1.2 oz)	80	3	2
Connoisseur				
Asiago Spread	1 tbsp	90	7	4
Cracker Barrel				
Baby Swiss	1 oz	110	9	6
Cheddar Extra Sharp	1 oz	120	10	7
Cheddar Marbled Sharp	1 oz	110	9	6
Cheddar New York Aged	1 oz	120	10	7
Cheddar Sharp	1 oz	120	10	7
Cheddar Vermont Sharp	1 oz	110	9	6
Reduced Fat Cheddar Extra Sharp	1 oz	90	6	4
Reduced Fat Cheddar Sharp	1 oz	90	6	4
Reduced Fat Cheddar Vermont Sharp	1 oz	90	6	4
Whipped Spreadable Cream Cheese & Extra Sharp Cheddar	2 tbsp (0.9 oz)	80	8	5
Whipped Spreadable Cream Cheese & Sharp Cheddar	2 tbsp (0.9 oz)	80	8	5
Whipped Spreadable Cream Cheese & Sharp Cheddar w/ Herbs	2 tbsp (0.9 oz)	80	8	5
Di Giorno				
Parmesan Grated	2 tsp (5 g)	25	2	1
Parmesan Shredded	2 tsp (5 g)	20	2	1
Romano Grated	2 tsp (5 g)	25	2	1
Romano Shredded	2 tsp (5 g)	20	2	1
Fleurs De France				
Brie	3.5 oz	311	25	18
Friendship				
Farmer	2 tbsp (1 oz)	50	3	2
Handi-Snacks				
Cheez'n Breadsticks	1 pkg (1.1 oz)	120	6	3
Cheez'n Crackers	1 pkg (1.1 oz)	110	7	3
Cheez'n Pretzels	1 pkg (1 oz)	100	5	3
Mozzarella String Cheese	1 piece (1 oz)	80	6	4
Nacho Stix'n Cheez	1 pkg (1.1 oz)	110	6	3
Healthy Choice				
American Singles White	1 slice (0.7 oz)	30	0	0

FOOD	PORTION	CALS	FAT	SAT FAT
American Singles Yellow	1 slice (0.7 oz)	30	0	0
Cheddar Fancy Shreds	¼ cup (1 oz)	45	0	0
Cheddar Shreds	¼ cup (1 oz)	45	0	0
Loaf	1 in cube (1 oz)	35	0	0
Mexican Shreds	¼ cup (1 oz)	45	0	0
Mozzarella	1 oz	45	0	0
Mozzarella Fancy Shreds	¼ cup (1 oz)	45	0	0
Mozzarella Shreds	¼ cup (1 oz)	45	0	0
Mozzarella String Cheese	1 stick (1 oz)	45	0	0
Pizza Fancy Shreds	¼ cup (1 oz)	45	0	0
Pizza String	1 stick (1 oz)	45	0	0
Hollow Road Farms				
Sheep's Milk	1 oz	45	3	—
Kraft				
Cheddar Extra Sharp	1 oz	120	10	7
Cheddar Medium	1 oz	110	9	6
Cheddar Mild	1 oz	110	9	6
Cheddar Sharp	1 oz	120	10	7
Cheddary Melts Medium Cheddar	1 oz	110	9	6
Cheddary Melts Mild Cheddar	1 oz	110	9	6
Cheddary Melts Shreds Medium Cheddar	¼ cup (1.1 oz)	120	9	6
Cheddary Melts Shreds Mild Cheddar	¼ cup (1.1 oz)	120	9	6
Cheese Food w/ Garlic	1 oz	90	7	5
Cheese Food w/ Jalapeno Peppers	1 oz	90	7	5
Colby	1 oz	110	9	6
Colby Monterey Jack	1 oz	110	9	6
Deluxe American	1 oz	100	9	6
Deluxe American White	1 oz	100	9	6
Deluxe Singles American	1 (0.7 oz)	70	6	4
Deluxe Singles American	1 (1 oz)	110	9	6
Deluxe Singles Pimento	1 (1 oz)	100	8	6
Deluxe Singles Swiss	1 slice (0.7 oz)	70	5	4
Deluxe Singles Swiss	1 (1 oz)	90	7	5
Free Grated	2 tsp (5 g)	15	0	0
Free Shredded Cheddar	¼ cup (0.9 oz)	40	0	0
Free Shredded Mozzarella	¼ cup (1 oz)	45	0	0
Grated Parm Plus! Garlic Herb	2 tsp (5 g)	15	0	0
Grated Parm Plus! Zesty Red Pepper	2 tsp (5 g)	15	0	0
Grated Parmesan	2 tsp (5 g)	20	2	1

FOOD	PORTION	CALS	FAT	SAT FAT
Grated Romano	2 tsp (5 g)	20	2	1
Marbled Cheddar Mild	1 oz	110	9	6
Marbled Cheddar & Monterey Jack	1 oz	110	9	6
Marbled Cheddar & Whole Milk Mozzarella	1 oz	100	8	5
Marbled Colby Monterey Jack	1 oz	110	9	6
Monterey Jack	1 oz	110	9	6
Monterey Jack w/ Jalapeno Peppers	1 oz	110	9	6
Mozzarella Part Skim Low Moisture	1 oz	80	5	4
Mozzarella String Cheese Low Moisture Part Skim	1 piece (1 oz)	80	6	4
Pizza Shredded Four Cheese	¼ cup (0.9 oz)	90	7	5
Pizza Shredded Mozzarella & Cheddar	⅓ cup (1.1 oz)	120	9	6
Pizza Shredded Mozzarella & Provolone w/ Smoke Flavor	¼ cup (0.9 oz)	90	7	5
Reduced Fat Cheddar Mild	1 oz	90	6	4
Reduced Fat Cheddar Sharp	1 oz	90	6	4
Reduced Fat Colby	1 oz	80	6	4
Reduced Fat Monterey Jack	1 oz	80	6	4
Shredded Cheddar Medium	¼ cup (0.9 oz)	100	8	6
Shredded Cheddar Mild	¼ cup (0.9 oz)	100	8	6
Shredded Cheddar Sharp	1 oz (0.9 oz)	110	9	6
Shredded Cheddar & Monterey Jack	¼ cup (0.9 oz)	100	8	6
Shredded Colby & Monterey Jack	¼ cup (0.9 oz)	100	8	6
Shredded Hearty Italian	⅓ cup (1.1 oz)	100	8	5
Shredded Italian Style Classic Garlic	⅓ cup (1.1 oz)	100	8	5
Shredded Italian Style Mozzarelle & Parmesan	⅓ cup (1.1 oz)	100	8	5
Shredded Lower Fat Cheddar Mild	¼ cup (0.9 oz)	80	6	4
Shredded Lower Fat Cheddar Sharp	¼ cup (0.9 oz)	80	6	4
Shredded Lower Fat Colby & Monterey Jack	¼ cup (0.9 oz)	80	5	4
Shredded Lower Fat Mozzarella	⅓ cup (1.1 oz)	80	5	3
Shredded Lower Fat Pizza Cheese	⅓ cup (1.1 oz)	90	6	4
Shredded Mexican Style Cheddar & Monterey Jack	⅓ cup (1.1 oz)	120	10	7
Shredded Mexican Style Cheddar & Monterey Jack w/ Jalapeno Peppers	⅓ cup (1.1 oz)	120	10	6
Shredded Mexican Style Four Cheese	⅓ cup (1.1 oz)	120	10	7
Shredded Mexican Style Taco Cheese	⅓ cup (1.1 oz)	120	10	7

FOOD	PORTION	CALS	FAT	SAT FAT
Shredded Monterey Jack	¼ cup (0.9 oz)	100	8	6
Shredded Parmesan	2 tsp (5 g)	20	2	1
Shredded Part Skim Mozzarella	¼ cup (1.1 oz)	90	6	4
Shredded Swiss	¼ cup (0.9 oz)	100	8	5
Shredded Whole Milk Mozzarella	¼ cup (1.1 oz)	100	8	5
Shredded Finely Cheddar Mild	¼ cup (1.1 oz)	120	10	6
Shredded Finely Cheddar Sharp	¼ cup (1.1 oz)	120	10	7
Shredded Finely Colby & Monterey Jack	¼ cup (1 oz)	110	9	6
Shredded Finely Lower Fat Cheddar Mild	⅓ cup (1.1 oz)	100	7	5
Shredded Finely Lower Fat Cheddar Sharp	⅓ cup (1.1 oz)	100	7	5
Shredded Finely Part Skim Mozzarella	¼ cup (1.1 oz)	90	6	4
Shredded Finely Swiss	¼ cup (0.9 oz)	110	8	6
Singles American	1 (1.2 oz)	110	8	6
Singles American	1 (0.6 oz)	60	5	3
Singles American	1 (0.7 oz)	60	5	3
Singles Mild Mexican	1 (0.7 oz)	70	5	4
Singles Monterey	1 slice (0.7 oz)	70	5	4
Singles Pimento	1 (0.7 oz)	60	5	3
Singles Reduced Fat American	1 (0.7 oz)	50	3	2
Singles Reduced Fat American White	1 (0.7 oz)	50	3	2
Singles Sharp	1 slice (0.7 oz)	70	6	4
Singles Swiss	1 slice (0.7 oz)	70	5	4
Singles Nonfat American	1 (0.7 oz)	30	0	0
Singles Nonfat American White	1 (0.7 oz)	30	0	0
Singles Nonfat Sharp Cheddar	1 (0.7 oz)	35	0	0
Singles Nonfat Swiss	1 slice (0.7 oz)	30	0	0
Slices Cheddar Mild	1 (1 oz)	110	9	6
Slices Colby	1 (1.6 oz)	180	14	10
Slices Part Skim Mozzarella	1 (1.6 oz)	130	8	6
Slices Part Skim Mozzarella	1 (1.5 oz)	120	8	5
Slices Provolone Smoke Flavor	1 (1.5 oz)	150	11	8
Slices Swiss	1 (1.6 oz)	180	14	9
Slices Swiss	1 (1.3 oz)	150	12	8
Slices Swiss	1 (0.8 oz)	90	7	5
Slices Swiss	1 (1.5 oz)	170	13	9
Slices Swiss Aged	1 (1.5 oz)	170	13	9
Slices Deli-Thin Part Skim Mozzarella	1 (1 oz)	80	5	4

FOOD	PORTION	CALS	FAT	SAT FAT
Slices Deli-Thin Swiss	1 (0.8 oz)	90	7	5
Slices Deli-Thin Swiss Aged	1 (0.8 oz)	90	7	5
Slices Reduced Fat Swiss	1 (1.3 oz)	130	9	6
Spread Bacon	2 tbsp (1.1 oz)	90	8	5
Spread Olive & Pimento	2 tbsp (1.1 oz)	70	6	4
Spread Pimento	2 tbsp (1.1 oz)	80	6	4
Spread Pineapple	2 tbsp (1.1 oz)	70	5	4
Spread Roka Brand Blue	2 tbsp (1.1 oz)	90	8	5
Swiss	1 oz	110	9	6
Land O Lakes				
American	1 slice (0.7 oz)	80	6	5
American Jalapeno	1 slice (0.6 oz)	70	6	4
American Light	1 oz	70	5	3
American Reduced Salt	1 oz	110	9	6
American Sharp	2 slices (1 oz)	100	9	6
American & Swiss	1 slice (0.6 oz)	70	5	4
Baby Swiss	1 oz	110	9	6
Chedarella	1 oz	100	8	5
Cheddar	1 oz	100	9	5
Cheddar Extra Sharp	1 oz	110	8	6
Cheddar Sharp	1 oz	110	9	5
Cheese Spread Golden Velvet	1 oz	80	6	4
Colby	1 oz	110	9	6
Jalapeno Light	1 oz	70	4	3
Monterey Jack	1 oz	110	8	5
Monterey Jack Hot Pepper	1 oz	110	8	5
Mozzarella	1 oz	80	6	4
Muenster	1 oz	100	8	5
Parmesan Grated	1 tbsp	35	4	2
Provolone	1 oz	100	8	5
Swiss	1 oz	110	8	6
Swiss Light	1 oz	80	4	3
Lifetime				
Cheddar Fat Free	1 oz	40	0	0
Cheddar Fat Free Lactose Free	1 oz	40	0	0
Garden Vegetable Fat Free	1 oz	40	0	0
Jalapeno Jack Fat Free	1 oz	40	0	0
Jalapeno Jack Fat Free Lactose Free	1 oz	40	0	0
Mild Mexican Fat Free	1 oz	40	0	0
Monterey Jack Fat Free	1 oz	40	0	0

FOOD	PORTION	CALS	FAT	SAT FAT
Mozzarella Fat Free	1 oz	40	0	0
Mozzarella Fat Free Lactose Free	1 oz	40	0	0
Onions & Chives Fat Free	1 oz	40	0	0
Sharp Cheddar Fat Free	1 oz	40	0	0
Smoked Cheddar Fat Free	1 oz	40	0	0
Swiss Fat Free	1 oz	40	0	0
Light N'Lively				
Singles American	1 (0.7 oz)	45	3	2
Northfield				
Naturally Slender	1 oz	90	7	–
Old English				
American Sharp	1 slice (1 oz)	100	9	6
Organic Valley				
Aged Swiss Unpasteurized	1 oz	100	8	5
Cheddar Reduced Fat Low Sodium	1 oz	90	6	4
Cheddar Sharp & Mild	1 oz	110	9	6
Cheddar Sharp & Mild Unpasteurized	1 oz	110	9	6
Colby	1 oz	110	9	5
Colby Unpasteurized	1 oz	110	9	5
Farmer Reduced Fat	1 oz	90	6	4
Feta	1 oz	90	7	5
Monterey Jack	1 oz	100	8	6
Monterey Jack Reduced Fat	1 oz	80	5	3
Mozzarella Part Skim	1 oz	80	5	3
Muenster	1 oz	100	8	5
Pepper Jack	1 oz	110	9	6
Provolone	1 oz	100	8	4
String Part Skim	1 oz	80	5	3
Wisconsin Raw Milk Cheese	1 oz	100	8	6
Polly-O				
String Lite	1 piece (1 oz)	60	3	2
President				
Feta	1 inch cube (1 oz)	90	7	5
Rouge Et Noir				
Breakfast	1 oz	86	7	4
Brie	1 oz	86	7	4
Camembert	1 oz	86	7	4
Schloss	1 oz	86	7	4
Sargento				
Blue Crumbled	¼ cup (1 oz)	100	8	5

FOOD	PORTION	CALS	FAT	SAT FAT
Cheddar Extra Sharp	1 oz	110	9	5
Cheddar Shredded	¼ cup (1 oz)	110	9	6
Cheese For Nachos & Tacos Shredded	¼ cup (1 oz)	110	9	5
Cheese For Pizza Shredded	¼ cup (1 oz)	90	6	4
Cheese For Tacos Shredded	¼ cup (1 oz)	110	9	6
Colby	1 slice (1 oz)	110	9	6
Colby-Jack Shredded	¼ cup (1 oz)	110	9	6
Jarlsberg	1 slice (1.2 oz)	120	9	5
Monterey Jack	1 slice (1 oz)	100	9	5
Monterey Jack Shredded	¼ cup (1 oz)	100	9	6
MooTown Snackers Cheddar	1 piece (0.8 oz)	100	8	5
MooTown Snackers Cheddar Mild Light	1 piece (0.8 oz)	60	4	3
MooTown Snackers Cheese & Pretzels	1 pkg (0.9 oz)	90	3	2
MooTown Snackers Colby-Jack	1 piece (0.8 oz)	90	8	5
MooTown Snackers Pizza Cheese & Sticks	1 pkg (1 oz)	100	4	3
MooTown Snackers String	1 piece (0.8 oz)	70	5	3
MooTown Snackers String Light	1 piece (0.8 oz)	60	3	2
Mozzarella	1 slice (1.5 oz)	130	9	6
Mozzarella Shredded	¼ cup (1 oz)	80	6	4
Muenster	1 slice (1 oz)	100	9	6
Parmesan Grated	1 tbsp (5 g)	25	2	1
Parmesan Shredded	¼ cup (1 oz)	110	7	5
Parmesan & Romano Shredded	¼ cup (1 oz)	110	7	5
Parmesan & Romano Grated	1 tbsp (5 g)	25	2	1
Pizza Double Cheese Shredded	¼ cup (1 oz)	90	6	5
Preferred Light Cheddar Mild Shredded	¼ cup (1 oz)	70	5	3
Preferred Light Mozzarella	1 slice (1.5 oz)	90	5	3
Preferred Light Mozzarella Shredded	¼ cup (1 oz)	70	3	2
Preferred Light Swiss	1 slice (1 oz)	80	4	3
Provolone	1 slice (1 oz)	100	8	5
Recipe Blend 4 Cheese Mexican Shredded	¼ cup (1 oz)	110	9	6
Recipe Blend 6 Cheese Italian Shredded	¼ cup (1 oz)	90	7	4
Reduced Fat 4 Cheese Mexican Shredded	¼ cup (1 oz)	80	6	3
Ricotta Light	¼ cup (2.2 oz)	60	3	2

FOOD	PORTION	CALS	FAT	SAT FAT
Ricotta Old Fashioned	¼ cup (2.2 oz)	90	6	4
Ricotta Part-Skim	¼ cup (2.2 oz)	80	5	3
Swiss	1 slice (0.7 oz)	80	6	4
Swiss Shredded	¼ cup (1 oz)	110	8	5
Swiss Wafer Thin	2 slices (1 oz)	110	9	5
Smart Beat				
American Fat Free	1 slice (0.6 oz)	25	0	0
Lactose Free Fat Free	1 slice (0.6 oz)	25	0	0
Mellow Cheddar Fat Free	1 slice (0.6 oz)	25	0	0
Sharp Cheddar Fat Free	1 slice (0.6 oz)	25	0	0
Sorrento				
Mozzarella Part Skim Jalapeno	1 oz	80	5	3
Pizza Cheese Shredded	¼ cup	90	7	5
Suisse Delicat				
Healthy Swiss	1 oz	90	6	5
Tree Of Life				
Cheddar 33% Reduced Fat Organic Milk	1 oz	90	6	4
Colby	1 oz	110	9	6
Colby Organic Milk	1 oz	120	10	6
Farmer Part-Skim Organic Milk	1 oz	90	6	4
Jalapeno Organic Milk	1 oz	110	9	6
Monterey Jack 35% Reduced Fat Organic Milk	1 oz	80	5	3
Monterey Jack Organic Milk	1 oz	100	8	6
Mozzarella Organic Milk	1 oz	80	5	3
Muenster Organic Milk	1 oz	100	8	5
Provolone	1 oz	100	8	5
Velveeta				
Light	1 oz	60	3	2
Shredded	¼ cup (1.3 oz)	130	9	6
Shredded Mild Mexican w/ Jalapeno Pepper	¼ cup (1.3 oz)	120	9	6
Spread	1 oz	90	6	4
Spread Hot Mexican	1 oz	90	6	4
Spread Mild Mexican	1 oz	90	6	4
Weight Watchers				
Cheddar Mild Yellow	1 oz	80	5	3
Cheddar Sharp Yellow	1 oz	80	5	3
Fat Free Grated Italian Topping	1 tbsp	20	0	0

FOOD	PORTION	CALS	FAT	SAT FAT
Fat Free Reduced Sodium Yellow	2 slices (0.75 oz)	30	0	0
Fat Free Sharp Cheddar	2 slices (0.75 oz)	30	0	0
Fat Free Swiss	2 slices (0.75 oz)	30	0	0
Fat Free White	2 slices (0.75 oz)	30	0	0
Fat Free Yellow	2 slices (0.75 oz)	30	0	0
Wholesome Valley				
Organic American Reduced Fat	1 slice (0.7 oz)	50	3	2

CHEESE DISHES
FROZEN
Banquet

Mozzarella Nuggets	6	260	18	8
Fillo Factory				
Tyropita Cheese Fillo Appetizers	5 (5 oz)	340	12	7
Health Is Wealth				
Mozzarella Stick	2 (1.3 oz)	120	5	3
Stouffer's				
Welsh Rarebit	½ cup (2.5 oz)	120	9	4
TAKE-OUT				
fondue	½ cup (3.8 oz)	247	15	9
souffle	1 serv (7 oz)	504	38	17
welsh rarebit	1 slice	228	16	–

CHEESE SUBSTITUTES

mozzarella	1 oz	70	3	1
Sargento				
Cheddar Shredded	¼ cup (1 oz)	90	7	2
Mozzarella Shredded	¼ cup (1 oz)	80	6	1
Yves				
Good Slice American	1 slice (0.7 oz)	35	2	0
Good Slice Cheddar	1 slice (0.7 oz)	35	2	0
Good Slice Jalapeno Jack	1 slice (0.7 oz)	35	2	0
Good Slice Mozzarella	1 slice (0.7 oz)	30	2	0
Good Slice Swiss	1 slice (0.7 oz)	35	2	0

CHERIMOYA

fresh	1	515	2	–

CHERRIES
CANNED

sour in heavy syrup	½ cup	232	tr	tr
sour in light syrup	½ cup	189	tr	tr

FOOD	PORTION	CALS	FAT	SAT FAT
sour water packed	1 cup	87	tr	tr
sweet in heavy syrup	½ cup	107	tr	tr
sweet in light syrup	½ cup	85	tr	tr
sweet juice pack	½ cup	68	tr	tr
sweet water pack	½ cup	57	tr	tr
Del Monte				
Dark Pitted In Heavy Syrup	½ cup (4.2 oz)	100	0	0
Sweet Dark Whole Unpitted In Heavy Syrup	½ cup (4.2 oz)	120	0	0
DRIED				
bing unsulfured	¼ cup	130	0	0
montmorency tart pitted	⅓ cup	160	1	0
yogurt covered	¼ cup	170	6	6
Sonoma				
Pitted	¼ cup (1.4 oz)	140	0	0
FRESH				
sour	1 cup	51	tr	tr
sweet	10	49	1	tr
Chiquita				
Cherries	21	90	1	0
FROZEN				
sour unsweetened	1 cup	72	1	tr
sweet sweetened	1 cup	232	tr	tr
CHERRY JUICE				
After The Fall				
American Pie Cherry	1 can (12 oz)	190	0	0
Black Cherry	1 can (12 oz)	170	0	0
Capri Sun				
Wild Cherry Drink	1 pkg (7 oz)	100	0	0
Eden				
Montmorency Juice	8 oz	140	1	0
Juicy Juice				
Drink	1 box (8.5 oz)	140	0	0
Drink	1 box (4.23 oz)	70	0	0
Kool-Aid				
Black Cherry Drink as prep w/ sugar	1 serv (8 oz)	100	0	0
Bursts Cherry Drink	1 (7 oz)	100	0	0
Cherry as prep	1 serv (8 oz)	60	0	0
Splash Drink	1 serv (8 oz)	110	0	0
Sugar Free Drink Mix as prep	1 serv (8 oz)	5	0	0

FOOD	PORTION	CALS	FAT	SAT FAT
Mott's				
Cherry	1 box (8 oz)	120	0	0
Ocean Spray				
Black Cherry Blast	8 oz	140	0	0
Squeezit				
Cherry Cola	1 bottle (7 oz)	110	0	0
Chucklin' Cherry	1 bottle (7 oz)	110	0	0
Veryfine				
Juice-Ups	8 fl oz	130	0	0
CHERVIL				
seed	1 tsp	1	tr	—
CHESTNUTS				
chinese cooked	1 oz	44	tr	tr
chinese dried	1 oz	103	tr	tr
chinese raw	1 oz	64	tr	tr
chinese roasted	1 oz	68	tr	tr
cooked	1 oz	37	tr	tr
creme de marrons	1 oz	73	tr	tr
dried peeled	1 oz	105	1	tr
japanese cooked	1 oz	16	tr	tr
japanese dried	1 oz	102	tr	tr
japanese raw	1 oz	44	tr	tr
japanese roasted	1 oz	57	tr	tr
raw peeled	1 oz	56	tr	tr
roasted	2 to 3 (1 oz)	70	1	tr
roasted	1 cup	350	3	1
CHEWING GUM				
bubble gum	1 block (8 g)	27	0	0
stick	1 (3 g)	10	0	0
Aquafresh				
Peppermint	2 pieces	5	0	0
Arm & Hammer				
Dental Care Spearmint or Peppermint	2 pieces (2.5 g)	5	0	0
Bazooka				
Gum	1 piece (6 g)	25	0	0
Gum	1 piece (4 g)	15	0	0
Beech-Nut				
Peppermint	1 stick (3 g)	10	0	0
Spearmint	1 stick (3 g)	10	0	0

FOOD	PORTION	CALS	FAT	SAT FAT
Big Red				
Stick	1	10	tr	—
Bubble Yum				
Bananaberry Split	1 piece (0.3 oz)	25	0	0
Cotton Candy	1 piece (0.3 oz)	25	0	0
Grape	1 piece (0.3 oz)	25	0	0
Luscious Lime	1 piece (0.3 oz)	25	0	0
Regular	1 piece (0.3 oz)	25	0	0
Sour Apple	1 piece (0.3 oz)	25	0	0
Sour Cherry	1 piece (0.3 oz)	25	0	0
Sugarless	1 piece (0.2 oz)	15	0	—
Sugarless Grape	1 piece (0.2 oz)	15	0	—
Sugarless Peppermint	1 piece (0.2 oz)	15	0	—
Sugarless Strawberry	1 piece (0.2 oz)	15	0	—
Sugarless Variety	1 piece (0.2 oz)	15	0	—
Variety Pack	1 piece (0.3 oz)	25	0	0
Watermelon	1 piece (0.3 oz)	25	0	0
Wild Strawberry	1 piece (0.3 oz)	25	0	0
CareFree				
Koolerz Lemonade	1 piece	5	0	0
Sugarless Bubble Gum	1 stick (3 g)	10	0	—
Sugarless Cinnamon	1 piece (3 g)	5	0	—
Sugarless Peppermint	1 piece (3 g)	5	0	—
Sugarless Spearmint	1 piece (3 g)	5	0	—
Sugarless Wild Cherry	1 stick (3 g)	10	0	0
Dentyne				
Ice Peppermint	2 pieces (3 g)	5	0	0
Doublemint				
Chewing Gum	1 piece	10	tr	—
Eclipse				
Spearmint	2 pieces	5	0	0
Extra Sugar Free				
Cinnamon	1 piece	8	tr	—
Spearmint & Peppermint	1 stick	8	tr	—
Winter Fresh	1 piece	8	tr	—
Freedent				
Spearmint Peppermint & Cinnamon	1 stick	10	tr	—
Fruit Stripe				
Bubble Gum Jumbo Pack	1 stick (3 g)	10	0	0
Variety Pack Chewing & Bubble Gum	1 stick (3 g)	10	0	0

FOOD	PORTION	CALS	FAT	SAT FAT
Hubba Bubba				
Bubble Gum Cola	1 piece	23	tr	—
Bubble Gum Sugarfree Grape	1 piece	13	tr	—
Bubble Gum Sugarfree Original	1 piece	14	tr	—
Original	1 piece	23	tr	—
Strawberry Grape Raspberry	1 piece	23	tr	—
Juicy Fruit				
Stick	1	10	tr	—
Lance				
Big Red Cinnamon	1 piece (3 g)	10	0	0
Double Bubble	1 piece (7 g)	25	0	0
Double Mint	1 piece (3 g)	10	0	0
Speakeasy				
Natural Rainforest All Flavors	2 pieces	10	0	0
StickFree				
Sugarless Peppermint	1 stick (3 g)	10	0	—
Sugarless Spearmint	1 stick (3 g)	10	0	—
Winterfresh				
Stick	1 stick (3 g)	10	0	0
Wrigley's				
Orbit	1 piece	5	0	0
Spearmint	1 stick	10	tr	—
Xylichew				
Licorice	2 pieces	4	0	0
CHIA SEEDS				
dried	1 oz	134	7	3
CHICKEN (see also CHICKEN DISHES, CHICKEN SUBSTITUTES, DINNER, HOT DOGS)				
CANNED				
chicken spread	1 tbsp	25	2	—
chicken spread	1 oz	55	3	—
chicken spread barbeque flavored	1 oz	55	3	—
w/ broth	½ can (2.5 oz)	117	6	2
w/ broth	1 can (5 oz)	234	11	3
FRESH				
broiler/fryer breast w/ skin batter dipped & fried	2.9 oz	218	11	3
broiler/fryer breast w/ skin batter dipped & fried	½ breast (4.9 oz)	364	18	5
broiler/fryer breast w/ skin roasted	2 oz	115	5	1

FOOD	PORTION	CALS	FAT	SAT FAT
broiler/fryer breast w/ skin roasted	½ breast (3.4 oz)	193	8	2
broiler/fryer breast w/ skin stewed	½ breast (3.9 oz)	202	8	2
broiler/fryer breast w/o skin fried	½ breast (3 oz)	161	4	1
broiler/fryer breast w/o skin roasted	½ breast (3 oz)	142	3	1
broiler/fryer breast w/o skin stewed	2 oz	86	2	tr
broiler/fryer drumstick w/ skin batter dipped & fried	1 (2.6 oz)	193	11	3
broiler/fryer drumstick w/ skin floured & fried	1 (1.7 oz)	120	7	2
broiler/fryer drumstick w/ skin roasted	1 (1.8 oz)	112	6	2
broiler/fryer drumstick w/ skin stewed	1 (2 oz)	116	6	2
broiler/fryer drumstick w/o skin fried	1 (1.5 oz)	82	3	1
broiler/fryer drumstick w/o skin roasted	1 (1.5 oz)	76	2	1
broiler/fryer drumstick w/o skin stewed	1 (1.6 oz)	78	3	1
broiler/fryer leg w/ skin batter dipped & fried	1 (5.5 oz)	431	26	7
broiler/fryer leg w/ skin floured & fried	1 (3.9 oz)	285	16	4
broiler/fryer leg w/ skin roasted	1 (4 oz)	265	15	4
broiler/fryer leg w/ skin stewed	1 (4.4 oz)	275	16	4
broiler/fryer leg w/o skin fried	1 (3.3 oz)	195	9	2
broiler/fryer leg w/o skin roasted	1 (3.3 oz)	182	8	2
broiler/fryer leg w/o skin stewed	1 (3.5 oz)	187	8	2
broiler/fryer neck w/ skin stewed	1 (1.3 oz)	94	7	2
broiler/fryer neck w/o skin stewed	1 (.6 oz)	32	1	tr
broiler/fryer skin batter dipped & fried	from ½ chicken (6.7 oz)	748	55	14
broiler/fryer skin floured & fried	from ½ chicken (2 oz)	281	24	7
broiler/fryer skin roasted	from ½ chicken (2 oz)	254	23	6
broiler/fryer skin stewed	from ½ chicken (2.5 oz)	261	24	7
FRESH				
broiler/fryer thigh w/ skin batter dipped & fried	1 (3 oz)	238	14	4
broiler/fryer thigh w/ skin floured & fried	1 (2.2 oz)	162	9	3

FOOD	PORTION	CALS	FAT	SAT FAT
broiler/fryer thigh w/ skin roasted	1 (2.2 oz)	153	10	3
broiler/fryer thigh w/ skin stewed	1 (2.4 oz)	158	10	3
broiler/fryer thigh w/o skin fried	1 (1.8 oz)	113	5	1
broiler/fryer thigh w/o skin roasted	1 (1.8 oz)	109	6	2
broiler/fryer thigh w/o skin stewed	1 (1.9 oz)	107	5	1
broiler/fryer w/ skin floured & fried	½ chicken (11 oz)	844	47	13
broiler/fryer w/ skin fried	½ chicken (16.4 oz)	1347	81	22
broiler/fryer w/ skin roasted	½ chicken (10.5 oz)	715	41	11
broiler/fryer w/ skin stewed	½ chicken (11.7 oz)	730	42	12
broiler/fryer w/ skin neck & giblets batter dipped & fried	1 chicken (2.3 lbs)	2987	180	48
broiler/fryer w/ skin neck & giblets roasted	1 chicken (1.5 lbs)	1598	90	25
broiler/fryer w/ skin neck & giblets stewed	1 chicken (1.6 lbs)	1625	93	26
broiler/fryer w/o skin fried	1 cup	307	13	3
broiler/fryer w/o skin roasted	1 cup (5 oz)	266	10	3
broiler/fryer w/o skin stewed	1 cup (5 oz)	248	9	3
broiler/fryer w/o skin stewed	1 oz	54	3	1
broiler/fryer wing w/ skin batter dipped & fried	1 (1.7 oz)	159	11	3
broiler/fryer wing w/ skin floured & fried	1 (1.1 oz)	103	7	2
broiler/fryer wing w/ skin roasted	1 (1.2 oz)	99	7	2
broiler/fryer wing w/ skin stewed	1 (1.4 oz)	100	7	2
capon w/ skin neck & giblets roasted	1 chicken (3.1 lbs)	3211	165	46
cornish hen w/ skin roasted	1 hen (8 oz)	595	42	12
cornish hen w/o skin & bone roasted	½ hen (2 oz)	72	2	1
cornish hen w/o skin & bone roasted	1 hen (3.8 oz)	144	4	1
cornish hen w/skin roasted	½ hen (4 oz)	296	21	6
roaster dark meat w/o skin roasted	1 cup (5 oz)	250	12	3
roaster light meat w/o skin roasted	1 cup (5 oz)	214	6	2
roaster w/ skin neck & giblets roasted	1 chicken (2.4 lbs)	2363	140	39

FOOD	PORTION	CALS	FAT	SAT FAT
roaster w/ skin roasted	½ chicken (1.1 lbs)	1071	64	18
roaster w/o skin roasted	1 cup (5 oz)	469	28	3
stewing dark meat w/o skin stewed	1 cup (5 oz)	361	21	6
stewing w/ skin neck & giblets stewed	1 chicken (1.3 lbs)	1636	107	29
stewing w/ skin stewed	6.2 oz	507	34	9
stewing w/ skin stewed	½ chicken (9.2 oz)	744	49	13

Amish Select

Boneless Skinless Breast w/ Honey Dijon Mustard	1 serv (4 oz)	130	2	0

Perdue

Boneless Skinless Breasts Cooked	3 oz	110	2	tr
Boneless Breast Roasted Garlic Herb	1 piece (3 oz)	90	1	—
Breaded Breast Strips Barbecue	3 oz	120	1	—
Breaded Breast Strips Hot & Spicy	3 oz	110	1	—
Breaded Breast Strips Original	3 oz	120	1	—
Burger Cooked	1 (3 oz)	160	10	3
Chicken Breast Seasoned Italian Cooked	1 piece (3 oz)	90	1	tr
Chicken Breast Seasoned Teriyaki Cooked	1 piece (3 oz)	90	1	tr
Ground Cooked	3 oz	170	11	4
Ground Breast Cooked	3 oz	80	1	—
Honey Rotisserie Dark Meat	3 oz	200	16	5
Honey Rotisserie White Meat	3 oz	140	8	3
Oven Stuffer Dark Meat Roasted	3 oz	210	15	5
Oven Stuffer Drumstick Roasted	1 (3.6 oz)	190	11	4
Oven Stuffer White Meat Roasted	3 oz	170	9	3
Oven Stuffer Wingette Roasted	3 (3.4 oz)	220	15	5
Ovenables Breast Lemon Pepper Cooked	1 piece (3 oz)	90	1	—
Seasoned Roasting Chicken Toasted Garlic Dark Meat	3 oz	190	14	4
Seasoned Roasting Chicken Toasted Garlic White Meat	3 oz	160	9	3
Seasoned Strips Parmesan Garlic cooked	3 oz	100	2	1

FOOD	PORTION	CALS	FAT	SAT FAT
Seasoned Strips Savory Classic cooked	3 oz	90	1	tr
Seasoned Strips Spicy Fiesta cooked	3 oz	140	7	2
Split Breast Cooked	1 piece (6.8 oz)	370	20	6
Thin Sliced Breast Rosemary Garlic Thyme	1 piece (3 oz)	90	2	1
Thin Sliced Breast Tomato Herb	1 piece (3 oz)	90	2	—
Whole Dark Meat cooked	3 oz	150	16	5
Whole White Meat Cooked	3 oz	170	10	3
Wings Roasted	2 (3.2 oz)	210	15	5
Tyson				
Broth Marinated Breast Filet	1 (4.7 oz)	140	4	1
Broth Marinated Drums	2 (4 oz)	140	7	2
Broth Marinated Thighs	1 (4.9 oz)	380	34	10
Broth Marinated Wings	4 pieces (4.2 oz)	240	18	5
Chicken Broccoli & Cheese	1 piece (5.9 oz)	320	16	5
Chicken Stuffed w/ Wild Rice & Mushroom	1 piece (5.9 oz)	300	12	3
Cordon Bleu	1 piece (5.9 oz)	350	17	6
Cornish Hen	1 serv (4 oz)	180	12	4
Kiev	1 piece (5.9 oz)	460	32	16
Wampler				
Breast Tenders	4 oz	130	2	1
FROZEN				
Banquet				
Breast Nuggets	7	280	20	5
Breast Patties Grilled Honey BBQ	1	110	5	2
Breast Patties Grilled Honey Mustard	1	120	5	2
Breast Tenders Our Original	3	250	15	4
Breast Tenders Southern	3 pieces	260	16	4
Country Fried	1 serv (3 oz)	270	18	5
Fat Free Baked Breast Patties	1	100	0	0
Fried Our Original	1 serv (3 oz)	280	18	5
Honey BBQ Skinless Fried	1 serv (3 oz)	230	13	3
Hot 'n Spicy Fried	1 serv (3 oz)	260	18	5
Nuggets Our Original	6	270	19	4
Nuggets Southern Fried	5	270	18	4
Patties Our Original	1	190	14	3
Patties Southern Fried	1	190	12	3
Skinless Fried	1 serv (3 oz)	220	13	3

FOOD	PORTION	CALS	FAT	SAT FAT
Smokehouse Big Wings	2	200	17	4
Southern Fried	1 serv (3 oz)	280	18	5
Wings Firehouse Big	2	190	14	4
Wings Honey BBQ	4	380	24	10
Wings Hot & Spicy	4 pieces	280	20	5
Bell & Evans				
Breaded Breast Nuggets	1 serv (4 oz)	190	6	1
Breaded Whole Breast Tenders	1 (4 oz)	190	6	1
Burgers	1 (3 oz)	120	6	2
Chicken Sandwich Steaks	1 serv (2 oz)	60	1	tr
Country Skillet				
Bites	5	270	16	3
Breast Tenders	3	240	14	4
Chunks	5	270	18	3
Fried	3 oz	270	18	5
Nuggets	10	280	17	4
Patties	1	190	12	3
Southern Fried Chunks	5	270	18	4
Southern Fried Patties	1	190	12	3
Health Is Wealth				
Nuggets	4 (3 oz)	150	6	2
Patties	1 (3 oz)	150	6	2
Tenders	3 (3 oz)	130	3	1
Kid Cuisine				
Dino Mite Nuggets	4 pieces	300	23	6
Radical Racin' Nuggets w/ Cheese	4 pieces	300	23	7
Sensible Chef				
Fried Breast	1 (3 oz)	200	10	3
Weaver				
Breast Strips	3 pieces (3.3 oz)	210	11	2
Breast Tenders	5 pieces (3 oz)	220	15	3
Croquettes	1 serv (3.5 oz)	290	18	5
Dutch Frye Nuggets	5 pieces (3.3 oz)	280	20	5
Honey Battered Tenders	5 pieces (2.9 oz)	230	15	3
Hot Wings Buffalo Style	3 pieces (2.7 oz)	190	13	4
Mini Drums Crispy	5 pieces (3.3 oz)	250	16	3
Nuggets	4 pieces (2.7 oz)	210	15	4
Patties	1 (2.6 oz)	180	11	3
Rondelet	1 (2.6 oz)	170	10	3
Rondelet Dutch Frye	1 (2.6 oz)	230	16	4

FOOD	PORTION	CALS	FAT	SAT FAT
Rondelet Italian	1 (2.6 oz)	210	14	3
READY-TO-EAT				
chicken roll light meat	2 oz	90	4	1
chicken roll light meat	1 pkg (6 oz)	271	13	3
poultry salad sandwich spread	1 tbsp (13 g)	109	2	tr
poultry salad sandwich spread	1 oz	238	4	1
Banquet				
Fat Free Baked Breast Tenders	3	120	0	0
Boar's Head				
Breast Hickory Smoked	2 oz	60	1	0
Breast Oven Roasted	2 oz	50	1	0
Breast Bar B Q Sauce Basted	2 oz	60	1	0
Butterball				
Crispy Baked Breasts Italian Style Herb	1 piece (0.5 oz)	190	6	2
Crispy Baked Breasts Lemon Pepper	1 piece (0.5 oz)	200	7	3
Crispy Baked Breasts Original	1 piece (0.5 oz)	180	6	2
Crispy Baked Breasts Parmesan	1 piece (0.5 oz)	200	7	3
Crispy Baked Breasts Southwestern	1 piece (0.5 oz)	170	6	2
Tenders Baked Breast	3 pieces	170	6	2
Tenders Hickory Smoked Grilled	4 pieces + sauce	160	5	2
Tenders Oriental Grilled	4 pieces + sauce	160	5	2
Carl Buddig				
Chicken Sliced	1 pkg (2.5 oz)	110	7	2
Lean Slices Honey Smoked Breast	1 pkg (2.5 oz)	70	1	1
Lean Slices Roasted Breast	1 pkg (2.5 oz)	60	1	1
Chicken By George				
Cajun	1 breast (4 oz)	130	4	1
Caribbean Grill	1 breast (4 oz)	150	4	1
Garlic & Herb	1 breast (4 oz)	120	3	1
Italian Bleu Cheese	1 breast (4 oz)	130	5	1
Lemon Herb	1 breast (4 oz)	120	3	1
Lemon Oregano	1 breast (4 oz)	130	4	1
Mesquite Barbecue	1 breast (4 oz)	130	3	1
Mustard Dill	1 breast (4 oz)	140	5	1
Roasted	1 breast (4 oz)	110	3	1
Teriyaki	1 breast (4 oz)	130	3	1
Tomato Herb With Basil	1 breast (4 oz)	140	5	1
Healthy Choice				
Deli-Thin Oven Roasted Breast	6 slices (2 oz)	45	0	0
Deli-Thin Smoked Breast	6 slices (2 oz)	60	2	1

FOOD	PORTION	CALS	FAT	SAT FAT
Fresh-Trak Oven Roasted Breast	1 slice (1 oz)	30	1	0
Oven Roasted Breast	1 slice (1 oz)	25	0	0
Smoked Breast	1 slice (1 oz)	35	1	0
Louis Rich				
Carving Board Classic Baked	2 slices (1.6 oz)	45	1	0
Carving Board Grilled	2 slices (1.6 oz)	45	1	0
Deli-Thin Oven Roasted Breast	4 slices (1.8 oz)	50	1	1
Oven Roasted Deluxe Breast	1 slice (1 oz)	30	1	0
Oscar Mayer				
Free Oven Roasted Breast	4 slices (1.8 oz)	45	0	0
Perdue				
Breast Cutlets Homestyle	1 (2.9 oz)	110	1	–
Breast Cutlets Italian Style	1 (2.9 oz)	120	2	1
Breast Fillets In Barbecue Sauce	1 piece + 3 tbsp sauce (5.9 oz)	200	1	–
Breast Strips In Garlic & Herb Sauce	1 serv (5 oz)	100	1	–
Breast Strips In Marinara Sauce	1 serv (5 oz)	120	3	1
Breast Strips In Teriyaki Sauce	1 serv (5 oz)	190	1	–
Carved Breast Honey Roasted	½ cup (2.5 oz)	100	2	1
Carved Breast Original Roasted	½ cup (2.5 oz)	90	2	1
Cutlets Cooked	1 (3.5 oz)	220	11	3
Nuggets	5 (3.4 oz)	210	11	3
Nuggets Chicken & Cheese	5 (3.4 oz)	230	13	5
Short Cuts Entrees In Teriyaki Sauce	5 oz	190	1	–
Short Cuts Italian	½ cup (2.5 oz)	100	3	1
Short Cuts Lemon Pepper	½ cup (2.5 oz)	100	3	1
Short Cuts Southwestern	½ cup (2.5 oz)	100	3	1
Shady Brook				
Slow Roasted Breast	2 oz	60	1	0
Tyson				
Breaded Breast Chunks	6 pieces (2.9 oz)	230	16	5
Breaded Breast Fillet	2 pieces (2.8 oz)	180	8	2
Breaded Breast Pattie	1 (2.6 oz)	190	12	3
Breaded Breast Tenders	5 pieces (3 oz)	220	15	3
Breaded Chicken Chunks	6 pieces (3 oz)	220	14	3
Chick'n Quick Chick'n Cheddar	1 patty (2.6 oz)	220	14	4
Chicken Bits Southern Fried	6 pieces (2.9 oz)	260	19	5
Chicken Strips Southwestern	1 serv (3 oz)	110	3	1
Country Fried Chicken Fritter	5 pieces (2.9 oz)	260	18	4
Drumsticks Hot BBQ Style	2 (3.5 oz)	160	7	2

FOOD	PORTION	CALS	FAT	SAT FAT
Glazed Grilled Breast Pattie	1 (2.7 oz)	120	7	2
Grilled Breast Strips	1 serv (3 oz)	110	3	1
Grilled Chicken Pattie	1 (2.9 oz)	170	12	4
Nuggets Breaded White Meat	6 pieces (2.9 oz)	250	18	5
Patties Southern Fried	1 (2.9 oz)	260	19	5
Roasted Drumsticks	3 (5.6 oz)	320	15	5
Roasted Drumsticks w/o Skin	2 (3.3 oz)	140	5	2
Roasted Half Chicken	1 serv (3 oz)	160	11	4
Roasted Whole Chicken	1 serv (3 oz)	160	11	4
Roasted Breast Boneless w/o Skin	1 (3.7 oz)	130	3	1
Roasted Breast Half w/o Skin	1 (4.3 oz)	150	3	1
Roasted Half Breast w/ Skin	1 (5.1 oz)	260	13	4
Roasted Half Chicken w/o Skin	1 serv (3 oz)	120	6	2
Roasted Tabasco Wings	3 (3 oz)	190	13	4
Roasted Thigh w/ Skin	1 (3.6 oz)	270	21	7
Roasted Thigh w/o Skin	1 (2.9 oz)	150	8	3
Roll White Meat	2 oz	90	6	2
Southern Fried Breaded Breast Pattie	1 (2.6 oz)	180	12	3
Southern Fried Breast Fillets	2 pieces (3.4 oz)	210	11	2
Southern Fried Chunks	6 pieces (2.9 oz)	260	19	5
Tenders Breaded Honey Battered	5 pieces (2.9 oz)	230	15	3
Tenders Breaded Pattie	3 pieces (3.2 oz)	100	0	0
Thick'n Crispy Pattie	1 (2.6 oz)	200	14	3
Wings BBQ	3 pieces (3.2 oz)	200	13	4
Wings Hot N'Spicy	4 (3.2 oz)	210	14	4
Wings Teriyaki	4 pieces (3.4 oz)	190	12	3
Wings Of Fire	4 pieces (3.4 oz)	220	15	4
TAKE-OUT				
oven roasted breast of chicken	2 oz	60	1	0

CHICKEN DISHES
CANNED
Bumble Bee

Chicken Salad	1 pkg (3.5 oz)	230	10	2

Dinty Moore

Noodles & Chicken	1 can (7.5 oz)	180	8	2
Stew	1 cup (8.5 oz)	220	11	3

FROZEN
White Castle

Grilled Chicken Sandwich	2 (4 oz)	250	9	3

FOOD	PORTION	CALS	FAT	SAT FAT
Grilled Chicken Sandwich w/ Sauce	2 (4.8 oz)	290	9	3
MIX				
Chicken Skillet Helper				
Stir-Fried Chicken as prep	1 cup	270	9	2
Hamburger Helper				
Reduced Sodium Cheddar Spirals Chicken Recipe as prep	1 cup	240	6	2
Reduced Sodium Italian Herb Chicken Recipe as prep	1 cup	200	2	1
Reduced Sodium Southwestern Beef Chicken Recipe as prep	1 cup	220	3	1
Tyson				
Mandarin Wrap Kit	1½ wraps (14.6 oz)	630	15	4
REFRIGERATED				
salad low fat	⅓ cup	90	2	–
Lloyd's				
Barbecue Shredded Chicken	¼ cup (2 oz)	90	2	1
Oscar Mayer				
Lunchables Chicken Wraps	1 pkg	440	13	5
Shady Brook				
Chicken Breast w/ Rice Pilaf	1 serv (12 oz)	350	13	4
Teriyaki Breast	1 serv (12 oz)	490	3	1
Tyson				
Chicken Breast Medallions In Tomato & Herb Sauce	1 serv (5 oz)	120	4	1
Wampler				
Cacciatore	1 cup	260	9	–
Fajitas	1 cup	210	7	–
Salad	⅓ cup	200	14	–
Salad Lite	⅓ cup	130	7	–
Smokey Barbecue Chicken	1 cup	430	15	–
Sweet-n-Sour	1 cup	250	4	–
SHELF-STABLE				
Dinty Moore				
Microwave Cup Chicken & Dumpling	1 pkg (7.5 oz)	200	6	2
Microwave Cup Stew	1 pkg (7.5 oz)	180	8	2
Lunch Bucket				
Chicken Fiesta	1 pkg (7.5 oz)	160	2	1
Dumplings'n Chicken	1 pkg (7.5 oz)	140	5	2

FOOD	PORTION	CALS	FAT	SAT FAT
TastyBite				
Chicken Moglai	1 pkg (9.5 oz)	300	16	3
TAKE-OUT				
b'stilla chicken pie	1 serv	926	227	21
boneless breaded & fried w/ barbecue sauce	6 pieces (4.6 oz)	330	18	6
boneless breaded & fried w/ honey	6 pieces (4 oz)	339	18	5
boneless breaded & fried w/ mustard sauce	6 pieces (4.6 oz)	323	17	6
boneless breaded & fried w/ sweet & sour sauce	6 pieces (4.6 oz)	346	18	6
boneless breast w/ apple stuffing	1 serv (5 oz)	260	9	2
breast & wing breaded & fried	2 pieces (5.7 oz)	494	30	8
chicken & dumplings	¾ cup	256	12	4
chicken & noodles	1 cup	365	18	5
chicken a la king	1 cup	470	34	13
chicken cacciatore	¾ cup	394	24	6
chicken paprikash	1½ cups	296	10	—
chicken pie w/ top crust	1 slice (5.6 oz)	472	31	—
chicken cordon bleu	1 serv (5 oz)	280	13	4
drumstick breaded & fried	2 pieces (5.2 oz)	430	27	7
grilled breast strips	4 strips (3 oz)	100	2	1
groundnut stew hkatenkwan	1 serv (15.7 oz)	576	40	10
jamaican jerk wings	4 wings (9.9 oz)	709	51	14
kobete turkish chicken w/ pastry	1 serv	513	13	4
sancocho de pollo dominican chicken stew	1 serv	702	30	8
souvlaki	1 serv	392	54	3
thigh breaded & fried	2 pieces (5.2 oz)	430	27	7

CHICKEN SUBSTITUTES
Health Is Wealth

Buffalo Wings	3 pieces (2.2 oz)	100	2	0
Chicken-Free Nuggets	3 pieces (2.25 oz)	90	1	0
Chicken-Free Patties	1 (3 oz)	120	2	0
Loma Linda				
Chicken Supreme Mix not prep	⅓ cup (0.9 oz)	90	1	0
Chik Nuggets	5 pieces (3 oz)	240	16	3
Fried Chik'n w/ Gravy	2 pieces (2.8 oz)	160	10	2

FOOD	PORTION	CALS	FAT	SAT FAT
Morningstar Farms				
Chik Nuggets	4 pieces (3 oz)	160	4	1
Chik Patties	1 (2.5 oz)	150	6	1
Meatless Buffalo Wings	5 pieces (3 oz)	200	9	2
Quorn				
Cutlets	1 (3.5 oz)	200	8	1
Naked Cutlets	1 (2.4 oz)	80	3	1
Nuggets	3-4 pieces (3 oz)	180	8	1
Patties	1 patty (2.6 oz)	160	7	1
Tenders	1 cup (3 oz)	90	2	1
Soy Is Us				
Chicken Not!	½ cup (1.75 oz)	140	2	1
Worthington				
Chic-Ketts	2 slices (1.9 oz)	120	7	1
Chicken Sliced or Roll	2 slices (2 oz)	80	5	1
Chicken Sliced	2 slices (2 oz)	80	5	1
ChikStiks	1 (1.6 oz)	110	7	1
CrispyChik Patties	1 (2.5 oz)	150	6	1
Cutlets	1 slice (2.1 oz)	70	1	0
Diced Chik	¼ cup (1.9 oz)	40	0	0
FriChik	2 pieces (3.2 oz)	120	8	1
FriChik Low Fat	2 pieces (3 oz)	80	3	0
Golden Croquettes	4 pieces (3 oz)	210	10	2
Yves				
Veggie Chicken Burgers	1 (3 oz)	120	3	0

CHICKPEAS
CANNED
chickpeas	1 cup	285	3	tr
Green Giant				
Garbanzo	½ cup (4.4 oz)	110	2	0
Old El Paso				
Garbanzo	½ cup (4.6 oz)	120	3	0
Progresso				
Chick Peas	½ cup (4.6 oz)	120	3	0
Garbanzo	½ cup (4.4 oz)	110	2	0

DRIED
cooked	1 cup	269	4	tr

CHICORY
greens raw chopped	½ cup	21	tr	tr

FOOD	PORTION	CALS	FAT	SAT FAT
root raw	1 (2.1 oz)	44	tr	tr
roots raw cut up	½ cup (1.6 oz)	33	tr	tr
witloof head raw	1 (1.9 oz)	9	tr	tr
witloof raw	½ cup (1.6 oz)	8	tr	tr
CHILI				
chile pepper paste	1 tbsp	6	1	–
chili w/ beans	1 cup	286	14	6
dried ancho	1 tsp	3	tr	–
dried casabel	1 tsp	3	tr	–
dried guajillo	1 tsp	3	tr	–
dried mulato	1 tsp	3	tr	–
dried pasilla	1 tsp	3	tr	–
dried smoked chipotle	1 tsp	3	tr	–
powder	1 tsp	8	tr	–
Amy's				
Chili & Cornbread	1 pkg (10.5 oz)	320	6	2
Organic Black Bean	1 cup	200	2	0
Organic Medium	1 cup	190	6	1
Organic Medium w/ Vegetables	1 cup	190	6	1
Armour				
Chili No Beans	1 cup (8.7 oz)	390	29	13
Chili W/ Beans Western Style	1 cup (8.8 oz)	370	22	10
Chili w/ Beans	1 cup (8.9 oz)	370	21	9
Chili w/ Beans Hot	1 cup (8.9 oz)	370	21	9
Vienna Sausage & Chili	1 cup (8.7 oz)	410	27	11
Carroll Shelby's				
Original Texas Chili Kit	2 tbsp	60	1	0
Chef Boyardee				
Chili Mac	½ can (7 oz)	260	11	–
Chili Man				
Seasoning Mix	1 tbsp (7 g)	25	1	–
Del Monte				
Sauce	1 tbsp (0.6 oz)	20	0	0
Dennison's				
Chili Beans In Chili Gravy	7.5 oz	180	1	–
Chili Con Carne w/ Beans	7.5 oz	300	19	–
Chili Con Carne w/ Beans	7.5 oz	310	15	–
Chunky Chili w/ Beans	7.5 oz	310	14	–
Cook-off Chili w/ Beans	7.5 oz	340	19	–

FOOD	PORTION	CALS	FAT	SAT FAT
Hot Chili Con Carne w/ Beans	7.5 oz	310	16	—
Gebhardt				
Chili Powder	¼ tsp (0.3 g)	1	tr	0
Chili Quik Seasoning	1 tbsp (0.3 oz)	43	1	0
Plain	1 cup (9.4 oz)	232	19	7
With Beans	1 cup (9.4 oz)	322	15	6
Gringo Billy's				
Chili Mix	1 tbsp	24	1	0
Health Valley				
Burrito	1 cup	160	1	—
Enchilada	1 cup	160	1	—
Fajita	1 cup	80	0	0
In A Cup Black Bean Mild	¾ cup	120	1	—
In A Cup Texas Style Spicy	¾ cup	120	1	—
Vegetarian Lentil Mild	1 cup	160	1	—
Vegetarian Lentil No Salt	1 cup	80	0	—
Vegetarian Mild	1 cup	160	1	—
Vegetarian Mild No Salt	1 cup	160	1	—
Vegetarian Spicy	1 cup	160	1	—
Vegetarian Spicy No Salt	1 cup	160	1	—
Vegetarian w/ 3 Beans Mild	1 cup	160	1	—
Vegetarian w/ Black Beans Mild	1 cup	160	1	—
Vegetarian w/ Black Beans Spicy	1 cup	160	1	—
Healthy Choice				
Bowls Chili & Cornbread	1 meal (9.5 oz)	350	8	3
Hormel				
Chunky w/ Beans	1 cup (8.7 oz)	270	7	3
Hot No Beans	1 cup (8.3 oz)	210	9	3
Hot With Beans	1 cup (8.7 oz)	270	7	3
Microcup Meals Chili Mac	1 cup (7.5 oz)	200	9	4
Microcup Meals Hot With Beans	1 cup (7.3 oz)	220	6	3
Microcup Meals No Beans	1 cup (7.3 oz)	190	8	3
Microcup Meals With Beans	1 cup (7.3 oz)	220	6	3
No Beans	1 cup (8.3 oz)	210	9	3
Turkey No Beans	1 cup (8.3 oz)	190	3	1
Turkey w/ Beans	1 cup (8.7 oz)	210	3	1
Vegetarian	1 cup (8.7 oz)	200	1	0
With Beans	1 cup (8.7 oz)	270	7	3

FOOD	PORTION	CALS	FAT	SAT FAT
Hunt's				
Chili Beans	½ cup (4.5 oz)	87	1	0
Chili Sauce	2 tbsp (1.2 oz)	35	tr	0
Hurst				
HamBeens Chili Beans	1 serv	130	1	0
Instant India				
Chili Ginger Paste	2 tbsp (1 oz)	90	7	1
Just Rite				
With Beans	1 cup (9 oz)	379	27	13
Lean Cuisine				
Everyday Favorites Three Bean Chili w/ Rice	1 pkg (10 oz)	250	6	2
Lunch Bucket				
Chili With Beans	1 pkg (7.5 oz)	260	12	5
Manwich				
Homestyle Fixins	½ cup (4.6 oz)	84	1	tr
Marie Callender's				
Chili & Cornbread	1 meal (16 oz)	560	21	9
McCormick				
Mexican Style Chili Powder	¼ tsp	0	0	0
Original Chili Seasoning	1⅓ tbsp (9 g)	30	1	–
Natural Choice				
Organic Vegan Three Bean	½ cup (4.6 oz)	140	1	0
Natural Touch				
Vegetarian	1 cup (8.1 oz)	170	1	0
Nature's Entree				
Texas Chili	1 pkg (12 oz)	320	7	2
Old El Paso				
Chili Seasoning Mix	1 tbsp (0.3 oz)	25	1	–
Chili With Beans	1 cup (8 oz)	200	7	2
Open Range				
Plain	1 cup (8.8 oz)	353	26	12
With Beans	1 cup (9 oz)	281	16	7
Soy7				
Chili Mix as prep	1 cup	150	2	0
Stouffer's				
With Beans	1 pkg (8.75 oz)	270	10	4
Ultimate				
No Beans Hot	1 cup (8.7 oz)	420	30	13
Turkey w/ Beans	1 cup (8.7 oz)	260	9	3

FOOD	PORTION	CALS	FAT	SAT FAT
W/ Beans	1 cup (8.7 oz)	320	16	7
W/ Beans Hot	1 cup (8.7 oz)	320	16	7
Van Camp				
Beanee Weenee Chilee	1 cup (7.7 oz)	240	12	3
Chili With Beans	1 cup (8.9 oz)	350	21	8
Mexican Style Chili Beans	½ cup (4.6 oz)	110	2	1
Wampler				
Turkey	1 cup	250	7	–
Wick Fowler's				
2 Alarm Chili Kit	3 tbsp	60	2	0
False Alarm Chili Kit	2 tbsp	50	2	0
Worthington				
Chili	1 cup (8.1 oz)	290	15	3
Low Fat	1 cup (8.1 oz)	170	1	0
Yves				
Veggie Chili	1 pkg (10.5 oz)	230	1	0
TAKE-OUT				
con carne w/ beans	8.9 oz	254	8	3

CHILI PEPPER (see PEPPERS)

CHINESE FOOD (see ASIAN FOOD)

CHINESE PRESERVING MELON

cooked	½ cup	11	tr	tr

CHIPS

barbecue	1 bag (7 oz)	971	64	16
barbecue	1 oz	139	9	2
corn	1 bag (7 oz)	1067	66	9
corn	1 oz	153	10	1
corn barbecue	1 bag (7 oz)	1036	65	9
corn barbecue	1 oz	148	9	1
corn cones	1 oz	145	8	6
corn cones nacho	1 oz	152	9	8
corn onion	1 oz	142	6	1
potato	1 oz	152	10	3
potato	1 bag (8 oz)	1217	79	25
potato cheese	1 oz	140	8	2
potato cheese	1 bag (6 oz)	842	46	15
potato light	1 bag (6 oz)	801	35	7
potato light	1 oz	134	6	1

FOOD	PORTION	CALS	FAT	SAT FAT
potato sour cream & onion	1 bag (7 oz)	1051	67	18
potato sour cream & onion	1 oz	150	10	3
potato sticks	½ cup (0.6 oz)	94	6	2
potato sticks	1 oz	148	10	3
potato sticks	1 pkg (1 oz)	148	10	3
taco	1 oz	136	7	1
taco	1 bag (8 oz)	1089	55	11
taro	10 (0.8 oz)	115	6	1
taro	1 oz	141	7	2
tortilla	1 bag (7.5 oz)	1067	56	11
tortilla	1 oz	142	7	1
tortilla nacho	1 bag (8 oz)	1131	58	11
tortilla nacho	1 oz	141	7	1
tortilla nacho light	1 oz	126	4	1
tortilla nacho light	1 bag (6 oz)	757	26	5
tortilla ranch	1 oz	139	7	1
tortilla ranch	1 bag (7 oz)	969	47	9
Atkins				
Cruncher Barbeque	1 pkg (1 oz)	100	3	0
Crunchers Nacho Cheese	1 pkg (1 oz)	100	3	0
Crunchers Original	1 pkg (1 oz)	90	3	0
Crunchers Sour Cream & Onion	1 pkg (1 oz)	100	4	1
Barbara's Bakery				
Potato	1¼ cups (1 oz)	150	10	1
Potato No Salt Added	1¼ cups (1 oz)	150	10	1
Potato Ripple	1¼ cups (1 oz)	150	10	1
Potato Yogurt & Green Onion	1¼ cups (1 oz)	150	9	1
Tortilla Blue Corn	15 chips (1 oz)	140	7	tr
Tortilla Blue Corn No Salt	15 chips (1 oz)	140	7	tr
Tortilla Pinta Salsa	15 chips (1 oz)	130	6	1
Bruno & Luigi's				
Pasta Chips Garlic & Herb	1 oz	117	1	0
Cape Cod				
Potato Golden Russet	1 pkg (0.5 oz)	70	4	1
Chester's				
Flamin'Hot	1 oz	140	8	2
Salsa	1 oz	140	7	2
Deliciously Slim				
Tortilla Black Bean & Sour Cream	1 oz	140	9	2
Tortilla Lightly Salted	1 oz	140	8	2

FOOD	PORTION	CALS	FAT	SAT FAT
Tortilla Ranch	1 oz	140	9	2
Doritos				
3D's Cooler Ranch	27 (1 oz)	140	6	2
3D's Nacho Cheesier	27 (1 oz)	140	7	2
Cooler Ranch	12 (1 oz)	140	7	2
Flamin' Hot	11 (1 oz)	140	7	2
Nacho Cheesier	11 (1 oz)	140	7	1
Salsa Verde	12 (1 oz)	150	7	2
Smokey Red	12 (1 oz)	150	7	2
Spicy Nacho	12 (1 oz)	140	6	2
Toasted Corn	13 (1 oz)	140	7	2
Wow Nacho Cheesier	1 pkg (0.75 oz)	70	1	0
Durangos				
Tortilla	15 (1 oz)	150	7	1
Eden				
Brown Rice Chips	1 oz	150	7	2
Sea Vegetable Chips	1 oz	140	5	2
Fritos				
Chili Cheese	31 (1 oz)	160	10	2
Corn Chips BBQ	29 (1 oz)	150	9	1
Corn Chips King Size	12 (1 oz)	150	10	2
Corn Chips Sabrositas Flamin' Hot	30 (1 oz)	150	9	2
Corn Chips Sabrositas Lime'N Chile	28 (1 oz)	150	9	2
Corn Chips Wild N'Mild Ranch	28 (1 oz)	160	10	2
Original	32 (1 oz)	160	10	2
Scoops	11 (1 oz)	160	10	1
Texas Grill Honey BBQ	15 (1 oz)	150	9	2
GeniSoy				
Soy Crisps	1 oz	110	2	0
Soy Crisps Apple Cinnamon Crunch	1 oz	120	2	0
Soy Crisps Creamy Ranch	1 oz	110	2	0
Soy Crisps Deep Sea Salt	1 oz	110	2	0
Soy Crisps Rich Cheddar Cheese	1 oz	110	2	0
Soy Crisps Roasted Garlic & Onion	1 oz	100	2	0
Soy Crisps Zesty Barbeque	1 oz	110	2	0
Guiltless Gourmet				
Tortilla Baked Chili Lime	18 (1 oz)	110	2	0
Tortilla Baked Mucho Nacho	18 (1 oz)	110	2	0
Tortilla Baked Organic Blue Corn	18 (1 oz)	110	2	0
Tortilla Baked Picante Ranch	18 (1 oz)	110	2	0

FOOD	PORTION	CALS	FAT	SAT FAT
Tortilla Baked Red Corn	18 (1 oz)	110	2	0
Tortilla Baked Spicy Black Bean	18 (1 oz)	110	2	0
Tortilla Baked Sweet White Corn	18 (1 oz)	110	2	0
Tortilla Baked Yellow Corn	18 (1 oz)	110	2	0
Tortilla Baked Yellow Corn Unsalted	18 (1 oz)	110	1	0
Herr's				
Potato	1 oz	140	8	3
Tortilla Restaurant Style White Corn	10 chips (1 oz)	140	6	1
Husman's				
Deli Style Tortilla	11 chips	150	7	1
Potato	18 (1 oz)	160	11	3
Potato Sour Cream & Onion	18 (1 oz)	150	9	3
Potato Sweet N'Sassy	18 (1 oz)	155	10	3
Keto				
Low Carb Tortilla All Flavors	1 oz	150	8	1
Lance				
BBQ	22 (1 oz)	160	10	3
Cajun	15 (1 oz)	150	10	3
Corn Chips	39 (1.25 oz)	200	11	3
Corn Chips Hot BBQ	35 (1.25 oz)	210	13	4
Hot Fries	1 pkg (0.9 oz)	140	10	3
Mesquite BBQ	22 (1 oz)	150	10	3
Potato	23 (1 oz)	160	10	3
Ripple	15 (1 oz)	160	11	3
Salt & Vinegar	22 (1 oz)	160	10	3
Sour Cream & Onion	22 (1 oz)	160	10	3
Tortilla Fiesta Salsa Triangles	16 (1 oz)	140	7	2
Tortilla Nacho Mini Round	46 (1.5 oz)	180	9	3
Tortilla Nacho Triangles	15 (1 oz)	140	14	4
Lay's				
Adobadas	16 (1 oz)	170	10	3
Baked KC Masterpiece BBQ	11 (1 oz)	120	3	0
Baked Original	11 (1 oz)	110	2	0
Baked Roasted Herb	12 (1 oz)	130	3	1
Baked Sour Cream & Onion	12 (1 oz)	120	2	0
Classic	20 (1 oz)	150	10	3
Deli Style Hot N'Tangy BBQ	18 (1 oz)	150	10	3
Deli Style Jalapeno	17 (1 oz)	150	10	3
Deli Style Original	17 (1 oz)	140	10	3
Deli Style Salt & Vinegar	16 (1 oz)	90	10	3

FOOD	PORTION	CALS	FAT	SAT FAT
Flamin' Hot	17 pieces (1 oz)	150	10	3
KC Masterpiece BBQ	15 (1 oz)	150	10	3
Onion & Garlic	19 (1 oz)	150	9	3
Original Baked	1 pkg 1⅛ oz	130	2	0
Salt & Vinegar	17 pieces (1 oz)	150	10	3
Sour Cream & Onion	17 pieces (1 oz)	160	11	3
Toasted Onion & Cheese	17 pieces (1 oz)	160	10	3
Wavy Au Gratin	13 (1 oz)	150	10	3
Wavy Original	11 pieces (1 oz)	160	10	3
Wavy Ranch	11 (1 oz)	160	11	3
Wow Mesquite BBQ	20 (1 oz)	75	0	0
Wow Original	20 (1 oz)	75	0	0
Wow Original	1 pkg (0.75 oz)	55	0	0
Wow Sour Cream & Chive	19 (1 oz)	80	0	0
Met-Rx				
Pro Chips Bar-B-Que	1 pkg (2 oz)	260	9	1
Pro Chips Nacho	1 pkg (2 oz)	260	10	2
Old Dutch Foods				
Potato	12-15 chips (1 oz)	150	8	1
Potato BBQ	12-15 chips (1 oz)	150	9	1
Potato BBQ Ripples	12-15 chips (1 oz)	150	9	1
Potato Cajun Ripples	12-15 chips (1 oz)	150	10	1
Potato Cheddar & Sour Cream Ripples	12-15 chips (1 oz)	160	9	2
Potato Cheddar & Sour Cream Ripples	12-15 chips (1 oz)	150	9	2
Potato Dill	12-15 chips (1 oz)	140	8	1
Potato Dutch Crunch	15-20 chips (1 oz)	130	6	1
Potato French Onion Ripples	12-15 chips (1 oz)	150	10	1
Potato Jalapeno & Cheddar Dutch Crunch	15-20 chips (1 oz)	130	6	2
Potato Jalapeno Cheese	12-15 chips (1 oz)	150	9	1
Potato Mesquite BBQ Dutch Crunch	15-20 chips (1 oz)	130	6	1
Potato Onion & Garlic	12-15 chips (1 oz)	140	8	1
Potato Outback Spicy BBQ	12-15 chips (1 oz)	150	10	1
Potato Ripples	12-15 chips (1 oz)	150	9	1
Potato Salt & Vinegar Dutch Crunch	15-20 chips (1 oz)	130	6	1
Potato Sour Cream & Onion	12-15 chips (1 oz)	150	9	1
Tortilla Bite Size White Corn	20 chips (1 oz)	150	8	1
Tortilla Nacho Cheese	15 chips (1 oz)	150	7	1

FOOD	PORTION	CALS	FAT	SAT FAT
Tortilla Restaurant Style White	9 chips (1 oz)	140	7	1
Tostados White Corn	11 chips (1 oz)	140	7	1
Tostados Yellow	11 chips (1 oz)	140	6	1
Old El Paso				
Tortilla NACHIPS	9 chips (1 oz)	150	8	2
Tortilla White Corn	11 chips (1 oz)	140	8	1
Pita-Snax				
Cheddar Cheese	34 (1 oz)	110	2	0
Chili & Lime	34 (1 oz)	120	2	0
Cinnamon	34 (1 oz)	120	2	0
Dill Ranch	34 (1 oz)	120	2	0
Garlic	34 (1 oz)	120	2	0
Lightly Salted	34 (1 oz)	110	1	0
Planters				
Corn Chips	34 chips (1 oz)	170	10	2
Corn Chips King Size	17 chips (1 oz)	160	10	2
Corn Chips Snacks To Go	1 pkg (1.5 oz)	240	15	2
Pringles				
BBQ	14 chips (1 oz)	150	10	3
Cheese & Onion	14 chips (1 oz)	160	11	2
Cheez-ums	14 chips (1 oz)	150	10	3
Original	14 chips (1 oz)	160	11	3
Pizzalicious	14 chips (1 oz)	160	11	3
Ranch	14 chips (1 oz)	150	10	3
Salt & Vinegar	14 chips (1 oz)	160	11	3
Sour Cream & Onion	14 chips (1 oz)	160	10	3
Racquet				
Wheat Chips All Flavors	6 chips	30	1	0
Revival				
Baked Soy Pasta Chips Lightly Salted Sunshine	1 bag (0.9 oz)	100	2	0
Baked Soy Pasta Chips Naturally Nice	1 bag (0.9 oz)	80	1	0
Baked Soy Pasta Chips Rev It Up Ranch	1 bag (0.9 oz)	105	3	0
Robert's American Gourmet				
Spirulina Spirals	1 oz	120	2	0
Ruffles				
Baked	10 (1 oz)	110	2	0
Baked Cheddar & Sour Cream	9 (1 oz)	120	3	0
Buffalo Style	11 chips (1 oz)	160	10	3
Cheddar & Sour Cream	11 chips (1 oz)	160	10	3

FOOD	PORTION	CALS	FAT	SAT FAT
French Onion	11 (1 oz)	150	10	3
MC Masterpiece Mesquite BBQ	11 (1 oz)	150	10	3
Original	12 chips (1 oz)	150	10	3
Original	1 pkg (1.5 oz)	240	16	4
Ranch	13 (1 oz)	150	9	3
Reduced Fat	16 (1 oz)	130	7	1
The Works	12 (1 oz)	160	11	3
Wow Cheddar & Sour Cream	15 (1 oz)	75	0	0
Wow Cheddar & Sour Cream	15 (1 oz)	75	0	0
Wow Original	17 (1 oz)	75	0	0
Santitas				
100% White Corn	6 (1 oz)	130	6	1
Restaurant Style Chips	7 (1 oz)	130	6	1
Restaurant Style Strips	10 (1 oz)	130	6	1
Skinny				
BBQ	1½ cups	90	2	1
Corn	1½ cups	90	2	1
Nacho Cheese	1½ cups	90	3	1
Sour Cream & Onion	1½ cups	90	2	1
Sticks Garden Veggie	1 oz	140	6	1
Sticks Island Lime Chili	1 oz	140	6	1
Sticks Maui Wowie	1 oz	140	6	1
Sticks Original Spud	1 oz	140	6	1
Snyder's Of Hanover				
BBQ Rib	1 oz	140	7	2
Barbeque Corn	1.5 oz	230	14	2
Cheddar Bacon	1 oz	150	6	2
Corn Chips	1.5 oz	230	15	2
Grilled Steak & Onion	1 oz	140	6	2
Hot Buffalo	1 oz	150	7	2
Kosher Dill	1 oz	140	6	2
No Salt	1 oz	140	6	2
Potato	1 oz	140	6	2
Ripple	1 oz	140	6	2
Salt & Vinegar	1 oz	140	6	2
Sausage Pizza	1 oz	150	6	2
Sour Cream & Onion	1 oz	150	7	2
Tasty Veggie Potato Chips	1 oz	150	6	2
Tortilla Nacho	1 oz	140	7	1
Tortilla No Salt Yellow Corn	1 oz	140	6	1

FOOD	PORTION	CALS	FAT	SAT FAT
Tortilla White Corn	1 oz	140	6	1
Tortilla Yellow Corn	1 oz	140	6	1
Tortilla Yellow Corn Mini	1 oz	160	8	1
Veggie Crisps	1 pkg (1.5 oz)	190	9	1
Soya King				
Soy Mongolian BBQ	23 chips (1 oz)	140	7	1
Soy Original	23 chips (1 oz)	140	7	1
Soy Sour Cream & Onion	23 chips (1 oz)	140	7	1
Soy Taco	23 chips (1 oz)	140	7	1
Stacy's				
Pita Chips Cinnamon Sugar	1 oz	130	4	0
Pita Chips Parmesan Garlic & Herb	1 oz	130	4	0
Pita Chips Simply Naked	1 oz	130	4	0
Twisted Pasta Low Fat	1 oz	110	2	0
State Line				
Chips	1 pkg (0.5 oz)	80	5	1
Sunchips				
French Onion	13 (1 oz)	140	7	1
Harvest Cheddar	13 (1 oz)	140	6	1
Original	14 (1 oz)	140	6	1
Terra Chips				
Sweet Potato	1 oz	140	7	1
Sweet Potato Spiced	1 oz	140	7	1
Taro Spiced	1 oz	130	5	1
Vegetable	1 oz	140	7	1
Torengos				
Chips	13 chips (1 oz)	140	9	1
Tostitos				
Baked Bite Size	20 (1 oz)	110	1	0
Baked Bite Size Salsa & Cream Cheese	16 (1 oz)	120	3	1
Baked Original	13 (1 oz)	110	1	0
Bite Size	15 (1 oz)	140	8	1
Crispy Rounds	13 (1 oz)	150	8	1
Nacho Style	6 (1 oz)	140	6	1
Restaurant Style	7 (1 oz)	140	6	1
Restaurant Style Hint Of Lime	6 (1 oz)	140	6	1
Santa Fe Gold	7 (1 oz)	140	6	1
Wow Original	6 (1 oz)	90	1	0
Tyson				
Tortilla Salted	13 (1 oz)	150	7	1

FOOD	PORTION	CALS	FAT	SAT FAT
Tortilla Yellow Corn Salted	13 (1 oz)	150	7	1
Utz				
Baked Crisps	12 (1 oz)	110	2	0
Carolina Barbeque	20 (1 oz)	150	9	2
Cheddar & Sour Cream	20 (1 oz)	160	10	3
Corn Chips	24 (1 oz)	160	10	2
Corn Chips Barbecue	24 (1 oz)	160	10	2
Grandma	20 (1 oz)	140	8	3
Grandma BBQ	20 (1 oz)	140	8	3
Home Style Kettle	20 (1 oz)	140	8	2
Home Style Kettle BBQ	20 (1 oz)	140	8	2
Kettle Classics Crunchy	20 (1 oz)	150	9	2
Kettle Classics Crunchy Mesquite BBQ	20 (1 oz)	150	9	2
No Salt Added	20 (1 oz)	150	9	2
Onion & Garlic	20 (1 oz)	150	9	2
Potato	20 (1 oz)	150	9	2
Reduced Fat BBQ	22 (1 oz)	140	6	2
Reducted Fat Ripple	24 (1 oz)	140	7	2
Ripple	20 (1 oz)	150	10	3
Ripple Sour Cream & Onion	20 (1 oz)	160	10	3
Ripple Barbeque	20 (1 oz)	150	10	3
Salt'N Vinegar	20 (1 oz)	150	9	2
The Crab Chip	20 (1 oz)	150	9	2
Tortilla Black Bean & Salsa	13 (1 oz)	150	7	1
Tortilla Low Fat Baked	10 (1 oz)	120	2	0
Tortilla Nacho	13 (1 oz)	150	8	1
Tortilla Restaurant Style	6 (1 oz)	140	7	1
Tortilla Spicy Nacho	13 (1 oz)	150	8	1
Tortilla White Corn	12 (1 oz)	140	7	1
Wavy	20 chips (1 oz)	150	9	2
Yes! Fat Free	20 (1 oz)	75	0	0
Yes! Fat Free Barbeque	20 (1 oz)	75	0	0
Yes! Fat Free Ripple	20 (1 oz)	75	0	0
Wise				
Dipsy Doodles	1 pkg (1.5 oz)	240	15	3

CHITTERLINGS

FOOD	PORTION	CALS	FAT	SAT FAT
pork cooked	3 oz	258	24	9

FOOD	PORTION	CALS	FAT	SAT FAT
CHIVES				
freeze-dried	1 tbsp	1	tr	tr
fresh chopped	1 tbsp	1	tr	tr
fresh chopped	1 tsp	0	tr	tr
CHOCOLATE (see also CANDY, COCOA, CHOCOLATE SYRUP, HOT COCOA, ICE CREAM TOPPINGS, MILK DRINKS)				
Twist				
Sugar Free Chocolate Spread	2 tbsp	170	12	2
BAKING				
baking	1 oz	145	15	9
grated unsweetened	1 cup	689	73	43
liquid unsweetened	1 oz	134	14	7
squares unsweetened	1 square (1 oz)	146	16	9
Baker's				
Bittersweet	½ square (0.5 oz)	70	6	3
German's Sweet	2 squares (0.5 oz)	60	4	2
Semi-Sweet	½ square (0.5 oz)	70	5	3
Unsweetened	½ square (0.5 oz)	70	7	5
White	½ square (0.5 oz)	80	5	3
Nestle				
Choco Bake	½ oz	80	8	5
Premier White Bar	½ oz	80	5	3
Premier White Morsels	1 tbsp	80	4	4
Semi-Sweet Bar	½ oz	70	4	3
Unsweetened Bar	½ oz	80	7	5
CHIPS				
milk chocolate	1 cup (6 oz)	862	52	31
semisweet	60 pieces (1 oz)	136	9	5
semisweet	1 cup (6 oz)	804	50	30
Baker's				
Real Milk Chocolate	½ oz	70	4	2
Real Semi-Sweet	½ oz	60	4	2
Semi-Sweet	½ oz	70	4	3
Cloud Nine				
Double Dark Chocolate	13 pieces (0.5 oz)	80	4	3
Ghirardelli				
Semi-Sweet	33 pieces (0.5 oz)	70	4	3
Hershey				
Almond Joy Bits	1 tbsp (0.5 oz)	60	4	2

FOOD	PORTION	CALS	FAT	SAT FAT
Chocolate & Peanut Butter Chips	1 tbsp (0.5 oz)	70	3	2
Holiday Baking Bits	1 tbsp (0.5 oz)	70	3	2
Milk Chocolate	1 tbsp (0.5 oz)	80	5	3
Mini Kisses For Baking	11 pieces (0.5 oz)	80	5	3
Mint Chocolate	1 tbsp (0.5 oz)	80	4	3
Premier White Milk Chips	1 tbsp (0.5 oz)	80	4	3
Raspberry Chips	1 tbsp (0.5 oz)	80	4	3
Semi-Sweet	1 tbsp (0.5 oz)	80	4	3
Semi-Sweet Mini	1 tbsp (0.5 oz)	80	4	3
Skor English Toffee Baking Bits	1 tbsp (0.5 oz)	70	5	3
M&M's				
Baking Bits Milk Chocolate	0.5 oz	70	3	2
Baking Bits Semi-Sweet	0.5 oz	70	4	2
Nestle				
Crunch Baking Pieces	1½ tbsp	80	4	2
Milk Chocolate Morsels	1 tbsp	70	4	3
Mint Chocolate Morsels	1 tbsp	70	4	3
Morsels Semi-Sweet	1 tbsp	70	4	3
Semi-Sweet Mega Morsels	1 tbsp	70	4	3
Semi-Sweet Mini Morsels	1 tbsp	70	4	3
Sunspire				
Chocolate Sundrops	47 pieces (1.4 oz)	190	5	3
Dark Chocolate Grain Sweetened	13 pieces (0.5 oz)	70	4	3
Organic	13 pieces (0.5 oz)	70	5	3
Toll House				
Mint-Chocolate	2 tbsp (1.5 oz)	130	3	2
Semi-Sweet	2 tbsp (1.5 oz)	130	4	2
Tropical Source				
Espresso Roast Dairy Free	13 pieces (1.5 oz)	70	4	4
Semi-Sweet Dairy Free	13 pieces (1.5 oz)	80	4	3
MIX				
powder	2-3 heaping tsp	75	1	tr
powder as prep w/ whole milk	9 oz	226	9	5
Quik				
Chocolate Powder	2 tbsp (0.8 oz)	90	1	1
Chocolate Powder No Sugar	2 tbsp (0.4 oz)	40	1	1

CHOCOLATE MILK (see MILK DRINKS)

FOOD	PORTION	CALS	FAT	SAT FAT
CHOCOLATE SYRUP				
chocolate fudge	1 cup (11.9 oz)	1176	46	19
chocolate fudge	1 tbsp (0.7 oz)	73	3	1
syrup	1 cup	653	3	2
syrup	2 tbsp	82	tr	tr
syrup as prep w/ whole milk	9 oz	232	9	5
Ah!Laska				
Organic	2 tbsp	85	0	0
Colac				
Chocolate Topping	1 tbsp	37	1	tr
DaVinci Gourmet				
Sugar Free	2 tbsp	15	0	0
Estee				
Chocolate	2 tbsp	15	0	0
Hershey				
Chocolate Fudge	1 tbsp (0.7 oz)	70	3	2
Chocolate Malt	2 tbsp (1.4 oz)	100	0	0
Lite	2 tbsp (1.2 oz)	50	0	0
Syrup	2 tbsp (1.4 oz)	100	0	0
Quik				
Chocolate	2 tbsp (1.3 oz)	100	1	0
Smucker's				
Plate Scapers Chocolate	2 tbsp	100	5	–
Toll House				
Mint Chocolate	2 tbsp (1.5 oz)	130	3	2
Semi-Sweet	2 tbsp (1.5 oz)	130	4	2
Walden Farms				
Sugar Free	2 tbsp	0	0	0
CHUTNEY				
apple	1.2 oz	68	0	–
apple cranberry	1 tbsp	16	0	–
coconut	¼ cup	74	7	6
mango	1 tbsp	54	2	–
tomato	1 tbsp	32	tr	–
Sonoma				
Dried Tomato	1 tbsp (0.7 g)	35	0	0
Wild Thyme Farms				
Apricot Cranberry Walnut	1 tbsp	15	0	0
Pineapple Peach Lime	1 tbsp	14	0	0

FOOD	PORTION	CALS	FAT	SAT FAT
CILANTRO				
fresh	1 tsp (2 g)	tr	tr	0
fresh	1 cup (1.6 oz)	11	tr	tr
CINNAMON				
ground	1 tsp	6	tr	tr
sticks	0.5 oz	39	tr	tr
Gringo Billy's				
Cinnamon Sweetener	½ tsp	0	0	0
CISCO				
raw	3 oz	84	2	tr
smoked	1 oz	50	3	tr
smoked	3 oz	151	10	1
CLAMS				
CANNED				
liquid only	1 cup	6	tr	—
liquid only	3 oz	2	tr	—
meat only	1 cup	236	3	tr
meat only	3 oz	126	2	tr
Bumble Bee				
Baby	2 oz	50	1	1
Progresso				
Creamy Clam Sauce	½ cup (4.2 oz)	110	6	2
Minced	¼ cup (2.1 oz)	25	0	0
Red Clam Sauce	½ cup (4.4 oz)	60	1	0
White Clam Sauce	½ cup (4.4 oz)	150	10	2
FRESH				
cooked	3 oz	126	2	tr
cooked	20 sm	133	2	tr
raw	9 lg (6.3 oz)	133	2	tr
raw	20 sm (6.3 oz)	133	2	tr
raw	3 oz	63	1	tr
TAKE-OUT				
breaded & fried	20 sm	379	21	5
CLEMENTINES				
Haddon House				
In Light Syrup	½ cup	80	0	0

FOOD	PORTION	CALS	FAT	SAT FAT
CLOVES				
ground	1 tsp	7	tr	tr
COCOA (see also HOT COCOA)				
powder unsweetened	1 tbsp (5 g)	11	1	tr
powder unsweetened	1 cup (3 oz)	197	12	7
Ah!Laska				
Organic	2 tbsp	100	0	0
Organic Bakers Cocoa	1 tbsp	20	0	0
Hershey				
Cocoa	1 tbsp (5 g)	20	1	0
European Cocoa	1 tbsp (5 g)	20	1	0
Nestle				
Cocoa	1 tbsp	15	1	0
COCONUT				
coconut water	1 tbsp	3	tr	tr
coconut water	1 cup	46	tr	tr
cream canned	1 cup	568	52	47
cream canned	1 tbsp	36	3	3
dried sweetened flaked	1 cup	351	24	21
dried sweetened flaked	7 oz pkg	944	64	57
dried sweetened flaked canned	1 cup	341	24	22
dried sweetened shredded	7 oz pkg	997	71	63
dried sweetened shredded	1 cup	466	33	29
dried toasted	1 oz	168	13	12
dried unsweetened	1 oz	187	18	16
fresh	1 piece (1.5 oz)	159	15	13
fresh shredded	1 cup	283	27	24
milk canned	1 cup	445	48	43
milk canned	1 tbsp	30	3	3
milk frozen	1 cup	486	50	44
milk frozen	1 tbsp	30	3	3
Baker's				
Angel Flake	1 tbsp (0.5 oz)	70	5	5
Angel Flake (canned)	2 tbsp (0.5 oz)	70	6	5
Premium Shred	2 tbsp (0.5 oz)	70	5	5
Thai Kitchen				
Milk	2 oz	124	12	7

FOOD	PORTION	CALS	FAT	SAT FAT
COD				
atlantic canned	3 oz	89	1	tr
atlantic canned	1 can (11 oz)	327	3	1
atlantic dried	3 oz	246	2	tr
atlantic fresh cooked	1 fillet (6.3 oz)	189	2	tr
atlantic fresh cooked	3 oz	89	1	tr
atlantic fresh raw	3 oz	70	1	tr
pacific fresh baked	3 oz	95	1	tr
roe canned	1 oz	34	1	—
roe raw	1 oz	37	tr	—
roe tarama	3.5 oz	547	55	—
Van De Kamp's				
Lightly Breaded Fillets	1 (4 oz)	220	10	2
TAKE-OUT				
roe baked w/ butter & lemon juice	1 oz	36	1	—
COFFEE (see also COFFEE BEVERAGES, COFFEE SUBSTITUTES)				
INSTANT				
decaffeinated	1 rounded tsp	4	0	0
decaffeinated as prep	6 oz	4	0	0
regular as prep	1 cup (6 oz)	4	0	0
regular w/ chicory	1 rounded tsp	6	0	0
regular w/ chicory as prep	6 oz	6	0	0
Nescafe				
Decafe	1 tsp (2 g)	0	0	0
Decafe w/ Chicory	1 tsp (2 g)	0	0	0
French Vanilla	1 tsp (2 g)	5	0	0
French Vanilla Decaf	1 tsp (2 g)	5	0	0
Hazelnut	1 tsp (2 g)	5	0	0
Irish Creme	1 tsp (2 g)	5	0	0
Regular	1 tsp (2 g)	0	0	0
With Chicory	1 tsp (2 g)	5	0	0
REGULAR				
brewed	8 oz	2	0	0
roasted beans	1 oz	64	4	—
Folgers				
Colombian Supreme	1 tbsp	16	tr	—
Custom Roast	1 tbsp	16	tr	—
Decaffeinated	1 tbsp	17	tr	—
French Roast	1 tbsp	16	tr	—

FOOD	PORTION	CALS	FAT	SAT FAT
Gourmet Supreme	1 tbsp	16	tr	—
Instant	1 tsp	8	tr	—
Instant Decaffeinated	1 tsp	8	tr	—
Singles	1 bag	21	tr	—
Singles Decaffeinated	1 bag	21	tr	—
Special Roast	1 tbsp	16	tr	—
Vacuum Pack	1 tbsp	16	tr	—
Maryland Club				
Ground	1 tbsp	16	tr	—
Nescafe				
Caffe Mocha	1 can (10 oz)	140	3	3
Caffe Latte	1 can (10 oz)	130	3	2
Caffe Latte Decaffeinated	1 can (10 oz)	130	3	2
Espresso	1 tsp (2 g)	0	0	0
Espresso Caffe Latte	1 pkg (0.6 oz)	70	2	1
Espresso Caffe Mocha	1 pkg (1 oz)	110	3	2
Espresso Cappuccino	1 pkg (0.6 oz)	80	3	2
Espresso Roast	1 can (10 oz)	90	1	1
French Vanilla	1 can (10 oz)	150	4	3
Hazelnut	1 can (10 oz)	130	3	2
Roasted Ground Decaffeinated as prep	1 cup (6 oz)	0	0	0
Roasted Ground as prep	1 cup (6 oz)	0	0	0
Revival				
Soy Caramel Corn	1 cup (8 oz)	0	0	0
Soy Hazelnut	1 cup (8 oz)	0	0	0
Soy Original Roast	1 cup (8 oz)	0	0	0
TAKE-OUT				
caffe amaretto w/ alcohol	1 serv	192	9	6
caffe au lait	1 cup (8 fl oz)	77	4	3
caffe brulot	1 cup	48	0	0
caffe brulot w/ alcohol	1 serv	130	tr	tr
cappuccino	1 cup (8 fl oz)	77	4	3
coffee con leche	1 cup (8 fl oz)	77	4	3
espresso	1 cup (3 fl oz)	2	0	0
irish coffee	1 serv	226	11	7
latte w/ skim milk	13 oz	88	tr	tr
latte w/ whole milk	13 oz	152	8	5
mocha	1 mug (9.6 fl oz)	202	15	9

FOOD	PORTION	CALS	FAT	SAT FAT
COFFEE BEVERAGES				
cappuccino mix as prep	7 oz	62	2	2
french mix as prep	7 oz	57	3	3
mocha mix as prep	7 oz	51	2	2
AchievONE				
All Flavors	1 bottle (9.5 oz)	120	0	–
Arizona				
Iced Latte Supreme	8 oz	110	2	1
Iced Mocha Latte	8 oz	110	2	1
Chock full o'Nuts				
New York Cappuccino French Vanilla	1 pkg (0.9 oz)	90	2	2
New York Cappuccino Hazelnut	1 pkg. (0.9 oz)	90	2	2
Coffee House USA				
All Flavors	1 bottle (9.5 oz)	100	4	3
Flavour Creations				
Coffee Flavoring Tablets All Flavors	1 tablet	0	0	0
Gehl's				
Iced Cappuccino	1 can (11 oz)	190	2	1
General Foods				
Cappuccino Coolers French Vanilla as prep w/ 2% milk	1 serv	180	5	3
International Coffee Sugar Free Cafe Vienna as prep	1 serv (8 oz)	30	2	1
International Coffee Sugar Free Fat Free Suisse Mocha as prep	1 serv (8 oz)	25	0	0
International Coffees Cafe Francais as prep	1 serv (8 oz)	60	4	1
International Coffees Cafe Vienna as prep	1 serv (8 oz)	70	3	1
International Coffees Decaffeinated French Vanilla Cafe as prep	1 serv (8 oz)	60	3	1
International Coffees Decaffeinated Suisse Mocha as prep	1 serv (8 oz)	60	2	1
International Coffees French Vanilla Cafe as prep	1 serv (8 oz)	60	3	1
International Coffees Hazelnut Belgian Cafe as prep	1 serv (8 oz)	70	2	1
International Coffees Irish Creme Cafe as prep	1 serv (8 oz)	60	2	1

FOOD	PORTION	CALS	FAT	SAT FAT
International Coffees Italian Cappuccino as prep	1 serv (8 oz)	60	2	1
International Coffees Kahlua Cafe as prep	1 serv (8 oz)	60	2	1
International Coffees Orange Cappuccino as prep	1 serv (8 oz)	70	2	1
International Coffees Suisse Mocha as prep	1 serv (8 oz)	60	2	1
International Coffees Viennese Chocolate Cafe as prep	1 serv (8 oz)	50	2	1
International Coffees Sugar Free Fat Free Decaffeinated French Vanilla	1 serv (8 oz)	25	0	0
International Coffees Sugar Free Fat Free Decaffeinated Suisse Mocha	1 serv (8 oz)	25	0	0
International Coffees Sugar Free Fat Free French Vanilla Cafe as prep	1 serv (8 oz)	25	0	0
Jakada				
Latte Mocha	1 bottle (10.5 oz)	180	3.5	0
Latte Vanilla	1 bottle (10.5 oz)	180	4	2
Maxwell House				
Cafe Cappuccino Amaretto as prep	1 serv (8 oz)	90	1	0
Cafe Cappuccino Decaffeinated Mocha as prep	1 serv (8 oz)	100	3	1
Cafe Cappuccino Decaffeinated Vanilla as prep	1 serv (8 oz)	90	1	0
Cafe Cappuccino Irish Cream as prep	1 serv (8 oz)	90	1	0
Cafe Cappuccino Mocha as prep	1 serv (8 oz)	100	3	1
Cafe Cappuccino Sugar Free Mocha as prep	1 serv (8 oz)	60	3	1
Cafe Cappuccino Sugar Free Vanilla as prep	1 serv (8 oz)	60	3	1
Iced Cappuccino as prep w/ 2% milk	1 serv (8 oz)	180	5	3
Silk				
Coffee Soylatte	1 bottle (11 oz)	220	5	1
Sipper Sweets				
Sugar Free Low Carb Cappuccino	1 serv	50	3	0
Starbucks				
Frappuccino	1 bottle (9.5 oz)	190	3	2
Frappuccino Mocha	1 bottle (9.5 oz)	190	3	2
Frappuccino Vanilla	1 bottle (9.5 oz)	190	3	2

FOOD	PORTION	CALS	FAT	SAT FAT
COFFEE SUBSTITUTES				
powder	1 tsp	9	tr	tr
powder as prep	6 oz	9	tr	tr
powder as prep w/ milk	6 oz	121	6	4
Natural Touch				
Kaffree Roma	1 tsp (2 g)	10	0	0
Roma Cappuccino	3 tbsp (0.4 oz)	50	3	3
Pero				
Instant Grain Beverage	1 tsp (1.5 g)	5	0	0
Postum				
Instant Coffee Flavor as prep	1 serv (8 oz)	10	0	0
Instant as prep	1 serv (8 oz)	10	0	0
COFFEE WHITENERS				
liquid nondairy frzn	1 tbsp (0.5 oz)	20	2	tr
powder nondairy	1 tsp	11	tr	1
N-Rich				
Coffee Creamer	1 tsp (2 g)	10	1	tr
Silk				
Creamer	1 tbsp	15	1	0
Creamer French Vanilla	1 tbsp	20	1	0
Creamer Hazelnut	1 tbsp	15	1	0
COLESLAW				
TAKE-OUT				
coleslaw w/ dressing	½ cup	42	2	tr
vinegar & oil coleslaw	3.5 oz	150	9	1
COLLARDS				
fresh cooked	½ cup	17	tr	–
frzn chopped cooked	½ cup	31	tr	–
raw chopped	½ cup	6	tr	–
Birds Eye				
Chopped Greens frzn	1 cup	30	0	0
COOKIES				
MIX				
chocolate chip	1 (0.56 oz)	79	4	1
oatmeal	1 (0.6 oz)	74	3	1
oatmeal raisin	1 (0.6 oz)	74	3	1

FOOD	PORTION	CALS	FAT	SAT FAT
Aunt Paula's				
Low Carb Chef Chocolate Chip as prep	1	66	4	1
Low Carb Chef Peanut Butter as prep	1	66	4	1
Betty Crocker				
Chocolate Peanut Butter as prep	1 bar	180	9	2
Date Bar as prep	1 bar	150	6	2
Oatmeal as prep	2	150	6	1
GoldnBrown				
Fat Free	1 (1.1 oz)	120	0	0
Keto				
Chocolate Chip as prep	1	47	2	–
Oatmeal Raisin as prep	2	59	3	–
MiniCarb				
All Flavors as prep	1	110	2	0
READY-TO-EAT				
animal	11 crackers (1 oz)	126	4	1
animal crackers	1 box (2.4 oz)	299	9	4
animal crackers	1 (2.5 g)	11	tr	tr
australian anzac biscuit	1	98	3	1
butter	1 (5 g)	23	1	1
chocolate chip	1 (0.4 oz)	48	2	1
chocolate chip	1 box (1.9 oz)	233	12	5
chocolate chip low fat	1 (0.25 oz)	45	2	tr
chocolate chip low sugar low sodium	1 (0.24 oz)	31	1	1
chocolate chip soft-type	1 (0.5 oz)	69	4	1
chocolate w/ creme filling	1 (0.35 oz)	47	2	tr
chocolate w/ creme filling chocolate coated	1 (0.60 oz)	82	5	1
chocolate w/ creme filling sugar free low sodium	1 (0.35 oz)	46	2	1
chocolate w/ extra creme filling	1 (0.46 oz)	65	3	1
chocolate wafer	1 (0.2 oz)	26	1	tr
cream cheese	1 (1.1 oz)	141	9	6
digestive biscuits plain	2	141	7	–
fig bars	1 (0.56 oz)	56	1	tr
fortune	1 (0.28 oz)	30	tr	tr
fudge	1 (0.73 oz)	73	1	tr
gingersnaps	1 (0.24 oz)	29	1	tr

FOOD	PORTION	CALS	FAT	SAT FAT
graham	1 squares (0.24 oz)	30	1	tr
graham chocolate covered	1 (0.49 oz)	68	3	2
graham honey	1 (0.24 oz)	30	1	tr
hermits	1 (1 oz)	117	5	2
jumbles coconut	1 (1 oz)	121	7	5
ladyfingers	1 (0.38 oz)	40	1	tr
macaroons	1 (0.8 oz)	97	3	3
madeleines	1 (0.8 oz)	86	5	3
marshmallow chocolate coated	1 (0.46 oz)	55	2	1
marshmallow pie chocolate coated	1 (1.4 oz)	165	7	2
meringue	1 (0.3 oz)	20	0	0
molasses	1 (0.5 oz)	65	2	tr
neapolitan tri-color cookie	1 (0.6 oz)	79	5	2
oatmeal	1 (0.6 oz)	81	3	1
oatmeal	1 (0.52 oz)	71	4	1
oatmeal soft-type	1 (0.5 oz)	61	2	tr
oatmeal raisin	1 (0.6 oz)	81	3	1
oatmeal raisin low sugar no sodium	1 (0.24 oz)	31	1	1
oatmeal raisin soft-type	1 (0.5 oz)	61	2	tr
peanut butter sandwich	1 (0.5 oz)	67	3	1
peanut butter sandwich sugar free low sodium	1 (0.35 oz)	54	3	1
peanut butter soft-type	1 (0.5 oz)	69	4	1
pinenut cookies	1 (1.1 oz)	134	9	1
raisin soft-type	1 (0.5 oz)	60	2	1
reginette queen'a biscuit	1 (0.8 oz)	86	3	1
shortbread	1 (0.28 oz)	40	2	tr
shortbread pecan	1 (0.49 oz)	79	5	1
spritz	1 (0.4 oz)	42	2	1
sugar	1 (0.52 oz)	72	3	1
sugar low sugar sodium free	1 (0.24 oz)	30	1	tr
sugar wafers w/ creme filling	1 (0.12 oz)	18	1	tr
sugar wafers w/ creme filling sugar free sodium free	1 (0.14 oz)	20	1	tr
toll house original	1 (0.8 oz)	105	6	2
vanilla sandwich	1 (0.35 oz)	48	2	tr
vanilla wafers	1 (0.21 oz)	28	1	tr
zeppole	1 (0.8 oz)	78	6	2

FOOD	PORTION	CALS	FAT	SAT FAT
Alternative Baking				
Vegan Chocolate Chip	1 serv (2.5 oz)	280	10	4
Vegan Expresso Chocolate Chip	1 serv (2 oz)	230	9	3
Vegan Lemon	1 serv (2.25 oz)	250	7	2
Vegan Oatmeal	1 serv (2.25 oz)	250	10	2
Vegan Peanut Butter	1 serv (2.25 oz)	270	10	2
Vegan Pumpkin	1 serv (2 oz)	200	6	2
Vegan Wheat Free Choco Cherry Chunk	1 serv (1.75 oz)	190	6	2
Vegan Wheat Free Hula Nut	1 serv (1.75 oz)	190	6	2
Vegan Wheat Free P-nut Fudge Fusion	1 serv (1.75 oz)	190	7	2
Vegan Wheat Free Snickerdoodle	1 serv (1.75 oz)	170	3	0
Amay's				
Chinese Style Almond	1 (0.5 oz)	80	4	2
Archway				
Alpine Fudge	1 (1.3 oz)	160	6	4
Carrot Cake	1 (1 oz)	130	5	2
Chocolate Chip	1 (0.9 oz)	120	6	2
Chocolate Chip Sugar Free	1 (0.8 oz)	110	5	2
Coconut Macaroon	2 (1.4 oz)	180	11	9
Devils Food Chocolate Drop Fat Free	1 (0.7 oz)	60	0	0
Dutch Cocoa	1 (0.9 oz)	100	4	1
Frosty Lemon	1 (0.9 oz)	100	4	2
Fruit & Honey Bar	1 (0.9 oz)	110	3	1
Fruit Bar Fat Free	1 (0.9 oz)	90	0	0
Fruit Filled Apricot	1 (0.8 oz)	90	3	1
Fruit Filled Raspberry	1 (0.8 oz)	90	3	1
Ginger Snaps	5 (1 oz)	120	5	1
Homestyle Chocolate Chip	3 (1 oz)	130	7	2
Iced Spice	1 (1 oz)	120	5	2
Oatmeal	1 (0.9 oz)	100	4	1
Oatmeal Apple Filled	1 (0.9 oz)	90	3	1
Oatmeal Pecan	1 (0.9 oz)	110	4	1
Oatmeal Raisin Bran	1 (0.9 oz)	100	3	1
Oatmeal Raspberry Fat Free	1 (1.1 oz)	100	0	0
Oatmeal Sugar Free	1 (0.8 oz)	110	5	1
Oatmeal Raisin	1 (0.9 oz)	100	4	1
Oatmeal Raisin Fat Free	1 (1.1 oz)	100	0	0
Old Dutch Apple	1 (0.9 oz)	110	4	1

FOOD	PORTION	CALS	FAT	SAT FAT
Peanut Butter	1 (1 oz)	150	9	2
Peanut Butter Fudge	1 (1.3 oz)	220	13	5
Peanut Butter Sugar Free	1 (0.8 oz)	110	6	2
Pecan Crunch	3 (1.2 oz)	180	10	2
Rocky Road	1 (0.8 oz)	110	5	2
Rocky Road Sugar Free	1 (0.8 oz)	100	5	1
Shortbread Sugar Free	1 (0.8 oz)	110	5	2
Arnott's				
Raspberry Tartlets	2	100	4	2
Atkins				
Endulge Wafer Bars Chocolate Creme	2 bars (1 oz)	120	9	5
Endulge Wafer Bars Mint	2 bars (1 oz)	120	9	5
Endulge Wafer Bars Peanut Butter	2 bars (1 oz)	120	9	4
BP Gourmet				
Biscotti Fat Free Cinnamon Crunch	6 (1 oz)	110	0	0
Biscotti Fat Free Vanilla Crunch	4 (1 oz)	80	0	0
Chocolate Fudge Chip Sugar Free	5 (1 oz)	100	6	3
Dreams Chocolate	7 (1 oz)	120	3	2
Dreams Fat Free Chocolate Fudge	13 (1 oz)	100	0	0
Dreams Fat Free Vanilla	19 (1 oz)	100	0	0
Tangos Fat Free Chocolate Fudge Chip	4 (1 oz)	100	0	0
Bahlsen				
Afrika	8 (1.1 oz)	170	10	6
Butter Leaves	7 (1 oz)	140	7	4
Choco Leibniz	2 (1 oz)	140	7	4
Choco Star Dark Chocolate	3 (1.1 oz)	170	12	6
Choco Star Milk Chocolate	3 (1.1 oz)	180	12	6
Chocolate Hearts	4 (1 oz)	160	9	6
Delice	6 (1 oz)	140	6	2
Deloba	4 (0.9 oz)	130	5	2
Hanover Waffelin	5 (1 oz)	160	10	9
Hit Chocolate Vanilla Filled	2 (1 oz)	140	8	6
Hit Vanilla Chocolate Filled	2 (1 oz)	140	7	5
Kipferl	4 (1 oz)	150	9	3
Leibniz	6 (1 oz)	130	4	2
Nuss Dessert	3 (1.1 oz)	180	11	5
Probiers	6 (1.1 oz)	150	6	3
Twingo	6 (1.1 oz)	170	11	9
Waffeletten	4 (1 oz)	160	9	6

FOOD	PORTION	CALS	FAT	SAT FAT
Baker's Breakfast Cookie				
Apple Pie	1 (3 oz)	204	2	tr
Banana Walnut	1 (3 oz)	274	8	1
Chocolate Chunk Raisin	1 (3 oz)	260	5	1
Double Chocolate Chunk	1 (3 oz)	250	5	1
Fruit & Nut	1 (3 oz)	270	5	1
Lemon Poppy Seed	1 (3 oz)	230	3	1
Mocha Chocolate Chunk	1 (3 oz)	250	5	1
Oatmeal Raisin	1 (3 oz)	250	4	1
Peanut Butter	1 (3 oz)	290	8	2
Peanut Butter & Jelly	1 (3 oz)	320	9	1
Pumpkin Spice	1 (3 oz)	230	3	1
Vegan Chocolate Chunk	1 (3 oz)	260	6	2
Vegan Peanut Butter Chocolate Chunk	1 (3 oz)	310	10	2
Baker's Harvest				
Animal	12 (0.9 oz)	130	3	1
Chocolate Grahams	2 (0.9 oz)	130	3	1
Cinnamon Grahams	2 (0.9 oz)	130	5	1
Cinnamon Grahams Low Fat	2 (0.9 oz)	110	2	0
Fig Bars	2 (1.2 oz)	120	3	0
Graham	2 (0.9 oz)	120	4	1
Graham Low Fat	2 (0.9 oz)	110	2	0
Iced Oatmeal	1 (0.6 oz)	70	3	1
Pecan Shortbread	1 (0.5 oz)	80	5	1
Vanilla Wafers	7 (1.1 oz)	150	6	1
Barbara's Bakery				
Apple Cinnamon Bars Fat Free Whole Wheat	1 (0.7 oz)	60	0	0
Chocolate Chip	1 (0.6 oz)	80	4	2
Double Dutch Chocolate	1 (0.6 oz)	80	4	2
Fig Bars Fat Free Wheat Free	1 (0.7 oz)	60	0	0
Fig Bars Fat Free Whole Wheat	1 (0.7 oz)	60	0	0
Nature's Choice Coconut Almond	1 bar (1 oz)	120	5	3
Nature's Choice Expresso Bean	1 bar (1 oz)	120	3	3
Nature's Choice Lemon Yogurt	1 bar (1 oz)	120	4	3
Nature's Choice Roasted Peanut	1 bar (1 oz)	130	5	2
Old Fashioned Oatmeal	1 (0.6 oz)	70	3	1
Raspberry Bars Fat Free Wheat Free Raspberry	1 (0.7 oz)	60	0	0
Snackimals Chocolate Chip	8 (1 oz)	120	5	1

FOOD	PORTION	CALS	FAT	SAT FAT
Snackimals Oatmeal Wheat Free	8 (1 oz)	120	5	0
Snackimals Vanilla	8 (1 oz)	120	5	0
Traditional Blueberry Low Fat	1 (0.7 oz)	60	1	0
Traditional Fig Low Fat	1 (0.7 oz)	60	1	0
Traditional Shortbread	1 (0.6 oz)	80	4	3
Bed & Breakfast				
Cranberry Orange Oatmeal	1 (0.8 oz)	110	5	2
Enrobed Shortbread	2 (1.4 oz)	190	9	4
Fruit Center Key Lime	2 (1.1 oz)	140	6	2
Fruit Center Raspberry	2 (1.1 oz)	140	6	2
Beigel's				
Black & White	1 (1 oz)	100	3	1
Breaktime				
Chocolate Chip	1 (0.3 oz)	37	2	tr
Coconut	1 (0.3 oz)	35	1	tr
Ginger	1 (0.3 oz)	34	1	tr
Oatmeal	1 (0.3 oz)	35	1	tr
Sprinkles	1 (0.3 oz)	36	2	tr
Brent & Sam's				
Chocolate Chip Pecan	2 (0.5 oz)	80	5	1
Chocolate Chip Raspberry	2 (0.5 oz)	70	4	1
Chocolate Chips	2 (0.5 oz)	70	4	1
Key Lime White Chocolate	2 (0.5 oz)	70	4	2
Oatmeal Raisin Pecan	2 (0.5 oz)	70	7	1
Toffee Pecan	2 (0.5 oz)	80	5	1
White Chocolate Macadamia	2 (0.5 oz)	80	5	2
Bud's Best				
Caco Creme	7 (1 oz)	140	6	2
Chocolate Chip	6 (1 oz)	140	6	2
French Vanilla	7 (1 oz)	150	6	2
Oatmeal	6 (1 oz)	130	5	2
Cadbury				
Fingers	3	85	4	3
Cafe				
Cinnamony Twists Chocolate Chip	1 (0.5 oz)	40	2	0
Sugar Free California Almond	4 (1 oz)	110	4	1
Twists Cinnamony	1 (0.3 oz)	40	2	0
Carbolite				
Chocolate Chip	1 (1 oz)	120	9	2
Peanut Butter	1 (1 oz)	120	9	2

FOOD	PORTION	CALS	FAT	SAT FAT
Shortbread	1 (1 oz)	180	9	2
Carr's				
Ginger Lemon Cremes	2 (1 oz)	140	7	4
Carriage Trade				
Finnish Ginger Snaps	3	60	7	—
Chortles				
Cookies	½ pkg. (1 oz)	125	3	1
Cookie Lover's				
Chocolate Chip	1 (0.8 oz)	90	4	2
Creme Supremes	2 (0.9 oz)	120	5	0
Creme Supremes Mint	2 (0.9 oz)	120	5	0
Grahams	2 (1 oz)	100	1	0
Grahams Cinnamon	2 (1 oz)	110	1	0
Peanut Butter	1 (0.8 oz)	100	4	2
Shortbread	1 (0.8 oz)	120	7	4
Dare				
Blueberry Cheesecake	1 (0.6 oz)	90	5	1
Butter Shortbread	1 (0.5 oz)	63	4	2
Butter Creme	1 (0.6 oz)	85	4	1
Carrot Cake	1 (0.6 oz)	92	5	1
Chocolate Chip	1 (0.5 oz)	77	4	1
Chocolate Fudge	1 (0.7 oz)	97	5	3
Cinnamon Danish	1 (0.4 oz)	47	2	tr
Coconut Creme	1 (0.7 oz)	99	5	3
French Creme	1 (0.5 oz)	80	5	3
Harvest From The Rain Forest	1 (0.5 oz)	70	4	1
Key Lime Creme	1 (0.6 oz)	86	4	1
Lemon Creme	1 (0.7 oz)	95	5	1
Maple Leaf Creme	1 (0.6 oz)	83	4	1
Maple Walnut Fudge	1 (0.7 oz)	99	5	3
Milk Chocolate Fudge	1 (0.7 oz)	99	5	3
Oatmeal Raisin	1 (0.4 oz)	59	3	1
Social Tea	1 (0.2 oz)	26	1	tr
Sun Maid Raisin Oatmeal	1 (0.5 oz)	52	3	1
De Beukelaer				
Pirouline	8 (1 oz)	130	4	3
Pirouline Viennese Wafers	1 (1 oz)	150	7	5
Delarce				
Chocosprits	1 (0.6 oz)	90	5	3
Marquisettes	3 (0.9 oz)	140	7	4

FOOD	PORTION	CALS	FAT	SAT FAT
Roules d'Or	4 (1 oz)	180	8	6
Dunkaroos				
Chocolate Graham	1 pkg	120	5	1
Cinnamon Graham	1 pkg	130	5	2
Honey Graham	1 pkg	120	5	1
Dutch Mill				
Chocolate Chip	3 (1.1 oz)	160	10	3
Coconut Macaroons	3 (1 oz)	120	7	6
Oatmeal Raisin	3 (1 oz)	130	6	2
Eddyleon				
Jelly Graham Raspberry	1 (0.9 oz)	134	8	5
Pudding Cookies	1 (0.9 oz)	134	6	5
English Bay				
Strawberry Fruit Bar	1 (1.2 oz)	120	3	1
Entenmann's				
Little Bites Chocolate Chip	8 (1.8 oz)	240	12	3
Soft Baked Chocolate Chip	1 (0.7 oz)	100	5	2
Soft Baked Double Chocolate Chip	1 (0.7 oz)	100	5	2
Soft Baked Milk Chocolate Chip	1 (0.7 oz)	100	5	2
Soft Baked Original Chocolate Chip	3 (1 oz)	150	7	2
Soft Baked White Chocolate Macadamia Nut	1 (0.7 oz)	100	6	2
Soft Baked Light Chocolately Chip	2 (1 oz)	120	4	2
Soft Baked Light Oatmeal Raisin	2 (1 oz)	100	0	0
Estee				
Chocolate Chip	4	150	7	2
Coconut	4	140	6	2
Fig Bars	2	100	1	0
Fudge	4	150	7	2
Lemon Thins	4	140	6	1
Oatmeal Raisin	4	130	5	1
Sandwich Chocolate	3	160	6	2
Sandwich Original	3	160	6	2
Sandwich Peanut Butter	3	160	7	1
Sandwich Vanilla	3	160	5	1
Shortbread	4	130	4	1
Sugar Free Chocolate Chip	3	110	4	1
Sugar Free Chocolate Walnut	3	110	4	0
Sugar Free Coconut	3	110	4	1
Sugar Free Grahams Chocolate	2	110	2	0

FOOD	PORTION	CALS	FAT	SAT FAT
Sugar Free Grahams Cinnamon	2	90	2	0
Sugar Free Grahams Old Fashion	2	90	2	0
Sugar Free Lemon	3	110	3	0
Sugar Free Wafer Banana Split	5	155	9	2
Sugar Free Wafer Chocolate	5	150	9	2
Sugar Free Wafer Chocolate Peanut Butter Caramel	5	150	8	2
Sugar Free Wafer Lemon Creme	5	150	8	2
Sugar Free Wafer Peanut Butter Creme	5	150	8	2
Sugar Free Wafer Vanilla	5	150	8	2
Sugar Free Wafer Vanilla Strawberry	5	150	8	2
Vanilla Thins	4	140	6	1
Falcone's				
Sorrentini	1 (1 oz)	100	4	1
Famous Amos				
Butter Shortie	1 (0.5 oz)	80	5	2
Chocolate Chip	4 (1 oz)	140	7	2
Chocolate Chip & Pecan	4 (1 oz)	140	8	2
Chocolate Chip Toffee	4 (1 oz)	130	6	3
Chocolate Creme Sandwich	3 (1.2 oz)	140	6	2
Chunky Chocolate Chip	1 (0.5 oz)	70	4	2
Fat Free Fig Bar	2 (1 oz)	90	0	0
Fat Free Strawberry Fruit Bar	2 (1 oz)	90	0	0
Fig Bar	2 (1.1 oz)	120	3	1
Oatmeal Chocolate Chip Walnut	4 (1 oz)	140	7	2
Oatmeal Raisin	4 (1 oz)	130	6	1
Oatmeal Macaroon Creme Sandwich	3 (1.2 oz)	160	7	2
Peanut Butter Chocolate Chunk	1 (0.5 oz)	80	5	2
Peanut Butter Creme Sandwich	3 (1.2 oz)	160	8	2
Pecan Shortie	1 (0.5 oz)	80	5	1
Vanilla Creme Sandwich	3 (1.2 oz)	160	7	2
Frookie				
Animal Frackers	14 (1 oz)	130	5	0
Chocolate Chip Wheat & Gluten Free	3 (1.1 oz)	140	5	2
Double Chocolate Wheat & Gluten Free	3 (1.1 oz)	130	4	1
Dream Creams Strawberry	4 (1 oz)	140	8	2
Dream Creams Vanilla	4 (1 oz)	140	8	2
Funky Monkeys Chocolate	16 (1 oz)	120	4	1

FOOD	PORTION	CALS	FAT	SAT FAT
Funky Monkeys Vanilla	16 (1 oz)	120	4	1
Graham Cinnamon	2 (1 oz)	100	3	0
Graham Honey	2 (1 oz)	110	3	0
Lemon Wafers	8 (1 oz)	110	0	0
Old Fashioned Ginger Snaps	8 (1 oz)	120	2	0
Organic Chocolate Chip	3 (1.1 oz)	150	7	2
Organic Double Chocolate Chip	3 (1.1 oz)	140	6	2
Organic Iced Lemon	3 (1.3 oz)	165	6	1
Organic Oatmeal Raisin	3 (1.1 oz)	140	5	1
Peanut Butter Chunk Wheat & Gluten Free	3 (1.1 oz)	140	5	1
Sandwich Chocolate	2 (0.7 oz)	100	4	0
Sandwich Lemon	2 (0.7 oz)	100	4	0
Sandwich Peanut Butter	2 (0.7 oz)	100	4	0
Sandwich Vanilla	2 (0.7 oz)	100	4	0
Shortbread	5 (1 oz)	130	5	3
Vanilla Wafers	8 (1 oz)	110	0	0
General Henry				
Fruit Bars Apple	1 (0.6 oz)	60	1	0
Fruit Bars Blueberry	1 (0.6 oz)	60	1	0
Fruit Bars Fig	1 (0.6 oz)	60	1	0
Girl Scout				
Apple Cinnamon Reduced Fat	3 (1 oz)	120	5	1
Do-si-dos	3 (1.2 oz)	170	8	1
Lemon Drops	3 (1.2 oz)	160	8	2
Samoas	2 (1 oz)	160	9	6
Striped Chocolate Chip	3 (1.2 oz)	180	10	4
Tagalongs	2 (0.9 oz)	150	10	4
Thin Mints	4 (1 oz)	140	8	2
Trefoils	5 (1.1 oz)	160	8	1
Glenny's				
Soy Fudgies All Flavors	3	70	2	0
Godiva				
Biscotti Dipped In Milk Chocolate	1 (0.9 oz)	120	6	3
Gol D Lite				
Low Carb Pizzelle	1 (0.3 oz)	46	2	0
Golden Grahams Treats				
Chocolate Chunk	1 bar (0.8 oz)	90	3	1
Honey Graham	1 bar (0.8 oz)	90	2	0
King Size Chocolate Chunk	1 bar (1.6 oz)	190	5	1

FOOD	PORTION	CALS	FAT	SAT FAT
King Size Honey Graham	1 bar (1.6 oz)	180	4	1
Goody Man				
Marshmallow Crispy Squares	1 (1.17 oz)	130	3	1
Gourmet				
Chocolate Chip	2 (1.1 oz)	160	9	6
Lemon Creme	2 (1.4 oz)	210	10	5
Oatmeal Raisin	2 (0.9 oz)	120	6	4
Peanut Butter Chip	2 (1 oz)	150	8	4
Raspberry Center	2 (1.1 oz)	140	5	3
Grandma's				
Chocolate Chip	1 (1.4 oz)	190	9	3
Fudge Chocolate Chip	1 (1.4 oz)	170	7	3
Fudge Sandwich	3	180	5	2
Fudge Vanilla Sandwich	3	120	4	1
Mini Fudge	9	150	7	2
Mini Peanut Butter	9	150	7	2
Mini Vanilla	9	150	7	2
Oatmeal Raisin	1 (1.4 oz)	160	6	2
Old Time Molasses	1 (1.4 oz)	160	4	2
Peanut Butter	1 (1.4 oz)	190	9	2
Peanut Butter Chocolate Chip	1 (1.4 oz)	190	9	3
Peanut Butter Sandwich	5	210	10	3
Rich N'Chewy	1 pkg	270	12	4
Vanilla Sandwich	3	180	5	2
Vanilla Sandwich	5	210	10	3
Granny Oats				
Low Carb Oatmeal	4	98	6	4
Handi-Snack				
Cookie Jammers Cookies & Fruit Spread	1 pkg (1.3 oz)	130	3	0
Health Valley				
Apple Spice	3	100	0	0
Apricot Delight	3	100	0	0
Biscotti Amaretto	2	120	3	—
Biscotti Chocolate	2	120	3	—
Biscotti Fruit & Nut	2	120	3	—
Cheesecake Bars Blueberry	1 bar	160	2	—
Cheesecake Bars Raspberry	1 bar	160	2	—
Cheesecake Bars Strawberry	1 bar	160	2	—
Chips Double Chocolate	3	100	0	0

FOOD	PORTION	CALS	FAT	SAT FAT
Chips Old Fashioned	3	100	0	0
Chips Original	3	100	0	0
Chocolate Fudge Center	2	70	0	0
Chocolate Sandwich Bars Bavarian Creme	1 bar	150	0	0
Chocolate Sandwich Bars Caramel Creme	1 bar	150	0	0
Chocolate Sandwich Bars Vanilla Creme	1 bar	150	0	0
Date Delight	3	100	0	0
Graham Amaranth	8	100	0	0
Graham Oat Bran	8	100	0	0
Graham Original Amaranth	6	120	3	—
Hawaiian Fruit	3	100	0	0
Jumbo Apple Raisin	1	80	0	0
Jumbo Raisin Raisin	1	80	0	0
Jumbo Raspberry	1	80	0	0
Marshmallow Bars Chocolate Chip	1	90	0	0
Marshmallow Bars Old Fashioned	1	90	0	0
Marshmallow Bars Tropical Fruit	1	90	0	0
Oat Bran Fruit Bars Raisin Cinnamon	1 bar	160	1	—
Raisin Oatmeal	3	100	0	0
Raspberry Fruit Center	1	70	0	0
Tarts Baked Apple Cinnamon	1	150	0	0
Tarts California Strawberry	1	150	0	0
Tarts Chocolate Fudge	1	150	0	0
Tarts Cranberry Apple	1	150	0	0
Tarts Mountain Blueberry	1	150	0	0
Tarts Red Raspberry	1	150	0	0
Tarts Sweet Red Cherry	1	150	0	0
Heavenly				
Meringues All Flavors Sugar Free Fat Free	1	0	0	0
Hellema				
Almond	1 pkg (0.6 oz)	90	5	1
Hershey				
Cripsy Rice Snacks Peanut Butter	1 (0.6 oz)	70	3	1
Jacques Gourmet				
Palmier Cinnamon	3 (1 oz)	140	9	4
Palmier Vanilla	3 (1 oz)	140	9	4

FOOD	PORTION	CALS	FAT	SAT FAT
Joseph's				
Almond Sugar Free	2 (0.9 oz)	100	5	1
Chocolate Chip Sugar Free	2 (0.9 oz)	100	5	1
Chocolate Walnut Sugar Free	2 (0.9 oz)	100	6	1
Coconut Sugar Free	2 (0.9 oz)	105	5	1
Lemon Sugar Free	2 (0.9 oz)	95	4	1
Oatmeal Raisin Sugar Free	2 (0.9 oz)	100	5	1
Peanut Butter Sugar Free	2 (0.9 oz)	95	5	1
Pecan Shortbread Sugar Free	2 (0.9 oz)	100	5	1
Keebler				
Animal Crackers Chocolate Chip	7 (1 oz)	130	5	1
Animal Crackers Ernie's	1 box	250	9	2
Animal Crackers Iced	6 (1.1 oz)	150	5	1
Animal Crackers Sprinkled	6 (1.1 oz)	150	5	1
Butter	5 (1.1 oz)	150	6	2
Chips Deluxe	1 (0.5 oz)	80	5	2
Chips Deluxe Chocolate Lovers	1 (0.6 oz)	90	5	3
Chips Deluxe Coconut	1 (0.5 oz)	80	5	2
Chips Deluxe Rainbow	1 (0.6 oz)	80	4	2
Chips Deluxe Soft 'n Chewy	1 (0.6 oz)	80	4	1
Chips Deluxe w/ Peanut Butter Cups	1 (0.6 oz)	90	5	2
Classic Collection Chocolate Fudge Creme	1 (0.6 oz)	80	4	1
Classic Collection French Vanilla Creme	1 (0.6 oz)	80	4	1
Cookie Stix Butter	5 (1.2 oz)	160	6	3
Cookie Stix Chocolate Chip	4 (0.9 oz)	130	5	2
Cookie Stix Rainbow	5 (1.2 oz)	150	6	2
Danish Wedding	4 (0.9 oz)	120	5	2
Droxies	3 (1.1 oz)	140	6	1
Droxies Reduced Fat	3 (1.1 oz)	140	5	2
E.L. Fudge Butter w/ Fudge Filling	2 (0.9 oz)	120	6	1
E.L. Fudge Fudge w/ Fudge Filling	2 (0.9 oz)	120	6	1
E.L. Fudge w/ Peanut Butter Filling	2 (0.9 oz)	120	6	1
Fudge Shoppe Deluxe Grahams	3 (1 oz)	140	7	5
Fudge Shoppe Double Fudge 'n Caramel	2 (1 oz)	140	7	4
Fudge Shoppe Fudge Sticks	3 (1 oz)	150	8	5
Fudge Shoppe Fudge Sticks Peanut Butter	3 (1 oz)	150	8	4

FOOD	PORTION	CALS	FAT	SAT FAT
Fudge Shoppe Fudge Stripes	3 (1.1 oz)	160	8	5
Fudge Shoppe Fudge Stripes Reduced Fat	3 (1 oz)	140	5	3
Fudge Shoppe Grasshoppers	4 (1 oz)	150	7	5
Fudge Shoppe S'mores	3 (1.2 oz)	160	8	5
Ginger Snaps	5 (1.1 oz)	150	6	1
Golden Fruit Cranberry	1 (0.7 oz)	80	2	0
Golden Fruit Raisin	1 (0.7 oz)	80	2	1
Graham Cinnamon Crisp	8 (1 oz)	140	5	1
Graham Cinnamon Crisp Low Fat	8 (1 oz)	110	2	1
Graham Honey	8 (1.1 oz)	150	6	2
Graham Honey Low Fat	8 (1.1 oz)	120	2	1
Graham Original	8 (1 oz)	130	3	1
Lemon Coolers	5 (1 oz)	140	6	2
Oatmeal Country Style	2 (0.8 oz)	120	5	1
Sandies Almond Shortbread	1 (0.5 oz)	80	5	1
Sandies Pecan Shortbread	1 (0.5 oz)	80	5	1
Sandies Simply Shortbread	1 (0.5 oz)	80	5	2
Snack Size Chips Deluxe	1 pkg (2 oz)	300	16	5
Snack Size Chips Deluxe Chocolate Lovers	1 pkg (2 oz)	280	15	7
Snack Size Mini Fudge Stripes	1 pkg (2 oz)	280	14	9
Snack Size Rainbow Chips Deluxe	1 pkg (2 oz)	290	16	4
Snack Size Sandies w/ Pecans	1 pkg (2 oz)	300	17	4
Snackin' Grahams Cinnamon	21 (1 oz)	130	3	1
Snackin' Grahams Honey	23 (1 oz)	130	4	1
Soft Batch Chocolate Chip	1 (0.6 oz)	80	4	1
Soft Batch Homestyle Chocolate Chunk	1 (0.9 oz)	130	7	3
Soft Batch Homestyle Double Chocolate	1 (0.9 oz)	130	7	2
Soft Batch Homestyle Oatmeal Raisin	1 (0.9 oz)	130	5	1
Soft Batch Oatmeal Raisin	1 (0.5 oz)	70	3	1
Sugar Wafers Creme	3 (0.9 oz)	130	6	2
Sugar Wafers Lemon	3 (0.9 oz)	130	6	1
Sugar Wafers Peanut Butter	4 (1.1 oz)	170	9	2
Vanilla Wafers	8 (1.1 oz)	150	7	2
Vanilla Wafers Reduced Fat	8 (1.1 oz)	130	4	1
Vienna Fingers	2 (1 oz)	140	6	2
Vienna Fingers Lemon	2 (1 oz)	140	6	2

FOOD	PORTION	CALS	FAT	SAT FAT
Keto				
Low Carb Biscotti Chocolate	1 (1.2 oz)	157	9	9
Low Carb Biscotti Lemon Nut	1 (1.2 oz)	157	9	4
Low Carb Biscotti Vanilla Almond	1 (1.2 oz)	157	9	9
Knott's Berry Farm				
Shortbread Apricot	3 (1 oz)	120	5	1
Shortbread Boysenberry	3 (1 oz)	120	5	1
Shortbread Raspberry	3 (1 oz)	120	5	1
LU				
Chocolatier	3 (1 oz)	150	9	7
Le Bastogne	2 (0.8 oz)	120	5	3
Le Dore	4 (1 oz)	140	6	3
Le Fondant	4 (1.1 oz)	170	10	9
Le Palmier	4 (1.2 oz)	180	10	5
Le Petit Beurre	4 (1.2 oz)	150	4	3
Le Petit Ecolier Dark Chocolate	2 (0.9 oz)	130	6	4
Le Petit Ecolier Extra Dark Chocolate	2	120	7	4
Le Petit Ecolier Hazelnut Milk Chocolate	2 (0.9 oz)	130	7	3
Le Petit Ecolier Milk Chocolate	2 (0.9 oz)	130	6	4
Le Raisin Dore	4 (1.2 oz)	160	7	5
Le Truffe Coconut	4 (1.2 oz)	190	12	11
Le Truffe Praline Chocolate	4 (1.2 oz)	170	9	7
Les Varietes	3 (0.9 oz)	140	7	5
Pim's Orange	2 (0.9 oz)	90	3	2
Pim's Raspberry	2 (0.9 oz)	90	3	1
La Choy				
Fortune	4 (1 oz)	112	tr	tr
Lance				
Apple Bar Fat Free	1 (1.75 oz)	160	0	0
Apple Oatmeal Bar	1 (1.8 oz)	190	6	2
Big Town Banana	1 pkg (2 oz)	250	10	3
Big Town Chocolate	1 pkg (2 oz)	250	8	3
Big Town Vanilla	1 pkg (2 oz)	250	11	3
Choc-O-Lunch	1 pkg (1.5 oz)	200	8	2
Choc-O-Mint	1 pkg (1¼ oz)	190	9	4
Coated Graham	1 pkg (1.3 oz)	190	8	2
Fig Bar	1 (1.75 oz)	180	4	1
Fudge Chocolate Chip	1 (2 oz)	130	5	2
Gourmet Chocolate Chip	1 (2 oz)	130	6	3

FOOD	PORTION	CALS	FAT	SAT FAT
Lem-O-Lunch	1 pkg (3.4 oz)	240	11	3
Lemon Nekot	1 pkg (1.5 oz)	210	10	2
Nut-O-Lunch	1 pkg (3.3 oz)	240	11	3
Oatmeal	1 (2 oz)	130	6	1
Oatmeal Creme	1 (2 oz)	240	10	3
Peanut Butter	1 (2 oz)	140	8	2
Peanut Butter Creme Wafer	1 pkg (1.5 oz)	230	12	3
Van-O-Lunch	1 pkg (1.5 oz)	210	8	2
Landies Candies				
Sugar Free Dark Royal Pecan Shortbread	2	167	9	4
Sugar Free Milk Chocolate Chip	2	173	11	5
Sugar Free Milk Chocolate Peanut Butter	2	171	8	5
Sugar Free White Chocolate Lemon	2	177	11	8
Larzaroni				
Arancelli	8 (1 oz)	160	8	tr
Calypso	3 (1 oz)	150	8	6
Limonelli	5 (1 oz)	140	8	5
Malaika	5 (1 oz)	158	9	tr
Nanette	4 (1.2 oz)	170	9	6
Okla	3 (1 oz)	186	10	tr
Oskar	10 (1 oz)	150	9	5
Samba	5 (1 oz)	160	10	9
Velieri	3 (0.9 oz)	120	5	3
Linden's				
Lemon	1 (1 oz)	120	5	1
Little Debbie				
Apple Flips	1 (1.2 oz)	150	5	2
Caramel Bars	1 (1.2 oz)	160	8	2
Cherry Cordials	1 (1.3 oz)	170	8	2
Coconut Rounds	1 (1.2 oz)	150	7	3
Cookie Wreaths	1 (0.6 oz)	100	5	1
Easter Puffs	1 (1.2 oz)	140	6	2
Fig Bars	1 (1.5 oz)	150	4	1
Fudge Delights	1 (1.1 oz)	110	2	0
Fudge Rounds	1 (1.2 oz)	140	6	2
German Chocolate Ring	1 (1 oz)	140	8	4
Ginger	1 (0.7 oz)	90	3	1
Jelly Creme Pies	1 (1.2 oz)	160	7	2

FOOD	PORTION	CALS	FAT	SAT FAT
Marshmallow Crispy Bar	1 (1.3 oz)	140	4	1
Marshmallow Supremes	1 (1.1 oz)	130	5	1
Marshmallow Pie Banana	1 pkg (1.5 oz)	180	6	2
Marshmallow Pie Chocolate	1 (1.4 oz)	160	6	3
Nutty Bar	1 (2 oz)	310	18	3
Oatmeal Raisin	1 (1.3 oz)	160	7	2
Oatmeal Creme Pie	1 (1.3 oz)	170	7	2
Oatmeal Delights	1 (1.1 oz)	110	2	0
Oatmeal Lights	1 (1.3 oz)	130	3	1
Peanut Butter Bars	1 (1.9 oz)	270	15	3
Peanut Butter & Jelly Oatmeal Pie	1 (1.1 oz)	130	5	1
Peanut Clusters	1 (1.4 oz)	190	11	2
Pumpkin Delights	1 (1.2 oz)	150	5	2
Raisin Creme Pie	1 (1.2 oz)	140	5	1
Star Crunch	1 (1.1 oz)	140	6	2
Sugar Free Chocolate Chip	3 (1.1 oz)	140	7	3
Sugar Free Oatmeal	6 (1.1 oz)	120	4	1
Yo-Yo's	1 (1.2 oz)	130	6	2
Low Carb Creations				
Chocolate Chip	1 (1 oz)	140	10	4
Coconut	1 (1 oz)	140	10	5
Lemon	1 (1 oz)	140	11	5
Snickerdoodle	1 (1 oz)	140	11	4
M&M's				
Cookies & Milky Way	1 bar (1.20 oz)	180	11	3
Mamma Says'				
Biscotti Almond Pistachio	1 (0.5 oz)	50	3	1
Biscotti Chocolate Macadamia	1 (0.5 oz)	45	3	1
Biscotti Orange Citrine	1 (0.5 oz)	60	2	1
Manischewitz				
Macaroons Chocolate	2 (0.9 oz)	90	4	4
Meringue				
Minis Chocolate Chip	13 (1 oz)	120	2	1
Milk Lunch Brand				
New England Biscuits	4 (1.1 oz)	140	5	1
Miss Meringue				
Minis Chocolate Raspberry	13 (1 oz)	80	0	0
Minis Mint Chocolate Chip	13 (1 oz)	120	2	1
Minis Mochaccino	13 (1 oz)	80	0	0

FOOD	PORTION	CALS	FAT	SAT FAT
Minis Orange	13 (1 oz)	80	0	0
Minis Rainbow Vanilla	13 (1 oz)	110	0	0
Minis Toasted Coconut	13 (1 oz)	90	2	1
Minis Very Chocolate	13 (1 oz)	80	0	0
Minis Very Minty	13 (1 oz)	80	0	0
Minis Very Vanilla	13 (1 oz)	80	0	0
MoonPie				
Chocolate	1 (2.75 oz)	330	10	6
Mini Banana	1 (1.2 oz)	152	5	3
Mini Chocolate	1 (1.2 oz)	152	5	3
Mini Vanilla	1 (1.2 oz)	152	5	3
Mother's				
Almond Shortbread	3	180	11	4
Checkerboard Wafers	8	150	8	5
Chocolate Chip	2	160	8	3
Chocolate Chip Angel	3	180	9	4
Chocolate Chip Parade	4	130	5	2
Circus Animals	6	140	6	5
Classic Assortments	2	140	7	4
Cocadas	5	150	7	3
Cookie Parade	4	140	7	3
Dinosaur Grrrahams	2	130	3	1
Double Fudge	2	180	9	5
English Tea	2	180	7	4
Flaky Flix Fudge	2	140	7	5
Flaky Flix Vanilla	2	140	8	5
Gaucho Peanut Butter	2	190	10	3
Iced Oatmeal	2	130	4	2
Iced Raisin	2	180	8	7
MLB Double Header Duplex	3	170	8	4
Macaroon	2	150	8	4
Marias	3	170	6	2
Oatmeal	2	110	5	2
Oatmeal Chocolate Chip	2	120	5	2
Oatmeal Raisin	5	150	7	2
Oatmeal Walnut Chocolate Chip	2	130	6	2
Rainbow Wafers	8	150	8	5
Striped Shortbread	3	170	8	5
Sugar	2	140	6	2
Taffy	2	180	8	2

FOOD	PORTION	CALS	FAT	SAT FAT
Triplet Assortment	2	140	7	3
Vanilla Wafers	6	150	6	2
Wallops Boysenberry	1	80	2	1
Wallops Honey Crust Fig	1	80	2	5
Wallops Honey Graham Fig	1	80	2	1
Wallops Mixed Berry	1	80	2	1
Wallops Peach Apricot	1	80	2	1
Wallops Raspberry	1	80	2	1
Wallops Strawberry	1	80	2	1
Walnut Fudge	2	130	7	3
Zoo Pals	14	140	5	2
Mrs. Alison's				
Coconut Bar	2 (1 oz)	130	6	1
Creme Wafers	5 (1.1 oz)	170	10	2
Duplex Sandwich	3 (1 oz)	130	5	2
Fudge Fingers	3 (1 oz)	160	10	6
Ginger Snaps	4 (1 oz)	130	3	1
Jelly Tops	5 (1 oz)	140	7	2
Lemon Creme	3 (1 oz)	130	5	2
Macaroons	2 (1 oz)	140	7	3
Pecan	2 (1 oz)	140	7	2
Shortbread	5 (1 oz)	120	5	1
Vanilla Sandwich	3 (1 oz)	130	5	1
Murray's				
Sugar Free Double Fudge	3 (1.2 oz)	140	6	3
Sugar Free Ginger Snap	6 (1 oz)	110	4	2
Sugar Free Peanut Butter	6 (1 oz)	130	7	2
Sugar Free Vanilla Sandwich Creme	3 (1 oz)	120	5	2
Sugar Free Vanilla Wafers	9 (1.1 oz)	120	4	1
Nabisco				
Barnum's Animal Crackers	10 (1 oz)	130	4	1
Barnum's Animal Crackers Chocolate	10 (1 oz)	130	4	1
Biscos Sugar Wafers	8 (1 oz)	140	6	2
Cafe Cremes Cappuccino	2 (1.1 oz)	160	8	2
Cafe Cremes Vanilla	2 (1.1 oz)	160	7	2
Cafe Cremes Vanilla Fudge	2 (1.1 oz)	200	10	2
Cameo	2 (1 oz)	130	5	1
Chips Ahoy!	3 (1.1 oz)	160	8	3
Chips Ahoy! Chewy	3 (1.3 oz)	170	8	3
Chips Ahoy! Chunky	1 (0.5 oz)	80	4	2

FOOD	PORTION	CALS	FAT	SAT FAT
Chips Ahoy! Munch Size	6 (1.1 oz)	160	8	2
Chips Ahoy! Reduced Fat	3 (1.1 oz)	140	5	2
Family Favorites Iced Oatmeal	1 (0.6 oz)	80	3	0
Family Favorites Oatmeal	1 (0.6 oz)	80	3	1
Famous Chocolate Wafers	5 (1.1 oz)	140	4	2
Grahams	4 (1 oz)	120	3	1
Honey Maid Chocolate	8 (1 oz)	120	3	1
Honey Maid Cinnamon Grahams	8 (1 oz)	120	3	0
Honey Maid Honey Grahams	8 (1 oz)	120	3	0
Honey Maid Low Fat Cinnamon Grahams	8 (1 oz)	110	2	0
Honey Maid Low Fat Grahams	8 (1 oz)	110	2	0
Honey Maid Oatmeal Crunch	8 (1 oz)	120	3	0
Lorna Doone	4 (1 oz)	140	7	1
Mallomars	2 (0.9 oz)	120	5	3
Marshmallow Twirls	1 (1 oz)	130	6	1
Mystic Mint	1 (0.5 oz)	90	5	1
National Arrowroot	1 (5 g)	20	1	–
Newtons Fat Free Fig	2 (1 oz)	90	0	0
Newtons Fig	2 (1.1 oz)	110	3	0
Newtons Fat Free Apple	2 (1 oz)	90	0	0
Newtons Fat Free Cobblers Apple Cinnamon	1 (0.8 oz)	70	0	0
Newtons Fat Free Cobblers Peach Apricot	1 (0.8 oz)	70	0	0
Newtons Fat Free Cranberry	2 (1 oz)	100	0	0
Newtons Fat Free Raspberry	2 (1 oz)	100	0	0
Newtons Fat Free Strawberry	2 (1 oz)	90	0	0
Nilla Wafers	8 (1.1 oz)	140	5	1
Nilla Wafers Chocolate Reduced Fat	8 (1 oz)	110	2	0
Nilla Wafers Reduced Fat	8 (1 oz)	120	2	0
Nutter Butter Bites	10 (1 oz)	150	7	1
Nutter Butter Chocolate Peanut Butter Sandwich	2 (1 oz)	130	5	1
Nutter Butter Peanut Butter Sandwich	2 (1 oz)	130	6	1
Old Fashioned Ginger Snaps	4 (1 oz)	120	3	1
Oreo	3 (1.2 oz)	160	7	2
Oreo Double Stuff	2 (1 oz)	140	7	2
Oreo Mini	1 pkg (0.5 oz)	65	3	1
Oreo Reduced Fat	3 (1.1 oz)	130	4	1

FOOD	PORTION	CALS	FAT	SAT FAT
Oreo Halloween	2 (1 oz)	140	7	2
Pecanz	1 (0.5 oz)	90	5	1
Pinwheels Chocolate Marshmallow	1 (1 oz)	130	5	3
Rugrats Chocolate Frosted	8 (1.1 oz)	150	5	2
Rugrats Vanilla Frosted	8 (1.1 oz)	150	6	2
Social Tea	6 (1 oz)	120	4	1
Sweet Crispers Chocolate	18 (1.1 oz)	130	3	1
Sweet Crispers Chocolate Chip	18 (1.1 oz)	130	3	1
Teddy Grahams Chocolate	24 (1 oz)	130	5	1
Teddy Grahams Chocolately Chip	24 (1 oz)	130	5	1
Teddy Grahams Cinnamon	24 (1 oz)	130	4	1
Teddy Grahams Honey	24 (1 oz)	130	4	1
Nestle				
Flipz Crunchy Graham White Fudge Chocolate	8 (1 oz)	140	6	5
Newman's Own				
Fig Newman's Organic	2 (1.3 oz)	120	0	0
Nonni's				
Biscotti Cioccalati	1 (1 oz)	130	5	3
Biscotti Decadence	1 (1.1 oz)	130	5	3
Biscotti Original	1 (1 oz)	100	4	2
Biscotti Paradiso	1 (1.1 oz)	130	6	3
NutraBalance				
Fibre Oatmeal Raisin	1 (0.7 oz)	80	4	1
Protein Fortified	1 (2 oz)	260	14	5
ReNeph Spice	1 (2 oz)	210	7	0
Old Brussels				
Ginger Crisps	2 (0.9 oz)	140	4	1
Old London				
Coffee Toppers Chocolate Creme	3 (0.5 oz)	70	3	2
Coffee Toppers Vanilla Creme	3 (0.5 oz)	70	4	3
Olde World				
Pizzelle Almond	3 (1 oz)	90	4	1
Pizzelle Anise	3 (1 oz)	90	4	1
Pizzelle Chocolate	3 (1 oz)	100	5	1
Pizzelle Lemon	3 (1 oz)	90	4	1
Pizzelle Vanilla	3 (1 oz)	90	4	1
Otis Spunkmeyer				
Butter Sugar	1 med (1.3 oz)	160	8	3
Butter Sugar	1 (2 oz)	250	12	5

FOOD	PORTION	CALS	FAT	SAT FAT
Carnival	1 med (1.3 oz)	170	7	3
Chocolate Chip	1 bite size (0.75 oz)	100	5	2
Chocolate Chip	1 med (1.3 oz)	170	8	4
Chocolate Chip	1 (2 oz)	250	11	6
Chocolate Chip Pecan	1 med (1.3 oz)	170	9	4
Chocolate Chip Walnut	1 bite size (0.75 oz)	100	5	3
Chocolate Chip Walnut	1 med (1.3 oz)	180	9	4
Chocolate Chip Walnut	1 (2 oz)	270	14	6
Double Chocolate Chip	1 bite size (0.75 oz)	100	5	3
Double Chocolate Chip	1 med (1.3 oz)	180	9	5
Oatmeal Raisin	1 bite size (0.75 oz)	90	4	3
Oatmeal Raisin	1 med (1.3 oz)	160	7	5
Otis Express Chocolate Chunk	1 (2 oz)	280	13	6
Otis Express Double Chocolate Chip	1 (2 oz)	270	14	7
Otis Express Oatmeal Raisin	1 (2 oz)	240	10	7
Otis Express Peanut Butter	1 (2 oz)	270	15	6
Peanut Butter	1 med (1.3 oz)	180	10	4
Pinnacle Checkpoint Chocolate Almond Coconut	1 (2.4 oz)	320	18	10
Pinnacle Mach One Mocha Chocolate Chunk	1 (2.4 oz)	300	13	6
Pinnacle Passport Peanut Butter Chocolate Chunk	1 (2.4 oz)	300	13	5
Pinnacle Ripcord Rocky Road	1 (2.4 oz)	310	15	6
Pinnacle Takeoff Triple Chocolate	1 (2.4 oz)	300	14	6
Pinnacle Transatlantic Turtle	1 (2.4 oz)	310	16	6
Travel Lite Low Fat Apple Cinnamon	1 (1.3 oz)	130	2	0
Travel Lite Low Fat Chocolate Chip	1 (1.3 oz)	130	2	1
Travel Lite Low Fat Ginger Spice	1 (1.3 oz)	130	2	0
Travel Lite Low Fat Oatmeal Rum Raisin	1 (1.3 oz)	130	2	0
White Chocolate Macadamia Nut	1 med (1.3 oz)	180	10	4
White Chocolate Macadamia Nut	1 (2 oz)	280	15	7
Pally				
Butter	5 (1 oz)	140	3	2
Carnival	5 (1 oz)	130	3	1
Cinnamon Biscuit	5 (1 oz)	130	3	1
Mariel Biscuit	6 (1 oz)	150	4	1
Tea Biscuits	5 (1 oz)	150	4	1

FOOD	PORTION	CALS	FAT	SAT FAT
Pamela's				
Pecan Shortbread Rice Flour	1 (0.8 oz)	130	8	4
Parmalat				
Grisbi Lemon	1 (0.6 oz)	90	6	2
Peek Freans				
Arrowroot	4 (1.2 oz)	150	5	1
Assorted Creme	1 (1 oz)	130	6	3
Dream Puffs	2 (0.9 oz)	110	4	3
Fruit Creme	2 (0.9 oz)	130	5	2
Ginger Crisp	4 (1.2 oz)	150	4	1
Nice	4 (1.2 oz)	160	6	3
Petit Beret Creme Caramel	2 (0.8 oz)	110	5	4
Petit Beret Fudge Truffle	2 (0.8 oz)	110	5	4
Petit Beurre	4 (1 oz)	130	4	2
Rich Tea	4 (1.2 oz)	160	5	2
Shortcake	2 (0.9 oz)	140	7	3
Traditional Oatmeal	1 (0.7 oz)	90	3	1
Tropical Cremes Calypso Lime	2 (0.9 oz)	130	5	2
Pepperidge Farm				
Biscotti Almond	1 (0.7 oz)	90	4	1
Biscotti Chocolate Hazelnut	1 (0.7 oz)	90	5	1
Biscotti Cranberry Pistachio	1 (0.7 oz)	90	3	1
Bordeaux	4	130	5	3
Brussels	2	100	5	2
Chantilly Raspberry	2 (1 oz)	120	3	1
Chessman	3	120	8	3
Chocoate Chunk Soft Baked Double Chocolate	1 (0.9 oz)	130	7	3
Chocolate Chip	3	140	7	3
Chocolate Chunk Chesapeake	1 (0.7 oz)	140	8	3
Chocolate Chunk Minis Nantucket	1 pkg (1.75 oz)	260	13	5
Chocolate Chunk Minis Sausalito	4 (1 oz)	160	9	4
Chocolate Chunk Montauk	1 (0.9 oz)	130	7	3
Chocolate Chunk Nantucket	1 (0.9 oz)	140	7	3
Chocolate Chunk Sausalito	1 (0.7 oz)	140	8	3
Chocolate Chunk Soft Baked	1	130	6	3
Chocolate Chunk Soft Baked Milk Chocolate Macadamia	1	130	7	3

FOOD	PORTION	CALS	FAT	SAT FAT
Chocolate Chunk Soft Baked Reduced Fat	1	110	5	2
Chocolate Chunk Soft Baked White Chocolate Pecan	1	120	5	2
Chocolate Chunk Tahoe	1 (0.9 oz)	130	8	3
Fruitful Apricot Raspberry Cup	3	140	6	2
Fruitful Strawberry Cup	3	140	5	2
Geneva	3	160	9	4
Ginger Man	4 (1 oz)	130	4	1
Goldfish Grahams Cinnamon	1 pkg (1.75 oz)	240	10	4
Lemon Nut Crunch	3	170	9	2
Lido	1	90	5	2
Milano	3	180	10	4
Milano Endless Chocolate	3	180	10	5
Milano Milk Chocolate	3	170	9	4
Milano Double Chocolate	2 (0.7 oz)	140	8	3
Milano Mint	2	130	7	4
Milano Orange	2	130	7	3
Pirouettes Chocolate Laced	5 (1.1 oz)	180	10	3
Pirouettes Traditional	5 (1.2 oz)	170	9	3
Shortbread	2	140	7	—
Soft Baked Oatmeal Raisin	1 (0.9 oz)	130	7	3
Soft Baked Reduced Fat Oatmeal Raisin	1 (0.9 oz)	100	3	1
Spritzers Cool Key Lime	6 (1.1 oz)	140	7	2
Spritzers Ripe Red Raspberry	5 (1.1 oz)	140	7	2
Spritzers Zesty Lemon	5 (1.1 oz)	140	7	2
Sugar	3	140	6	2
Verona Strawberry	3 (1.1 oz)	140	5	2
Pure De-Lite				
High Protein Chocolate Fudge	1 (2.2 oz)	210	8	2
High Protein Peanut Butter Crunch	1 (2.2 oz)	210	8	2
Ralston				
Animal	12 (0.9 oz)	130	3	1
Chocolate Grahams	2 (0.9 oz)	130	3	1
Cinnamon Grahams	2 (0.9 oz)	130	5	1
Cinnamon Grahams Low Fat	2 (0.9 oz)	110	2	0
Fig Bars	2 (1.2 oz)	120	3	0
Vanilla Wafers	7 (1.1 oz)	150	6	1

FOOD	PORTION	CALS	FAT	SAT FAT
Real Torino				
Lady Fingers	3 (1 oz)	110	1	0
Reko				
Pizzelle Maple	5 (1 oz)	150	6	1
Pizzelle Vanilla	1 (6 g)	30	1	tr
Royal				
Apple Bars	1 (1.1 oz)	100	2	0
Apple Cake	1 (1.1 oz)	110	3	1
Brownie Rounds	1 (1.1 oz)	130	6	2
Chocolate Chip	1 (1.1 oz)	140	6	2
Devilfood	1 (1 oz)	110	5	1
Fig Bars	1 (1.1 oz)	100	2	0
Oatmeal	1 (1.1 oz)	130	6	1
Raisin	1 (1 oz)	110	5	1
Strawberry Bars	1 (1.1 oz)	100	2	0
Salerno				
Mini Butter	25 (1 oz)	180	6	3
Mini Dinosaur Chocolate Graham	16 (1.1 oz)	140	5	2
Scooter Pie	1 (1.2 oz)	140	5	3
Santa Fe Farms				
Chocolate Chocolate Chip Fat Free	2 (1 oz)	60	0	0
Chocolate Mint Fat Free	2 (1 oz)	60	0	0
Ginger Fat Free	2 (1 oz)	70	0	0
Sargento				
MooTown Snackers Honey Graham Sticks & Vanilla Creme w/ Sprinkles	1 pkg (1 oz)	140	7	1
MooTown Snackers Vanilla Sticks & Chocolate Fudge Creme	1 pkg (1 oz)	130	6	2
Savion				
Chocolate Biscuits	5 (1 oz)	120	3	1
Tea Biscuits	5 (1 oz)	120	3	1
Tea Biscuits Vanilla	5 (1 oz)	120	3	1
Scotto's				
Biscotti Fat Free French Vanilla	4 (1 oz)	80	0	0
Season				
Hamantashen Poppy	1 (1 oz)	150	7	4
Hamantashen Apricot	1 (1 oz)	150	7	4
Simple Pleasures				
Almond	1 (0.3 oz)	37	2	tr
Cinnamon Snaps	1 (0.2 oz)	31	1	tr

FOOD	PORTION	CALS	FAT	SAT FAT
Digestive	1 (0.3 oz)	46	2	tr
Encore Tea Cookie	1 (0.2 oz)	29	1	tr
Lemon Social Tea	1 (0.2 oz)	29	1	tr
Oatmeal	1 (0.5 oz)	74	3	1
Spice Snaps	1 (0.3 oz)	34	1	tr
Sugar	1 (0.4 oz)	45	2	1
SnackWell's				
Bite Size Chocolate Chip	13 (1 oz)	130	4	2
Bite Size Double Chocolate Chip	13 (1 oz)	130	4	2
Chocolate Sandwich	2 (0.8 oz)	110	3	1
Creme Sandwich	1 pkg (1.7 oz)	210	5	1
Fat Free Devil's Food	1 (0.5 oz)	50	0	0
Golden Devil's Food	1 (0.5 oz)	50	1	0
Mint Creme	2 (0.9 oz)	110	4	1
Oatmeal Raisin	2 (0.9 oz)	110	3	0
Sugar Free Chocolate Chip	3 (1.2 oz)	150	8	3
Sugar Free Oatmeal	1 (0.8 oz)	90	3	1
Soybite				
All Flavors	1	79	5	1
Stella D'Oro				
Almond Toast Mandel	2 (1 oz)	110	3	1
Angel Wings	2 (0.9 oz)	140	9	3
Angelica	1 (0.8 oz)	100	4	1
Anginetti	4 (1.1 oz)	140	4	1
Anisette Sponge	2 (0.9 oz)	90	1	0
Anisette Toast	3 (1.2 oz)	130	1	0
Biscotti Almond	1 (0.8 oz)	100	3	1
Biscotti Chocolate Almond	1 (0.8 oz)	90	3	1
Biscotti Chocolate Chunk	1 (0.8 oz)	90	3	1
Biscotti Hazelnut	1 (0.8 oz)	100	4	1
Biscottini Cashews	1 (0.7 oz)	110	6	1
Breakfast Treats	1 (0.8 oz)	100	3	1
Breakfast Treats Chocolate	1 (0.8 oz)	100	4	1
Breakfast Treats Viennese Cinnamon	1 (0.8 oz)	100	3	1
Chinese Dessert Cookies	1 (1.2 oz)	170	9	2
Chocolate Castelets	2 (1 oz)	130	6	2
Egg Jumbo	2 (0.8 oz)	90	1	0
Fruit Slices Fat Free	1 (0.6 oz)	50	0	0
Kichel Low Sodium	21 (1 oz)	150	9	2
Lady Stella Assortment	3 (1 oz)	130	5	2

FOOD	PORTION	CALS	FAT	SAT FAT
Margherite Chocolate	2 (1.1 oz)	140	6	2
Margherite Vanilla	2 (1.1 oz)	140	5	1
Roman Egg Biscuits	1 (1.2 oz)	140	5	2
Sesame Regina	3 (1.1 oz)	150	6	2
Swiss Fudge	2 (0.9 oz)	130	7	2
Stieffenhofer				
Choco Minis	4 (1 oz)	160	8	5
Snaky	3 (1 oz)	160	8	2
Streit's				
Wafers	3 (1 oz)	160	9	2
Suissette				
Swiss Chocolate Hearts	4 (1 oz)	170	10	6
Swiss Delight	4 (1 oz)	160	9	4
Swiss Praline	4 (1 oz)	150	9	6
Sunshine				
All American Butter	5 (1.1 oz)	140	6	2
All American Lemon Coolers	5 (1 oz)	140	6	2
All American Mini Chip-A-Roos	5 (1.1 oz)	160	8	3
Animal Crackers	14 (1.1 oz)	140	4	1
Ginger Snaps	7 (1 oz)	130	5	1
Golden Fruit Cranberry	1 (0.7 oz)	80	2	0
Golden Fruit Raisin	1 (0.7 oz)	80	2	1
Hydrox	3 (1.1 oz)	150	7	2
Hydrox Reduced Fat	3 (1.1 oz)	140	5	2
Oatmeal Country Style	2 (0.8 oz)	120	5	1
Sugar Wafers Peanut Butter Creme	4 (1.1 oz)	170	9	2
Sugar Wafers Vanilla Creme	3 (0.9 oz)	130	6	2
Vanilla Wafers	7 (1.1 oz)	150	7	2
Vienna Fingers	2 (1 oz)	140	6	2
Vienna Fingers Lemon	2 (1 oz)	140	6	2
Vienna Fingers Reduced Fat	2 (1 oz)	130	5	1
Super Chip				
Chocolate Chip	2 (0.9 oz)	100	7	–
Sweet'N Low				
Sugar Free Amaretto Biscotti	4 (1 oz)	120	6	1
Sugar Free Chocolate Chip	4 (1 oz)	135	8	1
Sugar Free Cinnamon Graham	7 (1 oz)	120	6	1
Sugar Free Morning Crunch Bars	2 (1 oz)	120	6	1
Sugar Free Vanilla Wafers	7 (1 oz)	120	6	1

FOOD	PORTION	CALS	FAT	SAT FAT
Sweetzels				
Chocolate Chip	7 (1 oz)	160	9	4
Ginger Snaps	4 (1.2 oz)	140	3	1
Vanilla Wafers	7 (1.1 oz)	137	5	1
Tastykake				
Chocolate Chip	1 (1.4 oz)	180	7	2
Chocolate Chip Bar	1 (2 oz)	270	12	4
Chocolate Fudge Iced	1 (1.4 oz)	170	7	2
Fudge Bar	1 (2 oz)	250	10	2
Lemon Bar	1 (2 oz)	260	10	1
Oatmeal Raisin Bar	1 (2 oz)	260	10	3
Oatmeal Raisin Boxed	3 (0.4 oz)	130	6	2
Oatmeal Raisin Iced	1 (1.4 oz)	170	6	2
Strawberry Bar	1 (2 oz)	260	10	1
Sugar Boxed	3 (0.4 oz)	120	6	2
The Source				
Barry's Raspberry Palmiers	1 (0.7 oz)	80	3	0
Tom's				
Animal Crackers	½ pkg (1 oz)	120	2	1
Big Cookie Chocolate Chip	1 pkg (2.75 oz)	340	16	5
Big Cookie Peanut Butter Chocolate Chip	1 pkg (2 oz)	280	15	5
Chocolate Chip	1 pkg (2 oz)	280	15	5
Confetti Chip	1 pkg (2 oz)	300	13	6
Fat Free Apple Bar	1 pkg (1.75 oz)	160	0	0
Fat Free Fig Bar	1 pkg (1.75 oz)	160	0	0
Vanilla Wafers	½ pkg (1 oz)	130	5	1
Tree Of Life				
Fat Free Almond Butter	1 (0.8 oz)	60	0	0
Fat Free Carrot Cake	1 (0.8 oz)	60	0	0
Fat Free Devil's Food Chocolate	1 (0.8 oz)	70	0	0
Fat Free Oatmeal Raisin	1 (0.8 oz)	70	0	0
Fruit Bars Fat Free Fig	1 (0.8 oz)	70	0	0
Fruit Bars Fat Free Peach Apricot	1 (0.8 oz)	70	0	0
Fruit Bars Fat Free Wildberry	1 (0.8 oz)	70	0	0
Monster Carob Chip	1 (4.7 oz)	700	35	10
Monster Granola	1 (4.7 oz)	700	30	10
Monster Macaroon	1 (4.7 oz)	750	45	20
Monster Peanut Butter	1 (4.7 oz)	700	35	10
Monster Fat Free Carrot Cake	1 cookie (3.8 oz)	240	0	0

FOOD	PORTION	CALS	FAT	SAT FAT
Monster Fat Free Devil's Food Chocolate	1 cookie (3.8 oz)	320	0	0
Monster Fat Free Gingerbread	1 cookie (3.8 oz)	320	0	0
Monster Fat Free Maple Pecan	1 cookie (3.8 oz)	360	0	0
Oatmeal	1 (0.8 oz)	100	4	2
Sandwich Royal Vanilla	2 (0.9 oz)	120	5	0
Wheat Free Carob	1 (0.8 oz)	100	5	0
Wheat Free Maple Walnut	1 (0.8 oz)	100	6	0
Wheat Free Oatmeal	1 (0.8 oz)	90	5	0
Wheat Free Peanut Butter	1 (0.8 oz)	109	6	0
Twix				
Bars Chocolate Caramel	1 (0.9 oz)	140	7	3
Voortman				
Almonette	2 (1 oz)	150	8	2
Chocolate Chip	1 (0.7 oz)	100	5	2
Chocolate Wafers Sugar Free	3 (1 oz)	160	11	3
Coconut Delight	1 (0.6 oz)	90	5	3
Peanut Delight	1 (0.9 oz)	130	7	2
Strawberry Wafers Sugar Free	3 (1 oz)	160	11	3
Sugar	1 (0.6 oz)	80	4	1
Turnovers Blueberry	1 (0.9 oz)	100	3	1
Turnovers Cherry	1 (0.9 oz)	100	3	1
Turnovers Strawberry	1 (0.9 oz)	100	3	1
Vanilla Wafers Sugar Free	3 (1 oz)	160	11	3
Windmill	1 (0.7 oz)	90	4	1
Walkers				
Shortbread Triangles	2 (0.7 oz)	100	6	4
Weight Watchers				
Apple Raisin Bar	1 (0.75 oz)	70	2	1
Chocolate Chip	2 (1.06 oz)	140	5	2
Chocolate Sandwich	2 (1.06)	140	4	1
Fruit Filled Fig	1 (0.7 oz)	70	0	0
Fruit Filled Raspberry	1 (0.7 oz)	70	0	0
Oatmeal Raisin	2 (1.06 oz)	120	2	0
Vanilla Sandwich	2 (1.06 oz)	140	3	1
White Eagle Bakery				
Chruscik	2 (1 oz)	140	8	3
Wortz				
Animal	9 (1.1 oz)	140	5	1
Chocolate Graham	2 (0.9 oz)	130	3	1

FOOD	PORTION	CALS	FAT	SAT FAT
Cinnamon Grahams	2 (0.9 oz)	130	5	1
Vanilla Wafers	7 (1.1 oz)	150	6	1
REFRIGERATED				
chocolate chip	1 (0.42 oz)	59	3	1
chocolate chip unbaked	1 oz	126	6	2
oatmeal	1 (0.4 oz)	56	3	1
oatmeal raisin	1 (0.4 oz)	56	3	1
peanut butter	1 (0.4 oz)	60	3	1
peanut butter dough	1 oz	130	7	2
sugar	1 (0.42 oz)	58	3	1
sugar dough	1 oz	124	6	2
Pillsbury				
Bunny	2	130	7	2
Chocolate Chip	1 (1 oz)	130	6	3
Chocolate Chip Reduced Fat	1 (1 oz)	110	3	2
Chocolate Chip w/ Walnuts	1 (1 oz)	140	7	2
Chocolate Chunk	1 (1 oz)	130	6	2
Christmas Tree	2	130	7	2
Double Chocolate	1 (1 oz)	130	6	2
Flag	2	130	7	2
Frosty	2	130	7	2
M&M's	1 (1 oz)	130	6	2
Oatmeal Chocolate Chip	1 (1 oz)	120	6	2
One Step Pan Chocolate Chip	⅛ pan (1 oz)	130	6	2
One Step Pan M&M's	⅛ pan (1 oz)	130	6	2
Peanut Butter	1 (1 oz)	120	6	2
Pumpkin	2	130	7	2
Reeses	1 (1 oz)	130	6	3
Shamrock	2	130	7	2
Sugar	2	130	3	2
Sugar Holiday Red & Green	2	130	6	2
Valentine	2	130	7	2
White Chocolate Chunk	1 (1 oz)	130	6	2
TAKE-OUT				
biscotti with nuts chocolate dipped	1 (1.3 oz)	117	6	3
black & white	1 lg (3 oz)	302	9	5
finikia	1 (1.2 oz)	171	5	5
koulourakia butter cookie twist	1 (0.9 oz)	113	6	3
linzer tart	1 (2.4 oz)	280	14	4

FOOD	PORTION	CALS	FAT	SAT FAT
CORIANDER				
leaf dried	1 tsp	2	tr	–
leaf fresh	¼ cup	1	tr	–
seed	1 tsp	5	tr	tr
Instant India				
Tomato Coriander Paste	2 tbsp (1 oz)	90	6	1
CORN				
CANNED				
cream style	½ cup	93	1	tr
w/ red & green peppers	½ cup	86	1	tr
white	½ cup	66	1	tr
yellow	½ cup	66	1	tr
Del Monte				
Cream Style Golden	½ cup (4.4 oz)	90	1	0
Cream Style Golden No Salt Added	½ cup (4.4 oz)	60	1	0
Cream Style White	½ cup (4.4 oz)	100	1	0
Fiesta	½ cup (4.4 oz)	50	1	0
Gold & White Supersweet	½ cup (4.4 oz)	80	1	0
Whole Kernel Golden	½ cup (4.4 oz)	90	1	0
Whole Kernel Golden Supersweet No Salt Added	½ cup (4.4 oz)	70	1	0
Whole Kernel Golden Supersweet No Salt Added	½ cup (4.4 oz)	60	1	0
Whole Kernel Golden Supersweet No Sugar	½ cup (4.4 oz)	60	1	0
Whole Kernel Golden Supersweet Vacuum Packed	½ cup (3.7 oz)	70	1	0
Whole Kernel White Sweet	½ cup (4.4 oz)	60	1	0
Green Giant				
Cream Style	½ cup (4.5 oz)	100	1	0
Mexicorn	⅓ cup (2.7 oz)	60	0	0
Niblets	⅓ cup (2.7 oz)	70	0	0
Niblets 50% Less Sodium	⅓ cup (2.7 oz)	60	0	0
Niblets Extra Sweet	⅓ cup (2.6 oz)	50	1	0
Niblets No Added Sugar or Salt	⅓ cup (2.7 oz)	60	0	0
White Shoepeg	⅓ cup	80	1	0
Whole Sweet	½ cup (4.3 oz)	80	1	0
Whole Sweet 50% Less Sodium	½ cup (4.2 oz)	80	1	0

FOOD	PORTION	CALS	FAT	SAT FAT
S&W				
Cream Style	½ cup (4.4 oz)	60	1	0
Whole Kernel	⅓ cup (3 oz)	70	2	0
Veg-All				
Whole Kernel	½ cup	80	1	0
DRIED				
Goya				
Giant White	⅓ cup (1.6 oz)	160	2	1
FRESH				
on-the-cob w/ butter cooked	1 ear	155	3	2
white cooked	½ cup	89	1	tr
white raw	½ cup	66	1	tr
yellow cooked	1 ear (2.7 oz)	83	1	tr
yellow cooked	½ cup	89	1	tr
yellow raw	½ cup	66	1	tr
yellow raw	1 ear (3 oz)	77	1	tr
FROZEN				
cooked	½ cup	67	tr	tr
on-the-cob cooked	1 ear (2.2 oz)	59	tr	tr
Birds Eye				
Cob Big Ear	1 ear	120	1	0
Cut	⅓ cup	70	1	0
Gold & White Blend	½ cup (3.5 oz)	60	1	0
Cut	3.5 oz	85	1	—
Fresh Like				
On The Cob	1 ear (3 in)	96	1	—
Green Giant				
Butter Sauce Niblets	⅔ cup (4.3 oz)	130	3	2
Butter Sauce Shoepeg White	¾ cup (4 oz)	120	3	2
Cream Corn	½ cup (4.1 oz)	110	1	0
Extra Sweet Niblets	⅔ cup (3.1 oz)	70	1	0
Harvest Fresh Niblets	⅔ cup (3.4 oz)	80	1	0
Harvest Fresh Shoepeg White	½ cup (2.6 oz)	70	1	0
Niblets	⅔ cup (2.9 oz)	80	1	0
On The Cob Extra Sweet	1 ear (4.4 oz)	120	2	0
On The Cob Nibblers	1 ear (2.1 oz)	70	1	0
On The Cob Niblets	1 ear (5 oz)	160	2	0
Select Extra Sweet White	⅔ cup (2.9 oz)	50	1	0
Select Shoepeg White	¾ cup (3.2 oz)	100	1	0

FOOD	PORTION	CALS	FAT	SAT FAT
Stouffer's				
Souffle	½ cup (6 oz)	170	7	2
Tree Of Life				
Corn	⅔ cup (3.2 oz)	80	1	0
TAKE-OUT				
fritters	1 (1 oz)	62	2	tr
scalloped	½ cup	258	7	1

CORN CHIPS (see CHIPS)

CORNISH HEN (see CHICKEN)

CORNMEAL

FOOD	PORTION	CALS	FAT	SAT FAT
corn grits cooked	1 cup	146	tr	tr
corn grits uncooked	1 cup	579	2	tr
white	1 cup (4.8 oz)	505	2	tr
whole grain	1 cup (4.3 oz)	442	4	1
yellow	1 cup (4.8 oz)	505	2	tr
yellow self-rising	1 cup (4.3 oz)	407	4	1
Albers				
White	3 tbsp	110	0	0
Yellow	3 tbsp	110	0	0
Expert Foods				
Low Carb Grits Mix	1½ tsp	15	0	0
Hodgson Mill				
Cornbread Mix Jalapeno Mexican	¼ cup (1 oz)	100	1	0
Yellow Organic	¼ cup (1 oz)	100	1	0
Yellow Self Rising	¼ cup (1 oz)	90	1	0
Kentucky Kernal				
Sweet Cornbread Mix	¼ cup (1 oz)	120	2	0
McKenzie's				
Hush Puppies	1 serv (1.9 oz)	190	10	3
Quaker				
Yellow	3 tbsp (1 oz)	90	1	—
TAKE-OUT				
hush puppies	1 (0.75 oz)	74	3	tr

CORNSTARCH

FOOD	PORTION	CALS	FAT	SAT FAT
cornstarch	1 cup (4.5 oz)	488	tr	tr
Argo				
Cornstarch	1 tbsp (8 g)	30	0	0
Cornstarch	1 cup (128 g)	460	tr	0

FOOD	PORTION	CALS	FAT	SAT FAT
Armour				
Cream Cornstarch	1 tbsp (0.4 oz)	40	0	0
COTTAGE CHEESE				
creamed	1 cup (7.4 oz)	217	9	6
creamed	4 oz	117	5	3
creamed w/ fruit	4 oz	140	4	2
dry curd	1 cup (5.1 oz)	123	1	tr
dry curd	4 oz	96	tr	tr
lowfat 1%	4 oz	82	1	1
lowfat 1%	1 cup (7.9 oz)	164	2	1
lowfat 2%	4 oz	101	2	1
lowfat 2%	1 cup (7.9 oz)	203	4	3
Breakstone's				
2% Fat Large Curd	½ cup (4.2 oz)	90	3	2
2% Fat Small Curd	½ cup (4.2 oz)	90	3	2
4% Fat Large Curd	½ cup (4.2 oz)	120	5	3
4% Fat Small Curd	½ cup (4.2 oz)	120	5	3
Cottage Doubles Peach	1 pkg (5.5 oz)	140	3	2
Dry Curd	¼ cup (1.9 oz)	45	0	0
Free	½ cup (4.4 oz)	80	0	0
Snack 2% Fat Small Curd	1 pkg (4 oz)	90	2	2
Snack 4% Fat Small Curd	1 pkg (4 oz)	110	5	3
Snack Free	1 pkg (4 oz)	70	0	0
Cabot				
Cottage Cheese	½ cup	100	5	3
No Fat	½ cup	70	0	0
Horizon Organic				
Cottage Cheese	½ cup (3.9 oz)	110	5	3
Knudsen				
1.5% Fat Small Curd Pineapple	½ cup (4.6 oz)	120	2	1
2% Fat Small Curd	½ cup (4.2 oz)	100	3	2
4% Fat Large Curd	½ cup (4.5 oz)	130	5	4
4% Fat Small Curd	½ cup (4.3 oz)	120	5	4
Free	½ cup (4.2 oz)	80	0	0
On The Go! 1.5% Fat Peach	1 pkg (4 oz)	110	2	1
On The Go! 1.5% Fat Pineapple	1 pkg (4 oz)	110	2	1
On The Go! 1.5% Fat Strawberry	1 pkg (4 oz)	110	2	1
On The Go! 1.5% Fat Tropical Fruit	1 pkg (4 oz)	110	2	2
On The Go! 2% Fat	1 pkg (4 oz)	90	2	2

FOOD	PORTION	CALS	FAT	SAT FAT
On The Go! Free	1 pkg (4 oz)	70	0	0
Light N'Lively				
1% Fat	½ cup (4 oz)	80	1	1
1% Fat Garden Salad	½ cup (4.2 oz)	80	2	1
1% Fat Peach & Pineapple	½ cup (4.3 oz)	110	1	1
Fat Free	½ cup (4.4 oz)	80	0	0
COTTONSEED				
kernels roasted	1 tbsp	51	4	1
COUGH DROPS				
Lifesavers				
Menthol	2 (0.5 oz)	60	0	0
COUSCOUS				
cooked	1 cup (5.5 oz)	176	tr	tr
dry	1 cup (6.1 oz)	650	1	tr
Kitchen Del Sol				
Spicy Vegetable as prep	½ cup (1.1 oz)	120	3	tr
Tomato & Olive	½ cup (1.1 oz)	120	4	1
Melting Pot				
Calypso Cranberry	1 cup	200	0	0
Lentil Curry	1 cup	170	0	0
Lucky Seven	1 cup	190	1	0
Mango Salsa	1 cup	190	0	0
Roasted Garlic	1 cup	170	0	0
Sesame Ginger	1 cup	180	1	0
Sun-Dried Tomatoes	1 cup	190	1	0
Wild Mushroom	1 cup	190	0	0
Near East				
Parmesan as prep	1 cup	220	4	2
COWPEAS				
catjang dried cooked	1 cup (2.9 oz)	200	1	tr
common canned	1 cup	184	1	tr
frozen cooked	½ cup	112	tr	tr
leafy tips chopped cooked	1 cup	12	tr	tr
leafy tips raw chopped	1 cup	10	tr	tr

FOOD	PORTION	CALS	FAT	SAT FAT
CRAB				
CANNED				
blue	1 cup	133	2	tr
blue	3 oz	84	1	tr
Bumble Bee				
Fancy Lump Meat	½ can (1.9 oz)	40	1	0
Fancy White Meat	½ can (1.9 oz)	28	0	0
FRESH				
alaska king cooked	1 leg (4.7 oz)	129	2	tr
alaska king cooked	3 oz	82	1	tr
alaska king raw	3 oz	71	1	—
alaska king raw	1 leg (6 oz)	144	1	—
blue cooked	1 cup	138	2	tr
blue cooked	3 oz	87	2	tr
blue raw	3 oz	74	1	tr
blue raw	1 crab (7 oz)	18	tr	tr
dungeness raw	1 crab (5.7 oz)	140	2	tr
dungeness raw	3 oz	73	1	tr
queen steamed	3 oz	98	1	tr
TAKE-OUT				
baked	1 (3.8 oz)	160	2	tr
cake	1 (2 oz)	160	10	2
kenagi korean crab cooked	1 serv (3 oz)	71	tr	—
mousse	¼ cup	364	20	—
soft-shell fried	1 (4.4 oz)	334	18	4
CRACKER CRUMBS				
chocolate wafer cookie crumbs	½ cup (5.9 oz)	728	25	6
cracker meal	1 cup (4 oz)	440	2	tr
graham cracker crumbs	½ cup (4.4 oz)	540	13	3
Baker's Harvest				
Graham	⅓ cup (1 oz)	130	4	1
Kellogg's				
Corn Flake Crumbs	2 tbsp (0.4 oz)	40	0	0
Nabisco				
Nilla Cookie Crumbs	2 tbsp (0.5 oz)	70	3	1
CRACKERS				
cheese	14 (½ oz)	71	4	1
cheese	1 (1 in sq) (1 g)	5	tr	tr
cheese low sodium	14 (½ oz)	71	4	1

FOOD	PORTION	CALS	FAT	SAT FAT
cheese low sodium	1 (1 in sq) (1 g)	5	tr	tr
cheese w/ peanut butter filling	1 (0.24 oz)	34	2	tr
crispbread	3	61	2	–
crispbread rye	1 (0.35 oz)	37	tr	tr
crispbread rye	3	77	1	–
melba toast plain	1 (5 g)	19	tr	tr
melba toast pumpernickel	1 (5 g)	19	tr	tr
melba toast rye	1 (5 g)	19	tr	tr
melba toast wheat	1 (5 g)	19	tr	tr
milk	1 (0.42 oz)	55	2	tr
oyster cracker	1 (1 g)	4	tr	tr
peanut butter sandwich	1 (7 g)	34	2	tr
rusk toast	1 (0.35 oz)	41	1	tr
rye w/ cheese filling	1 (0.24 oz)	34	2	tr
rye wafers plain	1 (0.9 oz)	84	tr	tr
rye wafers seasoned	1 (0.8 oz)	84	2	tr
saltines	1 (3 g)	13	tr	tr
saltines fat free low sodium	3 (0.5 oz)	59	tr	tr
saltines fat free low sodium	6 (1 oz)	118	tr	tr
saltines low salt	1 (3 g)	13	tr	tr
snack cracker	1 (3 g)	15	1	tr
snack cracker low salt	1 (3 g)	15	1	tr
snack cracker w/ cheese filling	1 (7 g)	33	2	tr
soup cracker	1 (1 g)	4	tr	tr
water biscuits	3	92	3	–
wheat w/ cheese filling	1 (0.24 oz)	35	2	tr
wheat w/ peanut butter filling	1 (0.24 oz)	35	2	tr
wheat thins	1 (2 g)	9	tr	tr
wheat thins	7 (0.5 oz)	67	3	1
wheat thins low salt	7 (0.5 oz)	67	3	1
whole wheat	1 (4 g)	18	1	tr
whole wheat low salt	1 (4 g)	18	1	tr
zwieback	1 oz	107	1	–
Ak-mak				
100% Whole Wheat	5 (1 oz)	116	2	tr
Armenian Cracker Bread	1 sheet (1 oz)	100	2	1
Armenian Cracker Bread Whole Wheat	1 sheet (1 oz)	116	2	tr
Round Cracker Bread No Seeds	1 (1 oz)	100	1	1

FOOD	PORTION	CALS	FAT	SAT FAT
Round Cracker Bread Seeded	1 (1 oz)	100	2	1
Round Cracker Bread Whole Wheat	1 (1 oz)	116	2	tr
American Vintage				
Wine Biscuits All Flavors	5	140	7	1
Andre's				
CarboSave Crackerbread All Flavors	1 oz	140	8	1
Austin				
Cracker Sandwich Cheese On Cheese	6 (1.3 oz)	170	7	2
Cracker Sandwich Cheese Peanut Butter	6 (1.3 oz)	170	7	2
Cracker Sandwich Toasty Peanut Butter	6 (1.3 oz)	170	7	2
Cracker Sandwich Whole Wheat Cheese	6 (1.3 oz)	170	7	2
Baker's Harvest				
Cheese	23 (1 oz)	150	6	2
Cheese Reduced Fat	29 (1 oz)	130	4	1
Oyster	35 (0.5 oz)	70	2	0
Saltines Unsalted	5 (0.5 oz)	70	2	—
Saltines Deluxe	5 (0.5 oz)	60	2	—
Snackers	9 (1.1 oz)	160	8	2
Snackers Reduced Fat	10 (1.1 oz)	140	4	1
Snackers Unsalted	9 (1.1 oz)	160	8	2
Wheat Snacks	16 (1 oz)	140	6	1
Wheat Snacks Reduced Fat	16 (1.1 oz)	140	4	1
Woven Wheats	7 (1.1 oz)	140	5	1
Woven Wheats Reduced Fat	8 (1.1 oz)	130	3	1
Barbara's Bakery				
Cheese Bites	26 (1 oz)	120	2	0
Right Lite Rounds Original	5 (0.5 oz)	55	5	tr
Rite Lite Rounds Savory Poppy	5 (0.5 oz)	70	2	0
Rite Lite Rounds Tamari Sesame	5 (0.5 oz)	70	2	0
Wheatines All Flavors	1 lg sq (0.5 oz)	50	2	0
Blue Diamond				
Nut Thins Almond	16 (1 oz)	130	5	0
Nut Thins Hazelnut	16 (1 oz)	120	4	0
Nut Thins Pecan	16 (1 oz)	130	5	0
Bran-A-Crisp				
Low Carb Wheat Bran	1	20	0	0

FOOD	PORTION	CALS	FAT	SAT FAT
Breton				
Cabaret	3 (5 g)	70	4	2
Light	1 (5 g)	20	1	tr
Minis	20 (0.6 oz)	89	4	2
Minis Cheddar Cheese	20 (0.6 oz)	87	4	3
Minis Garden Vegetable	20 (0.6 oz)	87	4	3
Multi-Grain	3	70	4	2
Original	3	60	3	2
Reduced Fat & Sodium	3	60	2	1
Sesame	3	60	3	2
Cheeters				
Low Carb All Flavors	1 pkg (1 oz)	104	8	1
Cheetos				
Bacon Cheddar	1 pkg	190	9	3
Cheddar Cheese	1 pkg	210	11	3
Golden Toast	1 pkg	240	14	4
Cheez It				
Big	13 (1 oz)	150	8	2
Big Reduced Fat	15 (1 oz)	140	5	1
Heads & Tails	37 (1 oz)	140	6	2
Hot & Spicy	26 (1 oz)	150	8	2
Low Sodium	27 (1 oz)	160	8	2
Nacho	28 (1 oz)	150	7	2
Original	27 (1 oz)	160	8	2
Party Mix	½ cup (1 oz)	140	5	1
Party Mix Nacho	½ cup (1 oz)	130	5	1
Party Mix Reduced Fat	½ cup (1 oz)	130	3	1
Peanut Butter	1 pkg (1.3 oz)	190	10	2
Reduced Fat	29 (1 oz)	140	5	1
Snack Mix	½ cup (1 oz)	130	5	1
Snack Mix Big Crunch	¾ cup (1 oz)	110	6	1
Snack Mix Double Cheese	¾ cup (1 oz)	110	5	1
White Cheddar	26 (1 oz)	150	7	2
Courtney's				
Sun-Dried Tomato Organic	4 (0.5 oz)	60	1	0
Crown Pilot				
Crackers	1 (0.5 oz)	70	2	0
Dare				
Vinta	1 (6 g)	30	1	1

FOOD	PORTION	CALS	FAT	SAT FAT
Doritos				
Jalapeno Cheese	1 pkg	230	14	4
Nacho Cheddar	1 pkg	240	14	3
Eden				
Nori Nori Rice	15 (1 oz)	110	0	0
Estee				
Sugar Free Cracked Pepper	18	120	2	0
Sugar Free Golden	10	130	2	0
Sugar Free Wheat	17	100	2	0
Frito Lay				
Cheddar Snacks	1 pkg	200	10	3
Frookie				
Cheddar	17 (1 oz)	140	4	1
Cracked Pepper	8 (0.7 oz)	70	0	0
Garden Vegetable	13 (1 oz)	130	4	0
Garlic & Herb	8 (0.7 oz)	70	0	0
Pizza	17 (1 oz)	130	3	0
Snack & Party	10 (1 oz)	140	5	0
Water Crackers	8 (0.7 oz)	70	0	0
Wheat & Onion	12 (1 oz)	120	4	0
Wheat & Rye	13 (1 oz)	120	4	0
Gold'n Krackle				
Cheese	½ oz	65	2	1
Cheese & Oregano	½ oz	65	2	1
Hot & Spicy	½ oz	58	1	0
Onion & Garlic	½ oz	58	1	0
Plain	½ oz	58	1	0
Health Valley				
Healthy Pizza Garlic & Herb	6	50	0	0
Healthy Pizza Italiano	6	50	0	0
Healthy Pizza Zesty Cheese	6	50	0	0
Low Fat Mild Jalapeno	6	60	2	—
Low Fat Mild Ranch	6	60	2	—
Low Fat Roasted Garlic	6	60	2	—
Original Oat Bran	6	120	3	—
Original Rice Bran	6	110	3	—
Whole Wheat	5	50	0	0
Whole Wheat Cheese	5	50	0	0
Whole Wheat Herb	5	50	0	0
Whole Wheat No Salt Vegetable	5	50	0	0

FOOD	PORTION	CALS	FAT	SAT FAT
Whole Wheat Onion	5	50	0	0
Whole Wheat Vegetable	5	50	0	0
Healthy Choice				
Bread Crisps Garlic Herb	11 (1 oz)	110	2	0
Heavenly				
All Flavors Cholesterol Free Sugar Free	1	16	4	1
Kashi				
TLC Country Cheddar	15 (1 oz)	130	3	0
TLC Honey Sesame	15 (1 oz)	130	3	0
TLC Natural Ranch	15 (1 oz)	130	3	0
TLC Original 7 Grain	15 (1 oz)	130	3	0
Keebler				
Club 33% Reduced Fat	5 (0.6 oz)	70	2	0
Club 50% Reduced Sodium	4 (0.5 oz)	70	3	1
Club Original	4 (0.5 oz)	70	3	1
Elfin	23 (1 oz)	130	2	0
Export Soda	3 (0.5 oz)	60	2	1
Harvest Bakery Multigrain	2 (0.6 oz)	70	3	1
Munch'ems Cheddar	39 (1 oz)	140	5	1
Munch'ems Cheddar	30 (1 oz)	130	4	1
Munch'ems Chili Cheese	28 (1.1 oz)	130	4	2
Munch'ems Mexquite BBQ	40 (1 oz)	140	5	1
Munch'ems Ranch	40 (1 oz)	140	5	2
Munch'ems Ranch	33 (1 oz)	130	4	1
Munch'ems Salsa	28 (1.1 oz)	130	4	1
Munch'ems Seasoned Original	30 (1 oz)	130	5	1
Munch'ems Sour Cream & Onion	39 (1 oz)	140	5	2
Munch'ems Sour Cream & Onion 55% Reduced Fat	33 (1 oz)	130	4	1
Paks Cheese & Peanut Butter	1 pkg	190	9	2
Paks Club & Cheddar	1 pkg	190	11	3
Paks Toast & Peanut Butter	1 pkg	190	9	2
Paks Wheat & Cheddar	1 pkg (1.3 oz)	180	10	3
Toasteds Buttercrisp	5 (0.6 oz)	80	4	1
Toasteds Buttercrisp	9 (1 oz)	140	7	2
Toasteds Onion	9 (1 oz)	140	6	1
Toasteds Sesame	5 (0.6 oz)	80	4	1
Toasteds Sesame	9 (1 oz)	140	6	1
Toasteds Sesame Reduced Fat	10 (1 oz)	120	3	1

FOOD	PORTION	CALS	FAT	SAT FAT
Toasteds Wheat	5 (0.6 oz)	80	4	1
Toasteds Wheat	9 (1 oz)	140	6	2
Toasteds Wheat Reduced Fat	5 (0.5 oz)	60	2	0
Toasteds Wheat Reduced Fat	10 (1 oz)	120	3	1
Town House	5 (0.6 oz)	80	5	1
Town House 50% Reduced Sodium	5 (0.6 oz)	80	5	1
Town House Reduced Fat	6 (0.6 oz)	70	2	1
Town House Wheat	5 (0.6 oz)	80	4	1
Wheatables Honey Wheat	12 (1 oz)	140	6	2
Wheatables Original	12 (1 oz)	140	6	2
Wheatables Seven Grain	12 (1 oz)	140	6	2
Zesta Saltine 50% Reduced Sodium	5 (0.5 oz)	60	2	1
Zesta Saltine Fat Free	5 (0.5 oz)	50	0	0
Zesta Saltine Original	5 (0.5 oz)	60	2	1
Zesta Saltine Unsalted Top	5 (0.5 oz)	70	2	1
Zesta Soup & Oyster	42 (0.5 oz)	80	3	1
Lance				
Bonnie	6 (1⅛ oz)	160	7	3
Captain Wafers w/ Cream Cheese & Chives	1 pkg (1.3 oz)	190	9	2
Cheese-On-Wheat	1 pkg (1.3 oz)	190	10	2
Cranberry Bar Fat Free	1 (1.75 oz)	160	0	0
Lanchee	1 pkg (1¼ oz)	190	11	2
Malt	1 pkg (1¼ oz)	190	10	2
Nekot	1 pkg (1.5 oz)	210	10	2
Nip-Chee	1 pkg (1.3 oz)	190	10	2
Peanut Butter Wheat	1 pkg (1.3 oz)	190	11	2
Rye-Chee	1 pkg (1.4 oz)	210	11	3
Sour Dough w/ Cheddar & Sour Cream	1 pkg (1.6 oz)	240	15	4
Toastchee	1 pkg (1.4 oz)	200	12	2
Toasty	1 pkg (1¼ oz)	190	11	2
Wheat Italian	¾ cup (1.4 oz)	200	11	2
Wheat Pizza	¾ cup (1.4 oz)	200	10	2
Little Debbie				
Cheese Crackers With Peanut Butter	1 (0.9 oz)	140	8	2
Cheese On Cheese Crackers	1 (0.9 oz)	140	8	2
Cream Cheese & Chive	1 (0.9 oz)	140	7	2
Toasty Crackers With Peanut Butter	1 (0.9 oz)	140	7	2
Wheat Crackers With Cheddar Cheese	1 (0.9 oz)	140	8	2

FOOD	PORTION	CALS	FAT	SAT FAT
Nabisco				
Royal Lunch	1 (0.4 oz)	60	2	0
Zwieback	1 (8 g)	35	1	–
No-Carb Kitchen				
Cheese	1	25	3	1
No-No				
Flatbreads Tortilla Corn Low Fat Sugar Free Everything	3 (1 oz)	95	1	0
Oysterettes				
Crackers	19 (0.5 oz)	60	3	1
Partners				
Walla Walla Sweet Onion Perservative Free	0.5 oz	65	3	2
Pepperidge Farm				
Butter Thins	4 (0.5 oz)	70	3	1
English Water Biscuits	4 (0.5 oz)	70	2	0
Giant Goldfish Peanut Butter Sandwich	1 pkg (1.4 oz)	190	9	2
Giant Goldfish Wheat	14	140	5	1
Goldfish Cheddar	55	140	6	2
Goldfish Cheddar 30% Less Sodium	60 (1.1 oz)	150	6	2
Goldfish Cheese Trio	58	140	6	2
Goldfish Original	55	140	6	2
Goldfish Parmesan Cheese	60	140	5	2
Goldfish Pizza Flavored	55 (1 oz)	140	6	2
Goldfish Pretzel	43 (1 oz)	120	3	1
Hearty Wheat	3 (0.6 oz)	80	4	0
Sesame	3 (0.5 oz)	70	3	0
Snack Mix Fat Free Goldfish	⅔ cup (0.9 oz)	90	0	0
Peter Pan				
Cheese Peanut Butter	1 pkg	210	10	3
Toast Peanut Butter	1 pkg	210	11	3
Planters				
Cheese Peanut Butter Sandwiches	1 pkg (1.4 oz)	190	10	2
Toast Peanut Butter Sandwiches	1 pkg (1.4 oz)	190	10	2
Premium				
Saltine Fat Free	5 (0.5 oz)	50	0	0
Saltine Low Sodium	5 (0.5 oz)	60	1	0
Saltine Multigrain	5 (0.5 oz)	60	2	0
Saltine Original	5 (0.5 oz)	60	2	0

FOOD	PORTION	CALS	FAT	SAT FAT
Saltine Unsalted Tops	5 (0.5 oz)	60	2	0
Soup & Oyster	23 (0.5 oz)	60	2	0
Ralston				
Cheese	23 (1 oz)	150	6	2
Cheese Reduced Fat	29 (1 oz)	130	4	1
Oyster	35 (0.5 oz)	70	2	0
Rich & Crisp	1 (0.5 oz)	70	3	1
Saltines Fat Free	5 (0.5 oz)	60	0	0
Saltines Deluxe	5 (0.5 oz)	60	2	–
Snackers	9 (1.1 oz)	160	8	2
Snackers Reduced Fat	10 (1.1 oz)	140	4	1
Snackers Unsalted	9 (1.1 oz)	160	8	2
Wheat Snacks	16 (1 oz)	140	6	1
Wheat Snacks Reduced Fat	16 (1.1 oz)	140	4	1
Woven Wheats	7 (1.1 oz)	140	5	1
Woven Wheats Reduced Fat	8 (1.1 oz)	130	3	1
RedOval Farms				
Stoned Wheat Thins Cracked Pepper	4 (0.6 oz)	70	3	1
Ritz				
Low Sodium	5 (0.5 oz)	80	4	1
Rykrisp				
Seasoned	2	60	2	0
Savory Thins				
Toasted Onion & Garlic	15 (1 oz)	110	1	0
Smucker's				
Snackers Grape	1 pkg (3.3 oz)	410	20	5
Snackers Strawberry	1 pkg (3.3 oz)	410	20	5
SnackWell's				
Salsa Cheddar	32 (1 oz)	120	2	0
Sunshine				
Hi Ho	4 (0.5 oz)	70	4	1
Hi Ho Reduced Fat	5 (0.5 oz)	70	3	1
Krispy	5 (0.5 oz)	60	2	0
Krispy Fat Free	5 (0.5 oz)	50	0	0
Krispy Mild Cheddar	5 (0.5 oz)	60	2	1
Krispy Soup & Oyster	17 (0.5 oz)	60	2	0
Krispy Unsalted Tops	5 (0.5 oz)	60	2	0
Krispy Whole Wheat	5 (0.5 oz)	60	2	0
Tree Of Life				
Bite Size Fat Free Cracked Pepper	12 (0.5)	55	0	0

FOOD	PORTION	CALS	FAT	SAT FAT
Bite Size Fat Free Garden Vegetable	12 (0.5 oz)	55	0	0
Bite Size Fat Free Garlic & Herb	12 (0.5 oz)	55	0	0
Bite Size Fat Free Toasted Onion	12 (0.5 oz)	55	0	0
Oyster	40 (0.5 oz)	60	0	0
Saltine Cracked Pepper Fat Free	4 (0.5 oz)	60	0	0
Saltine Fat Free	4 (0.5 oz)	50	0	0
Triscuit				
Crackers	7 (1.1 oz)	140	5	1
Uneeda Biscuit				
Unsalted Tops	2 (0.5 oz)	60	2	0
Venus				
Fat Free Cracked Pepper	11 (0.5 oz)	60	0	0
Fat Free Garden Vegetable	5 (0.5 oz)	60	0	0
Fat Free Garlic & Herb	11 (0.5 oz)	60	0	0
Fat Free Multi-Grain	5 (0.5 oz)	60	0	0
Fat Free Spicy Chili	10 (0.5 oz)	60	0	0
Fat Free Toasted Onion	5 (0.5 oz)	60	0	0
Fat Free Toasted Wheat	5 (0.5 oz)	60	0	0
Fat Free Tomato & Basil	10 (0.5 oz)	60	0	0
Fat Free Zesty Italian	10 (0.5 oz)	60	0	0
Garden Vegetable	6 (1 oz)	150	8	2
Honey Wheat	1 oz	140	5	0
Low Fat Cracker Bread	5 (0.5 oz)	60	2	0
Low Fat Water Crackers	4 (0.5 oz)	60	1	0
Sesame & Flaxseed	1 oz	130	3	0
Soup Original	0.5 oz	60	2	0
Toasted Wheat	6 (1 oz)	150	7	2
Wine Cheese Caviar Original	0.5 oz	60	2	0
Wine Cheese Caviar Pepper & Poppy	0.5 oz	60	2	0
Wasa				
Crisp	3 (0.5 oz)	50	0	–
Crisp'N Light Sourdough Rye	3 (0.6 oz)	60	0	0
Crisp'N Light Wheat	2 (0.5 oz)	50	0	0
Crispbread Cinnamon Toast	1 (0.6 oz)	60	1	0
Crispbread Fiber Rye	1 (0.4 oz)	30	1	0
Crispbread Gluten & Wheat Free Corn	1 (0.4 oz)	40	1	0
Crispbread Hearty Rye	1 (0.5 oz)	45	0	0
Crispbread Light Rye	1 (0.3 oz)	25	0	0
Crispbread Multi Grain	1 (0.5 oz)	45	0	0
Crispbread Organic Rye	1 (0.3 oz)	25	0	0

FOOD	PORTION	CALS	FAT	SAT FAT
Crispbread Sodium Free Rye	1 (0.3 oz)	30	0	0
Crispbread Sourdough Rye	1 (0.4 oz)	35	0	0
Crispbread Toasted Wheat	1 (0.5 oz)	50	2	0
Crispbread Whole Wheat	1 (0.5 oz)	50	1	0
Waverly				
Crackers	5 (0.5 oz)	70	4	1
Wheatsworth				
Crackers	5	80	4	1
Wisecrackers				
Low Fat Poblano Chili & Sweet Onion	4 (0.5 oz)	45	1	0
Wortz				
Cheese	23 (1 oz)	150	6	2
Oyster	35 (0.5 oz)	70	2	0
Rich & Crisp	1 (0.5 oz)	70	3	1
Saltines Fat Free	5 (0.5 oz)	60	0	0
Saltines Deluxe	5 (0.5 oz)	60	2	—
Wheat Snacks	16 (1 oz)	140	6	1
Wheat Snacks Reduced Fat	16 (1.1 oz)	140	4	1
Woven Wheats	7 (1.1 oz)	140	5	1

CRANBERRIES

FOOD	PORTION	CALS	FAT	SAT FAT
cranberry sauce sweetened	½ cup	209	tr	—
fresh chopped	1 cup	54	tr	—
Jok'n'Al				
Cranberry Sauce	1 tbsp	8	0	0
Ocean Spray				
Craisins	⅓ cup (1.4 oz)	130	0	0
Cran*Fruit Cranberry Orange	¼ cup	120	0	0
Cranberry Sauce Jellied	¼ cup	110	0	0
Fresh	2 oz	25	0	0
Whole Berry Sauce	¼ cup	110	0	0
Steel's				
Spiced Cranberry Sauce	⅓ cup	20	0	0
Wild Thyme Farms				
Cranberry Sauce	1 tbsp	19	0	0

CRANBERRY BEANS

FOOD	PORTION	CALS	FAT	SAT FAT
canned	1 cup	216	1	tr
dried cooked	1 cup	241	1	tr

FOOD	PORTION	CALS	FAT	SAT FAT
CRANBERRY JUICE				
cocktail	1 cup	147	tr	–
cranberry juice cocktail	6 oz	108	tr	–
cranberry juice cocktail low calorie	6 oz	33	0	0
cranberry juice cocktail frzn	12 oz can	821	0	0
cranberry juice cocktail frzn as prep	6 oz	102	0	0
After The Fall				
Cape Cod Cranberry	1 bottle (10 oz)	130	0	0
Cranberry Ginger Ale	1 can (12 oz)	140	0	0
Crystal Light				
Cranberry Breeze Drink	1 serv (8 oz)	5	0	0
Cranberry Breeze Drink Mix as prep	1 serv (8 oz)	5	0	0
Everfresh				
Cranberry Cocktail	1 can (8 oz)	140	0	0
Keto				
Kooler	½ tsp	0	0	0
Langers				
Cocktail	8 oz	140	0	0
Diet	8 oz	30	0	0
White	8 oz	120	0	0
Mott's				
Cocktail	8 fl oz	150	0	0
Nantucket Nectars				
Big Cran	8 oz	140	0	0
Ocean Spray				
Cocktail	8 oz	140	0	0
Cocktail Reduced Calorie	8 oz	50	0	0
Lightstyle Cranberry Juice Cocktail	8 oz	40	0	0
White Cranberry	1 cup (8 oz)	120	0	0
White Cranberry Peach	1 cup (8 oz)	120	0	0
White Cranberry Strawberry	1 cup (8 oz)	120	0	0
Tropicana				
Twister Ruby Red	1 bottle (10 oz)	160	0	0
Veryfine				
Cocktail	1 bottle (10 oz)	180	0	0
Wellfleet Farms				
Cranberry	8 oz	130	0	0
CRAYFISH				
cooked	3 oz	97	1	tr

FOOD	PORTION	CALS	FAT	SAT FAT
raw	3 oz	76	1	tr
raw	8	24	tr	tr
CREAM (see also WHIPPED TOPPINGS)				
clotted cream	2 tbsp (1 oz)	164	18	–
creme fraiche	2 tbsp (1 oz)	100	11	–
half & half	1 cup (8.5 oz)	315	28	17
half & half	1 tbsp (0.5 oz)	20	2	1
heavy whipping	1 tbsp (0.5 oz)	52	6	3
heavy whipping whipped	1 cup (4.1 oz)	411	44	27
light coffee	1 cup (8.4 oz)	496	46	29
light coffee	1 tbsp (0.5 oz)	29	3	2
light whipping	1 tbsp (0.5 oz)	44	5	3
light whipping cream whipped	1 cup (4.2 oz)	345	37	23
Cabot				
Whipped	2 tbsp	30	2	2
Land O Lakes				
Fat Free Half & Half	2 tbsp (1 oz)	20	0	0
Half & Half	2 tbsp (1 oz)	40	4	2
Heavy Whipping	1 tbsp (0.5 oz)	50	6	4
Organic Valley				
Half & Half	2 tbsp (1 oz)	40	3	2
CREAM CHEESE				
cream cheese	1 oz	99	10	6
cream cheese	1 pkg (3 oz)	297	30	19
Alpine Lace				
Reduced Fat Roasted Garlic & Herbs	1 tsp (1 oz)	60	4	3
Reduced Fat Sundried Tomato & Basil	2 tsp (1 oz)	70	5	4
Boar's Head				
Cream Cheese	2 tbsp (1 oz)	100	10	7
Breakstone's				
Temp-Tee Whipped	2 tbsp (0.8 oz)	80	8	5
Galaxy				
Slices	1 slice (1 oz)	50	3	2
Healthy Choice				
Herbs & Garlic	2 tbsp (1 oz)	25	0	0
Plain	2 tbsp (1 oz)	25	0	0
Strawberry	2 tbsp (1 oz)	30	0	0
Horizon Organic				
Spreadable	2 tbsp	100	10	7

FOOD	PORTION	CALS	FAT	SAT FAT
Organic Valley				
Cream Cheese	1 oz	100	9	6
Philadelphia				
Free	1 oz	30	0	0
Regular	1 oz	100	10	6
Soft	2 tbsp (1 oz)	100	10	7
Soft Apple Cinnamon	2 tbsp (1.1 oz)	100	8	5
Soft Cheesecake	2 tbsp (1 oz)	110	9	6
Soft Chives & Onions	2 tbsp (1.1 oz)	110	10	7
Soft Garden Vegetable	2 tbsp (1.1 oz)	110	11	7
Soft Honey Nut	2 tbsp (1.1 oz)	110	10	6
Soft Pineapple	2 tbsp (1.1 oz)	100	9	6
Soft Salmon	3 tbsp (1.1 oz)	100	9	6
Soft Strawberry	2 tbsp (1.1 oz)	100	9	6
Soft Free	2 tbsp (1.2 oz)	30	0	0
Soft Free Garden Vegetable	2 tbsp (1.2 oz)	30	0	0
Soft Free Strawberries	2 tbsp (1.2 oz)	45	0	0
Soft Light	2 tbsp (1.1 oz)	70	5	4
Soft Light Jalapeno	2 tbsp (1.1 oz)	60	5	3
Soft Light Raspberry	2 tbsp (1.1 oz)	70	5	3
Soft Light Roasted Garlic	2 tbsp (1.1 oz)	70	5	3
Whipped	2 tbsp (0.7 oz)	70	7	5
Whipped Chives	2 tbsp (0.7 oz)	70	6	4
Whipped Smoked Salmon	2 tbsp (0.7 oz)	70	6	4
With Chives	1 oz	90	9	6
CREAM OF TARTAR				
cream of tartar	1 tsp	8	0	0
CREAM SUBSTITUTES				
ExpertExtras				
RealCream	1 tsp	14	1	1
CREPES				
basic crepe unfilled	1	75	2	—
Frieda's				
Ready-To-Use	2 (0.8 oz)	50	1	0
CROAKER				
atlantic breaded & fried	3 oz	188	11	3
atlantic raw	3 oz	89	3	1

FOOD	PORTION	CALS	FAT	SAT FAT
CROCODILE				
cooked	3 oz	78	1	–
CROISSANT				
apple	1 (2 oz)	145	5	3
cheese	1 (2 oz)	236	12	5
plain	1 (2 oz)	232	12	7
plain	1 mini (1 oz)	115	6	3
Sara Lee				
Broccoli & Cheese	1 (3.7 oz)	280	13	4
French Style	1 (1.5 oz)	170	8	3
Ham & Swiss	1 (3.7 oz)	300	16	5
Petite	2 (2 oz)	230	11	4
TAKE-OUT				
w/ egg & cheese	1 (4.5 oz)	368	25	14
w/ egg cheese & bacon	1 (4.5 oz)	413	28	15
w/ egg cheese & ham	1 (5.3 oz)	474	34	17
w/ egg cheese & sausage	1 (5.6 oz)	523	38	18
CROUTONS				
plain	1 cup (1 oz)	122	2	tr
seasoned	1 cup (1.4 oz)	186	7	2
Pepperidge Farm				
Garlic	6 (0.2 oz)	30	1	0
Homestyle	6 (0.2 oz)	30	1	0
Sourdough	6 (0.2 oz)	35	2	1
Up Country Naturals				
Organic Whole Wheat Garlic & Herb	¼ cup (0.3 oz)	35	2	0
CUCUMBER				
fresh raw	1 (11 oz)	38	tr	tr
fresh raw sliced	½ cup (1.8 oz)	7	tr	tr
Chiquita				
Cucumber	⅓ med (3.5 oz)	15	0	0
TAKE-OUT				
cucumber salad	3.5 oz	50	tr	tr
kimchee	½ cup (1.8 oz)	36	2	tr
tzatziki	½ cup (3.4 oz)	72	6	1
CUMIN				
seed	1 tsp	8	tr	–

FOOD	PORTION	CALS	FAT	SAT FAT
CURRANT JUICE				
black currant nectar	7 oz	110	0	—
red currant nectar	7 oz	108	tr	—
CURRANTS				
black fresh	½ cup	36	tr	tr
zante dried	½ cup	204	tr	tr
CUSK				
fillet baked	3 oz	106	1	—
CUSTARD				
HOME RECIPE				
baked	1 recipe 4 serv (19.8 oz)	549	26	13
flan	1 recipe 10 serv (53.7 oz)	2206	63	30
MIX				
as prep w/ 2% milk	½ cup (4.7 oz)	148	4	2
as prep w/ 2% milk	1 recipe 4 serv (18.7 oz)	595	15	8
as prep w/ whole milk	1 recipe 4 serv (18.7 oz)	652	22	12
as prep w/ whole milk	½ cup (4.7 oz)	163	5	3
flan as prep w/ 2% milk	1 recipe 4 serv (18.7 oz)	542	9	6
flan as prep w/ 2% milk	½ cup (4.7 oz)	135	2	1
flan as prep w/ whole milk	1 recipe 4 serv (18.7 oz)	600	16	10
flan as prep w/ whole milk	½ cup (4.7 oz)	150	4	3
Betty Crocker				
Flan w/ Caramel Sauce as prep	1 serv	330	7	4
Jell-O				
Americana Custard Dessert as prep w/ 2% milk	½ cup (5 oz)	140	3	2
Flan as prep w/ 2% milk	½ cup (5.1 oz)	140	3	2
READY-TO-EAT				
Kozy Shack				
Flan	1 pkg (4 oz)	150	4	2
Swiss Miss				
Egg Custard	1 pkg (4 oz)	153	5	1

FOOD	PORTION	CALS	FAT	SAT FAT
TAKE-OUT				
baked	½ cup (5 oz)	148	7	3
flan	½ cup (5.4 oz)	220	6	3
zabaione	½ cup (57.2 g)	135	5	2
CUTTLEFISH				
steamed	3 oz	134	1	tr
DANDELION GREENS				
fresh cooked	½ cup	17	tr	—
raw chopped	½ cup	13	tr	—
DANISH PASTRY				
FROZEN				
Morton				
Honey Buns	1 (2.28 oz)	270	13	3
Honey Buns Mini	1 (1.3 oz)	160	8	2
READY-TO-EAT				
plain ring	1 (12 oz)	1305	71	22
Dolly Madison				
Danish Rollers	3 (2.8 oz)	290	10	2
Tastykake				
Cheese	1 (3 oz)	290	14	3
Lemon	1 (3 oz)	290	14	3
Raspberry	1 (3 oz)	290	14	3
TAKE-OUT				
almond	1 (4¼ in) (2.3 oz)	280	16	4
apple	1 (4¼ in) (2.5 oz)	264	13	3
cheese	1 (3.2 oz)	353	25	5
cheese	1 (4¼ in) (2.5 oz)	266	16	5
cinnamon	1 (3.1 oz)	349	17	3
cinnamon	1 (4¼ in) (2.3 oz)	262	15	4
cinnamon nut	1 (4¼ in) (2.3 oz)	280	16	4
fruit	1 (3.3 oz)	335	16	3
lemon	1 (4¼ in) (2.5 oz)	264	13	3
raisin	1 (4¼ in) (2.5 oz)	264	13	3
raisin nut	1 (4¼ in) (2.3 oz)	280	16	4
raspberry	1 (4¼ in) (2.5 oz)	264	13	3
strawberry	1 (4¼ in) (2.5 oz)	264	13	3
DATES				
deglet noor dried	10	240	0	—

FOOD	PORTION	CALS	FAT	SAT FAT
dried chopped	1 cup	489	1	—
dried whole	10	228	tr	—
jujube dried	1 oz	75	tr	—
jujube fresh	1 oz	30	tr	—
jujube preserved in sugar	1 oz	91	tr	—
medjool	2-3 (1.4 oz)	120	0	0
Calavo				
Dried Pitted	5-6 (1.4 oz)	120	0	0
California Redi-Date				
Deglet Noor Dried	5-6 (1.4 oz)	120	0	0
Dromedary				
Chopped Dried	¼ cup	130	0	0
Sonoma				
Dried	5-6 (1.4 oz)	110	0	0

DEER *(see VENISON)*

DELI MEATS/COLD CUTS *(see also BEEF, CHICKEN, HAM, MEAT SUBSTITUTES, TURKEY)*

FOOD	PORTION	CALS	FAT	SAT FAT
barbecue loaf pork & beef	1 slice	40	2	1
beerwurst beef	1 slice (2¾ in x 1/16 in)	20	2	1
beerwurst beef	1 slice (4 in x ⅛ in)	75	7	3
beerwurst pork	1 slice (2¾ in x 1/16 in)	14	1	tr
beerwurst pork	1 slice (4 in x ⅛ in)	55	4	1
berliner pork & beef	1 oz	65	4	2
blood sausage	1 oz	95	9	3
bologna beef	1 oz	88	8	3
bologna beef & pork	1 oz	89	8	3
bologna pork	1 oz	70	6	2
braunschweiger pork	1 slice (2½ in x ¼ in)	65	6	2
braunschweiger pork	1 oz	102	9	3
corned beef loaf	1 oz	43	2	1
dried beef	1 oz	47	1	—
dutch brand loaf pork & beef	1 oz	68	5	2
headcheese pork	1 oz	60	5	1
honey loaf pork & beef	1 oz	36	1	tr

FOOD	PORTION	CALS	FAT	SAT FAT
honey roll sausage beef	1 oz	42	2	1
lebanon bologna beef	1 oz	60	4	2
liver cheese pork	1 oz	86	7	3
liverwurst pork	1 oz	92	8	3
luncheon meat beef	1 oz	87	7	3
luncheon meat pork & beef	1 oz	100	9	3
luncheon meat pork canned	1 oz	95	9	3
luncheon sausage pork & beef	1 oz	74	6	2
luxury loaf pork	1 oz	40	1	tr
mortadella beef & pork	1 oz	88	7	3
mother's loaf pork	1 oz	80	6	2
new england sausage pork & beef	1 oz	46	2	1
olive loaf pork	1 oz	67	5	2
peppered loaf pork & beef	1 oz	42	2	1
pepperoni pork & beef	1 slice (0.2 oz)	27	2	1
pepperoni pork & beef	1 (9 oz)	1248	110	40
pickle & pimiento loaf pork	1 oz	74	6	2
picnic loaf pork & beef	1 oz	66	5	2
salami cooked beef & pork	1 oz	71	6	2
salami hard pork	1 pkg (4 oz)	460	38	13
salami hard pork	1 slice (⅓ oz)	41	4	1
salami hard pork & beef	1 slice (0.3 oz)	42	3	1
salami hard pork & beef	1 pkg (4 oz)	472	39	14
sandwich spread pork & beef	1 tbsp	35	3	1
sandwich spread pork & beef	1 oz	67	5	2
summer sausage thuringer cervelat	1 oz	98	8	3
Boar's Head				
Bologna Beef	2 oz	150	13	4
Bologna Garlic	2 oz	150	13	5
Bologna Lowered Sodium	2 oz	150	13	5
Bologna Pork & Beef	2 oz	150	13	5
Braunschweiger Lite	2 oz	120	8	5
Head Cheese	2 oz	90	5	3
Liverwurst Strassburger	2 oz	170	15	6
Olive Loaf	2 oz	130	12	5
Pastrami	2 oz	90	4	2
Prosciutto	1 oz	60	3	1
Red Pastrami	2 oz	90	4	2
Salami Beef	2 oz	120	9	4
Salami Cooked	2 oz	130	11	5

FOOD	PORTION	CALS	FAT	SAT FAT
Salami Genoa	2 oz	180	14	5
Salami Hard	1 oz	110	9	4
Spiced Ham	2 oz	120	10	5
Carl Buddig				
Beef	1 pkg (2.5 oz)	100	5	2
Corned Beef	1 pkg (2.5 oz)	100	5	2
Pastrami	1 pkg (2.5 oz)	100	5	2
Healthy Choice				
Bologna	1 slice (1 oz)	30	1	0
Bologna Beef	1 slice (1 oz)	35	1	0
Deli-Thin Bologna	4 slices (1.8 oz)	60	2	1
Well-Pack Bologna	1 slice (1 oz)	30	1	0
Hormel				
Liverwurst Spread	4 tbsp (2 oz)	130	10	4
Pepperoni Chunk	1 oz	140	13	6
Pepperoni Sliced	15 slices (1 oz)	140	13	6
Pepperoni Twin	1 oz	140	13	5
Pillow Pack Genoa Salami	2 oz	160	18	7
Pillow Pack Pepperoni	16 slices (1 oz)	140	13	6
Jordan's				
Healthy Trim 95% Fat Free Macaroni & Cheese Loaf	2 slices (1.6 oz)	50	2	1
Healthy Trim 95% Fat Free Olive Loaf	2 slices (1.6 oz)	50	2	1
Healthy Trim 95% Fat Free Pickle & Pepper Loaf	2 slices (1.6 oz)	50	2	1
Healthy Trim 97% Fat Free Corned Beef	2 slices (1.6 oz)	45	2	1
Healthy Trim Low Fat Cooked Salami	3 slices (2 oz)	70	3	1
Healthy Trim Low Fat German Brand Bologna	3 slices (2 oz)	70	3	1
Oscar Mayer				
Bologna	1 slice (1 oz)	90	8	3
Bologna Beef	1 slice (1 oz)	90	8	4
Bologna Garlic	1 slice (1.4 oz)	110	12	5
Bologna Wisconsin Made Ring	2 oz	180	16	6
Braunschweiger Spread	2 oz	190	17	6
Brunschweiger	1 slice (1 oz)	100	9	3
Free Bologna	1 slice (1 oz)	20	0	0
Light Bologna	1 slice (1 oz)	60	4	2
Light Bologna Beef	1 slice (1 oz)	60	4	2

FOOD	PORTION	CALS	FAT	SAT FAT
Liver Cheese	1 slice (1.3 oz)	120	10	4
Luncheon Loaf Spiced	1 slice (1 oz)	70	5	2
Old Fashioned Loaf	1 slice (1 oz)	70	5	2
Olive Loaf	1 slice (1 oz)	70	6	2
Pepperoni	15 slices (1 oz)	140	13	5
Salami Cotto	1 slice (1 oz)	70	5	2
Salami Cotto Beef	1 slice (1 oz)	60	5	2
Salami For Beer	1 slices (1.6 oz)	110	9	3
Salami Hard	3 slices (1 oz)	100	9	3
Sandwich Spread	2 oz	130	10	4
Summer Sausage	2 slices (1.6 oz)	140	13	5
Summer Sausage Beef	2 slices (1.6 oz)	140	12	5
Spam				
Less Salt	2 oz	170	16	6
Lite	2 oz	110	8	3
Original	2 oz	170	16	6
Smoked	2 oz	170	16	6
TAKE-OUT				
corned beef	2 oz	70	2	1
corned beef brisket	2 oz	90	5	2
DILL				
seed	1 tsp	6	tr	tr
sprigs fresh	1 cup	4	tr	tr
sprigs fresh	5	0	tr	tr
weed dry	1 tsp	3	tr	—

DINNER (see also ASIAN FOOD, PASTA DISHES, POT PIES, SPANISH FOOD)

Amy's

FOOD	PORTION	CALS	FAT	SAT FAT
Country Dinner Vegetable Salisbury Steak	1 pkg (11 oz)	380	12	4
Banquet				
Beef Patty w/ Country Style Vegetables	1 meal (9.5 oz)	310	20	8
Boneless Pork Rib	1 meal (10 oz)	400	19	8
Boneless White Fried Chicken	1 meal (8.25 oz)	540	34	9
Chicken Parmigiana	1 meal (9.5 oz)	320	18	7
Chicken Fingers Meal	1 meal (7.1 oz)	740	43	11
Chicken Fried Beef Steak	1 pkg (10 oz)	420	23	12
Chicken Nuggets Meal	1 meal (6.75 oz)	430	23	8
Extra Helping Boneless Pork Riblet	1 meal (15.25 oz)	720	40	15

FOOD	PORTION	CALS	FAT	SAT FAT
Extra Helping Fried Beef Steak	1 meal (16 oz)	820	50	23
Extra Helping Fried Chicken	1 meal (14.7 oz)	910	55	13
Extra Helping Meatloaf	1 meal (16 oz)	610	40	15
Extra Helping Salisbury Steak	1 meal (16.5 oz)	740	54	21
Extra Helping Turkey & Gravy w/ Dressing	1 meal (17 oz)	620	32	8
Extra Helping White Fried Chicken	1 meal (13 oz)	690	48	12
Extra Helping Yankee Pot Roast	1 meal (14.5 oz)	410	20	7
Family Size Brown Gravy & Salisbury Steak	1 serv	240	20	10
Family Size Brown Gravy & Sliced Beef	1 serv	140	8	4
Family Size Chicken & Broccoli Alfredo	1 serv	270	12	7
Family Size Country Style Chicken & Dumplings	1 serv	290	14	5
Family Size Creamy Broccoli Chicken Cheese & Rice	1 serv	280	14	7
Family Size Hearty Beef Stew	1 cup	170	7	3
Family Size Homestyle Gravy & Sliced Turkey	2 slices	140	10	4
Family Size Mushroom Gravy & Charbroiled Beef Patties	1 patty	250	20	9
Family Size Potato Ham & Broccoli Au Gratin	⅔ cup	210	13	5
Family Size Savory Gravy & Meatloaf	1 slice	120	13	7
Fish Sticks	1 meal (6.6 oz)	290	13	5
Grilled Chicken	1 meal (9.9 oz)	330	13	3
Honey Roast Turkey Breast	1 meal (9 oz)	270	12	3
Meatloaf	1 meal (9.5 oz)	280	16	6
Our Original Fried Chicken	1 meal (9 oz)	470	27	9
Pork Cutlet Meal	1 meal (10.25 oz)	420	25	7
Salisbury Steak	1 meal (9.5 oz)	380	24	12
Sliced Beef	1 meal (9 oz)	270	10	5
Turkey	1 meal (9.25 oz)	270	11	4
Veal Parmagiana	1 meal (8.75 oz)	330	14	5
Western Style Beef Patty	1 meal (9.5 oz)	360	21	10
White Meat Fried Chicken	1 meal (8.75 oz)	460	28	11
Yankee Pot Roast	1 meal (9.4 oz)	230	10	4
Birds Eye				
Easy Recipe Creations Sweet & Sour w/ Pineapple Tidbits	1⅓ cups	200	1	0

FOOD	PORTION	CALS	FAT	SAT FAT
Voila! Zesty Garlic Chicken	2 cups (6.2 oz)	260	11	3
Voila! Beef Sirloin Steak And Garlic Potatoes	1 cup	240	9	2
Voila! Chicken Alfredo	1 cup	230	8	2
Voila! Garden Herb Chicken	1 cup	310	15	5
Voila! Grilled Salsa Chicken w/ Rice	1 cup	240	5	1
Voila! Homestyle Turkey w/ Roasted Potatoes	1 cup	200	6	2
Voila! Teriyaki	2 cups (6.4 oz)	240	9	5
Fillo Factory				
Fillo Pie Broccoli & Cheese	¼ pie (4 oz)	350	12	5
Fillo Pie Spinach & Cheese	⅕ pie (4.8 oz)	210	7	3
Green Giant				
Create A Meal Broccoli Stir Fry as prep	1⅓ cups (9.9 oz)	290	13	3
Create A Meal Cheese & Herb Primavera as prep	1¼ cups (10 oz)	330	11	4
Create A Meal Garlic Herb as prep	1¼ cups (10 oz)	340	14	6
Create A Meal Hearty Vegetable Stew as prep	1¼ cups (10 oz)	280	9	2
Create A Meal Lemon Herb as prep	1½ cups (10 oz)	360	11	4
Create A Meal Mushroom & Wine as prep	1¼ cups (10 oz)	390	16	6
Create A Meal Vegetable Almond Stir Fry as prep	1⅓ cups (10 oz)	320	11	2
Healthy Choice				
Beef Pepper Steak Oriental	1 meal (9.5 oz)	260	5	3
Beef Pot Roast	1 meal (11 oz)	300	6	2
Beef Stroganoff	1 meal (11 oz)	320	8	3
Beef Tips Francais	1 meal (9.5 oz)	300	7	3
Beef Tips Portabello	1 meal (11.25 oz)	270	5	3
Bowls Chicken Teriyaki w/ Rice	1 meal (9.5 oz)	270	4	1
Bowls Country Chicken Bake	1 meal (9.5 oz)	230	8	3
Bowls Fiesta Chicken	1 meal (9.5 oz)	220	2	1
Bowls Garlic Lemon Chicken w/ Rice	1 meal (9.5 oz)	300	4	2
Bowls Roasted Potatoes w/ Ham	1 meal (8.5 oz)	210	4	2
Bowls Southwestern Chicken & Pasta	1 meal (9.5 oz)	320	4	2
Bowls Turkey Divan	1 meal (9.5 oz)	250	6	2
Charbroiled Beef Patty	1 meal (11 oz)	310	9	3
Chicken Cantonese	1 meal (10.75)	280	6	3
Chicken Parmigiana	1 meal (11.5 oz)	330	8	3

FOOD	PORTION	CALS	FAT	SAT FAT
Chicken & Vegetables Marsala	1 meal (11.5 oz)	240	4	2
Chicken Broccoli Alfredo	1 meal (11.5 oz)	300	7	3
Chicken Dijon	1 meal (11 oz)	270	5	2
Chicken Teriyaki	1 meal (11 oz)	270	6	3
Country Breaded Chicken	1 meal (10.25 oz)	350	9	2
Country Glazed Chicken Breast	1 meal (8.5 oz)	250	5	2
Country Herb Chicken	1 meal (12.15 oz)	320	8	3
Country Inn Roast Turkey	1 meal (10 oz)	250	6	2
Garlic Chicken Milano	1 meal (9.5 oz)	260	6	3
Grilled Chicken Sonoma	1 meal (9 oz)	230	4	1
Grilled Chicken w/ Mashed Potatoes	1 meal (8 oz)	180	4	2
Herb Baked Fish	1 meal (10.9 oz)	340	7	2
Herb Breaded Pork Patty	1 meal (8 oz)	280	6	3
Homestyle Chicken & Pasta	1 meal (9 oz)	270	6	3
Honey Glazed Chicken	1 meal (10 oz)	270	7	3
Honey Mustard Chicken	1 meal (9.5 oz)	290	6	3
Lemon Pepper Fish	1 meal (10.7 oz)	320	7	2
Mandarin Chicken	1 meal (10 oz)	280	3	0
Mesquite Beef w/ Barbecue Sauce	1 meal (11 oz)	320	9	3
Mesquite Chicken Barbecue	1 meal (10.5 oz)	310	5	2
Oriental Style Chicken & Vegetable Stir Fry	1 meal (11.9)	360	6	2
Oven Roasted Beef	1 meal (10.15 oz)	280	8	3
Roast Turkey Breast	1 meal (8.5 oz)	220	5	2
Roasted Chicken	1 meal (11 oz)	230	5	3
Sesame Chicken	1 meal (10.8 oz)	360	7	2
Shrimp & Vegetables	1 meal (11.8 oz)	270	6	3
Sweet & Sour Chicken	1 meal (11 oz)	360	7	3
Traditional Meatloaf	1 meal (12 oz)	330	7	4
Tradtional Breast Of Turkey	1 meal (10.5 oz)	290	5	2
Tradtional Salisbury Steak	1 meal (11.5 oz)	330	7	3
Tuna Casserole	1 meal (8 oz)	240	5	2
Kid Cuisine				
Circus Show Corn Dog	1 meal (8.8 oz)	490	20	7
Cosmic Chicken Nuggets	1 meal (9.1 oz)	500	25	10
Futuristic Fish Sticks	1 meal (8.25 oz)	410	16	4
Game Time Taco Roll Up	1 meal (7.35 oz)	420	18	7
High Flying Fried Chicken	1 meal (10.1 oz)	440	20	9
Parachuting Pork Ribettes	1 meal (7.55 oz)	390	19	8

FOOD	PORTION	CALS	FAT	SAT FAT
Lean Cuisine				
Cafe Classics Baked Chicken	1 pkg (8.6 oz)	240	5	2
Cafe Classics Baked Fish	1 pkg (9 oz)	290	6	3
Cafe Classics Beef Peppercorn	1 pkg (8.75 oz)	260	7	2
Cafe Classics Beef Portobello	1 pkg (9 oz)	220	7	4
Cafe Classics Beef Pot Roast	1 pkg (9 oz)	210	6	2
Cafe Classics Chicken Carbonara	1 pkg (9 oz)	280	7	2
Cafe Classics Chicken Medallions w/ Creamy Cheese Sauce	1 pkg (9.37 oz)	300	7	3
Cafe Classics Chicken Mediterranean	1 pkg (10.5 oz)	260	4	1
Cafe Classics Chicken & Vegetables	1 pkg (10.5 oz)	240	5	3
Cafe Classics Chicken In Peanut Sauce	1 pkg (9 oz)	260	6	1
Cafe Classics Chicken In Wine Sauce	1 pkg (8.1 oz)	220	5	3
Cafe Classics Chicken L'Orange	1 pkg (9 oz)	230	2	1
Cafe Classics Chicken Parmesan	1 pkg (10.9 oz)	300	6	2
Cafe Classics Chicken Piccata	1 pkg (9 oz)	300	9	3
Cafe Classics Chicken w/ Basil Cream Sauce	1 pkg (8.5 oz)	260	7	2
Cafe Classics Country Vegetables & Beef	1 pkg (9 oz)	210	4	1
Cafe Classics Fiesta Chicken	1 pkg (9.25 oz)	270	5	1
Cafe Classics Glazed Chicken	1 pkg (8.5 oz)	240	6	1
Cafe Classics Glazed Turkey Tenderloins	1 pkg (9 oz)	260	5	1
Cafe Classics Grilled Chicken	1 pkg (9.4 oz)	250	5	2
Cafe Classics Grilled Chicken Salsa	1 pkg (8.9 oz)	270	7	3
Cafe Classics Herb Roasted Chicken	1 pkg (8 oz)	190	4	1
Cafe Classics Honey Mustard Chicken	1 pkg (8 oz)	270	4	1
Cafe Classics Honey Roasted Chicken	1 pkg (8.5 oz)	270	6	2
Cafe Classics Honey Roasted Pork	1 serv (9.5 oz)	250	6	3
Cafe Classics Meatloaf w/ Whipped Potatoes	1 pkg (9.4 oz)	260	7	4
Cafe Classics Oriental Beef	1 pkg (9.25 oz)	210	4	2
Cafe Classics Oven Roasted Beef	1 pkg (9.25 oz)	260	8	3
Cafe Classics Roasted Turkey Breast	1 pkg (9.75 oz)	270	2	1
Cafe Classics Salisbury Steak	1 pkg (9.5 oz)	280	8	4
Cafe Classics Sirloin Beef Peppercorn	1 pkg (8.75 oz)	220	7	2
Cafe Classics Southern Beef Tips	1 pkg (8.75 oz)	270	6	3
Everyday Favorites Vegetable Lasagna	1 pkg (10.5 oz)	260	7	3
Everyday Favorites Chicken Florentine	1 pkg (8 oz)	220	5	2

FOOD	PORTION	CALS	FAT	SAT FAT
Everyday Favorites Chicken Chow Mein	1 pkg (9 oz)	240	4	1
Everyday Favorites Homestyle Turkey	1 pkg (9.4 oz)	240	5	1
Everyday Favorites Hunan Beef & Broccoli	1 pkg (8.5 oz)	240	4	1
Everyday Favorites Mandarin Chicken	1 pkg (9 oz)	260	5	1
Everyday Favorites Roasted Chicken	1 pkg (8.1 oz)	260	7	3
Everyday Favorites Stuffed Cabbage	1 pkg (9.5 oz)	210	8	4
Everyday Favorites Swedish Meatballs	1 pkg (9.1 oz)	290	7	3
Hearty Portions Cheese & Spinach Manicotti	1 serv	370	8	2
Hearty Portions Chicken & Barbecue Sauce	1 serv	370	6	1
Hearty Portions Homestyle Beef Stroganoff	1 serv	350	9	3
Hearty Portions Jumbo Rigatoni w/ Meatballs	1 serv	440	9	4
Hearty Portions Oriental Glazed Chicken	1 serv	370	2	1
Hearty Portions Roasted Chicken w/ Mushrooms	1 serv	330	4	1
Skillet Sensations Beef Teriyaki & Rice	1 serv	280	3	1
Skillet Sensations Chicken Primavera	1 serv	320	5	2
Skillet Sensations Chicken Oriental	1 serv	280	3	1
Skillet Sensations Fiesta Beef & Rice	1 serv	300	4	2
Skillet Sensations Garlic Chicken	1 serv	340	5	2
Skillet Sensations Herb Chicken & Roasted Potatoes	1 serv	270	5	2
Skillet Sensations Roasted Turkey	1 serv	220	2	1
Skillet Sensations Savory Beef & Vegetables	1 serv	290	7	3
Skillet Sensations Three Cheese Chicken	1 serv	370	10	4
Luzianne				
Cajun Creole Dirty Rice	1 serv	160	1	0
Cajun Creole Etouffee	1 serv	200	1	0
Cajun Creole Gumbo	1 serv	160	1	0
Cajun Creole Jambalaya	1 serv	200	1	0
Marie Callender's				
Beef Stroganoff w/ Noodles	1 meal (13 oz)	600	27	11
Beef Tips In Mushroom Sauce	1 meal (13 oz)	430	19	7

FOOD	PORTION	CALS	FAT	SAT FAT
Breaded Chicken Parmigiana	1 meal (16 oz)	860	32	8
Breaded Fish w/ Mac & Cheese	1 meal (12 oz)	550	28	9
Cheesy Rice w/ Chicken & Broccoli	1 meal (12 oz)	390	13	9
Chicken & Dumplings	1 meal (14 oz)	390	20	10
Chicken & Noodles	1 meal (13 oz)	520	30	11
Chicken Cordon Bleu	1 meal (13 oz)	610	28	9
Chicken Fried Beef Steak & Gravy	1 meal (15 oz)	650	37	13
Chicken Teriyaki	1 meal (13 oz)	510	12	3
Country Fried Chicken & Gravy	1 meal (16 oz)	620	30	9
Country Fried Pork Chop	1 meal (15 oz)	540	28	9
Escalloped Noodles & Chicken	1 meal (13 oz)	740	46	16
Glazed Chicken	1 meal (13 oz)	490	25	11
Grilled Southwestern Style Chicken	1 meal (14 oz)	410	11	6
Grilled Chicken & Mashed Potatoes	1 meal (10 oz)	340	16	6
Grilled Chicken Breast & Rice Pilaf	1 meal (11.75 oz)	360	14	4
Grilled Chicken In Mushroom Sauce	1 meal (14 oz)	480	15	6
Grilled Turkey Breast & Rice Pilaf	1 meal (11.75 oz)	310	10	4
Herb Roasted Chicken & Mashed Potatoes	1 meal (14 oz)	580	34	16
Homestyle Turkey & Noodles	1 meal (12 oz)	600	35	18
Honey Roasted Chicken	1 meal (14 oz)	440	17	7
Honey Smoked Ham Steak w/ Macaroni & Cheese	1 meal (14 oz)	490	13	7
Meatloaf & Gravy w/ Mashed Potatoes	1 meal (14 oz)	540	30	12
Old Fashioned Beef Pot Roast & Gravy	1 meal (15 oz)	500	17	6
Roast Beef	1 meal (14.5 oz)	390	19	8
Sirloin Salisbury Steak & Gravy	1 meal (14 oz)	550	25	11
Skillet Meal Au Gratin Potatoes	⅔ cup (5 oz)	190	10	7
Skillet Meal Beef Pot Roast	½ pkg	290	9	4
Skillet Meal Beef Stroganoff	½ pkg	310	11	7
Skillet Meal Chicken & Rice w/ Broccoli & Cheese	½ pkg	440	14	10
Skillet Meal Chicken Teriyaki	½ pkg	340	1	1
Skillet Meal Herb Chicken	½ pkg	290	4	2
Skillet Meal Roasted Chicken & Vegetables	½ pkg	260	6	2
Skillet Meal White & Wild Rice In Cheese Sauce	1 cup	300	13	8

FOOD	PORTION	CALS	FAT	SAT FAT
Swedish Meatballs	1 meal (12.5 oz)	520	26	12
Sweet & Sour Chicken	1 meal (14 oz)	570	15	3
Turkey w/ Gravy & Dressing	1 meal (14 oz)	500	19	9
Morton				
Breaded Chicken Pattie	1 meal (6.75 oz)	290	17	4
Chicken Nuggets	1 meal (7 oz)	340	19	5
Chili Gravy w/ Beef Enchilada & Tamale	1 meal (10 oz)	270	9	4
Fried Chicken	1 meal (9 oz)	470	30	10
Gravy & Charbroiled Beef Patty	1 meal (9 oz)	310	18	9
Gravy & Salisbury Steak	1 meal (9 oz)	310	20	8
Gravy & Turkey w/ Stuffing	1 meal (9 oz)	240	10	4
Tomato Sauce w/ Meat Loaf	1 meal (9 oz)	250	13	5
Veal Parmagiana w/ Tomato Sauce	1 meal (8.75 oz)	290	15	5
Nature's Choice				
Broccoli Parmesan Alfredo	1 pkg (12 oz)	270	9	3
Nature's Entree				
Hearty Stew	1 pkg (12 oz)	290	9	3
Tuscany White Bean	1 pkg (12 oz)	330	8	2
Patio				
Ranchera	1 pkg (13 oz)	470	22	10
Stouffer's				
Baked Chicken Breast w/ Mashed Potatoes	1 serv (12.2 oz)	330	14	5
Beef Stroganoff	1 pkg (9.75 oz)	390	20	7
Chicken A La King	1 pkg (9.5 oz)	350	13	4
Creamed Chicken	1 pkg (6.5 oz)	260	19	10
Creamed Chipped Beef	½ cup (5.5 oz)	160	11	3
Creamy Chicken & Broccoli	1 pkg (8.9 oz)	320	15	5
Escalloped Chicken & Noodles	1 pkg (10 oz)	430	27	5
Fish w/ Macaroni & Cheese	1 serv (9.5 oz)	460	20	6
Glazed Chicken w/ Rice	1 serv (11.8 oz)	290	6	1
Green Pepper Steak	1 pkg (10.5 oz)	330	9	3
Homestyle Baked Chicken & Gravy & Whipped Potatoes	1 pkg (8.9 oz)	270	12	3
Homestyle Beef Pot Roast & Browned Potatoes	1 pkg (8.9 oz)	250	8	3
Homestyle Fish Filet w/ Macaroni & Cheese	1 pkg (9 oz)	430	21	5

FOOD	PORTION	CALS	FAT	SAT FAT
Homestyle Fried Chicken & Whipped Potatoes	1 pkg (7.5 oz)	310	12	4
Homestyle Meatloaf & Whipped Potatoes	1 pkg (9.9 oz)	330	16	6
Homestyle Roast Turkey w/ Gravy Stuffing & Whipped Potatoes	1 pkg (9.6 oz)	320	13	4
Homestyle Salisbury Steak & Gravy & Macaroni & Cheese	1 pkg (9.6 oz)	350	16	7
Meatloaf	1 serv (5.5 oz)	210	12	4
Meatloaf w/ Whipped Potatoes	1 serv (11.5 oz)	380	18	7
Stuffed Pepper	1 pkg (10 oz)	200	5	2
Swedish Meatballs	1 pkg (10.25 oz)	480	24	9
Swanson				
Beef Pot Roast	1 pkg (14 oz)	320	8	3
Chicken Parmigiana w/ Spaghetti	1 pkg (11 oz)	380	17	4
Turkey Breast	1 pkg (11.7 oz)	330	6	1
Tamarind Tree				
Alu Chole	1 pkg (9.2 oz)	350	6	1
Channa Dal Masala	1 pkg (9.2 oz)	340	5	1
Dal Makhini	1 pkg (9.2 oz)	330	6	2
Dhingri Mutter	1 pkg (9.2 oz)	290	5	1
Navratan Korma	1 pkg (9.2 oz)	430	15	4
Palak Paneer	1 pkg (9.2 oz)	380	15	6
Saag Chole	1 pkg (9.2 oz)	370	10	2
Vegetable Jalfrazi	1 pkg (9.2 oz)	310	6	1
Tyson				
BBQ Chicken Potato & Vegetable Medley	1 pkg (14.7 oz)	560	21	5
Beef Stir Fry	1 pkg (14 oz)	430	5	2
Blackened Chicken Spanish Rice & Corn	1 pkg (8.8 oz)	260	5	1
Chicken Primavera	1 pkg (11.3 oz)	350	6	3
Chicken Divan Candied Carrots & Pasta	1 pkg (9.8 oz)	370	15	4
Chicken Francais Sliced Potatoes & Green Beans	1 pkg (8.8 oz)	260	10	3
Chicken Kiev Rice Pilaf & Broccoli Carrots	1 pkg (9.1 oz)	440	25	11
Chicken Marsala Carrots & Red Potatoes	1 pkg (8.8 oz)	180	5	2

FOOD	PORTION	CALS	FAT	SAT FAT
Chicken Mesquite Corn & Pea Medley & Au Gratin Potatoes	1 pkg (8.8 oz)	320	8	3
Chicken Picatta	1 pkg (8.8 oz)	190	6	2
Chicken Stir Fry Kit	2¾ cups (14 oz)	430	5	1
Chicken w/ Broccoli & Cheese Carrots & Pasta	1 pkg (8.8 oz)	270	12	5
Chicken w/ Mushroom Sauce Rice Pilaf & Candied Carrots	1 pkg (8.8 oz)	220	6	2
Chicken w/ Tabasco BBQ Sauce	1 pkg (8.8 oz)	260	7	2
Fried Chicken & Gravy w/ Mashed Potatoes & Corn	1 pkg (10.8 oz)	360	15	3
Grilled Chicken Corn O'Brien & Ranch Beans	1 pkg (8.8 oz)	230	4	1
Grilled Italian Chicken Pasta & Vegetable Medley	1 pkg (8.8 oz)	190	4	2
Honey Dijon Chicken Pasta & Pea Medley	1 pkg (11.3 oz)	340	7	2
Roasted Chicken w/ Garlic Sauce Pasta & Vegetable Medley	1 pkg (8.8 oz)	210	7	2
Weight Watchers				
Smart One Grilled Salisbury Steak	1 pkg (8.5 oz)	250	9	4
Smart Ones Chicken Mirabella	1 pkg (9.2 oz)	180	2	1
Smart Ones Fiesta Chicken	1 pkg (8.5 oz)	210	2	1
Smart Ones Honey Mustard Chicken	1 pkg (8.5 oz)	200	2	1
Smart Ones Lemon Herb Chicken Piccata	1 pkg (8.5 oz)	190	2	1
Smart Ones Pepper Steak	1 pkg (10 oz)	240	5	2
Smart Ones Risotto w/ Cheese & Mushrooms	1 pkg (10 oz)	290	7	3
Smart Ones Roast Turkey Medallions & Mushrooms	1 pkg (8.5 oz)	180	2	1
Smart Ones Shrimp Marinara	1 pkg (9 oz)	180	2	1
Smart Ones Stuffed Turkey Breast	1 pkg (10 oz)	260	7	2
Smart Ones Swedish Meatballs	1 pkg (9 oz)	280	70	4
Yves				
Veggie Country Stew	1 pkg (10.5 oz)	170	0	0
DIP				
Breakstone's				
Bacon & Onion	2 tbsp (1.1 oz)	60	5	3

FOOD	PORTION	CALS	FAT	SAT FAT
Chesapeake Clam	2 tbsp (1.1 oz)	50	4	3
Free Creamy Salsa	2 tbsp (1.1 oz)	20	0	0
Free French Onion	2 tbsp (1.1 oz)	25	0	0
Free Ranch	2 tbsp (1.1 oz)	25	0	0
French Onion	2 tbsp (1.1 oz)	50	5	3
Toasted Onion	2 tbsp (1.1 oz)	50	5	3
Cabot				
Bac'n Horseradish	2 tbsp	50	5	3
Clam	2 tbsp	50	5	3
French Onion	2 tbsp	50	5	–
Ranch	1 tbsp	50	5	3
Salsa Grande	2 tbsp	50	5	3
Veggie	2 tbsp	50	5	3
Cheez Whiz				
Medium Cheese & Salsa	2 tbsp (1.2 oz)	100	8	5
Mild Cheese & Salsa	2 tbsp (1.2 oz)	100	8	5
Chi-Chi's				
Fiesta Bean	2 tbsp (0.9 oz)	35	2	1
Fiesta Cheese	2 tbsp (0.9 oz)	40	3	1
Fritos				
Bean	2 tbsp (1.2 oz)	40	1	1
Chili Cheese	1.2 oz	45	3	1
French Onion	2 tbsp (1.1 oz)	60	5	3
Hot Bean	2 tbsp (1.2 oz)	40	1	0
Jalapeno & Cheddar Cheese	2 tbsp (1.2 oz)	50	4	1
Gringo Billy's				
Guacamole Mix	1 tsp	10	0	0
Guiltless Gourmet				
Black Bean Mild	2 tbsp (1 oz)	30	0	0
Black Bean Spicy	2 tbsp (1 oz)	30	0	0
Knudsen				
Free Creamy Salsa	2 tbsp (1.1 oz)	20	0	0
Free French Onion	2 tbsp (1.1 oz)	25	0	0
Free Ranch	2 tbsp (1.1 oz)	25	0	0
Kraft				
Avocado	2 tbsp (1.1 oz)	60	4	3
Bacon & Horseradish	2 tbsp (1.1 oz)	60	5	3
Clam	2 tbsp (1.1 oz)	60	4	3
Free French Onion	2 tbsp (1.1 oz)	25	0	0
Free Ranch	2 tbsp (1.1 oz)	25	0	0

FOOD	PORTION	CALS	FAT	SAT FAT
Free Salsa	2 tbsp (1.1 oz)	20	0	0
French Onion	2 tbsp (1.1 oz)	60	4	3
Green Onion	2 tbsp (1.1 oz)	60	4	3
Jalapeno Cheese	2 tbsp (1.1 oz)	60	4	3
Premium Sour Cream	2 tbsp (1.1 oz)	50	4	3
Premium Sour Cream Bacon & Horseradish	2 tbsp (1.1 oz)	60	5	3
Premium Sour Cream Bacon & Onion	2 tbsp (1.1 oz)	60	5	3
Premium Sour Cream Creamy Onion	2 tbsp (1.1 oz)	45	4	3
Premium Sour Cream French Onion	2 tbsp (1.1 oz)	45	4	3
Premium Sour Cream Ranch	2 tbsp (1.1 oz)	50	4	3
Ranch	2 tbsp (1.1 oz)	60	5	3
Old El Paso				
Black Bean	2 tbsp (1 oz)	20	0	0
Cheese 'n Salsa Medium	2 tbsp (1 oz)	40	3	1
Cheese 'n Salsa Mild	2 tbsp (1 oz)	40	3	1
Chunky Salsa Medium	2 tbsp (1 oz)	15	0	0
Chunky Salsa Mild	2 tbsp (1 oz)	15	0	0
Jalapeno	2 tbsp (1 oz)	30	1	0
Racquet				
Hot Cheddar Jalapeno	2 tbsp	30	3	1
Ruffles				
French Onion	2 tbsp	70	5	1
Ranch	2 tbsp (1.2 oz)	70	6	1
Snyder's Of Hanover				
Microwavable Hot Nacho Cheese	2 tbsp	48	3	1
Microwavable Mild Cheese	2 tbsp	45	3	2
Mustard Pretzel	2 tbsp	60	2	0
Sour Cream & Onion	2 tbsp	60	5	3
Taco Bell				
Fat Free Black Bean	2 tbsp (1.2 oz)	30	0	0
Salsa Con Queso Medium	2 tbsp (1.2 oz)	45	3	1
Salsa Con Queso Mild	2 tbsp (1.2 oz)	45	3	1
Tyson				
Bleu Cheese For Dipping Wings	2 tbsp (1.4 oz)	140	14	3
Utz				
Fat Free Sour Cream & Onion	2 tbsp (1.1 oz)	30	0	0
Jalapeno & Cheddar	2 tbsp (1 oz)	30	3	1
Low Fat Desert Garden	2 tbsp (1.1 oz)	40	2	0
Low Fat Salsa Con Queso	2 tbsp (1 oz)	40	2	0

FOOD	PORTION	CALS	FAT	SAT FAT
Mild Cheddar	2 tbsp (1 oz)	45	3	2
Sour Cream & Onion	2 tbsp (1 oz)	60	5	3
Walden Farms				
Low Carb Bruschetta	2 tbsp	35	3	—
Low Carb Pesto Bruschetta	1 tsp	10	1	—

DOCK
fresh cooked	3½ oz	20	1	—
raw chopped	½ cup	15	tr	—

DOLPHINFISH
fresh baked	3 oz	93	1	tr
fresh fillet baked	5.6 oz	174	1	tr

DOUGHNUTS
cake type unsugared	1 (1.6 oz)	198	11	2
chocolate glazed	1 (1.5 oz)	175	8	3
chocolate sugared	1 (1.5 oz)	175	8	3
chocolate coated	1 (1.5 oz)	204	13	4
creme filled	1 (3 oz)	307	21	6
french cruller glazed	1 (1.4 oz)	169	8	2
frosted	1 (1.5 oz)	204	13	4
honey bun	1 (2.1 oz)	242	14	3
jelly	1 (3 oz)	289	16	4
old fashioned	1 (1.6 oz)	198	11	2
sugared	1 (1.6 oz)	192	10	3
wheat glazed	1 (1.6 oz)	162	9	1
wheat sugared	1 (1.6 oz)	162	9	1
yeast glazed	1 (2.1 oz)	242	14	3
Dolly Madison				
Chocolate Frosted	1 (1.1 oz)	140	8	5
Donut Gems Chocolate	4 (2 oz)	260	15	9
Donut Gems Crunch	3 (2 oz)	220	10	4
Donut Gems Powdered	4 (2 oz)	230	11	5
English Cruller	1 (2 oz)	250	14	6
Glazed Whirl	1 (1.6 oz)	210	11	5
Glazed Yeast	1 (1.5 oz)	190	9	5
Old Fashioned	1 (2.1 oz)	280	16	8
Plain	1 (1.2 oz)	140	7	3
Powdered	1 (1 oz)	120	6	3

FOOD	PORTION	CALS	FAT	SAT FAT
Dutch Mill				
Cider	1 (2.1 oz)	240	10	2
Cinnamon	1 (1.8 oz)	210	11	5
Donut Holes Double-Dipped Chocolate	3 (1.4 oz)	220	16	6
Donut Holes Shootin' Stars	3 (1.4 oz)	190	10	3
Double-Dipped Chocolate	1 (2.1 oz)	280	17	7
Glazed	1 (2.1 oz)	250	12	3
Glazed Chocolate	1 (2.4 oz)	270	11	3
Plain	1 (1.8 oz)	210	12	5
Sugared	1 (1.8 oz)	220	11	5
Hostess				
Blueberry	1 (1.7 oz)	210	13	6
Donettes Crumb	3 (1.5 oz)	170	8	3
Donettes Frosted	3 (1.5 oz)	200	12	7
Donettes Powdered	3 (1.5 oz)	180	9	3
Frosted	1 (1.4 oz)	180	11	7
O's Raspberry Filled	1 (2.2 oz)	230	10	4
Old Fashioned Glazed	1 (2.1 oz)	260	13	6
Plain	1 (1.1 oz)	140	7	3
Powdered	1 (1.3 oz)	150	8	4
Little Debbie				
Donut Sticks	1 (1.6 oz)	210	12	3
Mini Powdered	1 pkg (2.5 oz)	290	14	4
Snack & Smile				
Mini Donuts Chocolate	6	370	19	10
Mini Donuts Glazed	6	340	16	40
Mini Donuts Powdered Sugar	6	320	13	4
Super				
Donut Chocolate	1 (2.2 oz)	210	11	3
Donut Honey Wheat	1 (2.2 oz)	230	11	2
Tastykake				
Mini Plain Glaze	1 pkg (2.5 oz)	260	11	2
Mini Powdered Sugar	1 pkg (2.5 oz)	260	12	2
Mini Rich Frosted	1 pkg (3 oz)	370	22	10
Tom's				
Chocolate Gem	1 pkg (2.5 oz)	320	18	5
Dunkin' Sticks	1 pkg (2.5 oz)	370	22	7
Powdered Gems	1 pkg (2.5 oz)	320	18	5

FOOD	PORTION	CALS	FAT	SAT FAT
DRINK MIXERS				
whiskey sour mix not prep	1 pkg (0.6 oz)	64	0	0
whiskey sour mix	2 oz	55	0	0
Baja Bob's				
Bloody Mary Mix Lean & Mean	4 oz	20	0	0
Pina Colada	4 oz	30	1	0
Sugar Free Margarita Mix	4 oz	10	0	0
Sugar Free Margarita Mix Desert Lime	4 oz	10	0	0
Sugar Free Margarita Mix Wild Strawberry	4 oz	10	0	0
Sweet-n-Sour Mix	4 oz	10	0	0
Daily's				
Bloody Mary Original	1 serv (6 oz)	50	0	0
Margarita Daiquiri Strawberry	1 serv (4 oz)	180	0	0
Margarita Green Demon	1 serv (3 oz)	80	0	0
Pina Colada	1 serv (3 oz)	160	2	1
Tabasco				
Bloody Mary Mix	1 serv (8.4 oz)	56	tr	tr
Bloody Mary Mix Extra Spicy	1 serv (8.4 oz)	58	tr	tr
DRUM				
freshwater fillet baked	5.4 oz	236	10	2
freshwater baked	3 oz	130	5	1
DUCK				
w/ skin roasted	1 cup (4.9 oz)	472	40	14
w/ skin w/ bone leg roasted	3 oz	184	10	3
w/ skin w/o bone breast roasted	3 oz	172	9	2
w/o skin roasted	1 cup (4.9 oz)	281	16	6
w/o skin w/ bone leg braised	1 cup (6.1 oz)	310	10	2
w/o skin w/o bone breast broiled	1 cup (6.1 oz)	244	4	1
wild w/ skin raw	½ duck (9.5 oz)	571	41	14
wild w/o skin breast raw	½ breast (2.9 oz)	102	4	1
Grimaud Farms				
Muscovy Duck Confit	1 serv (3 oz)	170	10	4
DUMPLING				
Health Is Wealth				
Potstickers Chicken Free	2 (1.6 oz)	80	4	1
Potstickers Pork Free	2 (1.6 oz)	80	4	1
Potstickers Vegetable	2 (1.6 oz)	90	3	1

FOOD	PORTION	CALS	FAT	SAT FAT
Steamed Dumpling	2 (1.6 oz)	50	2	0
Pepperidge Farm				
Apple	1 (3 oz)	230	11	3
Peach	1 (3 oz)	320	11	3
DURIAN				
fresh	3.5 oz	141	2	–
EEL				
fresh cooked	3 oz	200	13	3
fresh cooked	1 fillet (5.6 oz)	375	24	5
raw	3 oz	156	10	2
smoked	3.5 oz	330	28	7
EGG (see also EGG DISHES, EGG SUBSTITUTES)				
CHICKEN				
fresh	1	75	5	2
frozen	1 cup	363	24	8
frozen	1	75	5	2
hard cooked	1	77	5	2
hard cooked chopped	1 cup	210	14	4
poached	1	74	5	2
white only	1	17	0	0
white only	1 cup	121	0	0
Eggology				
100% Organic Egg Whites	¼ cup	30	0	0
EggsPlus				
Fresh	1 (1.8 oz)	70	5	2
Horizon Organic				
Medium	1 (1.5 oz)	70	4	2
Land O Lakes				
Brown Extra Large	1 (2 oz)	80	5	2
Organic Valley				
Brown Extra Large	1 (2.2 oz)	90	6	5
Brown Large	1 (2 oz)	80	6	4
Brown Medium	1 (1.8 oz)	70	5	3
OTHER POULTRY				
duck	1 (2.5 oz)	130	10	3
duck 100 year old	1 (1 oz)	49	3	–
duck preserved hard core	1 (1.8 oz)	80	6	2
duck preserved soft core	1 (1.8 oz)	80	6	2

FOOD	PORTION	CALS	FAT	SAT FAT
duck salted	1 (1 oz)	54	4	–
goose	1 (5 oz)	267	19	5
quail	1 (9 g)	14	1	tr
turkey	1 (2.7 oz)	135	9	3

EGG DISHES
FROZEN
Weight Watchers

Handy Ham & Cheese Omelet	1 (4 oz)	220	5	3

TAKE-OUT

cheese omelette as prep w/ 2 eggs	1 (6.8 oz)	519	44	–
deviled	2 halves	145	13	3
omelette plain	1 serv (3.5 oz)	172	13	4
salad	½ cup	307	28	6
scotch egg	1 (4.2 oz)	301	21	–
scrambled plain	2 (3.3 oz)	199	15	6
scrambled w/ whole milk & margarine	1 serv	365	27	8
sunny side up	1	91	7	2

EGG ROLLS

egg roll wrapper fresh	1	83	tr	tr

Chun King

Chicken Mini	6	210	9	3
Chicken Restaurant Style	1 (3 oz)	190	9	5
Pork & Shrimp Mini	6	210	9	3
Shrimp Mini	6	190	6	2
Shrimp Restaurant Style	1 (3 oz)	180	7	3

Health Is Wealth

Broccoli	1 (3 oz)	150	5	1
Oriental Vegetable	1 (3 oz)	160	4	1
Oriental Chicken Free	1 (3 oz)	120	4	1
Pizza	1 (3 oz)	200	9	1
Spinach	1 (3 oz)	180	8	1
Spring Rolls	1 (1.6 oz)	70	2	1
Veggie	1 (3 oz)	130	4	0

La Choy

Chicken Mini	6	210	9	3
Chicken Restaurant Style	1 (3 oz)	210	9	5
Pork Restaurant Style	1 (3 oz)	220	11	3
Pork & Shrimp Bite Size	12	210	10	3

FOOD	PORTION	CALS	FAT	SAT FAT
Pork & Shrimp Mini	6	210	9	3
Shrimp Mini	6	190	6	2
Shrimp Restaurant Style	1 (3 oz)	180	7	2
Sweet & Sour Chicken Restaurant Style	1 (3 oz)	220	9	2
Vegetable w/ Lobster Mini	6	190	7	2
Lo-An				
White Meat Chicken	1 (2.7 oz)	140	4r	1
Worthington				
Vegetarian Egg Rolls	1 (3 oz)	180	8	2
TAKE-OUT				
lobster	1 (4.8 oz)	270	7	2
lumpia vegetable & shrimp	2 (3 oz)	120	0	0
meat & shrimp	1 (4.8 oz)	320	12	3
pork & shrimp	1 (5 oz)	300	10	4
shrimp	1 (3 oz)	170	5	1
spicy pork	1 (3 oz)	200	9	2
vegetable	1 (3 oz)	170	4	1
EGG SUBSTITUTES				
frozen	¼ cup	96	7	1
frozen	1 cup	384	27	5
liquid	1 cup (8.8 oz)	211	8	2
liquid	1½ oz	40	2	tr
powder	0.35 oz	44	1	tr
powder	0.7 oz	88	3	1
Better'n Eggs				
Fat Free Cholesterol Free	¼ cup (2 oz)	30	0	0
Deb-El				
Just Whites	2 tsp	12	0	0
Egg Beaters				
Egg Substitute	¼ cup	30	0	0
Omelette Cheese	½ cup	110	5	2
Omelette Vegetable	½ cup	50	0	0
Morningstar Farms				
Breakfast Sandwich Bagel Scramblers Pattie Cheese	1 (5.9 oz)	320	5	1
Breakfast Sandwich English Muffin Scramblers Pattie	1 (5.1 oz)	240	3	1

FOOD	PORTION	CALS	FAT	SAT FAT
Breakfast Sandwich English Muffin Scramblers Pattie Cheese	1 (6 oz)	280	3	1
Scramblers	¼ cup (2 oz)	35	0	0
Quick Eggs				
Fat Free Cholesterol Free	¼ cup	30	0	0

EGGNOG

FOOD	PORTION	CALS	FAT	SAT FAT
eggnog	1 cup	342	19	11
eggnog	1 qt	1368	76	45
eggnog flavor mix as prep w/ milk	9 oz	260	8	5
Oberweis				
Egg Nog	½ cup	240	15	7
TAKE-OUT				
eggnog	1 cup	306	22	14

EGGNOG SUBSTITUTES
Silk

FOOD	PORTION	CALS	FAT	SAT FAT
Nog	½ cup	90	2	0

EGGPLANT

FOOD	PORTION	CALS	FAT	SAT FAT
cubed cooked	1 cup	28	tr	tr
raw cut up	½ cup (1.4 oz)	11	tr	tr
slices grilled	4 (7 oz)	38	0	0
whole peeled raw	1 (1 lb)	117	1	tr
Progresso				
Caponata	2 tbsp (1 oz)	25	2	0
TastyBite				
Punjab Eggplant	½ pkg (5 oz)	130	8	1
TAKE-OUT				
baba ghannouj	¼ cup	55	4	–
caponata	2 tbsp (1 oz)	30	2	–
iman bayildi eggplant w/ onion & tomato	1 serv (15.6 oz)	345	28	4
indian eggplant runi	1 serv	180	14	4
moussaka	1 cup	237	13	5
papoutsakis little shoes	1 serv (15.5 oz)	245	16	7

ELDERBERRIES

FOOD	PORTION	CALS	FAT	SAT FAT
fresh	1 cup	105	1	–

ELDERBERRY JUICE

FOOD	PORTION	CALS	FAT	SAT FAT
elderberry	7 oz	76	0	0

FOOD	PORTION	CALS	FAT	SAT FAT
ELK				
roasted	3 oz	124	2	1
ENDIVE				
fresh	3.5 oz	9	tr	–
raw chopped	½ cup	4	tr	tr
ENERGY BARS (see also CEREAL BARS, NUTRITION SUPPLEMENTS)				
AllGoode Organics				
Amazin' Peanut Raisin	1 bar	210	11	2
Banana Nut Nirvana	1 bar	190	8	4
Cashew Almond Passion	1 bar	210	9	1
Chocolate Peanut Pleasure	1 bar	200	9	3
Honey Nut Harvest	1 bar	210	9	1
Nutty Chocolate Apricot	1 bar	200	10	5
Atkins				
Advantage Almond Brownie	1 bar (1.6 oz)	220	8	4
Advantage Chocolate Coconut	1 bar (1.6 oz)	230	11	8
Advantage Chocolate Decadence	1 bar (1.6 oz)	220	11	7
Advantage Chocolate Mocha Crunch	1 bar (1.6 oz)	220	10	6
Advantage Chocolate Peanut Butter	1 bar (1.6 oz)	240	12	6
Advantage Cookies 'N Creme	1 bar (1.6 oz)	220	11	7
Advantage S'mores	1 bar (1.6 oz)	220	10	5
Morning Start Apple Crisp	1 bar	170	9	4
Morning Start Blueberry Muffin	1 bar	160	7	4
Morning Start Chocolate Chip Crisp	1 bar	160	7	3
Back To Nature				
10th Tee Chocolate Fudge	1 bar	200	6	4
10th Tee Peanut Honey	1 bar	260	6	4
1st Tee Chocolate Peanut	1 bar	290	8	5
1st Tee Oatmeal Raisin	1 bar	280	7	4
Balance				
Chocolate Raspberry Fudge	1 bar (1.76 oz)	180	6	–
Oasis Strawberry Cheesecake	1 bar (1.69 oz)	180	3	2
Be Natural				
Almond & Apricot	1 bar	218	14	7
Almond & Coconut	1 bar	248	18	6
Banana & Wheat Bran	1 bar	201	9	8
Fruit & Nut Delight	1 bar	225	14	2
Macadamia & Apricot	1 bar	224	15	8
Nut Delight	1 bar	266	20	3

FOOD	PORTION	CALS	FAT	SAT FAT
Sesame Nut Split	1 bar	256	17	2
Walnut & Date	1 bar	147	9	1
Yogurt Coated Almond & Apricot	1 bar	233	14	3
Yogurt Coated Fruit & Nut	1 bar	190	12	1
Benecol				
Chocolate Crisp	1 bar (1.2 oz)	130	3	2
Chocolate Crisp	1 bar (1.2 oz)	130	3	2
Peanut Crisp	1 bar (1.2 oz)	140	4	2
Better Bar				
Chocolate Coated Caramel Pecan	1 bar (1.8 oz)	180	4	2
Chocolate Coated Peanut	1 bar (1.8 oz)	180	4	2
Yogurt Coated Raspberry	1 bar (1.8 oz)	180	3	2
Boost				
Chocolate Crunch	1 bar (1.5 oz)	190	7	4
Breakthru				
Organic Chocolate Fudge	1 bar (2.1 oz)	230	3	2
Organic Cinnamon Crunch	1 bar (2.1 oz)	220	3	1
Organic Honey Graham	1 bar (2.1 oz)	220	3	1
Organic Mocha Fudge	1 bar (2.1 oz)	230	3	2
Carb Options				
Chocolate Chip	1 bar	200	8	4
Chocolate Peanut	1 bar	200	8	4
Cinnamon Delight	1 bar	200	8	4
CarbWise				
Chocolate S'Mores Crunch	1 bar	240	9	6
Carbolite				
Chocolate Peanut Butter Sugar Free	1 bar (1 oz)	144	12	4
Centrum				
Energy Chocolate Nougat	1 (1.98 oz)	220	5	4
Energy Chocolate Peanut Butter	1 (1.98 oz)	220	5	4
Choice				
Berry Almond Crispy	1 bar	50	1	0
Fudge Brownie	1 bar	140	5	3
Peanut Butter Crispy	1 bar	60	2	2
Peanutty Chocolate	1 bar	140	5	3
Clif Bar				
Apricot	1 bar (2.4 oz)	220	3	0
Carrot Cake	1 bar (2.4 oz)	240	4	2
Chocolate Brownie	1 bar (2.4 oz)	240	4	1
Chocolate Almond Fudge	1 bar (2.4 oz)	230	5	1

FOOD	PORTION	CALS	FAT	SAT FAT
Chocolate Chip	1 bar (2.4 oz)	240	4	1
Chocolate Chip Peanut Crunch	1 bar (2.4 oz)	240	5	1
Cookies'N Cream	1 bar (2.4 oz)	230	4	2
Cranberry Apple Cherry	1 bar (2.4 oz)	220	2	0
Crunchy Peanut Butter	1 bar (2.4 oz)	240	5	1
GingerSnap	1 bar (2.4 oz)	230	4	1
Deliciously Slim				
Chocolate Fudge Cake	1 bar (2.1 oz)	200	6	3
DrSoy				
Double Chocolate	1 bar (1.76 oz)	180	3	3
Ensure				
All Flavors	1 bar (2.1 oz)	230	6	4
Extend				
Chocolate Chip Crunch	1 bar (1.4 oz)	160	3	2
Peanut Butter Crunch	1 bar (1.4 oz)	160	3	0
Fast Fuel Up				
Natural Chocolate Espresso	1 bar (2.3 oz)	300	19	7
Natural Chocolate Crunch	1 bar (2.3 oz)	300	19	7
Organic Chocolate Espresso	1 bar (1.8 oz)	230	15	5
Organic Chocolate Crunch	1 bar (1.8 oz)	230	15	6
Gatorade				
All Flavors	1 bar (2.3 oz)	260	5	1
GeniSoy				
Soy Protein Arctic Frost Crispy Chocolate Mint	1 bar (2.2 oz)	230	5	4
Soy Protein Dutch Crunch Sour Apple Crisp	1 bar (2.2 oz)	230	5	3
Soy Protein Fair Trade Arabica Cafe Mocha Fudge	1 bar (2.2 oz)	220	4	3
Soy Protein New York Style Blueberry Cheesecake	1 bar (2.2 oz)	220	4	3
Soy Protein Obsession Fudge Cookies & Cream	1 bar (2.2 oz)	230	5	3
Soy Protein Pure Golden Honey Creamy Peanut Yogurt	1 bar (2.2 oz)	230	5	3
Soy Protein Southern Style Chunky Peanut Butter Fudge	1 bar (2.2 oz)	240	6	3
Soy Protein Ultimate Chocolate Fudge Brownie	1 bar (2.2 oz)	230	5	3
Xtreme Carrot Cake Quake	1 bar (1.6 oz)	190	7	3

FOOD	PORTION	CALS	FAT	SAT FAT
Xtreme Peanut Butter Fix	1 bar (1.6 oz)	200	8	3
Xtreme Raspberry Rush	1 bar (1.6 oz)	190	7	4
Xtreme Rocky Roadtrip	1 bar (1.6 oz)	190	7	3
Glucerna				
All Flavors	1 bar (1.3 oz)	140	4	1
Hansen's				
Chocolate Banana Crunch	1 bar	180	3	2
Chocolate Orchard Crunch	1 bar	170	3	2
Natural Bar Tropical Fruit Crunch	1 bar	170	3	2
Natural Bar Yogurt Strawberry Crunch	1 bar	190	3	2
HeartBar				
Cranberry	1 bar (1.8 oz)	190	3	1
Original	1 bar (1.76 oz)	180	3	1
Hi-Lo				
Chocolate Caramel	1 bar (1.76 oz)	200	8	5
Chocolate Mint	1 bar (2.1 oz)	200	6	4
Chocolate Peanut Butter	1 bar (2.1 oz)	210	7	4
Chocolate Raspberry	1 bar (2.1 oz)	200	6	3
Ideal				
Mixed Berry Tart	1 bar (1.7 oz)	200	7	3
Jenny Craig				
Meal Bar Chocolate Peanut	1 bar (2 oz)	220	5	4
Meal Bar Lemon Meringue	1 bar (2 oz)	210	5	3
Meal Bar Milk Chocolate	1 bar (2 oz)	210	5	4
Meal Bar Oatmeal Raisin	1 bar (1.97 oz)	210	3	0
Meal Bar Yogurt Peanut	1 bar (2 oz)	220	5	3
Kashi				
GoLean Chocolate Almond Toffee	1 (2.7 oz)	290	6	5
GoLean Cookies 'N Cream	1 (2.7 oz)	290	6	4
GoLean Frosted Spice Cake	1 (2.7 oz)	290	5	3
GoLean Honey Vanilla Yogurt	1 (2.7 oz)	290	5	4
GoLean Malted Chocolate Chip	1 (2.7 oz)	290	6	4
GoLean Mocha Java	1 (2.7 oz)	290	6	4
GoLean Oatmeal Raisin Cookie	1 (2.7 oz)	280	5	3
GoLean Peanut Butter & Chocolate	1 (2.7 oz)	290	6	5
GoLean Strawberries 'N Cream	1 (2.7 oz)	290	5	4
GoLean Strawberry Vanilla Yogurt	1 (2.7 oz)	280	4	—
GoLean Crunchy Chocolate Caramel Karma	1 (1.6 oz)	140	3	2

FOOD	PORTION	CALS	FAT	SAT FAT
GoLean Crunchy Chocolate Peanut Bliss	1 (1.8 oz)	270	4	2
GoLean Crunchy Sublime Lemon Lime	1 (1.8 oz)	670	3	2
Lean Body For Her				
Chocolate Honey Peanut	1 bar (1.76 oz)	190	7	4
Luna				
Chai Tea	1 bar (1.7 oz)	180	4	3
Chocolate Pecan Pie	1 bar (1.7 oz)	180	5	3
LemonZest	1 bar (1.7 oz)	180	4	3
Nutz Over Chocolate	1 bar (1.7 oz)	180	5	3
S'Mores	1 bar (1.7 oz)	180	4	3
Sesame Raisin Crunch	1 bar (1.7 oz)	170	3	1
Toasted Nuts 'n Cranberry	1 bar (1.7 oz)	170	3	0
Tropical Crisp	1 bar (1.7 oz)	180	5	4
Met-Rx				
Big 100 Gram Bar Peanut Butter	1 bar (3.5 oz)	340	4	2
Source/One Chocolate Cheesecake	1 bar (2.1 oz)	160	5	4
Moto Bar				
Bodacious Banana Split	1 bar	300	6	2
Charming Cherry Almond	1 bar (2.9 oz)	300	6	1
Cozy Pumpkin Pie	1 bar	300	6	1
Jazzy Peanut Butter & Jelly	1 bar	300	3	1
Kooky Cappuccino	1 bar	300	6	1
Luscious Lemon Blueberry	1 bar	300	5	1
Saucy Apple Cinnamon	1 bar	280	4	1
Zany Cranberry Orange	1 bar	300	5	1
New You				
Chocolate Crisp	1 bar (1.65 oz)	180	4	3
NiteBite				
Chocolate Fudge	1 bar (0.9 oz)	100	4	1
Peanut Butter	1 bar (0.9 oz)	100	4	1
NuGo				
Banana Chocolate Protein	1 bar	190	3	1
Blue Berry Boom	1 bar	180	3	2
Chocolate Blast	1 bar	180	3	2
Coffee Break	1 bar	180	3	2
Orange Smoothie Protein	1 bar	190	3	2
Peanut Butter Pleaser	1 bar	180	3	2

FOOD	PORTION	CALS	FAT	SAT FAT
Nutiva				
Flaxseed & Raisin Organic	1 bar (1.4 oz)	280	19	2
Hempseed Bar Organic	1 bar (1.4 oz)	210	14	2
Nutribar				
Chocolate Covered Belgian Chocolate	1 bar (2.3 oz)	252	8	3
Chocolate Covered Caramel	1 bar (2.3 oz)	261	8	3
Chocolate Covered Chocolate Fudge	1 bar (2.3 oz)	267	8	3
Chocolate Covered Hazelnut	1 bar (2.3 oz)	261	8	3
Chocolate Covered Mocha Almond	1 bar (2.3 oz)	261	8	3
Chocolate Covered Peanut	1 bar (2.3 oz)	262	9	3
Yogurt Covered Peach Apricot	1 bar (2.3 oz)	261	8	3
Yogurt Covered Raspberry	1 bar (2.3 oz)	261	8	3
Yogurt Covered Wildberry	1 bar (2.3 oz)	261	8	3
Odwalla Bar!				
Peanut Crunch	1 bar (2.2 oz)	260	7	2
Peacekeeper				
Nuts About Peace All Flavors	1 bar (1.4 oz)	180	9	2
PermaLean				
Protein Crunch Chocoholic Chocolate	1 bar (1.8 oz)	170	3	2
Protein Crunch Chocolate Raspberry	1 bar (1.8 oz)	180	2	2
Protein Crunch Stark Raving Peanutz	1 bar (1.8 oz)	180	4	2
PowerBar				
Apple Cinnamon	1 bar (2.3 oz)	230	3	1
Banana	1 bar (2.3 oz)	230	2	1
Chocolate	1 bar (2.3 oz)	230	2	1
Essentials Chocolate	1 bar (1.9 oz)	180	4	2
Harvest Apple Crisp	1 bar (2.3 oz)	240	4	—
Harvest Blueberry	1 bar (2.3 oz)	240	4	1
Harvest Strawberry	1 bar (2.3 oz)	240	4	1
Malt-Nut	1 bar (2.3 oz)	230	3	1
Mocha	1 bar (2.3 oz)	230	3	1
Oatmeal Raisin	1 bar (2.3 oz)	230	3	1
Peanut Butter	1 bar (2.3 oz)	230	3	1
Power Gel Strawberry Banana	1 pkg	110	0	0
Pria Chocolate Honey Graham	1 bar (1 oz)	110	3	2
Pria Chocolate Peanut Crunch	1 bar (1 oz)	110	4	2
Pria Double Chocolate Cookie	1 bar (1 oz)	110	3	3
Pria French Vanilla Crisp	1 bar (1 oz)	110	3	3
Vanilla Crisp	1 bar (2.3 oz)	230	3	1
Wild Berry	1 bar (2.3 oz)	230	3	1

FOOD	PORTION	CALS	FAT	SAT FAT
Pure Protein				
Blueberry Cheesecake	1 bar	190	3	2
Revival				
Soy Apple Cinnamon Celebration	1 bar	200	5	4
Soy Autumn Frost Low Carb	1 bar	200	5	4
Soy Chocolate Raspberry Zing Low Carb	1 bar	200	5	3
Soy Chocolate Temptation	1 bar	220	3	1
Soy Marshmallow Krunch	1 bar	220	3	1
Soy Peanut Butter Chocolate Pal	1 bar	240	5	1
Soy Peanut Butter Pal	1 bar	240	5	1
Slim-Fast				
Crispy Peanut Caramel	1 bar	120	4	3
Dutch Chocolate	1 bar	140	5	2
Meal On-The-Go Apple Cobbler	1 bar	220	5	4
Meal On-The-Go Chocolate Cookie Dough	1 bar	220	5	4
Meal On-The-Go Honey Peanut	1 bar	220	5	4
Meal On-The-Go Milk Chocolate Peanut	1 bar	220	5	3
Meal On-The-Go Oatmeal Raisin	1 bar	220	5	4
Meal On-The-Go Rich Chocolate Brownie	1 bar	220	5	3
Meal On-The-Go Toasted Oat & Spice	1 bar	220	5	4
Peanut Butter	1 bar	150	5	3
Peanut Butter Crunch	1 bar	130	4	2
Rich Chewy Caramel	1 bar	120	4	3
SoBe				
Milk Chocolate	1 bar (1.75 oz)	240	14	9
Strive				
Crunchy Chocolate Smores	1 bar (2.1 oz)	200	9	5
Sweet Success				
Chewy Chocolate Brownie	1 bar (1.2 oz)	120	4	2
Think!				
Apple Spice	1 bar (2 oz)	205	3	1
Chocolate Almond Coconut Raisin	1 bar (2 oz)	243	7	2
Chocolate Fruit Harvest	1 bar (2 oz)	217	3	1
Zoe				
Flax & Soy Apple Crisp	1 bar (1.83 oz)	180	6	–

FOOD	PORTION	CALS	FAT	SAT FAT
ZonePerfect				
Honey Peanut	1 bar (1.8 oz)	200	7	4
ENERGY DRINKS				
AMP				
Energy Drink	1 can (8.4 oz)	120	0	0
Arizona				
Extreme Energy Shot	1 bottle (8.3 oz)	130	0	0
Atkins				
Cafe Au Lait	1 can (11 oz)	170	9	2
Chocolate	1 can (11 oz)	170	9	2
Chocolate Royale	1 can (11 oz)	170	9	2
Strawberry	1 can (11 oz)	170	9	2
Vanilla	1 can (11 oz)	170	9	2
Boost				
High Protein Vanilla	1 can (8 oz)	240	6	1
Vanilla	8 oz	240	4	1
California Joe				
All Natural Protein Drink Mix as prep	1 serv (8 oz)	165	4	2
Calorie Shed				
Shake Fat Free No Sugar Caramel Ripple	½ cup (4 fl oz)	70	0	0
Shake Fat Free No Sugar Chocolate	½ cup (4 fl oz)	70	0	0
Shake Fat Free No Sugar Marshmellow Nougat	½ cup (4 fl oz)	70	0	0
Choice				
Chocolate	1 can (8 oz)	220	10	2
Chocolate Fudge Sugar Free	1 pkg (11 oz)	125	3	1
French Vanilla Sugar Free	1 pkg (11 oz)	100	3	0
Strawberries'n Cream Sugar Free	1 pkg (11 oz)	100	3	0
Vanilla	1 can (8 oz)	220	10	2
Crunk				
Energy Drink	1 can	120	0	0
Fat Burner				
Diet Fruit Punch	8 fl oz	0	0	0
Fuze				
Energize Blackberry Grape	8 oz	100	0	0
Energize Exotic Punch	8 oz	100	0	0
Energize Mojo Mango	8 oz	100	0	0
Essential Cranberry Grapefruit	8 oz	90	0	0

FOOD	PORTION	CALS	FAT	SAT FAT
Focus Orange Carrot	8 oz	90	0	0
Refresh Banana Colada	8 oz	90	0	0
Refresh Mixed Berry	8 oz	90	0	0
Refresh Peach Mango	8 oz	90	0	0
Replenish Agave Cactus	8 oz	90	0	0
Slenderize Tropical Punch	8 oz	10	0	0
Stamina Grape & Aronia Punch	8 oz	80	0	0
Vitaboost Citrus Starfruit Punch	8 oz	90	0	0
Gatorade				
All Flavors	1 cup (8 oz)	50	0	0
Energy Drink All Flavors	1 bottle (12 oz)	310	0	0
Nutrition Shake All Flavors	1 can (11 oz)	370	6	1
GeniSoy				
Soy Protein Shake Chocolate	1 scoop (1.2 oz)	120	0	0
Soy Protein Shake Vanilla	1 scoop (1.2 oz)	130	0	0
Soy Protein Shake Strawberry Banana	1 scoop	130	0	0
Hansen's				
Energy Kiwi Strawberry	8 oz	120	0	0
Energy Peach	8 oz	130	0	0
Energy Punch	8 oz	120	0	0
Healthy Start Carrot Orange Antioxidant Blend	8 oz	130	0	0
Healthy Start Citrus Punch Focus Blend	8 oz	130	0	0
Healthy Start Cranberry Grape Defense Blend	8 oz	110	0	0
Healthy Start Tropical Orange Vitamix Blend	8 oz	110	0	0
Healthy Pleasures				
Chocolate Irish Cream	1 bottle (10.5 oz)	260	2	1
Hype				
Classic Energy	1 can (8.3 oz)	110	0	0
Impulse				
Energy Drink	1 can (8.3 oz)	110	0	0
Sugar Free	1 can (8.3 oz)	5	0	0
Invigor8				
Energy Boost	1 can	110	0	0
Nutrition Boost	1 can	110	0	0
Jugular				
Energy Drink	1 can (8.3 oz)	49	0	0

FOOD	PORTION	CALS	FAT	SAT FAT
Kashi				
GoLean Shake Mix Vanilla	2 scoops	220	0	0
GoLean Shake Mix Woman Chocolate	2 scoops	220	1	0
Shake Chocolate	1 can	230	3	0
Shake Vanilla	1 can	220	3	0
Kindercal				
Vanilla	1 can (8 oz)	250	11	3
Nancy Grey's				
Shake Hi-Protein Black Raspberry	1 cup (8 fl oz)	340	16	10
Shake Hi-Protein Chocolate	1 cup (8 fl oz)	340	15	10
Shake Hi-Protein Vanilla	1 cup (8 fl oz)	340	16	10
Nantucket Nectars				
Super Nectars Ginkgo Mango	8 oz	150	0	0
Super Nectars Green Angel	8 oz	140	0	0
Super Nectars Protein Smoothie	8 oz	170	1	–
Super Nectars Red Guarana Tea	8 oz	110	0	0
Super Nectars Vital C	8 oz	130	0	0
New York Minute				
Energy Drink	1 can (8.4 oz)	130	0	0
Nitro2Go				
High Energy	1 can	110	0	0
High Energy Lite	1 can	20	0	0
NutraShake				
Citrus	1 pkg (4 oz)	200	0	0
Citrus Free	1 serv (4 oz)	200	0	0
Vanilla	1 serv (8 oz)	400	12	–
Vanilla No Added Sugar	1 serv (4 oz)	200	8	–
Odwalla				
Blueberry B Monster	8 fl oz	140	0	0
C Monster	8 fl oz	150	1	–
Femme Vitale	8 fl oz	130	0	0
Glorious Morning	8 fl oz	130	0	0
Mango Tango	8 fl oz	150	2	1
Mo Beta	8 fl oz	140	0	0
Serious Energy	8 fl oz	150	0	0
Strawberry C Monster	8 fl oz	150	0	0
Super Protein	8 fl oz	170	1	–
Superfood	8 fl oz	140	1	–
Wellness	8 fl oz	150	1	–

FOOD	PORTION	CALS	FAT	SAT FAT
Peep One				
Erotic Drink	1 can (8.3)	109	tr	–
Pimp Juice				
Energy Drink	1 can	140	0	0
Pink				
Diet	1 can	10	0	0
Piranha				
Phunky Fruit Punch	1 can (8.4 oz)	140	0	0
Pounds Off				
Dark Chocolate Ecstasy	1 can (11 oz)	200	3	0
French Vanilla	1 can (11 oz)	220	3	1
Powerade				
Fruit Punch	8 fl oz	70	0	0
Lemon Lime	8 fl oz	70	0	0
Mountain Blast	8 fl oz	70	0	0
Pure Power				
Energy Drink	1 can (8.4 oz)	110	0	0
Shotz	1 can (5.75 oz)	80	0	0
RESQ				
Energy Drink	1 can (8 oz)	126	0	0
Red Bull				
Energy Drink	1 can (8.3 oz)	110	0	0
Sugar Free	1 can	10	0	0
Resource				
Fruit Beverage	1 pkg (8 oz)	180	0	–
Slim-Fast				
Chocolate as prep w/ fat free milk	1 serv	190	1	1
Chocolate Malt as prep w/ fat free milk	1 serv	190	1	1
JumpStart Chocolate as prep w/ fat free milk	1 serv	240	2	1
Strawberry as prep w/ fat free milk	1 serv	190	1	1
Vanilla as prep w/ fat free milk	1 serv	190	1	1
Snapple				
Meal Replacement All Flavors	1 bottle (11.5 oz)	210	0	0
SoBe				
Adrenaline Rush	1 can (8.3 oz)	140	0	0
Black & Blue Berry Brew	8 oz	120	0	0
Courage Cherry Citrus	8 oz	110	0	0
Drive	8 oz	120	0	0
Elixir Cranberry Grapefruit	8 oz	110	0	0

FOOD	PORTION	CALS	FAT	SAT FAT
Elixir Orange Carrot 3C	8 oz	90	0	0
Elixir Pomegranate Cranberry	8 oz	100	0	0
Energy	8 oz	120	0	0
Fuerte	8 oz	130	0	0
Karma	8 oz	120	0	0
Long John Lizard's Grape Grog	8 oz	120	0	0
Power	8 oz	120	0	0
Synergy All Flavors	1 can (11.5 oz)	120	0	0
Tsunami	8 oz	110	0	0
Wisdom	8.5 oz	110	0	0
Zen Blend	8.5 oz	90	0	0
Stevita				
All Flavors	2 tsp	0	0	0
Sustacal				
Vanilla	8 oz	240	6	1
Sweet Success				
Creamy Milk Chocolate	1 can	200	3	1
Creamy Milk Chocolate as prep w/ skim milk	1 serv	180	1	1
The Pumper				
Body Building MilkShake Chocolate	1 serv (13.5 oz)	390	2	1
Body Building Milkshake Banana	1 serv (13.5 oz)	390	2	1
TwinLab				
Hydra Fuel	16 oz	132	0	0
Nitro Fuel	16 oz	460	0	0
Ultra Fuel	16 oz	400	0	0
XO				
Balance	8 oz	50	0	0
Berry	1 bottle	90	0	0
Citrus	1 bottle	90	0	0
Defense	8 oz	40	0	0
Diet	1 bottle	15	0	0
Endurance	8 oz	50	0	0
Energy	8 oz	40	0	0
Essential	8 oz	40	0	0
Focus	8 oz	40	0	0
Grape	1 bottle	90	0	0
Multi-V	8 oz	40	0	0
Original	1 bottle	110	0	0
Peach	1 bottle	90	0	0

FOOD	PORTION	CALS	FAT	SAT FAT
Power-C	8 oz	40	0	0
Rescue	8 oz	40	0	0
Revive	8 oz	50	0	0
Stress-B	8 oz	40	0	0
Vanilla	1 bottle	90	0	0
YET				
Your Energy Drink	1 can	8	0	0

ENGLISH MUFFIN
FROZEN
Weight Watchers

FOOD	PORTION	CALS	FAT	SAT FAT
Sandwich	1 (4 oz)	210	5	3
READY-TO-EAT				
apple cinnamon	1	138	2	tr
crumpets	1 (1.5 oz)	80	0	0
granola	1	155	1	tr
mixed grain	1	155	1	tr
plain	1	134	1	tr
plain toasted	1	133	1	tr
raisin cinnamon	1	138	2	tr
sourdough	1	134	1	tr
wheat	1	127	1	tr
whole wheat	1	134	1	tr
Milton's				
Multi-Grain	1 (2 oz)	150	1	0
Pepperidge Farm				
Original	1	130	1	0
Thomas'				
Blueberry	1	140	1	0
Honey Wheat	1	130	1	0
Original	1	120	1	0
Raisin Bran	1	150	2	0
Raisin Cinnamon	1	140	1	0
Sourdough	1	120	1	0
Super Size	1 (3.2 oz)	200	2	0
Wonder				
Cinnamon Raisin	1 (2.1 oz)	140	2	1
Original	1 (2 oz)	130	1	0
Sourdough	1 (2 oz)	130	1	0

FOOD	PORTION	CALS	FAT	SAT FAT
TAKE-OUT				
w/ butter	1 (2.2 oz)	189	6	2
w/ cheese & sausage	1 (4 oz)	393	24	10
w/ egg cheese & canadian bacon	1 (4.8 oz)	289	13	5
w/ egg cheese & sausage	1 (5.8 oz)	487	31	12
EPAZOTE				
fresh	1 tbsp (1 g)	tr	0	–
fresh sprig	1 (2 g)	1	tr	–
EPPAW				
raw	½ cup	75	1	–
FALAFEL				
TAKE-OUT				
falafel	1 (1.2 oz)	57	3	tr
FAT *(see also* BUTTER, BUTTER SUBSTITUTES, MARGARINE, OIL*)*				
beef cooked	1 oz	193	20	8
beef suet	1 oz	242	27	15
beef tallow	1 tbsp (13 g)	115	13	6
chicken	1 cup	1846	205	61
chicken	1 tbsp	115	13	4
cocoa butter	1 tbsp	120	14	8
duck	1 tbsp (13 g)	115	13	4
goose	1 tbsp	115	13	4
goose	1 oz	257	29	2
lamb new zealand	1 oz	182	19	10
lard	1 tbsp (13 g)	115	13	5
lard	1 cup (205 g)	1849	205	80
nutmeg butter	1 tbsp	120	14	12
pork backfat	1 oz	230	25	9
pork cooked	1 oz	178	18	7
salt pork	1 oz	212	23	8
shortening	1 cup	1812	205	41
shortening	1 tbsp	113	13	3
turkey	1 tbsp	115	13	4
ucuhuba butter	1 tbsp	120	14	12
Crisco				
Butter Flavor	1 tbsp	110	12	3
Shortening	1 tbsp (0.4 oz)	110	12	3
Sticks	1 tbsp (0.4 oz)	110	12	3

FOOD	PORTION	CALS	FAT	SAT FAT
Sticks Butter Flavor	1 tbsp (0.4 oz)	110	12	3

FAT SUBSTITUTES
Smucker's
Baking Healthy 100% Fat Free	1 tbsp	30	0	0

Soy Is Us
Fat Not! Organic	3 tbsp	66	1	tr

FAVA BEANS
Progresso
Fava Beans	½ cup (4.6 oz)	110	1	0

FEIJOA
fresh	1 (1.75 oz)	25	tr	–
puree	1 cup	119	2	–

FENNEL
fresh bulb	1 (8.2 oz)	72	tr	–
fresh sliced	1 cup	27	tr	–
leaves	1 oz	7	tr	–
seed	1 tsp	7	tr	tr

FENUGREEK
seed	1 tsp	12	tr	–

FIBER
Apple Fiber
Pure	2 tbsp (7 g)	16	0	0

Benefiber
Supplement	1 pkg (4 g)	20	0	0

Choice
Fiber Burst Lemon Lime	3 pieces	45	1	0
Fiber Burst Tropical Fruit	3 pieces	45	1	0

Metamucil
Fiber Wafers Apple Crisp	2	120	5	1

ND Labs
Pure Apple Fiber	1 tbsp (7 g)	16	0	0

FIDDLEHEAD FERNS
fresh	3.5 oz	34	tr	–

FIGS
calimyrna	3 (5.4 oz)	120	0	0
canned in heavy syrup	3	75	tr	tr

FOOD	PORTION	CALS	FAT	SAT FAT
canned in light syrup	3	58	tr	tr
canned water pack	3	42	tr	—
dried cooked	½ cup	140	1	tr
dried whole	10	477	2	tr
fresh	1 med	50	tr	tr
Sonoma				
Dried White Mission	3-4 (1.4 oz)	110	0	0
FIREWEED				
leaves chopped	1 cup (0.8 oz)	24	1	—
FISH *(see also individual names,* FISH SUBSTITUTES, SUSHI*)*				
FROZEN				
breaded fillet	1 (2 oz)	155	7	2
sticks	1 stick (1 oz)	76	3	1
Gorton's				
Baked Au Gratin	1 piece (4.6 oz)	130	5	2
Baked Broccoli Cheddar	1 piece (4.6 oz)	130	5	2
Baked Primavera	1 piece (4.6 oz)	120	5	3
Batter Dipped Portions	1 piece (2.5 oz)	170	11	1
Crunchy Golden Fillets Breaded	2 (3.8 oz)	250	14	4
Crunchy Golden Sticks	6 (3.8 oz)	250	13	4
Garlic & Herb	2 pieces (3.6 oz)	220	11	3
Garlic Butter Crumb	1 piece (4.6 oz)	170	9	2
Grilled Cajun Blackened	1 piece (3.8 oz)	120	6	1
Grilled Garlic Butter	1 piece (3.8 oz)	120	6	1
Grilled Italian Herb	1 piece (3.8 oz)	130	6	1
Grilled Lemon Butter	1 piece (3.8 oz)	120	6	1
Grilled Lemon Pepper	1 piece (3.8 oz)	120	6	1
Parmesan	2 pieces (3.6 oz)	260	15	4
Ranch	1 piece (3.6 oz)	240	13	4
Southern Fried Country Style	2 pieces (3.6 oz)	230	14	4
Tenders	3.5 pieces (4 oz)	250	14	4
Tenders Extra Crunchy	3.5 pieces (4 oz)	270	12	4
Van De Kamp's				
Battered Fish Fillets	1 (2.6 oz)	180	11	2
Battered Fish Nuggets	8 (4 oz)	280	18	3
Battered Fish Portions	2 pieces (5 oz)	350	22	4
Battered Fish Sticks	6 (4 oz)	260	16	3
Breaded Fillets	2 (3.5 oz)	280	19	3
Breaded Fish Portions	3 pieces (4.5 oz)	330	21	3

FOOD	PORTION	CALS	FAT	SAT FAT
Breaded Fish Sticks	6 (4 oz)	290	17	3
Breaded Mini Fish Sticks	13 (3.3 oz)	250	14	2
Crisp & Healthy Breaded Fillets	2 (3.5 oz)	150	3	1
Crisp & Healthy Fish Sticks	6 (4 oz)	180	3	1
Fish 'n Fries	1 pkg (6.6 oz)	380	18	3
TAKE-OUT				
fish cake	1 (4.7 oz)	166	7	2
jamaican brown fish stew	1 serv	426	22	5
kedgeree	5.6 oz	242	11	–
mousse	1 serv (3.5 oz)	185	14	–
stew	1 cup (7.9 oz)	157	4	2
taramasalata	2 tbsp	124	14	–
FISH OIL				
cod liver	1 tbsp	123	14	3
herring	1 tbsp	123	14	3
menhaden	1 tbsp	123	14	4
salmon	1 tbsp	123	14	3
sardine	1 tbsp	123	14	4
shark	1 oz	270	29	–
whale	1 oz	270	29	–
FISH PASTE				
fish paste	2 tsp	15	1	–
FISH SUBSTITUTES				
Loma Linda				
Ocean Platter not prep	⅓ cup (0.9 oz)	90	1	0
Worthington				
Fillets	2 (3 oz)	180	10	2
Tuno	½ cup (1.9 oz)	80	6	1
FLAXSEED				
Arrowhead				
Organic Flax Seeds	¼ cup	140	9	–
Bite Me				
Flax Bar	1 bar (1.8 oz)	242	11	2
Bob's Red Mill				
Flax Seed Meal	2 tbsp	60	5	–
Cracker Flax				
Organic Apple Raisin	1 oz	130	5	0

FOOD	PORTION	CALS	FAT	SAT FAT
Hodgson Mill				
Milled	2 tbsp	60	1	0
FLOUNDER				
FRESH				
cooked	1 fillet (4.5 oz)	148	2	tr
cooked	3 oz	99	1	tr
FROZEN				
Van De Kamp's				
Lightly Breaded Fillets	1 (4 oz)	230	11	2
Natural Fillets	1 (4 oz)	110	2	0
TAKE-OUT				
battered & fried	3.2 oz	211	11	3
FLOUR				
buckwheat whole groat	1 cup (4.2 oz)	402	4	1
corn masa	1 cup (4 oz)	416	4	1
cottonseed lowfat	1 oz	94	tr	tr
peanut defatted	1 cup	196	tr	tr
peanut defatted	1 oz	92	tr	tr
peanut lowfat	1 cup	257	13	2
potato	1 cup (6.3 oz)	628	1	tr
rice brown	1 cup (5.5 oz)	574	4	tr
rice white	1 cup (5.5 oz)	578	2	1
rye dark	1 cup (4.5 oz)	415	3	tr
rye light	1 cup (3.6 oz)	374	1	tr
rye medium	1 cup (3.6 oz)	361	2	tr
sesame lowfat	1 oz	95	tr	tr
triticale whole grain	1 cup (4.6 oz)	439	2	tr
white all-purpose	1 cup (4.4 oz)	455	1	tr
white bread	1 cup (4.8 oz)	495	2	tr
white cake unsifted	1 cup (4.8 oz)	496	1	tr
white self-rising	1 cup (4.4 oz)	443	1	tr
white unbleached	1 cup (4.4 oz)	455	1	tr
whole wheat	1 cup (4.2 oz)	407	2	tr
All Trump				
Flour	¼ cup (1 oz)	100	0	0
Arrowhead				
Whole Grain Oat	⅓ cup	120	3	—

FOOD	PORTION	CALS	FAT	SAT FAT
Betty Crocker				
Softasilk Velvet Cake Flour	¼ cup (1 oz)	100	0	0
Gold Medal				
All Purpose	¼ cup (1 oz)	100	0	0
Better For Bread	¼ cup (1 oz)	100	0	0
Organic All Purpose	¼ cup (1 oz)	100	0	0
Self Rising	¼ cup (1 oz)	100	0	0
Unbleached	¼ cup (1 oz)	100	0	0
Wondra	¼ cup	100	0	0
Heckers				
All Purpose Unbleached	¼ cup	100	0	0
Whole Wheat	¼ cup	100	1	0
Hodgson Mill				
White Unbleached Organic	¼ cup (1 oz)	100	0	0
Whole Wheat Graham Organic	¼ cup (1 oz)	100	1	0
La Pina				
Flour	¼ cup (1 oz)	100	0	0
Red Band				
All Purpose	¼ cup (1 oz)	100	0	0
Self-Rising	¼ cup (1 oz)	100	0	0
Robin Hood				
All Purpose	¼ cup (1 oz)	100	0	0
Self-Rising	¼ cup (1 oz)	100	0	0
Unbleached	¼ cup (1 oz)	100	0	0
Whole Wheat	¼ cup (1 oz)	90	1	–

FRENCH BEANS

FOOD	PORTION	CALS	FAT	SAT FAT
dried cooked	1 cup	228	1	tr

FRENCH FRIES (see POTATOES)

FRENCH TOAST

FOOD	PORTION	CALS	FAT	SAT FAT
FROZEN				
french toast	1 slice (2 oz)	126	4	1
TAKE-OUT				
plain	1 slice	151	7	2
sticks	5 (4.9 oz)	513	29	5
w/ butter	2 slices (4.7 oz)	356	19	8

FROG'S LEGS

FOOD	PORTION	CALS	FAT	SAT FAT
TAKE-OUT				
as prep w/ seasoned flour & fried	1 (0.8)	70	5	–

FOOD	PORTION	CALS	FAT	SAT FAT
FRUCTOSE				
Estee				
Fructose	1 tsp	15	0	0
Packet	1 pkg	10	0	0
FRUIT DRINKS *(see also individual names)*				
FROZEN				
Tree Of Life				
Organic Smoothie Banana Raspberry Strawberry	⅔ cup (5 oz)	90	0	0
Organic Smoothie Mango Strawberry Raspberry	⅔ cup (5 oz)	70	0	0
Organic Smoothie Strawberry Banana	⅔ cup (5 oz)	90	0	0
Organic Smoothie Strawberry Blueberry Banana	⅔ cup (5 oz)	90	0	0
MIX				
Crystal Light				
Fruit Punch as prep	1 serv (8 oz)	5	0	0
Lemon-Lime Drink as prep	1 serv (8 oz)	5	0	0
Passion Fruit Pineapple Drink as prep	1 serv (8 oz)	5	0	0
Pineapple Orange Drink as prep	1 serv (8 oz)	5	0	0
Strawberry Orange Banana as prep	1 serv (8 oz)	5	0	0
Strawberry Kiwi as prep	1 serv (8 oz)	5	0	0
Watermelon Strawberry as prep	1 serv (8 oz)	5	0	0
Kool-Aid				
Grape Berry Splash Drink as prep	1 serv (8 oz)	70	0	0
Grape Berry Splash Drink as prep w/ sugar	1 serv (8 oz)	100	0	0
Kickin' Kiwi Lime Drink as prep	1 serv (8 oz)	60	0	0
Kickin' Kiwi Lime Drink as prep w/ sugar	1 serv (8 oz)	100	0	0
Lemon-Lime Drink as prep w/ sugar	1 serv (8 oz)	100	0	0
Man-O-Mango Berry Drink as prep	1 serv (8 oz)	60	0	0
Man-O-Mango Berry Drink as prep w/ sugar	1 serv (8 oz)	100	0	0
Oh Yeah Orange Pineapple Drink as prep	1 serv (8 oz)	60	0	0
Oh Yeah Orange Pineapple Drink as prep w/ sugar	1 serv (8 oz)	100	0	0
Pina-Pineapple Drink as prep	1 serv (8 oz)	60	0	0

FOOD	PORTION	CALS	FAT	SAT FAT
Pina-Pineapple Drink as prep w/ sugar	1 serv (8 oz)	100	0	0
Roarin' Raspberry Cranberry Drink as prep	1 serv (8 oz)	70	0	0
Roarin' Raspberry Cranberry Drink as prep w/ sugar	1 serv (8 oz)	100	0	0
Slammin' Strawberry Kiwi Drink as prep	1 serv (8 oz)	70	0	0
Slammin' Strawberry Kiwi Drink as prep w/ sugar	1 serv (8 oz)	100	0	0
Strawberry Raspberry Drink as prep	1 serv (8 oz)	60	0	0
Strawberry Raspberry Drink as prep w/ sugar	1 serv (8 oz)	100	0	0
Sugar Free Tropical Punch as prep	1 serv (8 oz)	5	0	0
Tropical Punch as prep	1 serv (8 oz)	60	0	0
Tropical Punch as prep w/ sugar	1 serv (8 oz)	100	0	0
Watermelon Cherry Drink as prep	1 serv (8 oz)	60	0	0
Watermelon Cherry Drink as prep w/ sugar	1 serv (8 oz)	100	0	0
Tang				
Orange Pineapple as prep	1 serv (8 oz)	100	0	0
READY-TO-DRINK				
fruit punch	6 fl oz	87	tr	0
pineapple & orange drink	8 fl oz	125	0	0
After The Fall				
Amaretto Almond	1 can (12 oz)	170	0	0
Apple Apricot	1 cup (8 oz)	100	0	0
Apple Raspberry	1 bottle (10 oz)	110	0	0
Apple Strawberry	1 bottle (10 oz)	120	0	0
Banana Casablanca	1 bottle (10 oz)	120	0	0
Berrymeister	1 can (12 oz)	160	0	0
Cranberry Meets Raspberry	1 bottle (10 oz)	120	0	0
Georgia Peach Blend	1 bottle (10 oz)	130	0	0
Mango Montage	1 bottle (10 oz)	140	0	0
Maui Grove	1 bottle (10 oz)	120	0	0
Oregon Berry	1 bottle (10 oz)	130	0	0
Passion Of The Islands	1 bottle (10 oz)	125	0	0
Vanilla Bean Cream	1 can (12 oz)	170	0	0
Apple & Eve				
Apple Cranberry	8 oz	120	0	0

FOOD	PORTION	CALS	FAT	SAT FAT
Capri Sun				
Fruit Punch	1 pkg (7 oz)	100	0	0
Maui Punch	1 pkg (7 oz)	100	0	0
Mountain Cooler	1 pkg (7 oz)	90	0	0
Pacific Cooler	1 pkg (7 oz)	100	0	0
Red Berry	1 pkg (7 oz)	100	0	0
Safari Punch	1 pkg (7 oz)	100	0	0
Strawberry Kiwi Drink	1 pkg (7 oz)	100	0	0
Surfer Cooler Drink	1 pkg (7 oz)	100	0	0
Citrus Squeeze				
California Punch	8 oz	130	0	0
Florida Punch	8 oz	120	0	0
Coco Lopez				
Mango Kiwi	8 fl oz	130	0	0
Crystal Light				
Fruit Punch	1 serv (8 oz)	5	0	0
Kiwi Strawberry	1 serv (8 oz)	5	0	0
Orange Strawberry Banana Drink	1 serv (8 oz)	5	0	0
Del Monte				
Peach Raspberry	5.5 fl oz	160	0	0
Pineapple Banana Orange	5.5 fl oz	170	0	0
Strawberry Peach Banana	5.5 fl oz	150	0	0
Dole				
Apple Berry Burst	8 fl oz	120	0	0
Cranberry Apple	8 fl oz	120	0	0
Fruit Fiesta	8 fl oz	140	0	0
Fruit Punch	1 carton (10 oz)	160	0	0
Mountain Cherry	8 fl oz	150	0	0
Orange Peach Mango	8 oz	120	0	0
Orange Strawberry Banana	8 oz	120	0	0
Orchard Peach	8 oz	140	0	0
Pineapple Orange	8 oz	120	0	0
Pineapple Orange Strawberry	8 oz	130	0	0
Tropical Fruit	8 oz	160	0	0
Eden				
Organic Apple Cherry Juice	8 oz	120	0	0
Everfresh				
Cranberry-Apple Drink	1 can (8 oz)	120	0	0
Grape-Strawberry	1 can (8 oz)	120	0	0
Kiwi-Strawberry	1 can (8 oz)	120	0	0

FOOD	PORTION	CALS	FAT	SAT FAT
Mandarin Orange Mango Drink	1 can (8 oz)	120	0	0
Orange Banana Strawberry Drink	1 can (8 oz)	120	0	0
Tropical Fruit Punch	1 can (8 oz)	120	0	0
Wild Blackberry Lime Drink	1 can (8 oz)	120	0	0
Fresh Samantha				
Banana Strawberry	1 cup (8 oz)	130	0	0
Carrot Orange	1 cup (8 oz)	100	0	0
Desperately Seeking C	1 cup (8 oz)	110	0	0
Protein Blast	1 cup (8 oz)	160	1	0
Super Juice	1 cup (8 oz)	140	1	0
The Big Bang	1 cup (8 oz)	100	0	0
Fruitopia				
Fruit Integration	8 fl oz	110	0	0
Guzzler				
Citrus Punch	8 fl oz	140	0	0
Island Punch	8 fl oz	140	0	0
Hansen's				
Fruit Punch 100% Juice	1 box (4.23 oz)	60	0	0
Juice Slam Wild Berry	1 box	120	0	0
Smoothie Apricot Nectar	1 can	170	0	0
Smoothie Cranberry Twist	1 can	180	0	0
Smoothie Energy Island Blast	1 can	170	0	0
Smoothie Guava Strawberry	1 can	170	0	0
Smoothie Mango Pineapple	1 can	170	0	0
Smoothie Peach Berry	1 can	170	0	0
Smoothie Pineapple Coconut	1 can	180	0	0
Smoothie Strawberry Banana	1 can	180	0	0
Smoothie Tropical Passion	1 can	170	0	0
Smoothie Whipped Orange	1 can	180	0	0
Smoothie Lite Cranberry Raspberry	1 can	50	0	0
Juicy Juice				
Apple Grape	1 box (8.45 oz)	140	0	0
Berry	1 box (8.45 oz)	130	0	0
Punch	1 box (8.45 oz)	140	0	0
Punch	1 box (4.23 oz)	70	0	0
Tropical	1 box (8.45 oz)	140	0	0
Kool-Aid				
Bursts Great Bluedini	1 (7 oz)	100	0	0
Bursts Kickin' Kiwi Lime	1 (7 oz)	100	0	0
Bursts Oh Yeah Orange Pineapple	1 (7 oz)	100	0	0

FOOD	PORTION	CALS	FAT	SAT FAT
Bursts Slammin' Strawberry Kiwi	1 (7 oz)	100	0	0
Bursts Tropical Punch	1 (7 oz)	100	0	0
Splash Grape Berry Punch	1 serv (8 oz)	120	0	0
Splash Kiwi Strawberry Drink	1 serv (8 oz)	110	0	0
Splash Tropical Punch	1 serv (8 oz)	120	0	0
Langers				
100% Juice Pineapple Coconut	8 oz	140	3	3
Blueberry Cranberry	8 oz	135	0	0
Cranberry Berry	8 oz	135	0	0
Cranberry Fuji	8 oz	160	0	0
Cranberry Grape	8 oz	165	0	0
Cranberry Grape Cocktail	8 oz	165	0	0
Cranberry Orange	8 oz	130	0	0
Diet Cranberry Berry	8 oz	30	0	0
Diet Cranberry Grape	8 oz	30	0	0
Fruit Punch Cocktail	8 oz	120	0	0
Kiwi Raspberry Cocktail	8 oz	120	0	0
Kiwi Strawberry Cocktail	8 oz	120	0	0
Mango Orange	8 oz	130	0	0
Mixed Berry 100% Juice	8 oz	120	0	0
Pineapple Orange Guava	8 oz	130	0	0
Ruby Orange	8 oz	130	0	0
Tropical Ruby	8 oz	135	0	0
White Cranberry Raspberry	8 oz	120	0	0
Mauna La'i				
Island Guava	8 oz	130	0	0
Paradise Passion	8 oz	130	0	0
Mott's				
Berry	1 box (8 oz)	100	0	0
Fruit Punch	8 fl oz	130	0	0
Fruit Punch	1 box (8 oz)	110	0	0
Nantucket Nectars				
Apple Raspberry	8 oz	140	0	0
California Melonberry	8 oz	110	0	0
Cranberry Apple	8 oz	140	0	0
Fruit Punch	8 oz	130	0	0
Kiwi Berry	8 oz	120	0	0
Orange Passionfruit	8 oz	120	0	0
Orange Mango	8 oz	130	0	0
Peach Orange	8 oz	130	0	0

FOOD	PORTION	CALS	FAT	SAT FAT
Pineapple Orange Banana	8 oz	140	0	0
Pineapple Orange Guava	8 oz	120	0	0
Watermelon Strawberry	8 oz	120	0	0
Oberweis				
Fruit Punch	8 oz	120	0	0
Ocean Spray				
Cran*Blueberry	8 oz	160	0	0
Cran*Cherry	8 oz	160	0	0
Cran*Currant	8 oz	140	0	0
Cran*Grape	8 oz	170	0	0
Cran*Mango	8 oz	130	0	0
Cran*Raspberry	8 oz	140	0	0
Cran*Raspberry Reduced Calorie	8 oz	50	0	0
Cran*Strawberry	8 oz	140	0	0
Cran*Tangerine	8 oz	130	0	0
Cranapple	8 oz	160	0	0
Cranapple Reduced Calorie	8 oz	50	0	0
Cranicot	8 oz	160	0	0
Crazy Kiwi Passion	8 oz	130	0	0
Fruit Punch	8 oz	130	0	0
Kiwi Strawberry	8 oz	120	0	0
Lightstyle Cran*Grape	8 oz	40	0	0
Lightstyle Cran*Mango	8 oz	40	0	0
Lightstyle Cran*Raspberry	8 oz	40	0	0
Mandarin Magic	8 oz	120	0	0
Ruby Red & Tangerine Grapefruit	8 oz	130	0	0
Ruby Red & Mango	8 oz	130	0	0
Odwalla				
Blackberry Fruit Shake	8 fl oz	140	0	0
Carrot Orange Apple	8 fl oz	100	0	0
Orange Pina Smoothie	8 fl oz	140	0	0
Rooty Fruity	8 fl oz	110	1	–
Strawberry Banana	8 fl oz	120	1	–
Shasta Plus				
Apple-Strawberry	1 can (11.5 oz)	160	0	0
Fruit Punch	1 can (11.5 oz)	160	0	0
Pineapple-Cherry	1 can (11.5 oz)	160	0	0
Snapple				
Cranberry Raspberry	8 fl oz	120	0	0
Diet Cranberry Raspberry	8 fl oz	10	0	0

FOOD	PORTION	CALS	FAT	SAT FAT
Fruit Punch	8 fl oz	110	0	0
Kiwi Strawberry	8 fl oz	110	0	0
Snapricot Orange	8 fl oz	120	0	0
Squeezit				
Berry B. Wild	1 bottle (7 oz)	110	0	0
Lemon Lime	1 bottle (7 oz)	110	0	0
Rockin' Red Puncher	1 bottle (7 oz)	110	0	0
Tropical Punch	1 bottle (7 oz)	110	0	0
Tropicana				
Berry Punch	8 fl oz	130	0	0
Citrus Punch	8 fl oz	140	0	0
Fruit Punch	8 oz	130	0	0
Tangerine Orange Juice	8 fl oz	110	0	0
Tropics Orange Strawberry Banana	8 fl oz	110	0	0
Tropics Orange Kiwi Passion	8 fl oz	100	0	0
Tropics Orange Peach Mango	8 fl oz	110	0	0
Tropics Orange Pineapple	8 fl oz	110	0	0
Twister Apple Raspberry Blackberry	1 bottle (10 fl oz)	160	1	—
Twister Citrus Punch	1 bottle (10 oz)	180	0	0
Twister Cranberry Punch	1 bottle (10 oz)	170	0	0
Twister Fruit Punch	1 bottle (10 oz)	170	0	0
Twister Light Orange Strawberry Banana	1 bottle (10 oz)	45	0	0
Twister Orange Cranberry	1 bottle (10 fl oz)	160	0	0
Twister Orange Strawberry Banana	1 bottle (10 oz)	160	0	0
Twister Ruby Red Tangerine	1 bottle (10 oz)	160	0	0
Twister Strawberry Kiwi	1 bottle (10 oz)	160	0	0
V8				
Splash Berry Blend	8 oz	110	0	0
Veryfine				
Apple Cranberry	1 bottle (10 oz)	190	0	0
Apple Quenchers Black Cherry White Grape	8 fl oz	120	0	0
Apple Quenchers Cranberry Tangerine	8 fl oz	120	0	0
Apple Quenchers Peach Kiwi	8 fl oz	130	0	0
Apple Quenchers Peach Plum	8 fl oz	130	0	0
Apple Quenchers Pear Passionfruit	8 fl oz	120	0	0
Apple Quenchers Raspberry Cherry	8 fl oz	120	0	0
Apple Quenchers Raspberry Lime	8 fl oz	120	0	0

FOOD	PORTION	CALS	FAT	SAT FAT
Apple Quenchers Strawberry Banana	8 fl oz	120	0	0
Chillers Arctic Mango Tangerine	8 fl oz	110	0	0
Chillers Freezing Fruit Punch	8 fl oz	130	0	0
Chillers Lemon Lime Blizzard	8 fl oz	120	0	0
Chillers Shivering Strawberry Melon	1 can (11.5 oz)	160	0	0
Chillers Tropical Freeze	8 fl oz	120	0	0
Cranberry Raspberry	8 fl oz	160	0	0
Fruit Punch	1 bottle (10 oz)	170	0	0
Juice-Ups Berry	8 fl oz	140	0	0
Juice-Ups Fruit Punch	8 fl oz	140	0	0
Orange Strawberry	8 fl oz	120	0	0
Papaya Punch	1 bottle (10 oz)	160	0	0
Pineapple Orange	1 bottle (10 oz)	160	0	0
Strawberry Banana	1 can (11.5 oz)	160	0	0
Strawberry Banana Punch	1 can (11.5 oz)	190	0	0
Wellfleet Farms				
Cranberry & Georgia Peach	8 oz	140	0	0
Cranberry & Granny Smith Apple	8 oz	130	0	0
Cranberry & Key Lime	8 oz	140	0	0
FRUIT MIXED (see also individual names)				
CANNED				
fruit cocktail in heavy syrup	½ cup	93	tr	tr
fruit cocktail juice pack	½ cup	56	tr	tr
fruit cocktail water pack	½ cup	40	tr	tr
fruit salad in heavy syrup	½ cup	94	tr	tr
fruit salad in light syrup	½ cup	73	tr	tr
fruit salad juice pack	½ cup	62	tr	tr
fruit salad water pack	½ cup	37	tr	tr
mixed fruit in heavy syrup	½ cup	92	tr	tr
tropical fruit salad in heavy syrup	½ cup	110	tr	—
Del Monte				
Cherry Mixed Light Syrup	½ cup (4.4 oz)	90	0	0
Chunky Mixed Fruit Naturals	½ cup (4.4 oz)	60	0	0
Chunky Mixed In Extra Light Syrup	½ cup (4.4 oz)	60	0	0
Chunky Mixed In Heavy Syrup	½ cup (4.5 oz)	100	0	0
Citrus Salad	½ cup (4.4 oz)	80	0	0
Fruit Cocktail Fruit Naturals	½ cup (4.4 oz)	60	0	0
Fruit Cocktail In Extra Light Syrup	½ cup (4.4 oz)	60	0	0

FOOD	PORTION	CALS	FAT	SAT FAT
Fruit Cocktail In Heavy Syrup	½ cup (4.5 oz)	100	0	0
Fruit Cup Fruit Naturals Mixed	1 pkg (4 oz)	50	0	0
Fruit Cup Mixed In Extra Light Syrup	1 pkg (4 oz)	50	0	0
Fruit Salad In Extra Light Syrup	½ cup (4.5 oz)	70	0	0
Fruit To Go Fruity Combo	1 pkg (4 oz)	70	0	0
Fruit To Go Wild Berry Jumble	1 pkg (4 oz)	80	0	0
Orchard Select California Mixed	½ cup (4.5 oz)	80	0	0
Orchard Select Premium Mixed	½ cup (4.4 oz)	80	0	0
Snack Cups Strawberry Banana Peaches	1 pkg	70	0	0
Snack Cups Tropical Fruit	1 pkg	70	0	0
SunFresh Ambrosia Salad	½ cup	70	0	0
Tropical Fruit Salad	½ cup (4.3 oz)	60	0	0
Tropical Fruit Salad In Light Syrup	½ cup (4.4 oz)	80	0	0
Very Cherry Mixed Fruit	½ cup (4.4 oz)	90	0	0
Dole				
FruitBowls Tropical Fruit	1 pkg (4 oz)	60	0	0
Tropical Fruit Salad	½ cup (4.3 oz)	80	0	0
Mott's				
Fruitsations Banana	1 pkg (4 oz)	90	0	0
Fruitsations Cherry	1 pkg (4 oz)	70	0	0
Fruitsations Mango Peach	1 pkg (4 oz)	70	0	0
Fruitsations Mixed Berry	1 pkg (4 oz)	90	0	0
Fruitsations Pear	1 pkg (4 oz)	90	0	0
Fruitsations Strawberry	1 pkg (4 oz)	80	0	0
Fruitsations Tropical Fruit	1 pkg (4 oz)	70	0	0
Healthy Harvest Peach Medley	1 pkg (3.9 oz)	50	0	0
Ocean Spray				
Cran*Fruit Cranberry Raspberry	¼ cup	120	0	0
Cran*Fruit Cranberry Strawberry	¼ cup	120	0	0
SunFresh				
Ambrosia Salad	½ cup (4.5 oz)	70	0	0
Mixed Fruit In Light Syrup	½ cup (4.6 oz)	90	0	0
Tropical Salad In Extra Light Syrup	½ cup (4.5 oz)	80	0	0
White House				
Apple Banana Sauce	1 pkg (4 oz)	100	0	0
Apple Mixed Berry Sauce	1 pkg (4 oz)	110	0	0
Apple Peach Sauce	1 pkg (4 oz)	100	0	0
DRIED				
mixed	11 oz pkg	712	1	tr

FOOD	PORTION	CALS	FAT	SAT FAT
Del Monte				
Mixed	⅓ cup (1.4 oz)	110	0	0
Paradise				
Old English Fruit & Peel Mix	1 tbsp (0.8 oz)	70	0	0
Planters				
Fruit'n Nut Mix	1 oz	140	9	2
Sonoma				
Diced	⅓ cup (1.4 oz)	120	0	0
Mixed Fruit	5-8 pieces (1.4 oz)	120	0	0
Sun-Maid				
Tropical Medley	¼ cup (1.4 oz)	130	0	0
FROZEN				
mixed fruit sweetened	1 cup	245	tr	tr
Birds Eye				
Mixed Fruit	½ cup	90	0	0
Tree Of Life				
Organic Mixed Berries	¾ cup (5 oz)	60	0	0
FRUIT SNACKS				
fruit leather	1 bar (0.8 oz)	81	1	1
fruit leather pieces	1 oz	97	2	tr
fruit leather pieces	1 pkg (0.9 oz)	92	2	tr
fruit leather rolls	1 sm (0.5 oz)	49	tr	tr
fruit leather rolls	1 lg (0.7 oz)	73	1	tr
Betty Crocker				
Fruit By The Foot All Flavors	1 roll	80	2	–
CoolFruits				
Apple Grape	1 bar (0.5 oz)	51	tr	0
Apple Strawberry	1 bar (0.5 oz)	51	tr	0
Wild Blueberry	1 bar (0.5 oz)	51	tr	0
Favorite Brands				
Cherry Fruit Snack	1 pkg (0.9 oz)	80	0	0
Creepy Crawler Fruit Snacks	1 pkg (0.9 oz)	80	0	0
Dinosaur Fruit Snack	1 pkg (0.9 oz)	80	0	0
Grape Fruit Snack	1 pkg (0.9 oz)	80	0	0
Space Alien Fruit Snack	1 pkg (0.9 oz)	80	0	0
Sports Fruit Snacks	1 pkg (0.9 oz)	80	0	0
Strawberry Fruit Snack	1 pkg (0.9 oz)	80	0	0

FOOD	PORTION	CALS	FAT	SAT FAT
Teenage Mutant Ninja Turtle Fruit Snacks	1 pkg (0.9 oz)	80	0	0
The Mega Roll Strawberry	1 pkg (1 oz)	110	3	2
The Roll Cherry	1 pkg (0.75 oz)	80	2	1
The Roll Strawberry	1 pkg (0.75 oz)	80	2	1
Troll Fruit Snacks	1 pkg (0.9 oz)	80	0	0
Zoo Animal Fruit Snacks	1 pkg (0.9 oz)	80	0	0
Health Valley				
Bakes Apple	1 bar	70	0	0
Bakes Date	1 bar	70	0	0
Bakes Raisin	1 bar	70	0	0
Fruit Bars Apple	1	140	0	0
Fruit Bars Apricot	1	140	0	0
Fruit Bars Date	1	140	0	0
Fruit Bars Raisin	1	140	0	0
Seneca				
Apple Chips	12 chips (1 oz)	140	7	1
Sensible Foods				
Crackin' Fruit Cherry Berry	1 pkg (0.6 oz)	51	0	0
Crackin' Fruit Tropical Fruit	1 pkg (0.6 oz)	65	1	0
Sonoma				
Trail Mix	¼ cup (1.4 oz)	160	7	3
Sunbelt				
Fruit Jammers	1 pkg (1 oz)	100	1	1
Sunkist				
100% Fruit Roll All Flavors	1 (0.5 oz)	50	0	0
Weight Watchers				
Apple & Cinnamon	1 pkg (0.5 oz)	50	0	0
Apple Chips	1 pkg (0.75 oz)	70	0	0
Peach & Strawberry	1 pkg (0.5 oz)	50	0	0
GARLIC				
clove	1	4	tr	tr
fresh chopped	1 tsp	4	tr	tr
powder	1 tsp	9	tr	—
Dorot				
Frozen Crushed Cubes	1 cube (4 g)	5	0	0
McCormick				
Garlic Salt	¼ tsp	0	0	0

FOOD	PORTION	CALS	FAT	SAT FAT
GEFILTE FISH				
sweet	1 piece (1.5 oz)	35	1	tr
GELATIN				
MIX				
low calorie	½ cup	8	0	0
mix as prep	½ cup (4.7 oz)	80	0	0
mix not prep	1 pkg (3 oz)	324	0	0
mix w/ fruit	½ cup (3.7 oz)	73	tr	–
powder unsweetened	1 pkg (7 g)	23	0	tr
Jell-O				
1-2-3-Brand Strawberry as prep	⅔ cup (5.2 oz)	130	2	1
Apricot as prep	½ cup (5 oz)	80	0	0
Berry Black as prep	½ cup (5 oz)	80	0	0
Berry Blue as prep	½ cup (5 oz)	80	0	0
Black Cherry as prep	½ cup (5 oz)	80	0	0
Cherry as prep	½ cup (5 oz)	80	0	0
Cranberry Raspberry as prep	½ cup (5 oz)	80	0	0
Cranberry Strawberry as prep	½ cup (5 oz)	80	0	0
Cranberry as prep	½ cup (5 oz)	80	0	0
Grape as prep	½ cup (5 oz)	80	0	0
Lemon as prep	½ cup (5 oz)	80	0	0
Lime as prep	½ cup (5 oz)	80	0	0
Mango as prep	½ cup (5 oz)	80	0	0
Mixed Fruit as prep	½ cup (5 oz)	80	0	0
Orange as prep	½ cup (5 oz)	80	0	0
Peach as prep	½ cup (5 oz)	80	0	0
Peach Passion Fruit as prep	½ cup (5 oz)	80	0	0
Pineapple as prep	½ cup (5 oz)	80	0	0
Raspberry as prep	½ cup (5 oz)	80	0	0
Sparkling White Grape as prep	½ cup (5 oz)	80	0	0
Strawberry Banana as prep	½ cup (5 oz)	80	0	0
Strawberry Kiwi as prep	½ cup (5 oz)	80	0	0
Strawberry as prep	½ cup (5 oz)	80	0	0
Sugar Free Cherry as prep	½ cup (4.2 oz)	10	0	0
Sugar Free Cranberry as prep	½ cup (4.2 oz)	10	0	0
Sugar Free Lemon	½ cup (4.2 oz)	10	0	0
Sugar Free Lime as prep	½ cup (4.2 oz)	10	0	0
Sugar Free Mixed Fruit as prep	½ cup (4.2 oz)	10	0	0
Sugar Free Orange as prep	½ cup (4.2 oz)	10	0	0

FOOD	PORTION	CALS	FAT	SAT FAT
Sugar Free Raspberry as prep	½ cup (4.2 oz)	10	0	0
Sugar Free Strawberry Banana as prep	½ cup (4.2 oz)	10	0	0
Sugar Free Strawberry as prep	½ cup (4.2 oz)	10	0	0
Sugar Free Strawberry Kiwi as prep	½ cup (4.2 oz)	10	0	0
Sugar Free Watermelon as prep	½ cup (4.2 oz)	10	0	0
Watermelon as prep	½ cup (5 oz)	80	0	0
Wild Strawberry as prep	½ cup (5 oz)	80	0	0
Kojel				
Diet	1 serv	10	tr	—
READY-TO-EAT				
Handi-Snacks				
Gels Blue Raspberry	1 serv (4 oz)	80	0	0
Gels Cherry	1 serv (4 oz)	80	0	0
Gels Orange	1 serv (3.5 oz)	80	0	0
Gels Strawberry	1 serv (3.5 oz)	80	0	0
Hunt's				
Snack Pack Juicy Gels Mixed Fruit	1 (4 oz)	100	0	0
Snack Pack Gels Cherry	1 serv (3.5 oz)	100	0	0
Snack Pack Gels Raspberry Berry	1 serv (3.5 oz)	100	0	0
Snack Pack Gels Strawberry	1 serv (3.5 oz)	100	0	0
Snack Pack Gels Strawberry Orange	1 serv (3.5 oz)	100	0	0
Jell-O				
Berry Black	1 serv (3.5 oz)	70	0	0
Berry Blue	1 serv (3.5 oz)	70	0	0
Cherry	1 serv (3.5 oz)	70	0	0
Orange	1 serv (3.5 oz)	70	0	0
Orange Strawberry Banana	1 serv (3.5 oz)	70	0	0
Raspberry	1 serv (3.5 oz)	70	0	0
Rhymin' Lymon	1 serv (3.5 oz)	70	0	0
Strawberry	1 serv (3.5 oz)	70	0	0
Strawberry Kiwi	1 serv (3.5 oz)	10	0	0
Sugar Free Orange	1 serv (3.2 oz)	10	0	0
Sugar Free Raspberry	1 serv (3.2 oz)	10	0	0
Sugar Free Strawberry	1 serv (3.2 oz)	10	0	0
Tropical Berry	1 serv (3.5 oz)	10	0	0
Tropical Fruit Punch	1 serv (3.5 oz)	70	0	0
Wild Watermelon	1 serv (3.5 oz)	70	0	0
Kozy Shack				
Gel Treat Cherry	1 pkg (4 oz)	100	0	0

FOOD	PORTION	CALS	FAT	SAT FAT
Gel Treat Lemon Lime	1 pkg (4 oz)	100	0	0
Gel Treat Orange	1 pkg (4 oz)	100	0	0
Gel Treat Strawberry	1 pkg (4 oz)	100	0	0
Gel Treat Sugar Free Orange	1 pkg (4 oz)	10	0	0
Gel Treat Sugar Free Strawberry	1 pkg (4 oz)	10	0	0
Swiss Miss				
Gels Berry Strawberry	1 pkg (3.5 oz)	79	0	0
Gels Berry Lemon	1 pkg (3.5 oz)	79	0	0
Gels Raspberry Orange	1 pkg (3.5 oz)	79	0	0
Gels Strawberry Raspberry	1 pkg (3.5 oz)	79	0	0
GIBLETS				
capon simmered	1 cup (5 oz)	238	8	3
chicken floured & fried	1 cup (5 oz)	402	19	6
chicken simmered	1 cup (5 oz)	228	7	2
turkey simmered	1 cup (5 oz)	243	7	2
GINGER				
ground	1 tsp (1.8 g)	6	tr	tr
pickled	0.5 oz	5	0	0
root fresh	¼ cup	17	tr	tr
root fresh	5 slices	8	tr	tr
root fresh sliced	¼ cup	17	tr	tr
Eden				
Pickled w/ Shiso Leaves	1 tbsp	15	0	0
McCormick				
Crystallized	¼ tsp	15	0	0
GINKGO NUTS				
canned	1 oz	32	tr	tr
dried	1 oz	99	tr	tr
raw	1 oz	52	tr	tr
GINSENG				
dried	1 oz	90	tr	—
fresh	1 oz	28	tr	—
GIZZARDS				
chicken simmered	1 cup (5 oz)	222	5	2
turkey simmered	1 cup (5 oz)	236	6	2
Shady Brook				
Turkey	4 oz	130	4	1

FOOD	PORTION	CALS	FAT	SAT FAT
GNOCCHI				
Bellino				
W/ Potato	1 cup	240	1	0
GOAT				
roasted	3 oz	122	3	1
GOOSE				
w/ skin roasted	6.6 oz	574	41	13
w/ skin roasted	½ goose (1.7 lbs)	2362	170	53
w/o skin roasted	5 oz	340	18	7
w/o skin roasted	½ goose (1.3 lbs)	1406	75	27
GOOSEBERRIES				
canned in light syrup	½ cup	93	tr	tr
fresh	1 cup	67	1	tr
GRAPE JUICE				
bottled	1 cup	155	tr	tr
frzn sweetened as prep	1 cup	128	tr	tr
frzn sweetened not prep	6 oz	386	1	tr
grape drink	6 oz	84	0	0
Capri Sun				
Drink	1 pkg (7 oz)	100	0	0
Daily				
Drink	8 oz	110	0	0
Everfresh				
Juice	1 can (8 oz)	150	0	0
Hansen's				
White Grape 100% Juice	1 box (4.23 oz)	90	0	0
Juicy Juice				
Drink	1 box (8.45 oz)	140	0	0
Drink	1 box (4.23 oz)	70	0	0
Keto				
Kooler	½ tsp	0	0	0
Kool-Aid				
Bursts Grape Drink	1 (7 oz)	100	0	0
Drink as prep w/ sugar	1 serv (8 oz)	100	0	0
Drink Mix as prep	1 serv (8 oz)	60	0	0
Sugar Free Drink Mix as prep	1 serv (8 oz)	5	0	0

FOOD	PORTION	CALS	FAT	SAT FAT
Langers				
Cocktail	8 oz	160	0	0
Mott's				
100% Juice	1 box (8 oz)	130	0	0
Grape Juice	8 fl oz	130	0	0
Nantucket Nectars				
Grapeade	8 oz	130	0	0
Shasta Plus				
Grape Drink	1 can (11.5 oz)	160	0	0
Squeezit				
Grumpy Grape	1 bottle (7 oz)	110	0	0
Veryfine				
100% Juice	1 bottle (10 oz)	200	0	0
Chillers Glacial Grape	1 can (11.5 oz)	160	0	0
Grape Drink	1 bottle (10 oz)	160	0	0
Juice-Ups	8 fl oz	130	0	0
Welch's				
100% White	8 oz	160	0	0
GRAPE LEAVES				
canned	1 (4 g)	3	tr	tr
fresh raw	1 (3 g)	3	tr	tr
Cedar's				
Grape Leaves Stuffed With Rice	6 pieces (4.9 oz)	180	8	1
TAKE-OUT				
dolmas	5 (4.2 oz)	200	11	1
GRAPEFRUIT				
CANNED				
juice pack	½ cup	46	tr	tr
unsweetened	1 cup	93	tr	tr
water pack	½ cup	44	tr	tr
SunFresh				
Red & White	½ cup (4.4 oz)	45	0	0
FRESH				
pink	½	37	tr	tr
pink sections	1 cup	69	tr	tr
red	½	37	tr	tr
red sections	1 cup	69	tr	tr
white	½	39	tr	tr
white sections	1 cup	76	tr	tr

FOOD	PORTION	CALS	FAT	SAT FAT
Ocean Spray				
Fresh	2 oz	50	0	0
GRAPEFRUIT JUICE				
fresh	1 cup	96	tr	tr
frzn as prep	1 cup	102	tr	tr
frzn not prep	6 oz	302	1	tr
sweetened	1 cup	116	tr	tr
After The Fall				
Pink	1 bottle (10 oz)	100	0	0
Apple & Eve				
Made In The Shade Ruby Red	8 fl oz	130	0	0
Everfresh				
Juice	1 can (8 oz)	90	0	0
Ruby Red Cocktail	1 can (8 oz)	130	0	0
Fresh Samantha				
Juice	1 cup (8 oz)	90	0	0
Langers				
Diet Ruby Red	8 oz	40	0	0
Ruby Red	8 oz	130	0	0
Mott's				
100% Juice	8 fl oz	110	0	0
Nantucket Nectars				
100% Juice	8 oz	100	0	0
100% Ruby Red	8 oz	100	0	0
Ocean Spray				
100% Juice	8 oz	100	0	0
100% Juice Pink	8 oz	110	0	0
Ruby Red Drink	8 oz	130	0	0
Odwalla				
Juice	8 fl oz	90	0	0
Tropicana				
Golden	8 oz	90	0	0
Ruby Red	8 oz	90	0	0
Season's Best	8 oz	90	0	0
Twister Pink	1 bottle (10 oz)	140	0	0
W/ Double Vitamin C	8 fl oz	110	0	0
Veryfine				
100% Juice	1 bottle (10 oz)	110	0	0

FOOD	PORTION	CALS	FAT	SAT FAT
Pink	1 bottle (10 oz)	150	0	0
Ruby Red	8 fl oz	120	0	0
GRAPES				
fresh	10	36	tr	tr
thompson seedless in heavy syrup	½ cup	94	tr	tr
thompson seedless water pack	½ cup	48	tr	tr
Chiquita				
Grapes	1½ cups (4.8 oz)	90	1	0
GRAVY				
CANNED				
au jus	1 cup	38	tr	tr
beef	1 cup	124	6	3
beef	1 can (10 oz)	155	7	3
chicken	1 cup	189	14	3
mushroom	1 cup	120	6	1
turkey	1 cup	122	5	1
Campbell's				
Beef	¼ cup	29	1	tr
Brown	¼ cup	46	3	tr
Chicken	¼ cup	42	2	1
Turkey	¼ cup	29	1	tr
MIX				
au jus as prep w/ water	1 cup	32	1	1
brown as prep w/ water	1 cup	75	2	1
chicken as prep	1 cup	83	2	1
mushroom as prep	1 cup	70	1	1
onion as prep w/ water	1 cup	77	1	tr
pork as prep	1 cup	76	2	1
turkey as prep	1 cup	87	2	1
Bournvita				
Extract	2 heaping tsp	34	1	–
Bovril				
Extract	1 heaping tsp	9	0	–
Durkee				
Au Jus as prep	¼ cup	5	0	0
Brown as prep	¼ cup	10	1	0
Brown Mushroom as prep	¼ cup	15	0	0
Brown Onion as prep	¼ cup	15	0	0
Chicken as prep	¼ cup	20	1	0

FOOD	PORTION	CALS	FAT	SAT FAT
Country as prep	¼ cup	35	2	1
Homestyle as prep	¼ cup	15	1	0
Mushroom as prep	¼ cup	15	0	0
Onion as prep	¼ cup	10	0	0
Pork as prep	¼ cup	10	0	0
Sausage as prep	¼ cup	35	2	1
Swiss Steak as prep	¼ cup	15	0	0
Turkey as prep	¼ cup	20	0	0
French's				
Au Jus as prep	¼ cup	5	0	0
Brown as prep	¼ cup	10	1	0
Chicken as prep	¼ cup	25	1	0
Country as prep	¼ cup	35	2	1
Herb Brown as prep	¼ cup	15	1	0
Homestyle as prep	¼ cup	10	1	0
Mushroom as prep	¼ cup	10	1	0
Onion	¼ cup	15	1	0
Pork as prep	¼ cup	10	1	0
Turkey as prep	¼ cup	20	0	0
Loma Linda				
Gravy Quik Brown	1 tbsp (5 g)	20	0	0
Gravy Quik Chicken	1 tbsp (5 g)	20	0	0
Quik Gravy Country	1 tbsp (5 g)	25	1	0
Quik Gravy Mushroom	1 tbsp (5 g)	15	0	0
Quik Gravy Onion	1 tbsp (5 g)	20	0	0
Marmite				
Extract	1 heaping tsp	9	0	–
McCormick				
Au Jus Natural as prep	¼ cup	5	0	0
Beef & Herb as prep	¼ cup	30	1	–
Brown as prep	¼ cup	20	1	–
Chicken as prep	¼ cup	20	0	0
Onion as prep	¼ cup	20	1	–
Turkey as prep	¼ cup	20	0	–
GREAT NORTHERN BEANS				
canned	1 cup	299	1	tr
dried cooked	1 cup	20921	1	tr
Eden				
Organic	½ cup (4.6 oz)	110	1	0

FOOD	PORTION	CALS	FAT	SAT FAT
Green Giant				
Great Northern	½ cup (4.4 oz)	100	1	0
Hurst				
HamBeens w/ Ham	3 tbsp (1.2 oz)	120	1	0
GREEN BEANS				
CANNED				
green beans	½ cup	13	tr	tr
italian	½ cup	13	tr	tr
italian low sodium	½ cup	13	tr	tr
low sodium	½ cup	13	tr	tr
Del Monte				
Cut	½ cup (4.2 oz)	20	0	0
Cut Italian	½ cup (4.2 oz)	30	0	0
Cut No Salt Added	½ cup (4.2 oz)	20	0	0
French Style	½ cup (4.2 oz)	20	0	0
French Style No Salt Added	½ cup (4.2 oz)	20	0	0
French Style Seasoned	½ cup (4.2 oz)	20	0	0
Whole	½ cup (4.2 oz)	20	0	0
Green Giant				
Cut	½ cup (4.2 oz)	20	0	0
Cut 50% Less Sodium	½ cup (4.2 oz)	20	0	0
French Style	½ cup (4.1 oz)	20	0	0
Kitchen Sliced	½ cup (4.2 oz)	20	0	0
Whole	½ cup (4.1 oz)	25	0	0
S&W				
Blue Lake Cut	½ cup (4.2 oz)	20	0	0
French Style	½ cup (4.2 oz)	20	0	0
Whole Small	½ cup (4.2 oz)	20	0	0
Veg-All				
French Style	½ cup	20	0	0
FRESH				
cooked	½ cup	22	tr	tr
raw	½ cup	17	tr	tr
FROZEN				
cooked	½ cup	18	tr	tr
italian cooked	½ cup	18	tr	tr
Birds Eye				
Cut	½ cup	25	0	0
Italian	½ cup	35	0	0

FOOD	PORTION	CALS	FAT	SAT FAT
Fresh Like				
Cut	3.5 oz	29	tr	—
French Cut	3.5 oz	29	tr	—
Green Giant				
Cut	¾ cup (2.8 oz)	25	0	0
Harvest Fresh & Almonds	⅔ cup (2.8 oz)	60	3	0
Harvest Fresh Cut	⅔ cup (2.9 oz)	25	0	0
Stouffer's				
Green Bean Mushroom Casserole	1 serv (4 oz)	130	8	2
Tree Of Life				
Cut	⅔ cup (2.8 oz)	25	0	0
GROUNDCHERRIES				
fresh	½ cup	37	tr	—
GROUPER				
cooked	3 oz	100	1	tr
cooked	1 fillet (7.1 oz)	238	3	1
raw	3 oz	78	1	tr
GUAR GUM				
Bob's Red Mill				
Guar Gum	1 tbsp	20	0	0
GUAVA				
fresh	1	45	1	tr
guava sauce	½ cup	43	tr	tr
GUAVA JUICE				
Nantucket Nectars				
Guava	8 oz	130	0	0
GUINEA HEN				
w/ skin raw	½ hen (12.1 oz)	545	22	—
w/o skin raw	½ hen (9.3 oz)	292	7	—
HADDOCK				
fresh cooked	1 fillet (5.3 oz)	168	1	tr
fresh cooked	3 oz	95	1	tr
fresh raw	3 oz	74	1	tr
roe raw	1 oz	37	tr	—
smoked	1 oz	33	tr	tr
smoked	3 oz	99	1	tr

FOOD	PORTION	CALS	FAT	SAT FAT
Van De Kamp's				
Battered Fillets	2 (4 oz)	260	16	3
Breaded Fillets	2 (3.5 oz)	280	17	3
Lightly Breaded Fillets	1 (4 oz)	220	10	2
TAKE-OUT				
breaded & fried	1 piece (3.5 oz)	187	9	3
HAKE				
raw	3.5 oz	84	1	–
HALIBUT				
atlantic & pacific cooked	½ fillet (5.6 oz)	223	5	1
atlantic & pacific cooked	3 oz	119	2	tr
atlantic & pacific raw	3 oz	93	2	tr
greenland baked	3 oz	203	15	2
greenland baked	5.6 oz	380	28	5
Van De Kamp's				
Battered Fillets	3 (4 oz)	300	21	3
HALVA (see SESAME)				
HAM				
canned extra lean roasted	3 oz	116	4	1
center slice country style lean roasted	4 oz	220	9	3
chopped canned	1 oz	68	5	2
ham & cheese loaf	1 oz	73	6	4
ham & cheese spread	1 tbsp	37	3	1
ham salad spread	1 tbsp	32	2	1
minced	1 oz	75	6	2
patty cooked	1 patty (2 oz)	203	18	7
prosciutto	1 oz	55	2	–
sliced extra lean 5% fat	1 oz	37	1	tr
sliced regular 11% fat	1 oz	52	3	1
steak boneless extra lean	1 (2 oz)	69	2	1
westphalian smoked	1 oz	105	10	–
Alpine Lace				
Boneless Cooked 98% Fat Free	2 slices (2 oz)	60	1	1
Honey Ham 98% Fat Free	2 slices (2 oz)	60	1	1
Smoked Virginia 98% Fat Free	2 slices (2 oz)	60	1	1
Armour				
Chopped Ham canned	2 oz	130	11	4
Deviled Ham Spread	1 pkg (3 oz)	210	18	6

FOOD	PORTION	CALS	FAT	SAT FAT
Lean Slices Brown Sugar	1 pkg (2.5 oz)	90	2	1
Star Canned	1 oz	34	1	–
Boar's Head				
Black Forest Smoked	2 oz	60	1	0
Cappy	2 oz	60	2	1
Deluxe	2 oz	60	1	0
Deluxe Lowered Sodium	2 oz	50	1	0
Maple Glazed Honey	2 oz	60	1	0
Pepper	2 oz	60	1	0
Rosemary & Sundried Tomato	2 oz	70	3	1
Sweet Slice Smoked	3 oz	100	3	2
Virgina	2 oz	60	1	0
Virginia Smoked	2 oz	60	1	0
Carl Buddig				
Ham Sliced w/ Natural Juices	1 pkg (2.5 oz)	120	7	3
Honey Ham Sliced w/ Natural Juice	1 pkg (2.5 oz)	120	7	3
Lean Slices Oven Roasted Honey Ham	1 pkg (2.5 oz)	90	2	1
Lean Slices Smoked	1 pkg (2.5 oz)	80	2	1
Healthy Choice				
Baked Cooked	3 slices (2.2 oz)	70	2	1
Cooked	3 slices (2.2 oz)	70	2	1
Deli-Thin Baked Cooked With Natural Juices	6 slices (2 oz)	60	2	1
Deli-Thin Cooked	6 slices (2 oz)	60	2	1
Deli-Thin Honey With Natural Juices	6 slices (2 oz)	60	2	1
Deli-Thin Smoked With Natural Juices	6 slices (2 oz)	60	2	1
Fresh-Trak Cooked	1 slice (1 oz)	30	1	0
Fresh-Trak Honey	1 slice (1 oz)	30	1	0
Honey Boneless	3 oz	100	3	1
Smoked	3 slices (2.2 oz)	70	2	1
Hillshire				
Deli Select Honey Ham	6 slices (2 oz)	60	2	1
Hormel				
Black Label Canned (refrigerated)	3 oz	100	5	2
Black Label Canned (self stable)	3 oz	110	5	2
Cure 81 Half Ham	3 oz	100	5	2
Curemaster	3 oz	80	3	1
Deviled Ham	4 tbsp (2 oz)	150	12	4
Ham & Cheese Patties	1 patty (2 oz)	190	17	6
Ham Patties	1 (2 oz)	180	17	6

FOOD	PORTION	CALS	FAT	SAT FAT
Light & Lean 97 Sliced	1 slice (1 oz)	25	1	0
Primissimo Prosciutto	2 oz	120	7	3
Spiral Cure 81	3 oz	150	9	5
Jordan's				
Healthy Trim 97% Fat Free Cooked	1 slice (1 oz)	30	1	0
Healthy Trim 97% Fat Free EZ Serve	1 slice (1 oz)	30	1	1
Healthy Trim 97% Fat Free Virginia	1 slice (1 oz)	30	1	1
Louis Rich				
Carving Board Baked	2 slices (1.6 oz)	50	2	1
Carving Board Honey Glazed Thin	6 slices (2.1 oz)	70	2	1
Carving Board Honey Glazed Traditional	2 slices (1.6 oz)	50	2	1
Carving Board Smoked	1 slice (1.6 oz)	45	2	1
Dinner Slices Baked	1 slice (3.3 oz)	80	2	1
Oscar Mayer				
Baked	3 slices (2.2 oz)	70	3	1
Boiled	3 slices (2.2 oz)	60	3	1
Chopped	1 slice (1 oz)	50	3	2
Dinner Slice	3 oz	80	3	1
Dinner Steaks	1 (2 oz)	60	2	1
Free Baked	3 slices (1.6 oz)	35	0	0
Free Honey	3 slices (1.6 oz)	35	0	0
Free Smoked	3 slices (1.6 oz)	35	0	0
Honey	3 slices (2.2 oz)	70	3	1
Lower Sodium	3 slices (2.2 oz)	70	3	1
Lunchables Ham Bagels	1 pkg	410	10	5
Lunchables Ham Wraps	1 pkg	430	13	5
Smoked	3 slices (2.2 oz)	60	3	1
Spam				
Spread	4 tbsp (2 oz)	140	12	4
Wampler				
Black Forest	2 oz	60	2	–

HAM DISHES
TAKE-OUT

croquettes	1 (3.1 oz)	217	14	5
salad	½ cup	287	23	5

HAM SUBSTITUTES
Yves

Veggie Ham Deli Slices	1 serv (2.2 oz)	80	0	0

FOOD	PORTION	CALS	FAT	SAT FAT
HAMBURGER				
Kid Cuisine				
Buckaroo Beef Patty Sandwich w/ Cheese	1 meal (8.5 oz)	410	15	7
White Castle				
Cheeseburger	2 (3.6 oz)	310	17	9
Hamburger	2 (3.2 oz)	270	14	6
TAKE-OUT				
double patty w/ bun	1 reg	544	28	10
double patty w/ cheese & bun	1 reg	457	28	13
double patty w/ cheese & double bun	1 reg	461	22	10
double patty w/ cheese ketchup mayonnaise onion pickle tomato & bun	1 reg	416	21	8
double patty w/ ketchup mayonnaise onion pickle tomato & bun	1 reg	649	35	13
double patty w/ ketchup cheese mayonnaise mustard pickle tomato & bun	1 lg	706	44	18
double patty w/ ketchup mustard mayonnaise onion pickle tomato & bun	1 lg	540	27	11
double patty w/ ketchup mustard onion pickle & bun	1 reg	576	32	12
single patty w/ bacon ketchup cheese mustard onion pickle & bun	1 lg	609	37	16
single patty w/ bun	1 reg	275	12	4
single patty w/ bun	1 lg	400	23	8
single patty w/ cheese & bun	1 reg	320	15	6
single patty w/ cheese & bun	1 lg	608	33	15
single patty w/ ketchup cheese ham mayonnaise pickle tomato & bun	1 lg	745	48	21
single patty w/ ketchup mustard mayonnaise onion pickle tomato & bun	1 reg	279	13	4
triple patty w/ cheese & bun	1 lg	769	51	22
triple patty w/ ketchup mustard pickle & bun	1 lg	693	41	16

FOOD	PORTION	CALS	FAT	SAT FAT
HAMBURGER SUBSTITUTES (see also MEAT SUBSTITUTES)				
Amy's				
All American Burger	1 (2.5 oz)	120	3	0
California Burger	1 (2.5 oz)	130	5	1
Chicago Burger	1 (2.5 oz)	160	5	2
Boca Burgers				
Flame Grilled	1	120	4	1
Hint of Garlic	1 patty (2.5 oz)	110	2	1
Vegan Original	1 patty (2.5 oz)	84	0	0
Franklin Farms				
Veggiburger Portabella	1 (3 oz)	120	2	0
GardenVegan				
Fat-Free Patty	1 patty (2.5 oz)	140	0	0
Gardenburger				
Classic Greek	1 (2.5 oz)	120	3	2
Fire Roasted Vegetable	1 (2.5 oz)	120	3	2
Hamburger Style	1 (2.5 oz)	90	0	0
Hamburger Style w/ Cheese	1 (2.5 oz)	110	3	2
Savory Mushroom	1 (2.5 oz)	120	3	2
Green Giant				
Southwestern Style	1 patty (3.2 oz)	140	4	2
Harmony Farms				
Soy Burgers Onion	1 (2.5 oz)	90	3	0
Soy Burgers Garlic	1 (2.5 oz)	110	3	0
Soy Burgers Mushroom	1 (2.5 oz)	110	3	0
Soy Burgers Original	1 (2.5 oz)	110	3	0
Lightlife				
Barbecue Grilles	1 patty (2.7 oz)	120	4	2
Lemon Grilles	1 patty (2.7 oz)	140	6	2
Light Burgers	1 (3 oz)	130	1	0
Tamari Grilles	1 patty (2.7 oz)	120	5	2
Loma Linda				
Patty Mix not prep	⅓ cup (0.9 oz)	90	1	0
Redi-Burger	⅝ in slice (3 oz)	120	3	1
Vege-Burger	¼ cup (1.9 oz)	70	2	1
Morningstar Farms				
Better'n Burger	1 (2.7 oz)	80	0	0
Garden Grille	1 patty (2.5 oz)	120	3	1
Garden Veggie Patties	1 patty (2.4 oz)	100	3	1
Hard Rock Cafe Veggie Burger	1 (3 oz)	170	8	1

FOOD	PORTION	CALS	FAT	SAT FAT
Harvest Burger Italian Style	1 patty (3.2 oz)	140	5	2
Harvest Burger Original	1 (3.2 oz)	140	4	2
Harvest Burger Southwestern	1 (3.2 oz)	140	4	2
Spicy Black Bean Burger	1 (2.7 oz)	110	1	0
Natural Touch				
Garden Veggie Pattie	1 (2.4 oz)	110	3	1
Okara Pattie	1 (2.2 oz)	110	5	1
Original Veggie Burger Kit not prep	¼ pkg (0.8 oz)	80	0	0
Southwestern Veggie Burger Kit not prep	¼ pkg (0.9 oz)	90	0	0
Spicy Black Bean Burger	1 (2.7 oz)	100	1	0
Vegan Burger	1 (2.7 oz)	70	0	0
NewMenu				
VegiBurger	1 patty (3 oz)	110	1	0
Superburgers				
Vegan Organic Original	1 (3 oz)	98	2	1
Vegan Organic Smoked	1 (3 oz)	98	2	1
Vegan Organic TexMex	1 (3 oz)	110	1	1
V'dora				
Vegetable BurgerLites	1 (3.3 oz)	58	0	0
Veggie Patch				
Burgeriffics	1 (2.5 oz)	110	3	—
Worthington				
Granburger not prep	3 tbsp (0.6 oz)	60	1	0
Prosage Patties	1 (1.3 oz)	80	3	1
Vegetarian Burger	¼ cup (1.9 oz)	60	2	0
Yves				
Black Bean & Mushroom Burgers	1 (3 oz)	100	0	0
Garden Vegetable Patties	1 (3 oz)	90	0	0
Veggie Burger	1 (3 oz)	119	2	0
HAZELNUTS				
dried blanched	1 oz	191	19	1
dried unblanched	1 oz	179	18	1
dry roasted unblanched	1 oz	188	19	1
oil roasted unblanched	1 oz	187	18	1
Crumpy				
Chocolate Hazelnut Spread	1 tbsp (0.5 oz)	80	5	1
Low Carb Creations				
Soft Hazelnut Brittle	2 pieces (1 oz)	160	12	2

FOOD	PORTION	CALS	FAT	SAT FAT
Torras				
Hazelnut Chocolate Spread	1 tsp	27	2	2
Twist				
Sugar Free Chocolate Hazelnut Spread	2 tbsp	180	14	4
HEART				
beef simmered	3 oz	148	5	1
chicken simmered	1 cup (5 oz)	268	11	3
lamb braised	3 oz	158	7	3
pork braised	1 cup	215	7	2
pork braised	1	191	7	2
turkey simmered	1 cup (5 oz)	257	9	3
veal braised	3 oz	158	6	2
HEARTS OF PALM				
canned	1 cup (5.1 oz)	41	1	tr
canned	1 (1.2 oz)	9	tr	tr
HEMP				
HempNut				
Shelled Hempseed	1 oz	162	13	1
Nutiva				
Hempseed	1½ tbsp (0.5 oz)	70	5	1
HERBAL TEA (see TEA/HERBAL TEA)				
HERBS/SPICES (see also individual names)				
chinese five spice	1 tsp	7	tr	–
curry powder	1 tsp	6	tr	–
garam masala	1 tsp	8	tr	–
poultry seasoning	1 tsp	5	tr	–
pumpkin pie spice	1 tsp	6	tr	–
Chi-Chi's				
Seasoning Mix	1 tsp (3 g)	10	0	0
Eden				
Furikake Seasoning	½ tsp	5	0	0
Gringo Billy's				
Meat Rubs Chipotle	¼ tsp	0	0	0
Meat Rubs Ultimate	¼ tsp	0	0	0
Tuna Seasoning	1 tsp	5	1	0

FOOD	PORTION	CALS	FAT	SAT FAT
Instant India				
Curry Paste Cilantro Garlic	2 tbsp (1 oz)	110	3	1
Curry Paste Ginger Garlic	2 tbsp (1 oz)	90	3	1
McCormick				
Big'n Season Buffalo Wings	1 tbsp (8 g)	30	0	0
Big'n Season Chicken	1 tbsp (6 g)	20	0	0
Big'n Season Pot Roast	1 tsp	10	0	0
Blends Bon Appetit	¼ tsp	0	0	0
Cajun Seasoning	¼ tsp	0	0	0
Greek Seasoning	¼ tsp	0	0	0
Jamaican Jerk Seasoning	¼ tsp	0	0	0
Meat Loaf Seasoning	1 tsp (4 g)	15	0	0
Seafood Seasoning	¼ tsp	0	0	0
Mrs. Dash				
Classic Italian	¼ tsp	0	0	0
Extra Spicy	¼ tsp	0	0	0
Garlic & Herb	¼ tsp	0	0	0
Grilling Blend Mesquite	¼ tsp	0	0	0
Grilling Blend Original Chicken	¼ tsp	0	0	0
Grilling Blend Original Steak	¼ tsp	0	0	0
Lemon Pepper	¼ tsp	0	0	0
Minced Onion Medley	¼ tsp	0	0	0
Original Blend	¼ tsp	0	0	0
Table Blend	¼ tsp	0	0	0
Tomato Basil Garlic	¼ tsp	0	0	0
HERRING				
atlantic cooked	3 oz	172	10	2
atlantic cooked	1 fillet (5 oz)	290	17	4
atlantic raw	3 oz	134	8	2
pacific baked	3 oz	213	15	4
pacific fillet baked	5.1 oz	360	26	6
roe canned	1 oz	34	1	—
roe raw	1 oz	37	tr	—
smoked	3.5 oz	210	14	3
TAKE-OUT				
atlantic kippered	1 fillet (1.4 oz)	87	5	1
atlantic pickled	½ oz	39	3	tr
fried	1 serv (3.5 oz)	233	15	—

FOOD	PORTION	CALS	FAT	SAT FAT
HICKORY NUTS				
dried	1 oz	187	18	2
HOMINY				
CANNED				
white	1 cup (5.6 oz)	482	1	tr
Van Camp				
Golden	½ cup (4.3 oz)	80	1	0
White	½ cup (4.3 oz)	80	1	0
HONEY				
honey	1 cup (11.9 oz)	1031	0	0
honey	1 tbsp (0.7 oz)	64	0	0
orange blossom	1 tbsp	60	0	0
wild honey	1 tbsp	60	0	0
Steel's				
Sugar Free	1 tbsp	24	0	0
SueBee				
Clover	1 tbsp	60	0	0
HONEYDEW				
FRESH				
cubed	1 cup	60	tr	–
wedge	⅒	46	tr	–
Chiquita				
Wedge	⅒ melon (4.7 oz)	50	0	0
HORSE				
roasted	3 oz	149	5	2
HORSERADISH				
wasabi root raw	1 (5.9 oz)	184	1	–
wasabi root raw sliced	1 cup (4.6 oz)	142	1	–
Boar's Head				
Horseradish	1 tsp (5 g)	5	0	0
Eden				
Wasabi Powder	1 tsp	10	0	0
Kraft				
Cream Style	1 tsp (5 g)	0	0	0
Horseradish Sauce	1 tsp (5 g)	20	2	0
Prepared	1 tsp (5 g)	0	0	0

FOOD	PORTION	CALS	FAT	SAT FAT
HOT COCOA				
mix as prep w/ water	7 oz	103	1	1
mix w/ equal as prep w/ water	7 oz	48	tr	tr
Carnation				
Hot Cocoa 70 Calorie	1 pkg (0.7 oz)	70	0	0
Hot Cocoa Double Chocolate Meltdown	1 pkg (1.2 oz)	150	4	3
Hot Cocoa Fat Free Raspberry	1 pkg (0.3 oz)	30	0	0
Hot Cocoa Fat Free w/ Marshmallows	1 pkg (0.4 oz)	45	0	0
Hot Cocoa Lactose Free	1 pkg (1 oz)	120	2	0
Hot Cocoa Marshmallow Blizzard	1 pkg (1.5 oz)	180	2	0
Hot Cocoa Milk Chocolate	3 tbsp (1 oz)	110	1	0
Hot Cocoa Rich Chocolate	3 tbsp (1 oz)	110	1	0
Hot Cocoa Rich Chocolate Fat Free	1 pkg (0.3 oz)	25	0	0
Hot Cocoa Rich Chocolate No Sugar Added	3 tbsp (0.5 oz)	50	0	0
Hot Cocoa Rich Chocolate w/ Marshmallows	3 tbsp (1 oz)	110	1	0
Keto				
Hot Cocoa	1 tsp	12	0	0
Nestle				
Hot Cocoa Rich Chocolate	1 pkg (1 oz)	110	1	1
Hot Cocoa Rich w/ Marshmallows	1 pkg (1 oz)	110	1	1
Sipper Sweets				
Sugar Free Low Carb Mix	1 serv	50	3	0
Swiss Miss				
Caramel Cream	1 serv	110	3	0
Hot Cocoa And Cream	1 serv	153	5	3
Hot Cocoa Chocolate Sensation	1 serv	148	4	2
Hot Cocoa Diet	1 serv	22	tr	tr
Hot Cocoa Fat Free	1 serv	52	tr	0
Hot Cocoa Fat Free Marshmallow Lovers	1 serv	65	tr	0
Hot Cocoa Lite	1 serv	76	1	tr
Hot Cocoa Marshmallow Lovers	1 serv	142	3	1
Hot Cocoa Milk Chocolate	1 serv	118	3	1
Hot Cocoa Milk Chocolate No Sugar Added	1 serv	55	1	1
Hot Cocoa Milk Chocolate w/ Marshmallows	1 serv	118	3	1

FOOD	PORTION	CALS	FAT	SAT FAT
Hot Cocoa Rich Chocolate	1 serv	110	2	tr
Hot Cocoa White Chocolate	1 serv	109	1	tr
Hot Cocoa w/ Marshmallows No Sugar Added	1 serv	56	1	0
Premiere Hot Cocoa Almond Mocha	1 serv	144	3	1
Premiere Hot Cocoa Raspberry Truffle	1 serv	144	3	1
Premiere Hot Cocoa Suisse Truffle	1 serv	142	2	1
Rich Hot Cocoa No Sugar Added	1 serv	54	1	1
Sidewalk Cafe Cappuccino	1 serv	119	4	1
Sidewalk Cafe Cinnamon	1 serv	126	4	1
Sidewalk Cafe French Vanilla	1 serv	121	4	1
Sidewalk Cafe Mocha	1 serv	120	4	1
Weight Watchers				
Hot Cocoa Mix as prep	1 pkg	70	0	0
TAKE-OUT				
hot cocoa	1 cup	218	9	6
mexican hot chocolate	1 cup	173	6	4
HOT DOG				
beef	1 (2 oz)	180	16	7
beef	1 (1.5)	142	13	5
beef & pork	1 (2 oz)	183	17	6
beef & pork	1 (1.5 oz)	144	13	5
chicken	1 (1.5 oz)	116	9	2
pork cheesefurter smokie	1 (1.5 oz)	141	12	5
turkey	1 (1.5 oz)	102	8	—
Applegate Farms				
Chicken Natural Uncured	1 (1.5 oz)	120	5	2
Natural Turkey	1 (1.5 oz)	120	5	2
Armour				
Star Jumbo Beef	1	190	18	—
Boar's Head				
Beef	1 (2 oz)	160	14	6
Beef Lite	1 (1.6 oz)	90	6	3
Pork & Beef	1 (2 oz)	150	14	5
Health Is Wealth				
Uncured Beef	1 (1.5 oz)	80	6	3
Uncured Chicken	1 (1.5 oz)	100	8	2
Healthy Choice				
Beef Low Fat	1 (1.8 oz)	70	3	1

FOOD	PORTION	CALS	FAT	SAT FAT
Bunsize	1 (2 oz)	70	2	1
Jumbo	1 (2 oz)	70	2	1
Low Fat Turkey Pork Beef	1 (1.4 oz)	60	2	1
Hormel				
Fat Free	1 (1.8 oz)	45	0	0
Fat Free Beef	1 (1.8 oz)	45	0	0
Jordan's				
Healthy Trim Low Fat	1 (1.8 oz)	70	3	1
Healthy Trim Low Fat Skinless	1 (1.8 oz)	70	3	1
Kid Cuisine				
Mystical Mini Corn Dogs	4 pieces	230	14	4
Louis Rich				
Bun Length	1 (2 oz)	110	8	3
Cheese	1 (1.6 oz)	90	6	3
Franks	1 (1.6 oz)	80	6	2
Organic Valley				
All-Natural Beef	1 (1.6 oz)	90	6	3
Oscar Mayer				
Beef	1 (1.6 oz)	140	13	6
Big & Juicy Franks Deli Style	1 (2.7 oz)	230	22	10
Big & Juicy Franks Original	1 (2.7 oz)	240	22	9
Big & Juicy Franks Quarter Pound	1 (4 oz)	350	32	13
Big & Juicy Weiners Hot 'N Spicy	1 (2.7 oz)	220	20	8
Big & Juicy Weiners Smokie Links	1 (2.7 oz)	220	19	7
Big & Juicy Wieners Original	1 (2.7 oz)	240	22	9
Bun-Length Beef	1 (2 oz)	180	17	7
Cheese	1 (1.6 oz)	140	13	5
Fat Free Beef	1 (1.8 oz)	40	0	0
Fat Free Turkey & Beef	1 (1.8 oz)	40	0	0
Jumbo Beef	1 (2 oz)	180	17	7
Light Beef	1 (1.6 oz)	90	6	3
Wieners	1 (1.6 oz)	150	13	5
Wieners Bun-Length	1 (2 oz)	190	17	6
Wieners Jumbo	1 (2 oz)	180	17	6
Wieners Light	1 (2 oz)	110	8	4
Wieners Little	6 (2 oz)	180	17	6
Wampler				
Chicken	1 (2 oz)	120	11	3
TAKE-OUT				
corndog	1	460	19	5

FOOD	PORTION	CALS	FAT	SAT FAT
w/ bun chili	1	297	13	5
w/ bun plain	1	242	15	5

HOT DOG SUBSTITUTES
Lightlife
Smart Deli Jumbo's	1 link (2.7 oz)	80	0	0
Smart Dogs	1 (1.5 oz)	45	0	0
Tofu Pups	1 (1.4 oz)	60	3	1
Wonder Dogs	1 (1.5 oz)	60	2	1

Loma Linda
Big Franks	1 (1.8 oz)	110	7	1
Big Franks Low Fat	1 (1.8 oz)	80	3	1
Corn Dogs	1 (2.5 oz)	150	4	1

Morningstar Farms
America's Original Veggie Dog	1 (2 oz)	80	1	0
Meatfree Corn Dog	1 (2.5 oz)	150	4	1
Meatfree Mini Corn Dog	4 (2.7 oz)	170	5	1

Natural Touch
Vege Frank	1 (1.6 oz)	100	6	1

NewMenu
VegiDogs	1 (1.5 oz)	45	0	0

Quorn
Meat-Free Dogs	1 (1.5 oz)	70	4	0

Veggie Patch
Perfectly Franks	1 (1.7 oz)	70	2	–

Worthington
Veja Links Low Fat	1 (1.1 oz)	40	2	0

Yves
Good Dog	1 (1.8 oz)	70	2	0
Tofu Dogs	1 (1.3 oz)	45	1	0
Veggie Dogs	1 (1.6 oz)	60	0	0
Veggie Dogs Chili	1 (1.6 oz)	50	0	0
Veggie Dogs Jumbo	1 (2.7 oz)	100	2	0
Veggie Dogs Jumbo Hot N' Spicy	1 (2.7 oz)	106	2	0

HUMMUS
hummus	1 cup	420	21	3

Athenos
Roasted Red Pepper	2 tbsp (1.1 oz)	60	4	1

TAKE-OUT
hummus	⅓ cup	140	7	1

FOOD	PORTION	CALS	FAT	SAT FAT
HYACINTH BEANS				
dried cooked	1 cup	228	1	–
ICE CREAM AND FROZEN DESSERTS *(see also* ICES AND ICE POPS, PUDDING				
POPS, SHERBET, YOGURT FROZEN)				
chocolate	½ cup (4 fl oz)	143	7	4
dixie cup chocolate	1 (3.5 fl oz)	125	6	4
dixie cup strawberry	1 (3.5 fl oz)	112	5	–
dixie cup vanilla	1 (3.5 fl oz)	116	6	4
freeze dried ice cream chocolate	1 pkg (0.75 oz)	158	5	2
strawberry & vanilla				
strawberry	½ cup (4 fl oz)	127	6	–
vanilla	½ cup (4 fl oz)	132	7	4
vanilla soft serve	½ cup	111	2	1
Atkins				
Endulge Butter Pecan	½ cup	170	15	7
Endulge Chocolate	½ cup	140	12	7
Endulge Chocolate Peanut	½ cup	170	14	7
Butter Swirl				
Endulge Vanilla	½ cup	140	12	7
Endulge Vanilla Fudge	½ cup	140	10	6
Endulge Bars Chocolate Fudge	1 bar	130	11	6
Endulge Bars Chocolate Fudge Swirl	1 bar	180	16	12
Endulge Bars Peanut Butter Swirl	1 bar	180	17	12
Endulge Bars Vanilla Fudge Swirl	1 bar	180	16	12
Better Than Ice Creme				
Soy Vanilla as prep	½ cup	110	3	tr
Bon Bons				
Dark Chocolate	5 pieces	190	13	8
Milk Chocolate	5 pieces	200	14	8
Breyers				
Almond Joy	½ cup	140	5	3
Banana Fudge Chunk	½ cup	170	9	5
Butter Almond	½ cup	160	10	5
Butter Pecan	½ cup	170	11	5
Butter Pecan Homemade	½ cup	170	11	5
Butter Pecan No Sugar Added	½ cup	120	7	3
Caramel Praline Crunch	½ cup	180	9	5
Caramel Toffee Crunch	½ cup	180	9	6
CarbSmart Chocolate	½ cup	130	10	6

FOOD	PORTION	CALS	FAT	SAT FAT
CarbSmart Strawberry	½ cup	130	9	6
CarbSmart Vanilla	½ cup	130	9	6
Cherry Chocolate Chip	½ cup	150	8	5
Cherry Vanilla	½ cup	140	8	5
Chocolate	½ cup	150	8	5
Chocolate 98% Fat Free	½ cup	90	2	1
Chocolate Caramel No Sugar Added	½ cup	110	4	3
Chocolate Chip	½ cup	160	9	5
Chocolate Chip Cookie Dough	½ cup	170	9	6
Chocolate Rainbow	½ cup	140	7	5
Coffee	½ cup	140	8	5
Cookies & Cream	½ cup	160	8	5
Creamsicle	½ cup	130	5	3
Deep Chocolate Fudge	½ cup	200	12	8
Dulce De Leche	½ cup	150	7	4
French Vanilla	½ cup	150	8	5
French Vanilla Light	½ cup	120	4	2
French Vanilla No Sugar Added	½ cup	110	5	3
Fresa Banana	½ cup	140	5	4
Heath English Toffee	½ cup	190	9	5
Hershey w/ Almonds	½ cup	170	8	5
Ice Cream Cake Oreo	1 slice	190	10	5
Ice Cream Cake Vanilla	1 slice	190	11	7
Klondike Sandwich	½ cup	160	7	4
Mint Chocolate Chip	½ cup	160	9	5
Mint Chocolate Chip Light	½ cup	130	5	3
Mint Oreo	½ cup	170	7	4
Mocha Almond Fudge	½ cup	170	9	4
Oreo	½ cup	160	6	5
Peach	½ cup	130	6	4
Peanut Butter & Fudge	½ cup	170	10	5
Reese's Peanut Butter Cups	½ cup	180	9	5
Rocky Road	½ cup	160	8	5
SpongeBob Cookie Dough	½ cup	160	7	4
Strawberry	½ cup	120	6	4
Strawberry Shortcake	½ cup	160	6	4
Turtle Sundae	½ cup	190	11	6
Vanilla	½ cup	140	8	5
Vanilla Calcium Rich	½ cup	130	7	4
Vanilla Fudge Twirl	½ cup	140	7	5

FOOD	PORTION	CALS	FAT	SAT FAT
Vanilla Homemade	½ cup	140	8	5
Vanilla Lactose Free	½ cup	130	7	5
Vanilla Light	½ cup	110	3	2
Vanilla Light 2% Milk	½ cup	130	5	3
Vanilla No Sugar Added	½ cup	100	5	3
Vanilla Caramel Brownie	½ cup	170	9	5
Vanilla Fudge Brownie	½ cup	180	9	5
Vanilla Fudge Twirl No Sugar Added	½ cup	110	4	3
Wild Berry Swirl	½ cup	140	8	5
Butterfinger				
Bar	1 (2.5 oz)	190	13	8
California Joe				
Soft Serve Chocolate	½ cup (2.5 oz)	72	0	0
Soft Serve Vanilla	½ cup (2.5 oz)	70	0	0
Carnation				
Cup Chocolate	1 (3 oz)	140	8	5
Cup Chocolate Malt	1 (12 oz)	270	6	1
Cup Strawberry	1 (3 oz)	100	5	3
Cup Vanilla	1 (3 oz)	100	6	3
Cup Vanilla	1 (5 oz)	170	10	5
Cup Vanilla Malt	1 (12 oz)	260	6	0
Sundae Cup Strawberry	1 (5 oz)	200	8	5
Sunday Cup Chocolate	1 (5 oz)	210	9	6
Cool Creations				
Cookies & Cream Sandwich	1 (3.5 oz)	240	11	4
Mickey Mouse Bar	1 (2.5 oz)	120	8	4
Mini Sandwich	1 (2.3 oz)	110	5	2
Dippin' Dots				
Dipping Dots Chocolate	⅝ cup (3 oz)	190	9	6
Drumstick				
Cone Chocolate	1 (4.6 oz)	320	17	10
Cone Chocolate Dipped	1 (4.6 oz)	320	16	10
Cone Vanilla	1 (4.6 oz)	340	19	11
Cone Vanilla Caramel	1 (4.6 oz)	360	20	13
Cone Vanilla Fudge	1 (4.6 oz)	360	20	10
Edy's				
3 Musketeers	½ cup	160	7	4
Dreamery Banana Split	½ cup	240	11	7
Dreamery Black Raspberry Avalanche	½ cup	270	16	10
Dreamery Caramel Toffee Bar Heaven	½ cup	290	16	9

FOOD	PORTION	CALS	FAT	SAT FAT
Dreamery Cashew Praline Parfait	½ cup	280	16	9
Dreamery Chocolate Truffle Explosion	½ cup	280	15	55
Dreamery Chocolate Peanut Butter Chunk	½ cup	310	18	9
Dreamery Coney Island Waffle Cone	½ cup	310	18	12
Dreamery Cool Mint	½ cup	300	17	11
Dreamery Deep Dish Apple Pie	½ cup	280	15	9
Dreamery Dulce De Leche	½ cup	270	14	9
Dreamery Grandma's Cookie Dough	½ cup	300	17	9
Dreamery Harvest Peach	½ cup	230	13	7
Dreamery New York Strawberry Cheesecake	½ cup	260	15	9
Dreamery Nothing But Chocolate	½ cup	280	14	8
Dreamery Nuts About Malt	½ cup	290	17	9
Dreamery Raspberry Brownie A La Mode	½ cup	270	14	7
Dreamery Raspberry Brownie A La Mode	½ cup	130	14	7
Dreamery Strawberry Fields	½ cup	220	12	7
Dreamery Tiramisu	½ cup	260	13	8
Dreamery Vanilla	½ cup	260	15	9
Grand Black Cherry Vanilla	½ cup	140	7	4
Grand Blue Ribbon Chocolate Cake	½ cup	180	10	5
Grand Butter Pecan	½ cup	170	10	5
Grand Cherry Chocolate Chip	½ cup	160	8	5
Grand Chocolate	½ cup	150	8	5
Grand Chocolate Caramel Swirl	½ cup	170	9	6
Grand Chocolate Chips	½ cup	170	9	6
Grand Chocolate Fudge Mousse	½ cup	160	8	5
Grand Chocolate Fudge Sundae	½ cup	170	9	5
Grand Coffee	½ cup	140	8	5
Grand Cookie Dough	½ cup	180	9	5
Grand Cookies'N Cream	½ cup	160	8	5
Grand Double Fudge Brownie	½ cup	170	9	5
Grand Espresso Chip	½ cup	150	8	5
Grand French Vanilla	½ cup	160	9	5
Grand French Vanilla Fudge Pie	½ cup	160	8	5
Grand Mint Chocolate Chips	½ cup	170	9	6
Grand Neapolitan	½ cup	140	7	5
Grand Nutty Cone Crunch	½ cup	180	10	6

FOOD	PORTION	CALS	FAT	SAT FAT
Grand Real Strawberry	½ cup	130	6	4
Grand Rocky Road	½ cup	170	10	5
Grand Spumoni	½ cup	150	8	5
Grand Strawberry Cupcake	½ cup	140	6	4
Grand Tin Roof Sundae	½ cup	170	9	5
Grand Utimate Caramel Cup	½ cup	170	8	5
Grand Vanilla	½ cup	140	8	5
Grand Vanillaberry Bar	½ cup	130	5	3
Grand Light Butter Pecan	½ cup	120	5	2
Grand Light Chocolate Raspberry Escape	½ cup	130	5	3
Grand Light Chocolate Fudge Mousse	½ cup	120	4	2
Grand Light Cookie Dough	½ cup	130	5	3
Grand Light Cookies 'N Cream	½ cup	120	4	2
Grand Light Crazy For Caramel	½ cup	120	4	3
Grand Light French Silk	½ cup	130	5	3
Grand Light Mint Chocolate Chips	½ cup	120	5	3
Grand Light Peanut Butter Cups	½ cup	120	5	3
Grand Light Rocky Road	½ cup	120	4	2
Grand Light S'Mores & More	½ cup	130	4	2
Grand Light Strawberry Shortcake	½ cup	110	4	2
Grand Light Vanilla	½ cup	100	3	2
Homemade All Natural Vanilla	½ cup	130	7	5
Homemade Brownies A La Mode	½ cup	150	7	4
Homemade Chocolate Chip Cookie Jar	½ cup	180	10	7
Homemade Chocolate Chip Mousse	½ cup	170	9	6
Homemade Double Chocolate Chunk	½ cup	170	9	6
Homemade Mint Chocolate Chunk	½ cup	170	9	6
Homemade Old Fashioned Butter Pecan	½ cup	160	10	5
Homemade Strawberries & Cream	½ cup	120	6	4
Homemade Vanilla Custard	½ cup	150	8	5
M&M's Almond	½ cup	180	10	5
M&M's Chocolate Brownie Sundae	½ cup	180	9	5
M&M's Mint	½ cup	200	11	6
M&M's Vanilla	½ cup	180	9	5
Milky Way	½ cup	160	7	4
Snickers	½ cup	180	9	5
Snickers Cruncher	½ cup	190	10	6

FOOD	PORTION	CALS	FAT	SAT FAT
Twix	½ cup	190	9	5
Twix Peanut Butter	½ cup	190	11	5
Flintstones				
Cool Cream	1 (2.75 oz)	90	2	1
Push-Up Pebbles Treats	1 (2.75 oz)	120	6	4
Good Humor				
Bar Oreo	1 (4 oz)	250	15	8
Bar Reese's Peanut Butter	1 (4 oz)	310	21	13
Bar Toasted Almond	1 (3 oz)	180	10	3
Bar Vanilla Dark Chocolate	1 (3 oz)	190	13	9
Bar Vanilla Milk Chocolate	1 (3 oz)	180	13	9
Bar Candy Center Crunch	1 (4 oz)	310	23	17
Bar Strawberry Shortcake	1 (4 oz)	230	12	4
Chocolate Eclair Bar	1 (4 oz)	220	11	5
Cone Premium Sundae	1 (4.3 oz)	270	15	8
Cone Strawberry Shortcake	1 (4.3 oz)	230	10	5
Giant Sandwich Neapolitan	1 (6 oz)	250	10	5
Giant Sandwich Vanilla	1 (6 oz)	250	10	5
King Cone	1 (4.6 fl oz)	250	13	6
King Cone Giant	1 (8 oz)	190	21	11
Number 1 Bar	1 (4 oz)	200	11	8
Sandwich Chocolate Chip Cookie	1 (4.5 oz)	290	13	6
Sandwich Vanilla	1 (3.5 oz)	160	6	3
Sundae Twist Cup	1 (6 oz)	160	3	2
Häagen-Dazs				
Bars Chocolate & Almonds	1 (3.7 oz)	380	27	14
Bars Chocolate & Dark Chocolate	1 (3.6 oz)	350	24	15
Bars Chocolate Peanut Butter Swirl	1 (3 oz)	320	23	11
Bars Coffee & Almond Crunch	1 (3.7 oz)	370	27	15
Bars Cookies & Cream Crunch	1 (3.6 oz)	370	26	15
Bars Dulce De Leche Caramel	1 (3.7 oz)	370	24	15
Bars Tropical Coconut	1 (3.5 oz)	340	24	15
Bars Vanilla & Almonds	1 (3.7 oz)	380	28	14
Bars Vanilla & Dark Chocolate	1 (3.6 oz)	350	24	15
Bars Vanilla & Milk Chocolate	1 (3.5 oz)	340	24	14
Butter Pecan	½ cup	310	23	11
Cappuccino Commotion	½ cup	310	21	12
Cherry Vanilla	½ cup	240	15	9
Chocolate	½ cup	270	18	11
Chocolate Brownie w/ Walnuts	½ cup	290	19	9

FOOD	PORTION	CALS	FAT	SAT FAT
Chocolate Chocolate Fudge	½ cup	290	18	12
Chocolate Chocolate Chip	½ cup	300	20	12
Chocolate Swiss Almond	½ cup	300	20	11
Cinnamon	½ cup	250	17	10
Coffee	½ cup	270	18	11
Coffee Mocha Chip	½ cup	290	19	12
Cookie Dough Chip	½ cup	310	20	12
Cookies & Cream	½ cup	270	17	10
Creme Caramel Pecan	½ cup	320	20	10
Dulce De Leche Caramel	½ cup	290	17	10
Low Fat Chocolate	½ cup	170	3	2
Low Fat Coffee Fudge	½ cup	170	3	2
Low Fat Strawberry	½ cup	150	2	1
Low Fat Vanilla	½ cup	170	3	2
Macadamia Brittle	½ cup	300	20	12
Mango	½ cup	250	14	6
Mint Chip	½ cup	300	19	12
Pineapple Coconut	½ cup	230	12	8
Pistachio	½ cup	290	20	11
Rum Raisin	½ cup	270	17	10
Strawberry	½ cup	250	16	10
Vanilla	½ cup	270	18	11
Vanilla Chocolate Chip	½ cup	310	20	12
Vanilla Fudge	½ cup	290	18	12
Vanilla Swiss Almond	½ cup	300	20	11
Healthy Choice				
Butter Pecan Crunch	½ cup	120	2	1
Cappuccino Chocolate Chunk	½ cup	120	2	1
Cappuccino Mocha Crunch	½ cup	120	2	1
Cherry Chocolate Chunk	½ cup	110	2	1
Chocolate Chocolate Chunk	½ cup	120	2	1
Coconut Cream Pie	½ cup	120	2	1
Cookies 'N Cream	½ cup	120	2	1
Cookies Creme De Mint	½ cup	130	2	1
Fudge Brownie	½ cup	120	2	1
Mint Chocolate Chip	½ cup	120	2	1
Old Fashioned Blueberry Hill	½ cup	120	2	1
Old Fashioned Butterscotch Blonde	½ cup	140	2	1
Old Fashioned Cherry Vanilla	½ cup	120	2	1
Old Fashioned Strawberry	½ cup	110	2	1

FOOD	PORTION	CALS	FAT	SAT FAT
Peanut Butter Cup	½ cup	110	2	1
Praline & Caramel	½ cup	130	2	1
Praline Caramel Cluster	½ cup	130	2	1
Rocky Road	½ cup	140	2	1
Turtle Fudge Cake	½ cup	130	2	1
Vanilla	½ cup	100	2	1
Vanilla Bean	½ cup	110	2	1
Wild Raspberry Truffle	½ cup	120	2	1
Heaven				
Sundae Bars Chocolate Fudge	1 bar	150	9	—
Sundae Bars Vanilla Fudge	1 bar	150	9	—
Vanilla Caramel Nut	1 bar	225	15	—
Vanilla Nut Fudge	1 bar	222	15	—
Klondike				
Bar Almond	1	300	21	14
Bar Cappuccino	1	280	19	14
Bar Caramel & Peanut	1	290	19	12
Bar Caramel Crunch	1	270	17	13
Bar Chocolate	1	280	19	14
Bar Dark Chocolate	1	280	19	13
Bar Heath	1	300	20	14
Bar Krunch	1	260	17	12
Bar Oreo	1	160	10	3
Bar Original	1	280	19	14
Bar Peppermint Patty	1	280	19	13
Bar Reese's	1	220	15	9
Big Bear Sandwich Neapolitan	1	300	12	6
Big Bear Sandwich Vanilla	1	300	12	6
Big Bear Cone Vanilla	1	330	20	8
Big Bear Cone Vanilla Caramel	1	360	21	9
Big Bear Cone Vanilla Fudge	1	380	20	9
CarbSmart Fudge Bar	1	60	7	5
CarbSmart Ice Cream Bar	1	130	15	11
Choco Taco	1	290	16	8
Cone Oreo	1	250	12	6
Cone Reese's	1	290	15	7
Cookie Sandwich Chips	1	470	20	9
Cookie Sandwich Oreo	1	230	9	4
Minis	2 pieces	170	11	8

FOOD	PORTION	CALS	FAT	SAT FAT
Sandwich Double Decker	1	370	14	7
Slim-A-Bear 98% Fat Free Sandwich Vanilla	1	130	2	0
Slim-A-Bear No Sugar Added Cone Vanilla	1	270	15	5
Slim-A-Bear No Sugar Added Fudge Bar	1	90	2	1
Slim-A-Bear No Sugar Added Reduced Fat Bar Vanilla	1	160	9	7
Slim-A-Bear No Sugar Added Sandwich Vanilla	1	120	3	1
Sundae Cup	1	280	17	10
Nestle Crunch				
Chocolate	1 bar (3 oz)	200	14	11
Crunch King	1 (4 oz)	270	19	14
Nuggets	8 pieces	310	21	10
Reduced Fat	1 (2.5 oz)	130	7	5
Vanilla	1 bar (3 oz)	200	14	11
NutraShake				
High Calorie High Protein All Flavors	1 serv (4 oz)	200	10	—
Perry's				
No Fat No Sugar Added Caramel	½ cup (2.8 oz)	90	0	0
No Fat No Sugar Added Chocolate	½ cup (2.6 oz)	80	0	0
No Fat No Sugar Added Peach	½ cup (2.9 oz)	90	0	0
No Fat No Sugar Added Strawberry	½ cup (2.8 oz)	90	0	0
No Fat No Sugar Added Vanilla	½ cup (2.6 oz)	80	0	0
Popsicle				
Bar Col Crunch Chocolate Eclair	1 (3 oz)	160	8	3
Bar Col Crunch Strawberry Shortcake	1 (3 oz)	170	9	3
Bar Snoopy	1 (3.5 oz)	150	8	6
Bar Sprinklers	1 (2.1 oz)	130	6	3
Cone Crispy	1 (2.5 oz)	150	7	4
Creamsicle Pop	1 (1.75 oz)	70	2	1
Cup Cookies & Cream	1 (10 oz)	310	13	8
Fruit Juicee Cups	1 (4 oz)	80	0	0
Ice Cream Bar Vanilla	1 (3 oz)	160	11	9
Ice Cream Pops Minis	2 (2.8 oz)	190	13	9
Sandwich Cookie Rugrats	1 (2.5 oz)	140	6	4
Sandwiches Minis	1 (2 oz)	100	4	2

FOOD	PORTION	CALS	FAT	SAT FAT
Scribblers Ice Cream Pops	2 (2.4 oz)	130	5	4
Swirl Bar Bubble Gum	1 (2.6 oz)	60	0	0
WWE Bar	1 (3.6 oz)	180	8	5
X-Men Wolverine Bar	1 (4 oz)	100	0	0
Rice Dream				
Cappuccino	½ cup (3.2 oz)	150	6	1
Carob	½ cup (3.2 oz)	150	6	1
Carob Almond	½ cup (3.2 oz)	170	8	1
Cherry Vanilla	½ cup (3.2 oz)	150	6	1
Cocoa Marble Fudge	½ cup (3.2 oz)	150	6	1
Cookies N' Dream	½ cup (3.2 oz)	170	7	1
Mint Chocolate Chip	½ cup (3.2 oz)	170	8	2
Neapolitan	½ cup (3.2 oz)	150	6	1
Orange Vanilla Swirl	½ cup (3.2 oz)	250	6	1
Strawberry	½ cup (3.2 oz)	140	5	0
Vanilla Swiss Almond	½ cup (3.2 oz)	180	8	2
Rice Dream Supreme				
Cappuccino Almond Fudge	½ cup (3.2 oz)	170	8	1
Cherry Chocolate Chunk	½ cup (3.2 oz)	170	7	2
Chocolate Almond Chunk	½ cup (3.2 oz)	170	8	2
Chocolate Fudge Brownie	½ cup (3.2 oz)	170	7	1
Double Espresso Bean	½ cup (3.2 oz)	160	7	1
Mint Chocolate Cookie	½ cup (3.2 oz)	170	8	1
Peanut Butter Cup	½ cup (3.2 oz)	180	8	2
Pralines N' Dream	½ cup (3.2 oz)	180	9	1
Silhouette				
The Skinny Cow Low Fat Ice Cream Sandwich Vanilla	1	130	2	1
Slim-Fast				
Chocolate Fudge Bar	1 bar	110	2	1
Ice Cream Sandwich Chocolate	1	130	2	1
Ice Cream Sandwich Vanilla	1	130	1	1
Starbucks				
Caramel Cappuccino Swirl	½ cup	240	12	7
Classic Coffee	½ cup	230	12	7
Coffee Almond Fudge	½ cup	250	13	7
Frappuccino Bar Java Fudge	1 bar	130	2	1
Frappuccino Bar Mocha	1 bar	120	2	1
Java Chip	½ cup	250	13	8
Low Fat Latte	½ cup	170	3	2

FOOD	PORTION	CALS	FAT	SAT FAT
Mud Pie	½ cup	240	11	6
White Chocolate Latte	½ cup	280	15	6
Tofutti				
Cuties Chocolate	1 (1.4 oz)	130	5	1
Cuties Vanilla	1 (1.4 oz)	121	5	1
Monkey Bars Peanut Butter	1 bar (2.5 oz)	220	13	8
Turkey Hill				
Black Cherry	½ cup	140	7	5
Black Raspberry	½ cup	140	7	—
Butter Pecan	½ cup	170	11	5
Chocolate Marshmallow	½ cup	160	7	—
Chocolate Mint Chip	½ cup	180	11	—
Chocolate Peanut Butter Cup	½ cup	180	11	—
Colombian Coffee	½ cup	140	8	—
Cookies 'N Cream	½ cup	160	9	5
Death By Chocolate	½ cup	160	8	—
Dutch Chocolate	½ cup	150	8	—
Egg Nog	½ cup	150	8	—
Fat Free No Sugar Added Caramel Fudge Decadence	½ cup	100	0	0
Fat Free No Sugar Added Cherry Vanilla Fudge	½ cup	90	0	0
Fat Free No Sugar Added Dutch Chocolate	½ cup	90	0	0
Fat Free No Sugar Added Vanilla Bean	½ cup	90	0	0
Fudge Ripple	½ cup	140	7	—
Light Butter Pecan	½ cup	130	6	3
Light Choco Mint Chip	½ cup	140	5	4
Light Tin Lissie Sundae	½ cup	140	5	—
Light Vanilla & Chocolate	½ cup	110	3	2
Light Vanilla Bean	½ cup	110	3	2
Neapolitan	½ cup	150	8	5
Orange Swirl	½ cup	140	6	—
Original Vanilla	½ cup	140	8	—
Peanut Butter Ripple	½ cup	170	11	—
Philadelphia Style Butter Almond	½ cup	180	12	—
Philadelphia Style Chocolate	½ cup	170	10	—
Philadelphia Style Mint Chocolate Chip	½ cup	180	11	—

FOOD	PORTION	CALS	FAT	SAT FAT
Philadelphia Style Sweet Cherry Vanilla	½ cup	160	8	–
Philadelphia Style Vanilla Bean	½ cup	170	10	–
Rocky Road	½ cup	170	8	4
Rum Raisin	½ cup	150	7	–
Sandwich Choco Mint Chip	1	200	8	–
Sandwiches Vanilla	1	190	8	–
Strawberries 'N Cream	½ cup	140	6	–
Sundae Cones Rocky Road	1	340	19	–
Sundae Cones Tin Roof Sundae	1	290	17	–
Tin Roof Sundae	½ cup	160	9	5
Vanilla & Chocolate	½ cup	150	8	5
Vanilla Bean	½ cup	140	8	5
Weight Watchers				
Chocolate Chip Cookie Dough Sundae	1 (2.64 oz)	190	5	2
Chocolate Mousse	1 bar	40	1	1
Chocolate Treat	1 bar	100	1	0
English Toffee Crunch	1 bar	110	6	3
Orange Vanilla Treat	1 bar	40	1	0
Vanilla Sandwich	1 bar	150	3	1
TAKE-OUT				
cone vanilla light soft serve	1 (4.6 oz)	164	6	4
gelato chocolate hazelnut	½ cup (5.3 oz)	370	29	4
gelato vanilla	½ cup (3 oz)	211	15	8
sundae caramel	1 (5.4 oz)	303	9	5
sundae hot fudge	1 (5.4 oz)	284	9	5
sundae strawberry	1 (5.4 oz)	269	8	4

ICE CREAM CONES AND CUPS

FOOD	PORTION	CALS	FAT	SAT FAT
sugar cone	1	40	tr	tr
wafer cone	1	17	tr	tr
Comet				
Sugar Cones	1 (12 g)	50	0	–
Waffle Cone	1 (17 g)	70	1	0
Dutch Mill				
Chocolate Covered Wafer Cups	1 (0.5 oz)	80	5	2
Frookie				
Chocolate Crunch	1 (0.4 oz)	50	1	0
Honey Crunch	1 (0.4 oz)	45	1	0

FOOD	PORTION	CALS	FAT	SAT FAT
Pineapple	2 tbsp (1.4 oz)	110	0	0
Strawberry	2 tbsp (1.4 oz)	110	0	0
Planters				
Nut	2 tbsp (0.5 oz)	100	9	1
Smucker's				
Plate Scrapers Caramel	2 tbsp	100	0	0
Steel's				
Sugar Free Butterscotch	2 tbsp	60	0	0
Sugar Free Chocolate Fudge	2 tbsp	45	3	2
Sugar Free Hot Fudge	2 tbsp	65	3	0
Sugar Free Peanut Butter Fudge	2 tbsp	75	6	2

ICED TEA
MIX

FOOD	PORTION	CALS	FAT	SAT FAT
instant artifically sweetened lemon flavored as prep w/ water	8 oz	5	0	0
instant sweetened lemon flavor as prep w/ water	9 oz	87	tr	tr
instant unsweetened lemon flavor as prep w/ water	8 oz	4	0	0
Atkins				
Sugar Free Lemon not prep	2 tbsp	0	0	0
Carb Options				
Lemon as prep	1 serv	0	0	0
Crystal Light				
Decaffeinated as prep	1 serv (8 oz)	5	0	0
Iced Tea as prep	1 serv (8 oz)	5	0	0
Peach Tea as prep	1 serv (8 oz)	5	0	0
Raspberry Tea as prep	1 serv (8 oz)	5	0	0
Lipton				
100% Tea Decaffeinated as prep	1 serv	0	0	0
100% Tea Unsweetened as prep	1 serv	0	0	0
100% Tea as prep	1 serv	0	0	0
Calorie Free as prep	1 serv	0	0	0
Decaffeinated Ice Tea Brew as prep	1 serv (8 oz)	0	0	0
Decaffeinated Lemon as prep	1 serv	90	0	0
Diet Decaffeinated Lemon as prep	1 serv	5	0	0
Diet Lemon as prep	1 serv	5	0	0
Diet Peach as prep	1 serv	5	0	0
Diet Raspberry as prep	1 serv	5	0	0

FOOD	PORTION	CALS	FAT	SAT FAT
Diet Tea & Lemonade as prep	1 serv	10	0	0
Herbal Iced Collection	1 tea bag	0	0	0
Ice Tea Brew as prep	1 serv (8 oz)	0	0	0
Lemon as prep	1 serv	90	0	0
Lemon as prep	1 pkg (0.5 oz)	50	0	0
Natural Brew 100% Tea Decaffeinated as prep	1 serv	0	0	0
Natural Brew 100% Tea as prep	1 serv	0	0	0
Natural Brew Diet Lemon as prep	1 serv	5	0	0
Natural Brew Diet Peach as prep	1 serv	5	0	0
Natural Brew Diet Tropical as prep	1 serv	5	0	0
Natural Brew Tropical as prep	1 serv	90	0	0
Natural Brew Unsweetened Lemon as prep	1 serv	0	0	0
Peach as prep	1 serv	90	0	0
Raspberry as prep	1 serv	90	0	0
Tea & Lemonade as prep	1 serv	90	0	0
Nestea				
100% Tea	2 tsp (1 g)	0	0	0
100% Tea Decafe	2 tsp (1 g)	0	0	0
Ice Teasers Lemon	1 serv (0.5 oz)	5	0	0
Ice Teasers Orange	1 serv (0.5 oz)	5	0	0
Ice Teasers Wild Cherry	1 serv (0.5 oz)	5	0	0
Lemon	2 tsp (1 g)	5	0	0
Lemon & Sugar	2 tbsp (0.7 oz)	80	0	0
Lemonade Tea	2 tbsp (0.7 oz)	80	0	0
Sugar Free	2 tbsp (0.7 oz)	5	0	0
Sugar Free Decafe	1 tbsp (0.7 oz)	5	0	0
Sun Tea	1 tsp (1 g)	0	0	0
READY-TO-DRINK				
Apple & Eve				
Lemon Fruit	8 fl oz	100	0	0
Peach Fruit	8 fl oz	100	0	0
Raspberry Fruit	8 fl oz	100	0	0
Tangerine Fruit	8 fl oz	100	0	0
Arizona				
Lemon	1 bottle (16 oz)	180	0	0
Crystal Light				
Lemon	1 serv (8 oz)	5	0	0
Peach Tea	1 serv (8 oz)	5	0	0

FOOD	PORTION	CALS	FAT	SAT FAT
Raspberry Tea	1 serv (8 oz)	5	0	0
Fuze				
LemonAID	8 oz	70	0	0
Vitamin Tea Diet Peach	8 oz	5	0	0
Vitamin Tea Green Tea w/ Ginseng	8 oz	60	0	0
Vitamin Tea Lemon	8 oz	70	0	0
White Tea	8 oz	60	0	0
Hansen's				
Chai	8 oz	150	0	0
China Black	8 oz	90	0	0
Green	8 oz	70	0	0
Green Diet Lemon	8 oz	0	0	0
Green Diet Peach	8 oz	0	0	0
Green Lemon	8 oz	70	0	0
Green Peach	8 oz	70	0	0
Oolong	8 oz	70	0	0
Spice	8 oz	90	0	0
Honest Tea				
Assam	8 oz	170	0	0
Black Forest Berry	8 oz	17	0	0
Gold Rush Herbal Cinnamon	8 fl oz	9	0	0
Green Dragon	8 oz	30	0	0
Kashmiri Chai	8 oz	17	0	0
Lori's Lemon	8 oz	30	0	0
Moroccan Mint	8 oz	17	0	0
Peach Oo-La-Long	8 oz	30	0	0
Inko's				
White Tea	1 bottle (16 oz)	56	0	0
White Tea Hint O'Mint	1 bottle	0	0	0
Lipton				
Caribbean Cooler	1 can (12 oz)	130	0	0
Diet Lemon	8 oz	0	0	0
Diet Lemon	1 bottle (16 oz)	10	0	0
Green Tea & Passion Fruit	1 bottle (16 oz)	160	0	0
Lemon	8 oz	80	0	0
Lemon	1 can (12 oz)	120	0	0
Lemon	1 bottle (16 oz)	180	0	0
Natural Lemon	1 box (8 oz)	100	0	0
Peach	8 oz	80	0	0
Peach	1 bottle (16 oz)	220	0	0

FOOD	PORTION	CALS	FAT	SAT FAT
Raspberry	8 oz	80	0	0
Raspberry	1 bottle (16 oz)	220	0	0
Raspberry Blast	1 can (12 oz)	130	0	0
Southern Style Extra Sweet No Lemon	1 bottle (16 oz)	240	0	0
Southern Style Lemon	1 bottle (16 oz)	200	0	0
Southern Style Sweetened No Lemon	1 bottle (16 oz)	200	0	0
Sweet	8 oz	80	0	0
Sweetened No Lemon	1 bottle (16 oz)	140	0	0
Sweetened Lemon	8 oz	80	0	0
Tangerine Twist	1 can (12 oz)	120	0	0
Tea & Lemonade	1 bottle (16 oz)	220	0	0
Unsweetened No Lemon	1 bottle (16 oz)	0	0	0
Mad River				
Red Tea w/ Guarana	8 oz	90	0	0
Nantucket Nectars				
Diet	8 oz	5	0	0
Diet Green Tea	8 oz	5	0	0
Half & Half	8 oz	90	0	0
Iced Tea	8 oz	80	0	0
Matt Fee	8 oz	80	0	0
Raspberry	8 oz	90	0	0
Savannah	8 oz	80	0	0
Oregon Chai				
Original Latte	1 bottle (9.5 oz)	150	4	3
Republic Of Tea				
No Carb Unsweetened All Flavors	1 bottle (12 oz)	0	0	0
Snapple				
Diet Lemon	8 fl oz	0	0	0
Diet Peach	8 fl oz	0	0	0
Diet Raspberry	8 fl oz	0	0	0
Ginseng Tea	8 fl oz	80	0	0
Green Tea w/ Lemon	8 fl oz	100	0	0
Lemon	8 fl oz	100	0	0
Lemonade Ice Tea	8 fl oz	110	0	0
Peach	8 fl oz	100	0	0
Raspberry	8 fl oz	100	0	0
SoBe				
Lemon	8 oz	90	0	0
Turkey Hill				
Blueberry Oolong w/ Vitamins C & E	1 cup	100	0	0

FOOD	PORTION	CALS	FAT	SAT FAT
Decaffeinated	1 cup	80	0	0
Decaffeinated Orange	1 cup	10	0	0
Diet	1 cup	0	0	0
Diet Decaffeinated	1 cup	0	0	0
Diet Green Tea w/ Ginseng & Honey	1 cup	5	0	0
Green Tea w/ Ginseng & Honey	1 cup	70	0	0
Lemon	1 cup	100	0	0
Mint Tea w/ Chamomile	1 cup	90	0	0
Oolong w/ Ginkgo Biloba & Ginseng	1 cup	100	0	0
Orange	1 cup	100	0	0
Peach	1 cup	110	0	0
Raspberry Tea	1 cup	110	0	0
Regular	1 cup	90	0	0
ICES AND ICE POPS				
fruit & juice bar	1 (3 fl oz)	75	tr	–
gelatin pop	1 (1.5 oz)	31	0	0
ice coconut pineapple	½ cup (4 fl oz)	109	3	–
ice fruit w/ Equal	1 bar (1.7 oz)	12	0	0
ice lime	½ cup (4 fl oz)	75	0	0
ice pop	1 (2 fl oz)	42	0	0
Breyers				
Fruit Bars No Sugar Added	1 (1.75 oz)	25	0	0
Juice Bar Strawberry	1 (3.75 oz)	120	0	0
Soft Frozen Cup Lemonade	1 pkg (12 oz)	290	0	0
Soft Frozen Cup Strawberry	1 pkg (12 oz)	260	0	0
Carnation				
Cup Orange Sherbet	1 (5 oz)	150	2	1
Cup Orange Sherbet	1 (3 oz)	90	1	0
Cold Fusion				
Protein Juice Bar All Flavors	1 bar (3.8 oz)	130	0	0
Cool Creations				
Ice Pop	1 pop (2 oz)	50	0	0
Mickey Mouse Bar	1 (4 oz)	170	11	4
Surprise Pops	1 (2 oz)	60	0	0
CoolFruits				
Fruit Juice Freezer Pops Grape & Cherry	3 pops (3 oz)	70	0	0
Dole				
Fruit'n Juice Coconut	1 bar (4 oz)	210	7	5

FOOD	PORTION	CALS	FAT	SAT FAT
Fruit'n Juice Lemonade	1 bar (4 oz)	120	0	0
Fruit'n Juice Lime	1 bar (4 oz)	110	0	0
Fruit'n Juice Peach Passion	1 bar (2.5 oz)	70	0	0
Fruit'n Juice Pineapple Coconut	1 bar (4 oz)	150	4	4
Fruit'n Juice Pineapple Orange Banana	1 bar (2.5 oz)	70	0	0
Fruit'n Juice Pineapple Orange Banana	1 bar (4 oz)	110	0	0
Fruit'n Juice Raspberry	1 bar (2.5 oz)	70	0	0
Fruit'n Juice Strawberry	1 bar (2.5 oz)	70	0	0
Fruit'n Juice Strawberry	1 bar (4 oz)	110	0	0
Grape No Sugar Added	1 bar (1.75 oz)	25	0	0
Raspberry	1 bar (1.75 oz)	45	0	0
Raspberry No Sugar Added	1 bar (1.75 oz)	25	0	0
Strawberry	1 bar (1.75 oz)	45	0	0
Strawberry No Sugar Added	1 bar (1.75 oz)	25	0	0
Edy's				
Fruit Bars Strawberry	1 (3 oz)	80	0	0
Sherbet Berry Rainbow	½ cup	130	1	1
Sherbet Lime	½ cup	130	2	1
Sherbet Orange Cream	½ cup	120	2	1
Sherbet Raspberry	½ cup	130	1	1
Sherbet Starburst Orange & Cherry	½ cup	150	2	1
Sherbet Starburst Strawberry	½ cup	160	3	2
Sherbet Swiss Orange	½ cup	150	3	3
Sherbet Tropical Rainbow	½ cup	130	1	1
Sorbet Coconut	½ cup	140	3	3
Sorbet Lemon	½ cup	140	0	0
Sorbet Mandarin Orange	½ cup	130	0	0
Sorbet Peach	½ cup	130	0	0
Sorbet Raspberry	½ cup	130	0	0
Sorbet Strawberry	½ cup	120	0	0
Whole Fruit Bars Creamy Coconut	1 bar	120	3	3
Whole Fruit Bars Lemonade	1 bar	80	0	0
Whole Fruit Bars Lime	1 bar	80	0	0
Whole Fruit Bars Tangerine	1 bar	80	0	0
Whole Fruit Bars Wild Berry	1 bar	80	0	0
Flintstones				
Push-Up Sherbet Treats	1 (2.75 oz)	100	2	1

FOOD	PORTION	CALS	FAT	SAT FAT
Frozfruit				
Banana Cream	1 bar (4 oz)	150	7	5
Cantaloupe	1 bar (4 oz)	60	0	0
Cappuccino Cream	1 bar (3 oz)	140	6	4
Cherry	1 bar (4 oz)	70	0	0
Coconut Cream	1 bar (4 oz)	170	11	8
Kiwi Strawberry	1 bar (4 oz)	90	0	0
Lemon	1 bar (4 oz)	90	0	0
Lemon Iced Tea	1 bar (4 oz)	80	0	0
Lime	1 bar (4 oz)	90	0	0
Orange	1 bar (4 oz)	90	0	0
Pina Colada Cream	1 bar (4 oz)	170	8	6
Pineapple	1 bar (4 oz)	80	0	0
Raspberry	1 bar (4 oz)	80	0	0
Strawberry	1 bar (4 oz)	80	0	0
Strawberry Banana Cream	1 bar (4 oz)	140	6	3
Strawberry Cream	1 bar (4 oz)	130	5	3
Tropical	1 bar (4 oz)	90	0	0
Watermelon	1 bar (4 oz)	50	0	0
Good Humor				
Great White	1 (3 oz)	70	0	0
Hyper Stripe	1 (2.7 oz)	80	0	0
Häagen-Dazs				
Sorbet Chocolate	½ cup	120	0	0
Sorbet Mango	½ cup	120	0	0
Sorbet Orange	½ cup	120	0	0
Sorbet Orchard Peach	½ cup	130	0	0
Sorbet Raspberry	½ cup	120	0	0
Sorbet Strawberry	½ cup	120	0	0
Sorbet Zesty Lemon	½ cup	120	0	0
Sorbet Bar Chocolate	1 (2.7 oz)	80	0	0
Sorbet Bars Raspberry & Vanilla Yogurt	1 (2.5 oz)	90	0	0
Sorbet Bars Strawberry & Vanilla Ice Cream	1 (2.5 oz)	110	5	4
Lifesavers				
Ice Pops	1 (1.75 oz)	35	0	0
Mr. Freeze				
Assorted	2 bars (3 oz)	45	0	0
Tropical	2 bars (3 oz)	45	0	0

FOOD	PORTION	CALS	FAT	SAT FAT
Natural Choice				
Organic Banana	½ cup (3.6 oz)	110	0	0
Organic Blueberry	½ cup (3.6 oz)	100	0	0
Organic Kiwi	½ cup (3.6 oz)	110	0	0
Organic Lemon	½ cup (3.6 oz)	110	0	0
Organic Mango	½ cup (3.6 oz)	110	0	0
Organic Strawberry	½ cup (3.6 oz)	110	0	0
Organic Strawberry Kiwi	½ cup (3.6 oz)	110	0	0
Popsicle				
All Natural Ice Pops	1 (1.75 oz)	50	0	0
Bar Bart Simpson	1 (4 oz)	110	1	—
Bar Dora The Explorer	1 (4 oz)	100	0	0
Bar Fruti Holanda Lemon Lime	1 (3 oz)	90	0	0
Bar Fruti Holanda Strawberry	1 (3 oz)	90	0	0
Bar Incredible Hulk	1 (4 oz)	100	0	0
Bar Jimmy Neutron	1 (4 oz)	100	0	0
Bar Mega Warheads	1 (4 oz)	110	1	0
Bar Power Ranger	1 (4 oz)	100	0	0
Bar Spider Man	1 (4 oz)	100	0	0
Bar SpongeBob	1 (4 oz)	100	0	0
Big Stick Pops Big Reds	1 (3.5 oz)	70	0	0
Big Stick Pops Cherry Pineapple	1 (3.5 oz)	50	0	0
Bubble Play	1 (4 oz)	100	0	0
Creamsicle Bar	1 (2.5 oz)	100	3	2
Creamsicle Sugar Free	2 (3.3 oz)	40	2	2
Creamsicle Pop No Sugar Added	1 (1.75 oz)	25	0	0
Cup Cherry	1 (12 oz)	240	0	0
Cup Frostee Fudge	1 (10 oz)	280	11	7
Cup Lemon	1 (12 oz)	230	0	0
Cup Screwball	1 (3.75 oz)	110	0	0
Firecracker	1 (1.6 oz)	35	0	0
Fruita Holanda Coconut Bar	1 (3 oz)	120	3	2
Fudgsicle Bar	1 (2.5 oz)	90	2	1
Fudgsicle Bar Fat Free	1 (1.75 oz)	60	0	0
Fudgsicle Pop	1 (1.75 oz)	60	1	1
Fudgsicle Pops No Sugar Added	2 (1.75 oz)	90	1	0
Minis Fudge Bar	2 (2.4 oz)	80	2	2
Pop Great White	1 (1.75 oz)	45	0	0
Pop Lick-A-Color	1 (2 oz)	50	0	0
Pop Sherbet Cyclone	1 (1.8 oz)	50	1	0

FOOD	PORTION	CALS	FAT	SAT FAT
Pop Towering Tornado	1 (3.5 oz)	90	0	0
Pop Ups Orange Burst	1 (2.75 oz)	80	1	0
Pop Ups Reckless Rainbow	1 (2.75 oz)	90	1	0
Pop Ups SpongeBob	1 (2.75 oz)	90	2	1
Pops Tropical Sugar Free	1 (1.75 oz)	15	0	0
Pops Wild Bunch	2 (2.2 oz)	60	0	0
Rainbow Floats	1 (1.75 oz)	60	2	1
Rainbow Pops	1 (1.75 oz)	45	0	0
Scribblers Juice Pops	2 (2.4 oz)	60	0	0
Shots	1 serv (1.7 oz)	40	1	–
Snow Cone	1 (7 oz)	30	0	0
Sugar Free Pops Orange Cherry Grape	1 (1.75 oz)	15	0	0
Super Mario Bros Bar	1 (4 oz)	100	0	0
Swirl Bar Cotton Candy	1 (2.6 oz)	60	0	0
Tingle Twister Ice Pops	1 (1.75 oz)	45	0	0
Torpedo Pop Cherry	1 (1.75 oz)	35	0	0
Silhouette				
Fat Free Fudge Bars	1	90	0	0
JACKFRUIT				
fresh	3.5 oz	70	tr	–
JALAPENO (see PEPPERS)				
JAM/JELLY/PRESERVES				
all flavors jam	1 tbsp (0.7 oz)	48	0	0
all flavors jam	1 pkg (0.5 oz)	34	0	0
all flavors jelly	1 pkg (0.5 oz)	38	0	0
all flavors jelly	1 tbsp (0.7 oz)	52	0	0
all flavors preserve	1 pkg (0.5 oz)	34	0	0
all flavors preserve	1 tbsp (0.7 oz)	48	0	0
apple butter	1 cup (9.9 oz)	519	1	–
apple butter	1 tbsp (0.6 oz)	33	0	0
apple jelly	1 pkg (0.5 oz)	38	0	0
apple jelly	1 tbsp (0.7 oz)	52	0	0
apricot jam	0.5 oz	36	0	0
blackberry jam	0.5 oz	34	0	0
cherry jam	0.5 oz	36	0	0
linganberry jam	0.5 oz	23	tr	tr
orange jam	0.5 oz	35	0	0

FOOD	PORTION	CALS	FAT	SAT FAT
orange marmalade	1 tbsp (0.7 oz)	49	0	0
orange marmalade	1 pkg (0.5 oz)	34	0	0
plum jam	0.5 oz	34	0	0
quince jam	0.5 oz	43	0	0
raspberry jam	0.5 oz	35	0	0
raspberry jelly	0.5 oz	37	0	0
red currant jam	0.5 oz	34	0	0
red currant jelly	0.5 oz	38	0	0
rose hip jam	0.5 oz	36	0	0
strawberry jam	1 pkg (0.5 oz)	34	0	0
strawberry jam	1 tbsp (0.7 oz)	48	0	0
strawberry preserve	1 pkg (0.5 oz)	34	0	0
strawberry preserve	1 tbsp (0.7 oz)	48	0	0
Colac				
Jelly All Flavors	1 tbsp	37	0	0
Eden				
Cherry Butter	1 tbsp	35	0	0
Organic Apple Butter	1 tbsp	20	0	0
Estee				
Fruit Spread Apple Spice	1 tbsp	16	0	0
Fruit Spread Apricot	1 tbsp	16	0	0
Fruit Spread Grape	1 tbsp	16	0	0
Fruit Spread Peach	1 tbsp	16	0	0
Fruit Spread Red Raspberry	1 tbsp	16	0	0
Fruit Spread Strawberry	1 tbsp	16	0	0
Jok'n'Al				
Low Carb Fruit Spreads All Flavors	1 tbsp	10	0	0
Polaner				
All Fruit Peach	1 tbsp	40	0	0
All Fruit Raspberry	1 tbsp	40	0	0
Sarabeth's				
Spreadable Fruit Orange Apricot	1 tbsp	30	0	0
Spreadable Fruit Peach Apricot	1 tbsp	40	0	0
Spreadable Fruit Strawberry Raspberry	1 tbsp	40	0	0
Smucker's				
Concord Grape Jelly	1 tbsp	50	0	0
Peach Preserves	1 tbsp	50	0	0
Simply Fruit Red Raspberry	1 tbsp	40	0	0

FOOD	PORTION	CALS	FAT	SAT FAT
Tabasco				
Spicy Pepper Jelly	1 tbsp (0.6 oz)	50	0	0
Welch's				
Grape Jam	1 tbsp	50	0	0
White House				
Apple Butter	1 tbsp (0.6 oz)	35	0	0
Wild Thyme Farms				
Fruit Spreads Blackberry Currant Ginger	1 tsp	8	0	0
Fruit Spreads Mango Apricot	1 tsp	7	0	0

JAPANESE FOOD (see ASIAN FOOD, SUSHI)

JAVA PLUM

fresh	1 cup	82	tr	—
fresh	3	5	tr	—

JELLY (see JAM/JELLY/PRESERVES)

JUTE

cooked	1 cup	32	tr	tr

KALE

chopped cooked	½ cup	21	tr	tr
frzn chopped cooked	½ cup	20	tr	tr
raw chopped	½ cup	21	tr	tr
scotch chopped cooked	½ cup	18	tr	tr

KEFIR

kefir	7 oz	132	8	—

KETCHUP

banana	1 tsp	10	0	0
ketchup	1 tbsp	16	tr	tr
ketchup	1 pkg (0.2 oz)	6	tr	tr
low sodium	1 tbsp	16	tr	tr
Atkins				
Ketch-A-Tomato	1 tbsp	10	0	0
Del Monte				
Ketchup	1 tbsp (0.5 oz)	15	0	0
Estee				
Ketchup	1 tbsp	15	0	0

FOOD	PORTION	CALS	FAT	SAT FAT
Healthy Choice				
Ketchup	1 tbsp (0.5 oz)	9	tr	0
Heinz				
Ketchup	1 tbsp (0.6 oz)	15	0	0
Hunt's				
Ketchup	1 tbsp (0.6 oz)	16	tr	0
No Salt Added	1 tbsp (0.6 oz)	16	tr	0
Keto				
Ketchup	1 tbsp	4	0	0
McIlhenny				
Spicy	1 tbsp (0.6 oz)	20	0	0
Muir Glen				
Organic	1 tbsp (0.6 oz)	15	0	0
Smucker's				
Tomato	1 tbsp	25	0	0
Steel's				
Sugar Free	1 tbsp	10	0	0
Stokelys				
Tomato	1 tbsp	15	0	0
Tree Of Life				
Ketchup	1 tbsp (0.5 oz)	10	0	0
Walden Farms				
Calorie Free	1 tbsp	0	0	0
KIDNEY				
beef simmered	3 oz	122	3	1
lamb braised	3 oz	117	3	1
pork cooked	3 oz	128	4	1
pork cooked	1 cup	211	7	2
veal braised	3 oz	139	5	1
KIDNEY BEANS				
canned	1 cup	207	1	tr
dried cooked	1 cup	225	1	tr
B&M				
Red Baked Beans	½ cup (4.6 oz)	170	2	1
Eden				
Organic Cannellini	½ cup (4.6 oz)	100	1	—
Friend's				
Red Baked Beans	½ cup (4.6 oz)	160	1	0

FOOD	PORTION	CALS	FAT	SAT FAT
Green Giant				
Dark Red	½ cup (4.5 oz)	110	0	0
Light Red	½ cup (4.5 oz)	110	0	0
Hunt's				
Kidney Beans	½ cup (4.5 oz)	94	1	0
Progresso				
Dark Red	½ cup (4.5 oz)	110	0	0
Red	½ cup (4.6 oz)	110	1	0
S&W				
Dark Red Premium	½ cup (4.6 oz)	100	1	0
Van Camp				
Dark Red	½ cup (4.6 oz)	90	0	0
Light Red	½ cup (4.6 oz)	90	0	0
KIWI JUICE				
After The Fall				
Kiwi Bear	1 cup (8 oz)	100	0	0
KIWIS				
fresh	1 med	46	tr	—
Chiquita				
Fresh	2 med (5.2 oz)	100	1	0
Sonoma				
Dried	7-8 pieces (1 oz)	90	1	0
KNISH				
TAKE-OUT				
cheese & blueberry	1 (7 oz)	378	13	—
cheese & cherry	1 (7 oz)	378	13	—
everything	1 (7 oz)	221	8	—
kashe	1 (7 oz)	270	8	—
potato	1 lg (7 oz)	332	12	3
potato	1 med (3.5 oz)	166	6	2
potato w/ broccoli & cheese	1 (7 oz)	312	15	—
potato w/ spinach & mushroom	1 (7 oz)	214	8	—
KOHLRABI				
raw sliced	½ cup	19	tr	tr
sliced cooked	½ cup	24	tr	tr
KRILL				
fresh	1 oz	22	1	—

FOOD	PORTION	CALS	FAT	SAT FAT
KUMQUATS				
fresh	1	12	tr	—
LAMB				
cubed lean only braised	3 oz	190	7	3
cubed lean only broiled	3 oz	158	6	2
ground broiled	3 oz	240	17	7
leg lean & fat Choice roasted	3 oz	219	14	6
loin chop w/ bone lean & fat Choice broiled	1 chop (2.3 oz)	201	15	6
loin chop w/ bone lean only Choice broiled	1 chop (1.6 oz)	100	5	2
new zealand lean & fat cooked	3 oz	259	19	9
new zealand lean only cooked	3 oz	175	8	3
rib chop lean & fat Choice broiled	3 oz	307	25	11
rib chop lean only Choice broiled	3 oz	200	11	4
shank lean & fat Choice braised	3 oz	206	11	5
shank lean & fat Choice roasted	3 oz	191	11	4
shoulder chop w/ bone lean & fat Choice braised	1 chop (2.5 oz)	244	17	7
shoulder chop w/ bone lean only Choice braised	1 chop (1.9 oz)	152	8	3
sirloin lean & fat Choice roasted	3 oz	248	21	7
LAMB DISHES				
TAKE-OUT				
couscous lamb	1 serv	275	80	3
curry	¾ cup	345	17	3
lamb fattoush salad	1 serv	606	31	—
lamb tagine casserole	1 serv	261	12	5
moroccan pilaf w/ bulgur	1 serv	327	13	2
moussaka	5.6 oz	312	21	—
sambousa lamb & vegetable pocket	1	645	54	9
stew	¾ cup	124	5	1
LAMBSQUARTERS				
chopped cooked	½ cup	29	1	tr
LEEKS				
chopped cooked	¼ cup	8	tr	tr
cooked	1 (4.4 oz)	38	tr	tr
freeze dried	1 tbsp	1	0	0

FOOD	PORTION	CALS	FAT	SAT FAT
raw	1 (4.4 oz)	76	tr	tr
raw chopped	¼ cup	16	tr	tr
LEMON				
fresh	1 med	22	tr	tr
peel	1 tbsp	0	tr	tr
wedge	1	5	tr	tr
LEMON CURD				
lemon curd made w/ egg	2 tsp	29	1	—
LEMON EXTRACT				
Virginia Dare				
Extract	1 tsp	22	0	—
LEMON GRASS				
fresh	1 cup (2.4 oz)	66	tr	tr
fresh	1 tbsp (5 g)	5	tr	tr
LEMON JUICE				
bottled	1 tbsp	3	tr	tr
fresh	1 tbsp	4	0	—
frzn	1 tbsp	3	tr	tr
After The Fall				
Spicy Lemon	1 can (12 oz)	150	0	0
Canarino				
Italian Hot Lemon Beverage	1 cup (8 oz)	0	0	0
Realemon				
Juice	1 tsp (5 ml)	0	0	0
LEMONADE				
FROZEN				
as prep w/ water	1 cup	100	tr	tr
not prep	1 can (6 oz)	397	tr	tr
MIX				
powder as prep w/ water	9 fl oz	113	tr	tr
powder w/ equal	1 pitcher (67 oz)	40	0	0
Country Time				
Lem'n Berry Sippers Cranberry Raspberry Lemonade as prep	1 serv (8 oz)	90	0	0
Lem'n Berry Sippers Raspberry Lemonade as prep	1 serv (8 oz)	90	0	0

FOOD	PORTION	CALS	FAT	SAT FAT
Lem'n Berry Sippers Strawberry Lemonade as prep	1 serv (8 oz)	90	0	0
Lem'n Berry Sippers Wildberry Lemonade as prep	1 serv (8 oz)	90	0	0
Lem'n Berry Sippers Sugar Free Strawberry Lemonade as prep	1 serv (8 oz)	5	0	0
Lemonade as prep	1 serv (8 oz)	70	0	0
Pink as prep	1 serv (8 oz)	70	0	0
Sugar Free Pink as prep	1 serv (8 oz)	5	0	0
Sugar Free as prep	1 serv (8 oz)	5	0	0
Crystal Light				
Lemonade as prep	1 serv (8 oz)	5	0	0
Pink as prep	1 serv (8 oz)	5	0	0
Keto				
Kooler Pink	½ tsp	0	0	0
Kool-Aid				
Lemonade as prep	1 serv (8 oz)	70	0	0
Mix as prep w/ sugar	1 serv (8 oz)	100	0	0
Pink as prep w/ sugar	1 serv (8 oz)	100	0	0
Soarin' Strawberry Lemonade as prep	1 serv (8 oz)	70	0	0
Soarin' Strawberry Lemonade as prep w/ sugar	1 serv (8 oz)	100	0	0
Sugar Free Soarin' Strawberry Lemonade as prep	1 serv (8 oz)	5	0	0
Sugar Free Mix as prep	1 serv (8 oz)	5	0	0
Sipper Sweets				
Sugar Free Low Carb	1 serv	8	0	0
READY-TO-DRINK				
After The Fall				
Apple Raspberry	1 bottle (10 oz)	120	0	0
Crystal Light				
Lemonade	1 serv (8 oz)	5	0	0
Pink	1 serv (8 oz)	5	0	0
Everfresh				
Lemonade	1 can (8 oz)	120	0	0
Ruby Red	1 can (8 oz)	110	0	0
Hansen's				
Sparkling	8 fl oz	100	0	0
Sparkling Pink	8 fl oz	120	0	0

FOOD	PORTION	CALS	FAT	SAT FAT
Langers				
Raspberry Lemonade	8 oz	120	0	0
White Cranberry Lemonade	8 oz	120	0	0
Minute Maid				
Chilled	8 fl oz	110	0	0
Nantucket Nectars				
Authentic	8 oz	120	0	0
Pink	8 oz	120	0	0
Newman's Own				
Lemonade	1 bottle (10 oz)	140	0	0
Roadside Virginia	8 fl oz	110	0	0
Odwalla				
Pure Squeezed	8 fl oz	96	0	0
Strawberry Quencher	8 fl oz	110	0	0
Santa Cruz				
Organic	8 oz	100	0	0
Shasta Plus				
Lemonade	1 can (11.5 oz)	160	0	0
Snapple				
Diet Pink	8 fl oz	20	0	0
Lemonade	8 fl oz	120	0	0
Pink	8 fl oz	120	0	0
Turkey Hill				
Lemonade	1 cup	120	0	0
Raspberry	1 cup	120	0	0
Strawberry Kiwi	1 cup	120	0	0
Veryfine				
Chillers	1 can (11.5 oz)	190	0	0
Chillers Cherry	8 fl oz	120	0	0
Chillers Peach	8 fl oz	120	0	0
Chillers Pink	1 can (11.5 oz)	180	0	0
Chillers Strawberry	1 can (11.5 oz)	170	0	0
LENTILS				
dried cooked	1 cup	231	1	tr
Natural Touch				
Lentil Rice Loaf	1 in slice (3.2 oz)	170	9	3
Shiloh Farms				
Organic Green not prep	¼ cup (1.6 oz)	150	0	0

FOOD	PORTION	CALS	FAT	SAT FAT
TastyBite				
Bengal Lentils	½ pkg (5 oz)	190	5	1
Jodhpur Lentils	½ pkg (5 oz)	190	9	4
Madras Lentils	½ pkg (5 oz)	130	7	3
TAKE-OUT				
indian sambar	1 serv	236	5	2
middle eastern lentil salad	1 serv (4.5 oz)	158	3	tr
yemiser selatta ethiopian lentil salad	1 serv (3 oz)	115	7	1

LETTUCE (see also SALAD)

FOOD	PORTION	CALS	FAT	SAT FAT
arugula	½ cup (0.4 oz)	3	tr	—
bibb	1 head (6 oz)	21	tr	tr
boston	1 head (6 oz)	21	tr	tr
boston	2 leaves	2	tr	tr
cornsalad field salad	1 cup (1.9 oz)	7	tr	—
iceberg	1 leaf	3	tr	tr
iceberg	1 head (19 oz)	70	1	tr
looseleaf shredded	½ cup	5	tr	tr
romaine shredded	½ cup	4	tr	tr
Dole				
Iceberg	1 cup (3 oz)	15	0	0
Romaine	1½ cups (3 oz)	15	0	0
Shredded	1½ cup (3 oz)	15	0	0
Earthbound Farm				
Romaine Salad Organic	1½ cups (2.9 oz)	15	0	0
Western Express				
Hearts Of Romaine	6 leaves (3 oz)	20	1	0

LILY ROOT

FOOD	PORTION	CALS	FAT	SAT FAT
dried	1 oz	89	1	—
fresh	1 oz	32	tr	—

LIMA BEANS
CANNED

FOOD	PORTION	CALS	FAT	SAT FAT
large	1 cup	191	tr	tr
lima beans	½ cup	88	tr	tr
Del Monte				
Green	½ cup (4.4 oz)	80	0	0
Dennison's				
With Ham	7.5 oz	250	7	—

FOOD	PORTION	CALS	FAT	SAT FAT
Eden				
Organic Baby	½ cup (4.6 oz)	100	1	0
S&W				
Small Green	½ cup (4.4 oz)	80	0	0
Veg-All				
Baby Green	½ cup	90	1	0
DRIED				
baby cooked	1 cup	229	1	tr
cooked	½ cup	104	tr	tr
large cooked	1 cup	217	1	tr
Hurst				
HamBeens Baby Limas w/ Ham	1 serv	120	1	0
HamBeens Large Limas w/ Ham	1 serv	120	1	0
FROZEN				
cooked	½ cup	94	tr	tr
fordhook cooked	½ cup	85	tr	tr
Birds Eye				
Baby	½ cup	130	0	0
Fordhook	½ cup	100	0	0
Fresh Like				
Baby	3.5 oz	138	1	–
Green Giant				
Butter Sauce	⅔ cup (3.6 oz)	120	3	2
Harvest Fresh Baby	½ cup (2.7 oz)	80	0	0
LIME				
fresh	1	20	tr	tr
LIME JUICE				
bottled	1 tbsp	3	tr	tr
fresh	1 tbsp	4	tr	tr
limeade	1 can (6 oz)	408	tr	tr
After The Fall				
Caribbean Lime	1 can (12 oz)	170	0	0
Key West	1 cup (8 oz)	100	0	0
Odwalla				
Summertime Lime	8 fl oz	90	0	0
Realime				
Juice	1 tsp (5 ml)	0	0	0

FOOD	PORTION	CALS	FAT	SAT FAT
LING				
blue raw	3.5 oz	83	1	–
fresh baked	3 oz	95	1	–
fresh fillet baked	5.3 oz	168	1	–
LINGCOD				
baked	3 oz	93	1	tr
fillet baked	5.3 oz	164	2	tr
LIQUOR/LIQUEUR (see also BEER AND ALE, CHAMPAGNE, WINE)				
7&7	1 serv	178	0	0
alabama slammer	1 serv	103	tr	0
amaretto sour	1 serv	295	tr	tr
angel's kiss	1 serv	85	1	1
anisette	1 oz	111	0	0
antifreeze	1 serv	177	tr	tr
apricot brandy	1 oz	96	0	0
apricot sour	1 serv	164	tr	0
aquavit	1 oz	65	0	0
b 52	1 serv	247	4	2
b&b	1 serv	75	0	0
bahama breeze	1 serv	70	tr	0
bahama mama	1 serv	153	tr	tr
bailey's & amaretto	1 serv	184	5	3
banana colada	1 serv	376	1	tr
bay breeze	1 serv	173	tr	tr
bend me over	1 serv	242	tr	tr
benedictine	1 oz	104	0	0
betsy ross	1 serv	206	0	0
black devil	1 serv	220	tr	tr
black russian	1 serv	184	tr	tr
bloody mary	1 serv	150	tr	tr
blue whale	1 serv	222	tr	0
bourbon & soda	1 serv (4 oz)	105	0	0
bourbon sour	1 serv	166	tr	0
brandy alexander	1 serv	266	6	4
brandy sour	1 serv	164	tr	0
bushwacker	1 serv	286	5	2
coffee liqueur	1 serv (1.5 oz)	175	tr	tr
coffee w/ cream liqueur	1 serv (1.5 oz)	154	7	5

FOOD	PORTION	CALS	FAT	SAT FAT
Keebler				
Chocolatey Cone	1 (0.4 oz)	50	1	0
Fudge Dipped Cup	1 (0.3 oz)	35	2	1
Ice Creme Cup	1 (0.2 oz)	15	0	0
Sugar Cone	1 (0.4 oz)	50	1	0
Waffle Bowl	1 (0.4 oz)	50	1	0
Waffle Cone	1 (0.4 oz)	50	1	0
ICE CREAM TOPPINGS				
butterscotch	2 tbsp (1.4 oz)	103	tr	tr
caramel	2 tbsp (1.4 oz)	103	tr	tr
marshmallow cream	1 jar (7 oz)	615	tr	—
marshmallow cream	1 oz	88	tr	—
pineapple	2 tbsp (1.5 oz)	106	0	—
strawberry	2 tbsp (1.5 oz)	107	tr	—
strawberry	1 cup (11.5 oz)	863	1	—
walnuts in syrup	2 tbsp (1.4 oz)	167	9	1
Colac				
Passion Fruit	1 tbsp	31	0	0
Strawberry	1 tbsp	31	0	0
Hershey				
Chocolate Shop Double Chocolate	1 tbsp (0.7 oz)	50	0	0
Chocolate Shoppe Apple Pie A La Mode	2 tbsp (1.3 oz)	100	0	0
Chocolate Shoppe Butterscotch Caramel	1 tbsp (0.7 oz)	70	1	1
Chocolate Shoppe Caramel	2 tbsp (1.3 oz)	100	0	0
Chocolate Shoppe Chocolate Mini	1 tbsp (0.7 oz)	50	0	0
Chocolate Shoppe Double Chocolate	1 tbsp (0.6 oz)	60	1	1
Chocolate Shoppe Hot Fudge	1 tbsp (0.7 oz)	70	3	1
Chocolate Shoppe Hot Fudge Fat Free	2 tbsp (1.4 oz)	100	0	0
Chocolate Shoppe Sprinkles Milk Chocolate	1 tbsp (0.5 oz)	70	3	2
Chocolate Shoppe Sprinkles Reeses	1 tbsp (0.5 oz)	70	4	2
Chocolate Shoppe Sprinkles York	1 tbsp (0.6 oz)	80	4	3
Kraft				
Butterscotch	2 tbsp (1.4 oz)	130	2	1
Caramel	2 tbsp (1.4 oz)	120	0	0
Chocolate	2 tbsp (1.4 oz)	110	0	0
Hot Fudge	2 tbsp (1.4 oz)	140	5	2

FOOD	PORTION	CALS	FAT	SAT FAT
cognac	1 oz	67	0	0
cosmopolitan martini	1 serv	126	tr	0
creme de menthe	1 serv (1.5 oz)	186	tr	tr
curacao liqueur	1 oz	81	0	0
daiquiri	1 serv	187	0	0
daiquiri banana	1 serv	277	tr	tr
dark & stormy	1 serv	64	0	0
doctor pepper	1 serv	95	0	0
frozen daiquiri	1 serv	393	2	—
frozen daiquiri pineapple	1 serv	186	tr	tr
frozen tequila screwdriver	1 serv	159	tr	tr
fuzzy navel	1 serv	247	tr	tr
gimlet vodka	1 serv	150	tr	0
gin	1 serv (1.5 oz)	110	0	0
gin & tonic	1 serv (7.5 oz)	171	0	0
gin ricky	1 serv	114	tr	0
grasshopper	1 serv	275	5	3
happy hawaiian	1 serv	434	8	5
harvey wallbanger	1 serv	198	tr	tr
head banger	1 serv	165	0	0
hot buttered rum	1 serv	219	4	3
hot toddy	1 serv	188	1	tr
hurricane	1 serv	205	tr	0
kamikaze	1 serv	136	0	0
long island iced tea	1 serv	292	tr	0
lynchburg lemonade	1 serv	465	tr	tr
mai tai	1 serv	165	tr	tr
manhattan	1 serv	171	tr	0
margarita	1 serv	173	0	0
margarita strawberry	1 serv	106	tr	tr
martini apple	1 serv	147	tr	tr
martini rum	1 serv	131	0	0
martini vodka	1 serv	135	tr	tr
mellow yellow	1 serv	95	0	0
mexican grasshopper	1 serv	638	19	12
mint julep	1 serv	136	tr	tr
mississippi mud	1 serv	496	12	7
mudslide	1 serv	566	10	6
narragansett	1 serv	168	0	0

FOOD	PORTION	CALS	FAT	SAT FAT
nutcracker	1 serv	730	10	6
old fashioned	1 serv	223	tr	0
orange crush	1 serv	461	tr	tr
pain killer	1 serv	277	tr	tr
peppermint pattie	1 serv	344	tr	tr
pina colada	1 serv (4.5 oz)	262	3	1
planter's cocktail	1 serv	105	0	0
planter's punch	1 serv	233	tr	tr
presbyterian	1 serv	170	0	0
purple passion	1 serv	215	tr	tr
rob roy	1 serv	171	0	0
rum	1 serv (1.5 oz)	97	0	0
rum boogie	1 serv	134	tr	0
rum cola	1 serv	209	tr	0
rum highball	1 serv	170	0	0
rum punch	1 serv	448	1	tr
rusty nail	1 serv	159	0	0
salty dog	1 serv	210	tr	tr
scotch & soda	1 serv	104	0	0
screwdriver rum	1 serv	166	tr	tr
sea breeze	1 serv	207	tr	tr
sex on the beach	1 serv	190	tr	tr
slippery nipple	1 serv	142	2	2
sloe gin fizz	1 serv (2.5 oz)	132	0	0
snake bite	1 serv	362	0	0
sour rum	1 serv	156	tr	0
swizzle rum	1 serv	187	0	0
tequila gimlet	1 serv	150	tr	0
tequila sour	1 serv	156	tr	0
tequila stinger	1 serv	221	tr	0
tequila sunrise	1 serv (6.8 oz)	232	tr	tr
tom collins	1 serv (7.5 oz)	121	0	0
vermouth cassis	1 serv	97	tr	0
vodka	1 serv (1.5 oz)	97	0	0
vodka sour	1 serv	138	tr	0
vodka stinger	1 serv	378	tr	tr
whiskey	1 serv (1.5 oz)	105	0	0
whiskey sour	1 serv	159	0	0
white russian	1 serv	290	8	5
zombie	1 serv	235	tr	tr

FOOD	PORTION	CALS	FAT	SAT FAT
LIVER (see also PATE)				
beef braised	3 oz	137	4	2
beef pan-fried	3 oz	184	7	2
chicken stewed	1 cup (5 oz)	219	8	3
duck raw	1 (1.5 oz)	60	2	1
goose raw	1 (3.3 oz)	125	4	1
lamb braised	3 oz	187	7	3
lamb fried	3 oz	202	11	4
pork braised	3 oz	140	4	1
sheep raw	3.5 oz	131	4	–
turkey simmered	1 cup (5 oz)	237	8	3
veal braised	3 oz	140	6	2
veal fried	3 oz	208	10	4
Shady Brook				
Turkey	4 oz	160	5	2
LOBSTER				
northern cooked	3 oz	83	1	tr
northern cooked	1 cup	142	1	tr
northern raw	3 oz	77	1	–
northern raw	1 lobster (5.3 oz)	136	1	–
spiny steamed	1 (5.7 oz)	233	3	tr
spiny steamed	3 oz	122	2	tr
Progresso				
Lobster Sauce	½ cup (4.3 oz)	100	7	1
TAKE-OUT				
newburg	1 cup	485	27	–
LOGANBERRIES				
frzn	1 cup	80	tr	–
LONGANS				
fresh	1	2	0	0
LOQUATS				
fresh	1	5	tr	tr
LOTUS				
root raw sliced	10 slices	45	tr	tr
root sliced cooked	10 slices	59	tr	tr
seeds dried	1 oz	94	1	tr

FOOD	PORTION	CALS	FAT	SAT FAT
Eden				
Root	1 serv (0.3 oz)	35	0	0
LOX (see SALMON)				
LUPINES				
dried cooked	1 cup	197	5	1
LYCHEES				
fresh	1	6	tr	—
MACADAMIA NUTS				
dry roasted w/ salt	10-12 nuts (1 oz)	200	22	4
oil roasted	1 oz	204	22	3
Hawaiian Host				
Chocolate Covered	1 piece (0.5 oz)	53	6	3
Keto				
Chocolately Covered	1 oz	171	19	5
MacFarms of Hawaii				
Chocolate Covered	¼ cup (1.3 oz)	210	16	6
Dry Roasted Salted	¼ cup (1.3 oz)	220	23	4
Kona Coffee Dark Chocolate Covered	¼ cup (1.3 oz)	210	16	6
Maranatha				
Macadamia Butter	2 tbsp	230	24	—
MACE				
ground	1 tsp	8	1	tr
MACKEREL				
CANNED				
jack	1 cup	296	12	4
jack	1 can (12.7 oz)	563	23	7
DRIED				
Eden				
Bonito Flakes	2 tbsp	4	0	0
FRESH				
atlantic cooked	3 oz	223	15	4
atlantic raw	3 oz	174	12	3
jack baked	3 oz	171	9	2
jack fillet baked	6.2 oz	354	18	5
king baked	3 oz	114	2	tr
king fillet baked	5.4 oz	207	4	1

FOOD	PORTION	CALS	FAT	SAT FAT
pacific baked	3 oz	171	9	2
pacific fillet baked	6.2 oz	354	18	5
spanish cooked	1 fillet (5.1 oz)	230	9	3
spanish cooked	3 oz	134	5	2
spanish raw	3 oz	118	5	2
SMOKED				
atlantic	3.5 oz	296	24	5
MALANGA				
fresh	½ cup	137	tr	–
MALT				
nonalcoholic	12 fl oz	32	0	0
MALTED MILK				
chocolate as prep w/ milk	1 cup	229	9	6
chocolate flavor powder	3 heaping tsp (¾ oz)	79	1	tr
natural flavor as prep w/ milk	1 cup	237	10	6
natural flavor powder	3 heaping tsp (¾ oz)	87	2	1
Carnation				
Chocolate	3 tbsp (0.7 oz)	90	1	1
Original	3 tbsp (0.7 oz)	90	2	1
MAMMY-APPLE				
fresh	1	431	4	–
MANGO				
fresh	1	135	1	tr
Del Monte				
In Extra Light Syrup	½ cup (4.4 oz)	100	1	0
Rainforest Farms				
Slices Dried	6 slices (1.3 oz)	140	1	0
Sonoma				
Pieces Dried	8 pieces (2 oz)	180	1	0
MANGO JUICE				
After The Fall				
Hawaiian Mango	1 can (12 oz)	180	0	0
Mango Ginger	1 can (12 oz)	150	0	0

FOOD	PORTION	CALS	FAT	SAT FAT
Fresh Samantha				
Mango Mama	1 cup (8 oz)	120	0	0
Guzzler				
Mango Passion	8 fl oz	140	0	0
Langers				
Mongo Mango	8 oz	120	0	0
Ocean Spray				
Mango Mango	8 oz	130	0	0
Snapple				
Mango Madness	8 fl oz	110	0	0
Tang				
Drink Mix as prep	1 serv (8 oz)	100	0	0
MARGARINE				
squeeze	1 tsp	34	4	1
stick corn	1 tsp	34	4	1
stick corn	1 stick (4 oz)	815	91	15
tub corn	1 tsp	34	4	1
tub diet	1 tsp	17	2	tr
Benecol				
Single Serve Light	1 pkg (0.3 oz)	30	3	0
Tub Light	1 tbsp (0.5 oz)	45	5	1
Tub Regular	1 tbsp (0.5 oz)	80	9	1
Brummel & Brown				
Spread Made With Yogurt	1 tbsp (0.5 oz)	45	5	1
I Can't Believe Its Not Butter				
Spray	5 sprays	0	0	0
Parkay				
Squeeze	1 tbsp (0.5 oz)	80	9	2
Stick	1 tbsp (0.5 oz)	90	10	2
Whipped	1 tbsp (0.3 oz)	70	7	2
Promise				
Spread Soft	1 tbsp	80	8	2
Spread Stick	1 tbsp	90	10	3
Spread Light Soft	1 tbsp	50	6	1
Spread Light Stick	1 tbsp	50	6	2
Ultra Soft	1 tbsp	30	4	0
Ultra Spread Fat Free	1 tbsp	5	0	0
Smart Balance				
No Trans Fat	1 tbsp (0.5 oz)	120	14	4

FOOD	PORTION	CALS	FAT	SAT FAT
No Trans Fat Light	1 tbsp (0.5 oz)	45	5	2
No Trans Fat Spread	1 tbsp (0.5 oz)	80	9	3
Smart Beat				
Light Unsalted	1 tbsp (0.5 oz)	25	3	0
Squeeze Fat Free	1 tbsp (0.5 oz)	5	0	0
Super Light Trans Fat Free	1 tbsp (0.5 oz)	20	2	0
Take Control				
Light	1 tbsp	45	5	1
Spread	1 tbsp (0.5 oz)	80	8	1
Weight Watchers				
Light	1 tbsp	45	4	1
Light Sodium Free	1 tbsp	45	4	1
MARINADE *(see SAUCE)*				
MARJORAM				
dried	1 tsp	2	tr	—
MARLIN				
raw	3 oz	110	3	—
MARSHMALLOW				
marshmallow	1 reg (0.3 oz)	23	0	0
marshmallow	1 cup (1.6 oz)	146	tr	—
Gol D Lite				
Sugar Free	⅓ pkg (0.9 oz)	51	0	0
Joyva				
Twists Chocolate Covered	2 (1.5 oz)	190	4	2
Just Born				
Peeps	5 (1.5 oz)	160	0	0
MATZO				
egg	1 (1 oz)	111	1	tr
egg & onion	1 (1 oz)	111	1	tr
plain	1 (1 oz)	112	tr	tr
whole wheat	1 (1 oz)	99	tr	tr
Eddyleon				
Dark Chocolate Coated Egg Matzo	1 oz	97	3	2
Milk Chocolate Coated Egg Matzo	1 oz	97	4	3
Manischewitz				
Matzo Meal	¼ cup (1 oz)	130	0	0

FOOD	PORTION	CALS	FAT	SAT FAT
MAYONNAISE				
mayonnaise	1 cup	1577	175	26
mayonnaise	1 tbsp	99	11	2
reduced calorie	1 tbsp	34	3	1
reduced calorie	1 cup	556	46	8
sandwich spread	1 tbsp	60	5	1
Blue Plate				
Squeeze	1 tbsp	100	11	2
Hellman's				
Mayonnaise	1 tbsp	100	11	2
Kraft				
Fat Free	1 tbsp (0.6 oz)	10	0	0
Light	1 tbsp (0.5 oz)	50	5	1
Real	1 tbsp (0.5 oz)	100	11	2
Mother's				
Mayonnaise	1 tbsp	100	11	–
Smart Beat				
Fat Free	1 tbsp	10	0	0
Weight Watchers				
Fat Free	1 tbsp	10	0	0
Light	1 tbsp	25	2	0
Light Low Sodium	1 tbsp	25	2	0
MAYONNAISE TYPE SALAD DRESSING				
mayonnaise type salad dressing	1 cup	916	78	12
mayonnaise type salad dressing	1 tbsp	57	5	1
reduced calorie w/o cholesterol	1 tbsp	68	7	1
reduced calorie w/o cholesterol	1 cup	1084	107	17
Carb Options				
Whipped Dressing	1 tbsp	50	5	1
Miracle Whip				
Free	1 tbsp (0.5 oz)	15	0	0
Light	1 tbsp (0.5 oz)	35	3	0
Salad Dressing	1 tbsp (0.6 oz)	70	7	1
Nasoya				
Nayonaise	1 tbsp	35	4	1
Nayonaise Dijon	1 tbsp	30	3	1
Weight Watchers				
Fat Free Whipped Dressing	1 tbsp	15	0	0

FOOD	PORTION	CALS	FAT	SAT FAT
MEAT STICKS				
jerky beef	1 oz	96	4	1
jerky beef	1 lg piece (0.7 oz)	67	3	1
smoked	1 (0.7 oz)	109	10	4
smoked	1 oz	156	14	6
Big Ones				
BBQ	1 (1 oz)	130	12	5
Hot n'Spicy	1 (1 oz)	130	12	5
Original	1 (1 oz)	130	12	5
Teriyaki	1 (1 oz)	130	12	5
Jack Link's				
Kippered Beefsteak Teriyaki	1 oz	80	1	1
Lance				
Beef & Cheese	1 pkg (1.5 oz)	150	11	6
Beef Jerky	1 piece (0.25 oz)	30	2	1
Beef Snack	1 piece (0.63 oz)	100	8	4
Hot Sausage	1 piece (0.9 oz)	60	5	2
Lowrey's				
Smokehouse Tender Hickory Smoked	1 pkg (1 oz)	80	2	1
Smokehouse Tender Original	1 pkg (1 oz)	60	1	0
Smokehouse Tender Peppered	1 pkg (1 oz)	60	1	0
Oberto				
Beef Jerky	1 pkg (1.3 oz)	100	1	0
Pemmican				
Original Tender Kippered Beef Steak	1	110	5	3
Peppered Tender Kippered Beef Steak	1	110	5	3
Rough Cut				
Beef Steak Hot	1 pkg (1 oz)	70	1	0
Beef Steak Original	1 pkg (1 oz)	60	1	0
Beef Steak Peppered	1 pkg (1 oz)	60	1	0
Rustlers Roundup				
Beef Jerky	1 serv (5 g)	20	2	1
Flamin' Hot	1 serv (8 g)	40	3	2
Smoky Steak	1 serv (0.8 oz)	60	2	1
Spicy	1 serv (0.5 oz)	70	6	3
Slim Jim				
Spicy	1 (4½ in) (0.3 oz)	50	4	2
Spicy Big	1 (.44 oz)	70	6	3
Spicy Giant	1 (0.97 oz)	150	14	6
Spicy Super	1 (0.64 oz)	100	9	4

FOOD	PORTION	CALS	FAT	SAT FAT
MEAT SUBSTITUTES *(see also* BACON SUBSTITUTES, CANADIAN BACON SUBSTITUTES, CHICKEN SUBSTITUTES, HAMBURGER SUBSTITUTES, SAUSAGE SUBSTITUTES, TURKEY SUBSTITUTES*)*				
simulated meat product	1 oz	88	1	tr
Boca Burgers				
Chef Max's Original	1 patty (2.5 oz)	110	2	1
Frieda's				
SoyTaco	1 oz	50	3	1
Soyrizo	4 tbsp (1.9 oz)	120	9	1
Ken & Robert's				
Veggie Pockets	1 (4.5 oz)	250	8	1
Veggie Pockets Bar B Que	1 (4.5 oz)	290	8	1
Veggie Pockets Broccoli & Cheddar	1 (4.5 oz)	250	8	0
Veggie Pockets Greek	1 (4.5 oz)	250	8	0
Veggie Pockets Indian	1 (4.5 oz)	260	8	1
Veggie Pockets Pizza	1 (4.5 oz)	270	8	1
Veggie Pockets Pot Pie	1 (4.5 oz)	250	9	1
Veggie Pockets Potato & Cheddar	1 (4.5 oz)	260	8	1
Veggie Pockets Santa Fe	1 (4.5 oz)	250	8	1
Veggie Pockets Tex Mex	1 (4.5 oz)	260	8	1
Lightlife				
Foney Baloney	3 slices (1.5 oz)	60	3	1
Gimme Lean Beef	2 oz	70	0	0
Smart Deli Bologna	3 slices (1.5 oz)	50	0	0
Smart Deli Ham	3 slices (1.5 oz)	50	0	0
Smart Deli Peppercorn	3 slices (1.5 oz)	45	0	0
Smart Deli Sticks Soylami	1 oz	40	0	0
Smart Deli Sticks Pepperoni	1 oz	45	0	0
Smart Ground Original	⅓ cup (1.9 oz)	70	0	0
Smart Ground Taco	⅓ cup (2 oz)	60	0	0
Loma Linda				
Dinner Cuts	2 slices (3.2 oz)	90	2	1
Nuteena	⅜ in slice (1.9 oz)	160	13	5
Sandwich Spread	¼ cup (1.9 oz)	80	5	1
Savory Dinner Loaf Mix not prep	½ cup (0.9 oz)	90	2	0
Swiss Steak	1 piece (3.2 oz)	120	6	1
Tender Bits	6 pieces (3 oz)	110	5	1
Tender Rounds	6 pieces (2.8 oz)	120	5	1
Vita Burger Chunks not prep	¼ cup (0.7 oz)	70	1	0
Vita Burger Granules	3 tbsp (0.7 oz)	70	1	0

FOOD	PORTION	CALS	FAT	SAT FAT
Morningstar Farms				
Burger Style Recipe Crumbles	⅔ cup (1.9 oz)	80	3	0
Ground Meatless	½ cup (1.9 oz)	60	0	0
Harvest Burger Recipe Crumbles	½ cup (2 oz)	70	0	0
Quarter Prime	1 patty (3.4 oz)	140	2	0
Natural Touch				
Dinner Entree	1 patty (3 oz)	220	15	3
Loaf Mix not prep	4 tbsp (1 oz)	100	1	0
Stroganoff Mix not prep	4 tbsp (0.8 oz)	90	4	2
Taco Mix not prep	3 tbsp (0.6 oz)	60	1	0
Vegan Burger Crumbles	½ cup (1.9 oz)	60	0	0
Quorn				
Grounds	⅔ cup (3 oz)	80	3	1
Soy Is Us				
Beef Not!	½ cup (1.75 oz)	140	2	1
Soy7				
Burger Bits as prep	½ cup	60	1	0
Burger Mix as prep	1 serv (3.2 oz)	120	3	0
Recipe Strips as prep	¾ cup	70	1	1
Taco Mix as prep	¼ cup	70	1	0
Veggie Patch				
Veggie Rounds	1 (2.5 oz)	120	3	—
Veggitinos Meatballs	5 (2.8 oz)	120	4	—
Worthington				
Beef Style Meatless	⅜ in slice (1.9 oz)	110	7	1
Bolono	3 slices (2 oz)	80	4	1
Choplets	2 slices (3.2 oz)	90	2	1
Corned Beef Meatless	4 slices (2 oz)	140	9	2
Country Stew	1 cup (8.4 oz)	210	9	2
Dinner Roast	¾ in slice (3 oz)	180	12	2
FriPats	1 patty (2.2 oz)	130	6	1
Multigrain Cutlets	2 slices (3.2 oz)	100	2	1
Numete	⅜ in slice (1.9 oz)	130	10	3
Prime Steaks	1 piece (3.2 oz)	120	7	1
Prosage Roll	⅝ in slice (1.9 oz)	140	10	2
Protose	⅜ in slice (1.9 oz)	130	7	1
Salami Meatless	3 slices (2 oz)	130	8	1
Savory Slices	3 slices (2.9 oz)	150	9	4
Smoked Beef Meatless	6 slices (2 oz)	120	6	1
Stakelets	1 piece (2.5 oz)	140	8	2

FOOD	PORTION	CALS	FAT	SAT FAT
Veelets	1 patty (2.5 oz)	180	9	2
Vegetable Skallops	½ cup (3 oz)	90	2	1
Vegetable Steaks	2 pieces (2.5 oz)	80	2	1
Wham	2 slices (1.6 oz)	80	5	1
Yves				
Veggie Bologna	4 slices (2.2 oz)	70	0	0
Veggie Ground Italian	⅓ cup (2 oz)	60	0	0
Veggie Ground Round Italian	⅓ cup (1.9 oz)	60	0	0
Veggie Ground Round Original	2 oz	60	0	0
Veggie Pizza Pepperoni Slices	1 serv (1.7 oz)	70	0	0
Veggie Salami Deli Slices	1 serv (2.2 oz)	90	0	0
MELON				
melon balls frzn	1 cup	55	tr	—
SunFresh				
Melon Salad In Extra Light Syrup	½ cup (4.5 oz)	45	0	0
MELON JUICE				
Ocean Spray				
Mega Melon	8 oz	130	0	0

MEXICAN FOOD (see SALSA, SPANISH FOOD, TORTILLA)

FOOD	PORTION	CALS	FAT	SAT FAT
MILK				
CANNED				
condensed sweetened	1 oz	123	3	2
condensed sweetened	1 cup	982	27	17
evaporated	½ cup	169	10	6
evaporated skim	½ cup	99	tr	tr
Carnation				
Evaporated	2 tbsp	40	2	2
Evaporated Fat Free	2 tbsp	25	0	0
Sweetened Condensed	⅓ cup	330	8	5
Pet				
Evaporated	2 tbsp	40	2	2
DRIED				
buttermilk	1 tbsp	25	tr	tr
nonfat instantized	1 pkg (3.2 oz)	244	tr	tr
Carnation				
Nonfat	⅓ cup	80	0	0
Saco				
Cultured Buttermilk	4 tbsp (0.8 oz)	80	tr	0

FOOD	PORTION	CALS	FAT	SAT FAT
Sanalac				
Powder	¼ cup (0.8 oz)	85	tr	0
REFRIGERATED				
1%	1 cup	102	3	2
1%	1 qt	409	10	6
1% protein fortified	1 qt	477	12	7
1% protein fortified	1 cup	119	3	2
2%	1 cup	121	5	3
2%	1 qt	485	19	12
buffalo	7 oz	224	16	–
buttermilk	1 cup	99	2	1
buttermilk	1 qt	396	9	5
camel	7 oz	160	8	–
donkey	7 oz	86	2	–
goat	1 cup	168	10	7
goat	1 qt	672	40	26
human	1 cup	171	11	5
indian buffalo	1 cup	236	17	11
low sodium	1 cup	149	8	5
mare	7 oz	98	4	–
nonfat	1 cup	86	tr	tr
nonfat	1 qt	342	2	1
nonfat protein fortified	1 qt	400	2	2
nonfat protein fortified	1 cup	100	1	tr
sheep	1 cup	264	17	11
whole	1 cup	150	8	5
Cool Cow				
Low Fat	1 cup (8 oz)	110	3	1
Farmland				
Skim Plus	1 cup (8 oz)	110	0	0
Horizon Organic				
Fat Free	1 cup (8 oz)	80	0	0
Land O Lakes				
1% Lowfat	1 carton (10 oz)	120	3	2
Fat Free	1 carton (10 oz)	100	5	0
Whole	1 carton (10 oz)	180	10	7
NutraBalance				
LactaCare	1 pkg (8 oz)	500	18	–
Organic Valley				
Low Fat	1 cup	100	3	2

FOOD	PORTION	CALS	FAT	SAT FAT
Nonfat	1 cup	80	0	0
Reduced Fat	1 cup	130	5	3
Whole	1 cup	150	8	5
Stonyfield Farm				
Organic Whole Milk	1 cup (8 oz)	180	10	6
Organic Whole Milk Vanilla	1 cup (8 oz)	230	8	5
Turkey Hill				
Cool Moos 2% Reduced Fat	1 cup	130	5	3
Cool Moos Whole Milk	1 cup	160	8	5
MILK DRINKS				
chocolate milk	1 cup	208	8	5
chocolate milk	1 qt	833	34	21
chocolate milk 1%	1 cup	158	3	2
chocolate milk 1%	1 qt	630	10	6
chocolate milk 2%	1 cup	179	5	3
strawberry flavor mix as prep w/ whole milk	9 oz	234	8	5
Cocio				
Chocolate Milk	1 bottle	225	7	–
Garelick				
Colossal Coffee	1 cup	145	3	2
Ultimate Chocolate	1 cup	150	3	2
Horizon Organic				
Lowfat Chocolate Milk	1 cup (8 oz)	160	3	2
Keto				
Chocolate Milk Mix	1 scoop	36	1	–
Land O Lakes				
Chocolate	1 cup (8.4 oz)	200	7	5
Organic Valley				
Chocolate Milk Reduced Fat	1 cup	180	5	3
Quik				
Banana Lowfat	1 cup (8.4 oz)	200	5	3
Banana Powder	2 tbsp (0.8 oz)	90	0	0
Chocolate	1 cup (8.4 oz)	230	8	5
Chocolate Lowfat	1 carton (8.4 oz)	200	5	3
Cookies n Cream Powder	2 tbsp (0.8 oz)	100	1	1
Strawberry	1 cup (8.4 oz)	230	8	5
Strawberry Lowfat	1 carton (8.4 oz)	210	5	3
Strawberry Powder	2 tbsp (0.8 oz)	90	0	0

FOOD	PORTION	CALS	FAT	SAT FAT
Turkey Hill				
Cool Moos Chocolate 1% Lowfat	1 cup	180	3	2
Cool Moos Orange Cream 1% Lowfat	1 cup	190	3	2
Cool Moos Strawberry 1% Lowfat	1 cup	160	3	2
Cool Moos Vanilla 1% Lowfat	1 cup	160	3	2
MILK SUBSTITUTES				
imitation milk	1 cup	150	8	2
imitation milk	1 qt	600	33	7
8th Continent				
Soymilk Low Fat Chocolate	1 bottle (8 oz)	140	3	1
Soymilk Low Fat Original	1 bottle (8 oz)	80	3	0
Soymilk Low Fat Vanilla	1 bottle (8 oz)	90	3	0
Better Than Milk				
Rice Original	2 tbsp (0.66 oz)	78	2	tr
Rice Original Light	2 tbsp (0.66 oz)	66	0	0
Rice Vanilla	2 tbsp (0.66 oz)	78	2	tr
Rice Vanilla Light	2 tbsp (0.66 oz)	66	0	0
Soy Carob	2 tbsp (1 oz)	90	2	tr
Soy Chocolate	2 tbsp (1.1 oz)	112	2	tr
Soy Light	2 tbsp (0.66 oz)	73	2	tr
Soy Original	2 tbsp (0.8 oz)	100	3	0
Soy Vanilla	2 tbsp (0.7 oz)	77	2	tr
Blue Diamond				
Almond Breeze Chocolate	8 oz	120	3	0
Almond Breeze Original	8 oz	60	2	0
Almond Breeze Vanilla	8 oz	90	3	0
EdenBlend				
Organic	8 oz	120	3	1
Edensoy				
Organic Light	8 oz	93	2	tr
Organic Light Vanilla	8 oz	120	2	tr
Galaxy				
Veggie Milk Chocolate	1 cup (8 oz)	150	2	0
Veggie Milk Original	1 cup (8 oz)	110	3	0
Hansen's				
Soy Smoothie Lemon Chiffon	8 oz	150	0	0
Soy Smoothie Orange Dream	8 oz	150	0	0
Harmony Farms				
Original Rice Beverage	1 cup (8 oz)	90	0	0

FOOD	PORTION	CALS	FAT	SAT FAT
Harmony House				
Enriched Rice Beverage	1 cup (8 oz)	90	0	0
Enriched Soy Beverage	1 cup (8 oz)	90	0	0
Original Soy Beverage	1 cup (8 oz)	90	0	0
Health Valley				
Soy Moo	1 cup	110	0	—
Keto				
Low Carb Mix	1 scoop	54	2	—
NutraBalance				
NuTaste	1 pkg (8 oz)	80	2	tr
Rice Dream				
Carob	1 box (8 oz)	150	3	0
Chocolate	1 box (8 oz)	170	3	0
Chocolate Enriched	1 box (8 oz)	170	3	0
Organic Original	1 box (8 oz)	120	2	0
Organic Original Enriched	1 box (8 oz)	120	2	0
Vanilla	1 box (8 oz)	130	2	0
Vanilla Enriched	1 box (8 oz)	130	2	0
Silk				
Chocolate	1 cup	140	4	0
Organic Plain	1 cup	100	4	0
Vanilla	1 bottle (11 oz)	140	5	1
Soy Dream				
Carob	8 oz	210	5	1
Chocolate Enriched	8 oz	210	5	1
Original	8 oz	140	5	1
Original Enriched	8 oz	140	5	1
Vanilla	8 oz	170	5	1
Vanilla Enriched	8 oz	140	5	1
Tree Of Life				
Original Rice Beverage	1 cup	90	0	0
Vitamite				
Non-Dairy	1 cup (8 oz)	110	5	2
Vitasoy				
1% Low Fat Vanilla Delight	8 oz	90	2	0
Carob Supreme	8 fl oz	150	5	1
Creamy Unsweetened	8 oz	80	4	1
Creamy Original	8 fl oz	110	5	1
Enriched Light Original	8 fl oz	60	2	1
Enriched Light Vanilla	8 fl oz	90	2	1

FOOD	PORTION	CALS	FAT	SAT FAT
Green Tea Soymilk	8 oz	130	4	1
Original Creamy	8 fl oz	110	4	1
Original Light	8 fl oz	60	2	1
Rich Chocolate	8 fl oz	160	4	1
Rich Cocoa	8 fl oz	150	5	1
Vanilla Light	8 fl oz	90	2	1
Vanilla Delite	8 fl oz	120	4	1
White Wave				
Mocha	1 cup	140	4	0
MILKFISH				
baked	3 oz	162	7	–
MILKSHAKE				
chocolate	10 oz	360	11	7
strawberry	10 oz	319	8	–
thick shake chocolate	10.6 oz	356	8	5
thick shake vanilla	11 oz	350	10	6
vanilla	10 oz	314	8	5
Breyers				
Quick Vanilla	1 serv (10 oz)	320	17	11
Carb Options				
Chocolate Delite	1 can (11 oz)	190	9	2
Creamy Vanilla	1 can (11 oz)	190	9	2
D'Frosta Shake				
Vanilla	1 serv (13.5 oz)	340	9	6
Freeze Flip				
Fruit Shake No Fat Lactose Free Black Raspberry	1 serv (6 oz)	150	0	0
Hood				
Shake Up Chocolate	1 cup (8 oz)	240	6	4
Shake Up Strawberry	1 cup (8 oz)	220	5	3
Shake Up Vanilla	1 cup (8 oz)	220	5	3
Parmalat				
Shake A Shake Chocolate	1 box (6 oz)	180	4	2
Shake A Shake Orange Vanilla	1 box (6 oz)	110	3	2
Shake A Shake Vanilla	1 box (6 oz)	170	3	2
MILLET				
cooked	1 cup (6.1 oz)	207	2	tr

MINERAL WATER *(see WATER)*

FOOD	PORTION	CALS	FAT	SAT FAT
MISO				
dried	1 oz	86	3	–
miso	½ cup	284	8	1
Eden				
Organic Genmai	1 tbsp	25	1	0
Eden				
Tekka	1 tsp	5	0	0
MOLASSES				
blackstrap	1 tbsp (0.7 oz)	47	0	0
blackstrap	1 cup (11.5 oz)	771	tr	–
molasses	1 tbsp (0.7 oz)	53	0	0
molasses	1 cup (11.5 oz)	873	1	–
Brer Rabbit				
Dark	1 tbsp	60	0	0
Mott's				
Sulphured	1 tbsp	50	0	0
Unsulphured	1 tbsp	50	0	0
MONKFISH				
baked	3 oz	82	2	–
MOOSE				
roasted	3 oz	114	1	tr
MOTH BEANS				
dried cooked	1 cup	207	1	tr
MOUSSE				
FROZEN				
Sara Lee				
Chocolate	⅓ pkg (4.3 oz)	400	25	20
Weight Watchers				
Chocolate Mousse	1 (2.75 oz)	190	5	2
TAKE-OUT				
chocolate	½ cup (7.1 oz)	447	33	19
orange	½ cup	87	5	–
MUFFIN				
FROZEN				
Pepperidge Farm				
Blueberry	1 (2 oz)	180	7	1
Bran w/ Raisins	1 (2 oz)	180	6	1

FOOD	PORTION	CALS	FAT	SAT FAT
Corn	1 (2 oz)	190	7	1
Orange Cranberry	1 (2 oz)	180	6	1
Sara Lee				
Blueberry	1 (2.2 oz)	220	11	2
Blueberry	1 (2.2 oz)	220	11	2
Corn	1 (2.2 oz)	260	14	3
Weight Watchers				
Chocolate Chocolate Chip	1 (2.5 oz)	190	2	1
Fat Free Banana	1 (2.5 oz)	170	0	0
Fat Free Blueberry	1 (2.5 oz)	160	0	0
MIX				
blueberry	1 (1¾ oz)	149	4	1
corn	1 (1.75 oz)	160	5	1
wheat bran as prep	1 (1¾ oz)	138	5	1
Betty Crocker				
Apple Cinnamon as prep	1	170	7	2
Apple Streusel as prep	1	210	8	1
Banana Nut as prep	1	170	6	1
Cranberry Orange as prep	1	150	5	1
Double Chocolate as prep	1	220	11	4
Golden Corn as prep	1	160	5	1
Lemon Poppyseed as prep	1	180	8	1
Sunkist Lemon Poppyseed as prep	1	190	7	1
Twice The Blueberries as prep	1	140	3	1
Wild Blueberry as prep	1	170	5	1
Carbsense				
Honey Bran not prep	1 serv (1.3 oz)	120	4	0
Flako				
Corn	⅓ cup (1.4 oz)	160	4	1
Gold Medal				
Corn	1	160	6	2
Hodgson Mill				
Bran	¼ cup (1.3 oz)	130	1	0
Cornbread	¼ cup (1.3 oz)	130	1	0
Whole Wheat	¼ cup (1.3 oz)	130	1	0
Ketogenics				
Apple Cinnamon Bran as prep	1	190	10	0
Chocolate Chip as prep	1	215	14	0
Wild Blueberry as prep	1	190	14	0

FOOD	PORTION	CALS	FAT	SAT FAT
MiniCarb				
Apple Cinnamon as prep	1	225	16	2
Sweet Corn as prep	1	225	16	1
Robin Hood				
Apple Cinnamon	1	170	8	2
Banana Nut	1	170	8	2
Blueberry	1	160	6	2
Caramel Nut	1	170	7	2
Sweet Rewards				
Low Fat Apple Cinnamon as prep	1	140	2	0
Wanda's				
Blue Corn	¼ cup mix per serv (1.2 oz)	130	1	0
READY-TO-EAT				
blueberry	1 (2 oz)	158	4	1
corn	1 (2 oz)	174	5	1
oat bran wheat free	1 (2 oz)	154	4	1
toaster type blueberry	1	103	3	tr
toaster type corn	1	114	4	1
toaster type wheat bran w/ raisins	1 (1.3 oz)	106	3	1
Dolly Madison				
Blueberry	1 (1.75 oz)	170	7	3
Mega Banana Nut	1 (5.9 oz)	620	31	5
Mega Blueberry	1 (5.9 oz)	590	28	4
Mega Chocolate Chip	1 (5.9 oz)	620	29	5
Mega Cranberry Orange	1 (5.9 oz)	590	28	5
Mega Cream Cheese	1 (5.9 oz)	620	33	7
Dutch Mill				
Apple Oat Bran	1 (2 oz)	180	5	1
Banana Walnut	1 (2 oz)	220	6	2
Carrot	1 (2 oz)	190	7	2
Corn	1 (2 oz)	190	6	3
Cranberry Orange	1 (2 oz)	170	6	3
Raisin Bran	1 (2 oz)	230	5	3
Freihofer's				
Corn Toasters	1 (1.3 oz)	130	6	1
Hostess				
Banana Bran Low Fat	1 (2.7 oz)	240	3	1
Blueberry Low Fat	1 (2.7 oz)	230	3	1
Hearty Banana Nut	1 (5.9 oz)	620	31	5

FOOD	PORTION	CALS	FAT	SAT FAT
Hearty Blueberry	1 (5.9 oz)	590	28	4
Hearty Chocolate Chip	1 (5.9 oz)	620	29	2
Hearty Cranberry Orange	1 (5.9 oz)	590	28	5
Hearty Cream Cheese	1 (5.9 oz)	620	33	7
Mini Banana Walnut	3 (1.2 oz)	160	9	1
Mini Blueberry	3 (1.2 oz)	150	8	1
Mini Chocolate Chip	3 (1.2 oz)	160	9	3
Mini Cinnamon Apple	3 (1.2 oz)	160	9	2
Mini Cinnamon Bites	3 (1.1 oz)	130	6	1
Mini Rocky Road	3 (1.2 oz)	160	9	3
Muffin Loaf Apple Spice	1 (3.7 oz)	430	18	4
Muffin Loaf Banana Nut	1 (3.8 oz)	460	20	3
Muffin Loaf Blueberry	1 (3.8 oz)	440	19	3
Muffin Loaf Chocolate Chocolate Chip	1 (3.8 oz)	400	17	4
Muffin Loaf Raspberry	1 (3.8 oz)	440	19	3
Oat Bran	1 (1.5 oz)	160	8	1
Otis Spunkmeyer				
Apple Cinnamon	1 (2 oz)	220	11	2
Low Fat Wild Blueberry	1 (2.25 oz)	200	4	1
Mayport Almond Poppy Seed	½ muffin (2 oz)	210	12	3
Mayport Banana Nut	1 (2.25 oz)	270	14	3
Mayport Cheese Streusel	½ muffin (2 oz)	220	10	3
Mayport Chocolate Chocolate Chip	1 (2.25 oz)	260	13	3
Mayport Chocolate Chip	½ muffin (2 oz)	240	13	3
Mayport Cinnamon Spice	½ muffin (2 oz)	230	13	3
Mayport Corn	½ muffin (2 oz)	230	13	2
Mayport Harvest Bran	1 (2.25 oz)	240	10	2
Mayport Lemon	½ muffin (2 oz)	230	13	3
Mayport Orange	½ muffin (2 oz)	230	13	3
Mayport Pineapple	½ muffin (2 oz)	210	12	3
Mayport Wild Blueberry	1 (2.25 oz)	230	13	3
Mayport Low Fat Apple Cinnamon	1 (4 oz)	380	6	1
Mayport Low Fat Banana Nut	1 (4 oz)	350	6	1
Mayport Low Fat Chocolate Chocolate Chip	1 (4 oz)	370	6	2
Uncle Wally's				
Chocolate Passion	1 (2 oz)	130	0	0
Cranberry Orange Supreme	1 (2 oz)	130	0	0
Fat Free Apple Cinnamon Delight	1 (2 oz)	110	0	0
Fat Free Wild Blueberry Bliss	1 (2 oz)	120	0	0

FOOD	PORTION	CALS	FAT	SAT FAT
Golden Waves Of Corn	1 (2 oz)	120	0	0
Honey Raisin Bran	1 (2 oz)	130	0	0
No Nut Banana	1 (2 oz)	130	0	0
VitaMuffin				
Blue Bran	1 (2 oz)	100	0	0
Cran Bran	1 (2 oz)	100	0	0
Deep Chocolate	1 (4 oz)	200	3	2
Multi Bran	1 (2 oz)	100	0	0
VitaTops Apple Berry Bran	1 (2 oz)	100	0	0
VitaTops Blue Bran	1 (2 oz)	100	0	0
VitaTops Cran Bran	1 (2 oz)	100	0	0
VitaTops Deep Chocolate	1 (2 oz)	100	2	1
VitaTops MultiBran	1 (2 oz)	100	0	0
Weight Watchers				
Fat Free Apple Crisp	1 (2.5 oz)	160	0	0
Fat Free Cranberry Orange	1 (2.5 oz)	160	0	0
Fat Free Double Chocolate	1 (2.5 oz)	180	0	0
Fat Free Wild Blueberry	1 (2.5 oz)	160	0	0
Low Fat Apple Cinnamon	1 (2.5 oz)	170	3	0
Low Fat Blueberry	1 (2.5 oz)	180	3	0
Low Fat Carrot	1 (2.5 oz)	160	3	0
Low Fat Chocolate Chip	1 (2.5 oz)	180	3	1
Low Fat Cranberry Orange	1 (2.5 oz)	180	3	0
Low Fat Lemon Poppy	1 (2.5 oz)	190	3	0
TAKE-OUT				
raisin bran lowfat	1 (4 oz)	270	1	0
MULBERRIES				
fresh	1 cup	61	1	–
MULLET				
striped cooked	3 oz	127	4	1
striped raw	3 oz	99	3	1
MUNG BEANS				
dried cooked	1 cup	213	1	tr
MUNGO BEANS				
dried cooked	1 cup	190	1	tr

FOOD	PORTION	CALS	FAT	SAT FAT
MUSHROOMS				
CANNED				
chanterelle	3.5 oz	12	1	–
pieces	½ cup	19	tr	tr
straw	1 cup (6.4 oz)	58	1	tr
whole	1 (0.4 oz)	3	tr	tr
BinB				
Pieces & Stems	1 can (4.2 oz)	30	0	0
Sliced	1 can (4.2 oz)	30	0	0
Sliced With Garlic	1 can (4.2 oz)	35	1	0
Whole	1 can (4.2 oz)	30	0	0
Green Giant				
Pieces & Stems	½ cup (4.2 oz)	30	0	0
Sliced	½ cup (4.2 oz)	30	0	0
Whole	½ cup (4.2 oz)	30	0	0
DRIED				
chanterelle	1 oz	25	tr	–
cloud ear	1 (5 g)	13	tr	–
cloud ears	1 cup (1 oz)	80	tr	–
shitake	4 (½ oz)	44	tr	tr
straw	1 piece (6 g)	2	tr	0
tree ear	½ cup (0.4 oz)	36	tr	–
wood ear mok yee	½ cup (0.4 oz)	25	tr	–
Eden				
Shitake	6 (0.4 oz)	35	0	0
FRESH				
chanterelle	3.5 oz	11	tr	–
enoki raw	1 (4 in)	2	tr	tr
morel	3.5 oz	9	tr	–
oyster raw	1 lg (5.2 oz)	55	1	–
oyster raw	1 sm (0.5 oz)	6	tr	–
portabella	1 serv (2 oz)	14	tr	0
raw	1 (½ oz)	5	tr	tr
raw sliced	½ cup	9	tr	tr
shitake cooked	4 (2.5 oz)	40	tr	tr
sliced cooked	½ cup	21	tr	tr
whole cooked	1 (0.4 oz)	3	tr	tr
Mother Earth				
Organic	4 oz	35	1	–

FOOD	PORTION	CALS	FAT	SAT FAT
MUSKRAT				
roasted	3 oz	199	10	–
MUSSELS				
blue raw	3 oz	73	2	tr
blue raw	1 cup	129	3	1
fresh blue cooked	3 oz	147	4	1
MUSTARD				
dry mustard	1 tsp	15	1	tr
yellow ready-to-use	1 tsp	5	tr	tr
Boar's Head				
Delicatessen Style	1 tsp (5 g)	0	0	0
Honey	1 tsp (5 g)	10	0	0
Country Cupboard				
Smokey Garlic or Horseradish	1 tsp	10	0	0
Eden				
Organic Stone Ground	1 tsp	0	0	0
French's				
Classic Yellow	1 tsp	0	0	0
Gulden's				
Spicy Brown	1 tsp	5	0	0
Hunt's				
Mustard	1 tsp (5 g)	3	tr	0
Kosciuszko				
Spicy Brown	1 tsp	5	tr	–
Kraft				
Horseradish Mustard	1 tsp (5 g)	0	0	0
Mustard	1 tsp (5 g)	0	0	0
Luzianne				
Creole Mustard	1 tbsp	10	0	0
Tree Of Life				
Dijon	1 tsp (5 g)	0	0	0
Dijon Imported	1 tsp (5 g)	5	0	0
Stone Ground	1 tsp (5 g)	0	0	0
Yellow	1 tsp (5 g)	0	0	0
Watkins				
Country Mill	1 tsp (7 g)	15	1	0
Dusseldorf	1 tsp (7 g)	10	0	0
Horseradish	1 tsp (7 g)	10	0	0
Jalapeno	1 tsp (7 g)	10	0	0

FOOD	PORTION	CALS	FAT	SAT FAT
Onion	1 tsp (7 g)	10	0	0
Parisienne	1 tsp (7 g)	10	0	0
Wild Thyme Farms				
Chili Pepper Garlic	1 tsp	5	0	0
Dill Horseradish	1 tsp	5	0	0
MUSTARD GREENS				
fresh chopped cooked	½ cup	11	tr	tr
fresh raw chopped	½ cup	7	tr	tr
frozen chopped cooked	½ cup	14	tr	tr
Birds Eye				
Chopped	1 cup	30	0	0
NATTO				
natto	½ cup	187	10	1
NAVY BEANS				
CANNED				
navy	1 cup	296	1	tr
DRIED				
cooked	1 cup	259	1	tr
Hurst				
HamBeens w/ Ham	3 tbsp (1.2 oz)	120	1	0
NECTARINE				
fresh	1	67	1	–
Chiquita				
Fresh	1 med (4.9 oz)	70	1	0
NEUFCHATEL				
neufchatel	1 oz	74	7	4
neufchatel	1 pkg (3 oz)	221	20	13
Horizon Organic				
Neufchatel	2 tbsp	70	6	4
Organic Valley				
Neufchatel	1 oz	70	6	4
Philadelphia				
Neufchatel	1 oz	70	6	4
NOODLE DISHES (see also PASTA DINNERS)				
Hormel				
Microcup Meals Noodles & Chicken	1 cup (7.5 oz)	200	9	3

FOOD	PORTION	CALS	FAT	SAT FAT
Hunt's				
Noodles & Chicken	1 cup (8.7 oz)	176	6	2
Noodles & Beef	1 cup (8.7 oz)	151	4	2
Kraft				
Noodle Classics Cheddar Cheese as prep	1 cup (7.4 oz)	400	19	5
Noodle Classics Savory Chicken as prep	1 cup (8.5 oz)	340	13	3
Lipton				
Noodles & Sauce Alfredo Broccoli as prep	1 cup (2.2 oz)	340	14	6
Noodles & Sauce Alfredo as prep	1 cup (2.2 oz)	330	14	6
Noodles & Sauce Beef as prep	1 cup (2.1 oz)	280	10	2
Noodles & Sauce Butter as prep	1 cup (2.2 oz)	310	14	6
Noodles & Sauce Butter & Herb as prep	1 cup (2.2 oz)	300	13	5
Noodles & Sauce Chicken Broccoli as prep	1 cup (2.1 oz)	310	11	4
Noodles & Sauce Chicken Tetrazzini as prep	1 cup (2 oz)	300	12	4
Noodles & Sauce Chicken as prep	1 cup (2.1 oz)	290	11	3
Noodles & Sauce Creamy Chicken as prep	1 cup (2.1 oz)	320	13	5
Noodles & Sauce Parmesan as prep	1 cup (2.1 oz)	330	15	6
Noodles & Sauce Sour Cream & Chives as prep	1 cup (2.2 oz)	310	14	6
Noodles & Sauce Stroganoff as prep	1 cup (2 oz)	300	11	4
Luigino's				
Stroganoff	1 pkg (8 oz)	310	17	5
TAKE-OUT				
noodle pudding	½ cup	132	7	4
NOODLES				
cellophane	1 cup	492	tr	tr
chow mein	1 cup (1.6 oz)	237	14	2
egg	1 cup (38 g)	145	2	tr
egg cooked	1 cup (5.6 oz)	213	2	tr
japanese soba cooked	1 cup (4 oz)	113	tr	tr
japanese somen cooked	1 cup (6.2 oz)	231	tr	tr
korean acorn noodles not prep	2 oz	195	tr	—

FOOD	PORTION	CALS	FAT	SAT FAT
rice cooked	1 cup (6.2 oz)	192	tr	tr
spinach/egg cooked	1 cup (5.6 oz)	211	3	1
Annie Chun				
Chow Mein	2 oz	200	1	0
Rice	2 oz	210	0	0
Rice Hunan	2 oz	210	0	0
Rice Pad Thai	2 oz	210	0	0
Rice Pad Thai Basil	2 oz	210	0	0
Azumaya				
Spinach	1 cup	210	1	0
Thin Cut	1 cup	210	1	0
Wide Cut	1 cup	210	1	0
Chun King				
Chow Mein	½ cup (1 oz)	137	6	1
Eden				
Kudzu	2 oz	200	0	0
Hodgson Mill				
Four Color Veggie Egg	2 oz	200	2	1
Whole Wheat Egg not prep	2 oz	190	0	0
La Choy				
Chow Mein	½ cup (1 oz)	137	6	1
Chow Mein Crispy Wide	½ cup (1 oz)	148	8	2
Rice	½ cup (1 oz)	121	3	1
Manischewitz				
Fine Yolk Free	1½ cups	210	1	0
Fine Egg	1½ cups	220	3	1
Wide Yolk Free	1¾ cups	210	1	0
Nasoya				
Chinese	1 cup	210	1	0
Japanese	1 cup	210	1	0
Spinach	1 cup	210	1	0
NOPALES				
cooked	1 cup (5.2 oz)	23	tr	–
raw sliced	1 cup (3 oz)	14	tr	–
NUTMEG				
ground	1 tsp	12	1	1
Watkins				
Ground	¼ tsp (0.5 g)	0	0	0

FOOD	PORTION	CALS	FAT	SAT FAT
NUTRITION SUPPLEMENTS (see also CEREAL BARS, ENERGY BARS, ENERGY DRINKS)				
Boost				
High Protein Powder Vanilla as prep w/ water	1 serv (8 oz)	200	1	0
Enlive!				
Drink All Flavors	1 box (8.1 oz)	300	0	0
Ensure				
Supplement All Flavors	1 can (8 fl oz)	250	6	1
Essential				
Protein Powder	1 serv (0.6 oz)	70	tr	0
GeniSoy				
Soy Natural Protein Powder	1 scoop (1 oz)	100	0	0
Glucerna				
Shakes All Flavors	1 can (8 oz)	220	9	1
Juven				
Orange w/ HMB	1 pkg (0.8 oz)	90	0	0
Met-Rx				
Lite	1 pkg (1.6 oz)	170	1	1
Mass Action	1 scoop (0.9 oz)	60	4	–
Original	1 pkg (2.5 oz)	250	2	2
Protein Shake	1 can	200	3	1
Ultra	1 pkg (2.6 oz)	250	2	2
Nestle				
Additions	2⅓ tsp (0.7 oz)	100	5	1
NutraBalance				
EggPro	1 tbsp (7.5 g)	30	0	0
Nutribar				
Shake Chocolate Supreme as prep w/ 2% milk	1 serv (10 oz) (4.6 oz)	262	8	4
Shake Vanilla as prep w/ 2% milk	1 (10 oz)	259	7	4
PermaLean				
Protein Powder Bodacious Berry	1 scoop (1 oz)	104	tr	0
Protein Powder Chocoholic Chocolate	1 scoop (1 oz)	104	tr	0
Pounds Off				
All Flavors	1 bar (2.1 oz)	210	5	1
Resource				
Fructose Sweetened	1 pkg (8 oz)	250	11	–
Liquid Food	1 pkg (8 oz)	250	9	–
Plus Liquid Food	1 pkg (8 oz)	355	13	–

FOOD	PORTION	CALS	FAT	SAT FAT
Viactiv				
Calcium Chews	1	20	1	–
Chocolate	1	20	1	–
NUTS MIXED (see also individual names)				
dry roasted w/ peanuts	1 oz	169	15	2
dry roasted w/ peanuts salted	1 oz	169	15	2
mixed nuts chocolate covered	¼ cup (1.5 oz)	240	17	7
oil roasted w/ peanuts	1 oz	175	16	2
oil roasted w/ peanuts salted	1 oz	175	16	2
oil roasted w/o peanuts	1 oz	175	16	3
oil roasted w/o peanuts salted	1 oz	175	16	3
Estee				
Fruit & Nut Mix	¼ cup	210	12	7
Judy's				
Sugar Free Mixed Nut Brittle	¼ piece (1 oz)	120	7	2
Maranatha				
Cashew Macadamia Butter	2 tbsp	210	20	4
Tamari Organic	¼ cup	160	14	2
Tamari Roasted	¼ cup	160	14	2
Planters				
Cashews & Peanuts Honey Roasted	1 oz	150	12	2
Deluxe Oil Roasted	1 oz	170	16	2
Dry Roasted	1 oz	170	14	2
Honey Roasted	1 oz	140	13	2
Lightly Salted Oil Roasted	1 oz	170	15	2
No Brazils Lightly Salted Oil Roasted	1 oz	170	15	2
No Brazils Oil Roasted	1 oz	170	15	2
Oil Roasted	1 oz	170	15	3
Select Mix Cashews Almonds & Macadamias Oil Roasted	1 oz	170	16	3
Select Mix Cashews Almonds & Pecans Oil Roasted	1 oz	170	15	2
Unsalted Oil Roasted	1 oz	170	15	2
OCTOPUS				
fresh steamed	3 oz	140	2	tr
OHELOBERRIES				
fresh	1 cup	39	tr	–

FOOD	PORTION	CALS	FAT	SAT FAT
OIL				
almond	1 cup	1927	218	1
almond	1 tbsp	120	14	1
apricot kernel	1 tbsp	120	14	1
apricot kernel	1 cup	1927	218	14
avocado	1 tbsp	124	14	2
avocado	1 cup	1927	218	25
babassu palm	1 tbsp	120	14	11
butter oil	1 tbsp	112	13	8
butter oil	1 cup	1795	204	127
canola	1 cup	1927	218	15
canola	1 tbsp	124	14	2
coconut	1 tbsp	117	14	12
corn	1 tbsp	120	14	2
corn	1 cup	1927	218	28
cottonseed	1 cup	1927	218	56
cottonseed	1 tbsp	120	14	4
cupu assu	1 tbsp	120	14	7
grapeseed	1 tbsp	120	14	1
hazelnut	1 tbsp	120	14	1
hazelnut	1 cup	1927	218	1
mustard	1 tbsp	124	14	2
mustard	1 cup	1927	218	25
oat	1 tbsp	120	14	3
olive	1 cup	1909	216	26
olive	1 tbsp	119	14	2
palm	1 tbsp	120	14	7
palm	1 cup	1927	218	107
palm kernel	1 tbsp	117	14	11
palm kernel	1 cup	1879	218	178
peanut	1 cup	1909	216	36
peanut	1 tbsp	119	14	2
poppyseed	1 tbsp	120	14	2
pumpkin seed	1 oz	217	29	–
rice bran	1 tbsp	120	14	3
safflower	1 tbsp	120	14	1
safflower	1 cup	1927	218	20
sesame	1 tbsp	120	14	2
sheanut	1 tbsp	120	14	6
soybean	1 cup	1927	218	31

FOOD	PORTION	CALS	FAT	SAT FAT
soybean	1 tbsp	120	14	2
soybean organic	1 tbsp	120	14	2
sunflower	1 tbsp	120	14	1
sunflower	1 cup	1927	218	23
teaseed	1 tbsp	120	14	3
tomatoseed	1 tbsp	120	14	3
vegetable	1 cup	1927	218	2
vegetable	1 tbsp	120	14	2
walnut	1 cup	1927	218	20
walnut	1 tbsp	120	14	1
wheat germ	1 tbsp	120	14	3
Bertolli				
Classico	1 tbsp	120	14	—
Extra Light	1 tbsp	120	14	—
Extra Virgin	1 tbsp	120	14	—
Crisco				
Corn Canola	1 tbsp (0.5 fl oz)	120	14	2
Oil	1 tbsp (0.5 fl oz)	120	14	2
Puritan Canola	1 tbsp (0.5 fl oz)	120	14	1
Eden				
Olive Spanish Extra Virgin	1 tbsp	120	14	2
Safflower	1 tbsp (0.5 oz)	120	14	1
Enova				
Oil	1 tbsp	120	14	1
House Of Tsang				
Hot Chili Sesame	1 tsp (5 g)	45	5	1
Mongolian Fire	1 tsp (5 g)	45	5	1
Pure Sesame	1 tsp (5 g)	45	5	1
Singapore Curry	1 tsp (5 g)	45	5	1
Wok Oil	1 tbsp (0.5 oz)	130	14	3
Loriva				
5 Pepper Hot	1 tbsp	120	14	1
Avocado	1 tbsp	120	14	2
Basil Flavored	1 tbsp	120	14	1
Canola	1 tbsp	120	14	1
Canolive	1 tbsp	120	14	1
Garlic Flavored	1 tbsp	120	14	1
Grapeseed	1 tbsp	120	14	1
Olive	1 tbsp	120	14	2
Olive Organic Extra Virgin	1 tbsp	120	14	1

FOOD	PORTION	CALS	FAT	SAT FAT
Peanut	1 tbsp	120	14	2
Rice Bran	1 tbsp	120	14	2
Safflower	1 tbsp	120	14	1
Sesame	1 tbsp	120	14	2
Sunflower	1 tbsp	120	14	2
Toasted Sesame	1 tbsp	120	14	2
Walnut	1 tbsp	120	14	2
Mazola				
Oil	1 tbsp	120	14	2
Monini				
Olive Extra Virgin	1 tbsp	118	13	2
Orville Redenbacher's				
Popping	1 tbsp (0.5 oz)	120	14	2
Pam				
Butter	⅓ sec spray (0.3 g)	0	0	0
Cooking Spray	⅓ sec spray (0.3 g)	0	0	0
Olive Oil	⅓ sec spray (0.3 g)	0	0	0
Planters				
Peanut	1 tbsp (0.5 oz)	120	14	3
Popcorn	1 tbsp (0.5 oz)	120	14	3
Pompeian				
Olive	1 tbsp	130	14	–
Progresso				
Olive Extra Mild	1 tbsp (0.5 oz)	120	14	2
Olive Extra Virgin	1 tbsp (0.5 oz)	120	14	2
Olive Riviera Blend	1 tbsp (0.5 oz)	120	14	2
Smart Beat				
Canola	1 tbsp	120	14	1
Tree Of Life				
Olive Extra Virgin Organic	1 tbsp (0.5 g)	130	14	1
Weight Watchers				
Butter Spray	⅓ sec spray	0	0	0
Cooking Spray	⅓ sec spray	0	0	0
Wesson				
Canola	1 tbsp	120	14	4

FOOD	PORTION	CALS	FAT	SAT FAT
OKRA				
FRESH				
raw	8 pods	36	tr	tr
raw sliced	½ cup	19	tr	tr
sliced cooked	½ cup	25	tr	tr
sliced cooked	8 pods	27	tr	tr
FROZEN				
sliced cooked	1 pkg (10 oz)	94	1	tr
sliced cooked	½ cup	34	tr	tr
Birds Eye				
Cut	¾ cup	25	0	0
Whole	9 pods	25	0	0
McKenzie's				
Breaded Okra	1 serv (2.8 oz)	90	1	0
OLIVES				
green	3 extra lg	15	2	tr
green	4 med	15	2	tr
green olive tapenade	1 tbsp	25	3	0
ripe	1 sm	4	tr	tr
ripe	1 lg	5	tr	tr
ripe	1 jumbo	7	1	tr
ripe	1 colossal	12	1	tr
spanish stuffed	5 (0.5 oz)	15	1	0
Italia In Tavola				
Black Olives Paste	1 tbsp (0.5 oz)	20	2	–
Progresso				
Olive Salad (drained)	2 tbsp (0.8 oz)	25	3	0
Vlasic				
Ripe Colossal Pitted	2 (0.6 oz)	20	2	0
Ripe Jumbo Pitted	3 (0.6 oz)	25	2	0
Ripe Large Pitted	4 (0.5 oz)	25	3	0
Ripe Medium Pitted	5 (0.5 oz)	25	3	0
Ripe Sliced	¼ cup (0.5 oz)	25	3	0
Ripe Small Pitted	6 (0.5 oz)	25	3	0
ONION				
CANNED				
chopped	½ cup	21	tr	tr
whole	1 (2.2 oz)	12	tr	tr

FOOD	PORTION	CALS	FAT	SAT FAT
Boar's Head				
Sweet Vidalia In Sauce	1 tbsp	10	0	0
Watkins				
Liquid Spice	1 tbsp (0.5 oz)	120	14	2
DRIED				
flakes	1 tbsp	16	tr	tr
powder	1 tsp	7	tr	–
shallots	1 tbsp	3	0	0
Watkins				
Flakes	¼ tsp (1 g)	0	0	0
FRESH				
chopped cooked	½ cup	47	tr	tr
raw chopped	1 tbsp	4	tr	tr
raw chopped	½ cup	30	tr	tr
scallions raw chopped	1 tbsp	2	tr	tr
scallions raw sliced	½ cup	16	tr	tr
shallots raw chopped	1 tbsp	7	tr	tr
welsh raw	3½ oz	34	tr	tr
Antioch Farms				
Vidalia	1 med	60	0	–
FROZEN				
chopped cooked	1 tbsp	4	tr	tr
chopped cooked	½ cup	30	tr	tr
rings	7 (2.5 oz)	285	19	6
rings cooked	2 (0.7 oz)	81	5	2
whole cooked	3½ oz	28	tr	0
Birds Eye				
Diced	⅔ cup	30	0	0
Pearl Onions In Real Cream Sauce	½ cup	60	2	1
Small Whole	17	30	0	0
Kineret				
Rings	6 (3 oz)	200	10	3
McKenzie's				
Onion Rounds	1 serv (3.2 oz)	220	10	2
TAKE-OUT				
fried	½ cup (7.5 oz)	176	11	6
rings breaded & fried	8 to 9	275	16	7
OPOSSUM				
roasted	3 oz	188	9	–

FOOD	PORTION	CALS	FAT	SAT FAT
ORANGE				
CANNED				
Del Monte				
Mandarin In Light Syrup	½ cup (4.5 oz)	80	0	0
Dole				
FruitBowls Mandarin Oranges	1 pkg (4 oz)	70	0	0
FRESH				
california navel	1	65	tr	tr
california valencia	1	59	tr	tr
florida	1	69	tr	tr
peel	1 tbsp	6	tr	tr
sections	1 cup	85	tr	tr
ORANGE EXTRACT				
Virginia Dare				
Extract	1 tsp	22	0	–
ORANGE JUICE				
canned	1 cup	104	tr	tr
chilled	1 cup	110	1	tr
fresh	1 cup	111	tr	tr
frzn as prep	1 cup	112	tr	tr
frzn not prep	6 oz	339	tr	tr
mandarin orange	7 oz	94	tr	–
orange drink	6 oz	94	0	0
After The Fall				
Juice	1 bottle (10 oz)	110	0	0
Orange Icicle Cream	1 can (12 oz)	170	0	0
Big Juicy				
Drink	8 oz	110	0	0
Capri Sun				
Drink	1 pkg (7 oz)	100	0	0
Everfresh				
Juice	1 can (8 oz)	100	0	0
Ruby Red Orange Drink	1 can (8 oz)	130	0	0
Fresh Samantha				
Juice	1 cup (8 oz)	100	0	0
Hood				
From Concentrate	1 cup (8 oz)	120	0	0
Select	1 cup (8 oz)	120	0	0
With Calcium	1 cup (8 oz)	120	0	0

FOOD	PORTION	CALS	FAT	SAT FAT
Horizon Organic				
Juice Pulp Free	8 fl oz	110	0	0
Juicy Juice				
Punch	1 box (4.23 oz)	60	0	0
Punch	1 box (8.45 oz)	130	0	0
Kool-Aid				
Drink Mix Orange as prep	1 serv (8 oz)	60	0	0
Orange Drink as prep w/ sugar	1 serv (8 oz)	100	0	0
Minute Maid				
Original	8 fl oz	110	0	0
Original Calcium + Vitamin D	8 oz	110	0	0
Plus Calcium	8 fl oz	110	0	0
Simply Orange 100%	8 fl oz	110	0	0
Simply Orange Calcium Fortified	8 fl oz	110	0	0
Simply Orange Grove Made	8 fl oz	110	0	0
Mott's				
100% Juice	1 box (8 oz)	130	0	0
100% Juice	8 fl oz	130	0	0
Nantucket Nectars				
100% Juice	8 oz	120	0	0
NutraShake				
Fortified	1 pkg (4 oz)	50	0	0
Ocean Spray				
100% Juice	8 oz	120	0	0
Odwalla				
Organic	8 fl oz	110	0	0
Shasta Plus				
Orange Drink	1 can (11.5 oz)	160	0	0
Simply Orange				
Pulp Free w/ Calcium	8 oz	110	0	0
Snapple				
Juice	10 fl oz	130	0	0
Orangeade	8 fl oz	120	0	0
Squeezit				
Smarty Arty Orange	1 bottle (7 oz)	110	0	0
Tang				
Orange Drink as prep	1 serv (8 oz)	90	0	0
Sugar Free Orange as prep	1 serv (8 oz)	5	0	0

FOOD	PORTION	CALS	FAT	SAT FAT
Tropicana				
Double Vitamin C	8 fl oz	110	0	0
Light'N Healthy	8 oz	70	0	0
Original No Pulp	8 oz	110	0	0
Ruby Red	8 oz	110	0	0
Season's Best	8 oz	110	0	0
Season's Best Homestyle	8 fl oz	110	0	0
With Calcium + Vitamin D	8 oz	110	0	0
Turkey Hill				
Orangeade	1 cup	120	0	0
Veryfine				
100% Juice	1 bottle (10 oz)	150	0	0
Chillers Arctic Orange	8 fl oz	130	0	0
Juice Blend	1 can (11.5 oz)	160	0	0
Juice-Ups Orange Punch	8 fl oz	140	0	0
Orange Drink	1 bottle (10 oz)	160	0	0
TAKE-OUT				
orange julius	1 serv (24 oz)	443	tr	tr

OREGANO

ground	1 tsp	5	tr	tr
Watkins				
Liquid Spice	1 tbsp (0.5 oz)	120	14	2

ORGAN MEATS (see BRAINS, GIBLETS, GIZZARD, HEART, KIDNEY, LIVER, SWEETBREADS)

OSTRICH

cooked	3 oz	120	3	–

OYSTERS

canned eastern	3 oz	58	2	1
canned eastern	1 cup	170	6	2
eastern cooked	6 med	58	2	1
eastern cooked	3 oz	117	4	1
eastern raw	6 med	58	2	1
eastern raw	1 cup	170	6	2
pacific raw	1 med	41	1	tr
pacific raw	3 oz	69	2	tr
steamed	3 oz	138	4	1
steamed	1 med	41	1	tr

FOOD	PORTION	CALS	FAT	SAT FAT
Bumble Bee				
Fancy Whole	2 oz	70	3	1
Smoked	½ can (1.9 oz)	120	7	2
TAKE-OUT				
breaded & fried	6 (4.9 oz)	368	18	5
oysters rockefeller	3 oysters	66	2	–
stew	1 cup	278	18	10
PANCAKE/WAFFLE SYRUP				
low calorie	1 tbsp	12	0	0
maple	1 tbsp (0.8 oz)	52	0	–
maple	1 cup (11.1 oz)	824	1	–
pancake syrup	1 tbsp (0.7 oz)	57	0	0
pancake syrup	1 cup (11 oz)	903	0	0
pancake syrup light	1 oz	46	0	–
pancake syrup w/ butter	1 cup (11 oz)	933	5	3
pancake syrup w/ butter	1 tbsp (0.7 oz)	59	tr	tr
Atkins				
Sugar Free	¼ cup	0	0	0
Aunt Jemima				
Butter Rich	¼ cup (2.8 oz)	210	0	0
Butterlite	¼ cup (2.5 oz)	100	0	0
Lite	¼ cup (2.5 oz)	100	0	0
Original	¼ cup	210	0	0
Country Cupboard				
Boysenberry	¼ cup	0	0	0
Maple Butter	¼ cup	0	0	0
Strawberry	¼ cup	0	0	0
Estee				
Maple	¼ cup	80	0	0
Keto				
Maple Butter	¼ cup	0	0	0
Ketogenics				
Zero Carb	¼ cup	0	0	0
Log Cabin				
Original	¼ cup	210	0	0
Mrs. Butterworth's				
Lite	¼ cup	100	0	0
Original	¼ cup (2 oz)	230	0	0

FOOD	PORTION	CALS	FAT	SAT FAT
Mrs.Richardson's				
Lite	¼ cup (2.5 oz)	100	0	0
Original Recipe	¼ cup (2.8 oz)	210	0	0
Red Wing				
Lite	¼ cup (2 oz)	100	0	0
Syrup	¼ cup (2 oz)	210	0	0
Smucker's				
Breakfast Syrup Sugar Free	¼ cup (2 oz)	30	0	0
Stonewall Kitchen				
Maine Maple	¼ cup	210	0	0
PANCAKES				
FROZEN				
buttermilk	1 4 in diam	83	1	tr
plain	1 4 in diam	83	1	tr
Aunt Jemima				
Blueberry	3 (3.4 oz)	210	4	1
Buttermilk	3 (3 oz)	180	3	1
Lowfat	3 (3.4 oz)	130	2	0
Original	3 (3.4 oz)	200	3	1
Eggo				
Buttermilk	3 (4.1 oz)	270	8	2
Jimmy Dean				
Flapstick	1 (2.5 oz)	240	14	4
Flapstick Blueberry	1 (2.5 oz)	260	15	4
MIX				
buckwheat	1 (4 in diam)	62	2	1
buttermilk	1 (4 in diam)	74	1	tr
plain	1 (4 in diam)	74	1	tr
sugar free low sodium	1 (3 in diam)	44	tr	tr
whole wheat	1 (4 in diam)	92	3	1
Atkins				
Quick Quisine Buttermilk not prep	⅓ cup	100	0	0
Quick Quisine Original not prep	¼ cup	80	2	1
Aunt Jemima				
Buckwheat Pancake & Waffle Mix	¼ cup (1.4 oz)	120	1	0
Buttermilk Pancake & Waffle Mix	⅓ cup (1.9 oz)	190	2	1
Original Pancake & Waffle Mix	⅓ cup (1.6 oz)	150	1	0
Pancake & Waffle Mix Regular	⅓ cup (1.9 oz)	190	2	1
Pancake & Waffle Mix Whole Wheat	¼ cup (1.4 oz)	130	1	0

FOOD	PORTION	CALS	FAT	SAT FAT
Aunt Paula's				
Pancake & Waffle Mix as prep	2	132	8	—
Betty Crocker				
Buttermilk as prep	3	200	3	1
Original as prep	3	200	3	1
Bisquick				
Shake 'N Pour Blueberry as prep	3	210	4	1
Bruce				
Sweet Potato Pancakes	2	210	3	1
Carbolite				
Low Carb Mix not prep	⅓ cup	100	tr	—
Carbsense				
Buckwheat not prep	½ cup	140	3	0
Buttermilk not prep	½ cup	140	3	0
Estee				
Pancake Mix as prep	4 (4 in diam)	180	0	0
Hodgson Mill				
Buckwheat	⅓ cup (1.8 oz)	160	1	0
Hungry Jack				
Potato as prep	3 (3 in diam)	90	2	0
Keto				
Banana not prep	⅓ cup	114	2	—
Original not prep	⅓ cup	114	2	—
Ketogenics				
Low Carb not prep	⅔ cup	185	4	2
MiniCarb				
Apple Cinnamon as prep	2	150	6	1
Robin Hood				
Buttermilk as prep	3	230	6	2
Stone-Buhr				
Buckwheat	¼ cup (1.4 oz)	130	1	0
Oat Bran	¼ cup (1.4 oz)	130	0	0
Whole Wheat	¼ cup (1.4 oz)	120	1	0
Wanda's				
Blue Corn	⅓ cup mix per serv (1.7 oz)	170	2	0
TAKE-OUT				
blueberry	1 (4 in diam)	84	4	1
plain	1 (4 in diam)	86	4	1
potato	1 (4 in diam)	78	6	1

FOOD	PORTION	CALS	FAT	SAT FAT
w/ butter & syrup	2 (8.1 oz)	520	14	6
PAPAYA				
fresh	1	117	tr	tr
fresh cubed	1 cup	54	tr	tr
Sonoma				
Dried Pieces	2 pieces (2 oz)	200	4	0
SunFresh				
In Extra Light Syrup	½ cup (4.5 oz)	70	0	0
PAPAYA JUICE				
nectar	1 cup	142	tr	tr
Everfresh				
Premium Drink	1 can (8 oz)	140	0	0
Nantucket Nectars				
Cocktail	8 oz	120	0	0
PAPRIKA				
paprika	1 tsp	6	tr	tr
Watkins				
Ground	¼ tsp (0.5 oz)	0	0	0
PARSLEY				
dry	1 tsp	1	tr	–
dry	1 tbsp	1	tr	–
fresh chopped	½ cup	11	tr	tr
PARSNIPS				
fresh cooked	1 (5.6 oz)	130	tr	tr
fresh sliced cooked	½ cup	63	tr	tr
raw sliced	½ cup	50	tr	tr
PASSION FRUIT				
purple fresh	1	18	tr	–
PASSION FRUIT JUICE				
purple	1 cup	126	tr	–
yellow	1 cup	149	tr	–
Snapple				
Passion Supreme	10 fl oz	160	0	0
PASTA (see also NOODLES, PASTA DINNERS, PASTA SALAD)				
DRY				
corn cooked	1 cup (4.9 oz)	176	1	tr

FOOD	PORTION	CALS	FAT	SAT FAT
corn spaghetti	2 oz	180	2	0
elbows	1 cup	389	2	tr
elbows cooked	1 cup (4.9 oz)	197	1	tr
shells small cooked	1 cup (4 oz)	162	1	tr
shells small protein fortified cooked	1 cup (4 oz)	189	tr	tr
spaghetti cooked	1 cup (4.9 oz)	197	1	tr
spaghetti protein fortified cooked	1 cup (4.9 oz)	230	tr	tr
spinach spaghetti cooked	1 cup (4.9 oz)	182	1	tr
spirals cooked	1 cup (4.7 oz)	189	tr	tr
vegetable cooked	1 cup (4.7 oz)	172	tr	tr
whole wheat cooked	1 cup (4.9 oz)	174	tr	tr
whole wheat spaghetti cooked	1 cup (4.9 oz)	174	1	tr
Annie Chun's				
Soba Noodles	2 oz	200	1	0
Atkins				
All Shapes not prep	2 oz	230	3	0
Quick Quisine All Shapes as prep	¾ cup	210	3	1
Barilla				
Conchiglie Rigate	1 cup (2 oz)	200	1	0
Gemelli as prep	1 cup (2 oz)	200	1	0
Pennette Rigate	1⅓ cups (2 oz)	200	1	0
Tortelloni Porcini Mushroom	¾ cup	240	8	5
Tortelloni Ricotta & Asparagus	¾ cup	240	8	5
Tortelloni Ricotta & Spinach	¾ cup	220	8	5
Bella Vita				
Low Carb Penne Rigate	2 oz	190	1	0
Classico				
Gnocchi Di Toscana	1 cup (2 oz)	210	1	0
Cuore				
Capellini cooked	1⅓ cups (2 oz)	190	1	0
Fusilli cooked	1⅓ cups (2 oz)	190	1	0
Tortiglioni cooked	1⅓ cups (2 oz)	190	1	0
DaVinci				
Rotini	1 cup	210	1	0
Spaghetti	2 oz	210	1	0
Darielle				
All Shapes not prep	2 oz	160	1	0
De Bole's				
Whole Wheat Organic Elbows	2 oz	210	2	0

FOOD	PORTION	CALS	FAT	SAT FAT
DeCecco				
Whole Wheat Linguine cooked	2 oz	180	2	0
Duc Amici				
Pasta Lite Low Carb Fusilli	2 oz	160	1	0
Eden				
Organic Extra Fine	2 oz	210	2	0
Organic Gemelli	2 oz	210	2	0
Organic Pesto Gemelli	2 oz	210	1	0
Organic Ribbons Saffron	2 oz	210	2	0
Organic Spaghetti Semolina	2 oz	200	1	0
Organic Spaghetti 50% Whole Grain	2 oz	210	1	0
Organic Spirals Kamut Vegetable	2 oz	210	2	0
Organic Spirals Sesame Rice	2 oz	200	2	0
Organic Spirals Mixed Grain	2 oz	210	2	0
Organic Spirals Spinach	2 oz	210	1	0
Organic Vegetable Alphabets	2 oz	200	1	0
Spirals Rye	2 oz	200	0	0
Goya				
Coditos not prep	½ cup	230	1	0
Hodgson Mill				
Four Color Veggie Bows	2 oz	200	1	0
Four Color Veggie Rotini Spirals	2 oz	200	1	0
Pastamania! Durum Wheat Fettuccine	2 oz	200	2	1
Pastamania! Fettuccine Garlic & Parsley	2 oz	200	2	1
Pastamania! Fettuccine w/ Jerusalem Artichoke	2 oz	210	2	0
Pastamania! Fettuccine w/ Mushroom	2 oz	210	2	1
Pastamania! Fusilli Tre Colore w/ Tomato & Spinach	2 oz	200	1	0
Pastamania! Sea Shell Mix	2 oz	200	1	0
Pastamania! Spinach Fettuccine	2 oz	200	2	1
Pastamania! Thin Linguine	2 oz	200	2	1
Pastamania! Tomato Spinach & Durum Wheat	2 oz	210	2	1
Spaghetti Whole Wheat not prep	2 oz	190	0	0
Whole Wheat Lasagne not prep	2 oz	190	0	0
Whole Wheat Spinach Spaghetti not prep	2 oz	190	1	0

FOOD	PORTION	CALS	FAT	SAT FAT
Keto				
Elbows not prep	1.6 oz	108	0	0
Spaghetti not prep	1.3 oz	130	1	0
Lundberg				
Spaghetti Organic Brown Rice	2 oz	210	2	1
Lupini				
Elbow uncooked	½ cup (2 oz)	190	2	0
Spaghetti Light uncooked	½ cup (2 oz)	190	2	0
Spaghetti With Triticale	½ pkg (2 oz)	190	3	1
Pastalia				
Heart Health Low Carb not prep	2 oz	176	2	–
Pritikin				
Spaghetti Whole Wheat	⅛ box (2 oz)	190	1	0
Spiral	⅔ cup (2 oz)	190	1	0
Real Torino				
Tirali not prep	1 cup (2 oz)	210	1	0
Revival				
Soy Penne	⅛ box	200	2	0
Soy Thin Spaghetti	⅛ box	200	2	0
Ronzoni				
Elbows not prep	½ cup (2 oz)	210	1	0
Lasagne	2½ pieces (2 oz)	210	1	0
Tradizione D'Italia All Shapes	2 oz	210	1	0
San Giorgio				
Healthy Harvest Whole Wheat Blend	2 oz	210	2	0
Soy7				
Pasta All Shapes	2 oz	200	1	0
Whey Cool				
High Protein Xtreme Rotini	1 serv (2 oz)	210	2	0
FRESH				
cooked	2 oz	75	1	tr
spinach cooked	2 oz	74	1	tr
Di Giorno				
Angel's Hair	1 cup	160	2	0
Beef & Roasted Garlic Tortellini	1 cup	340	11	4
Fettuccine	1 cup	200	2	0
Four Cheese Raviolo	1 cup	350	15	9
Herb Linguine	1 cup	200	2	0
Italian Sausage Ravioli In Green Bell Pepper Pasta	1¼ cups	350	12	6

FOOD	PORTION	CALS	FAT	SAT FAT
Lemon Chicken Tortellini In Cracked Black Pepper Pasta	1 cup	270	5	3
Light Cheese Ravioli	1 cup	280	7	4
Linguine	1 cup	200	2	0
Mozzarella Garlic Tortellini	1 cup	300	8	5
Pesto Tortellini	1 cup	320	8	5
Portabello Mushroom Tortellini	1 cup	310	7	5
Red Bell Pepper Fettuccine	1 cup	200	2	0
Spinach Fettuccine	1 cup	190	2	0
Sun-Dried Tomato Ravioli	1⅓ cups	380	14	8
Three Cheese Tortellini	¾ cup	250	7	4
Trios				
Ravioli Cracked Pepper Garlic Cheese	1 cup (4.3 oz)	340	9	5

PASTA DINNERS (see also PASTA SALAD)
CANNED
Chef Boyardee

FOOD	PORTION	CALS	FAT	SAT FAT
99% Fat Free Beef Ravioli	1 cup (8.6 oz)	210	1	0
99% Fat Free Cheese Ravioli	1 cup (8.8 oz)	210	1	0
Beef Ravioli	1 cup (8.6 oz)	230	5	3
Beefaroni	1 cup (8.7 oz)	260	7	3
Macaroni & Cheese	½ can (7.5 oz)	180	2	–
Mini Ravioli	1 cup (8.8 oz)	252	6	3
Spaghetti & Meat Balls	1 cup (8.4 oz)	240	10	4
Tortellini Cheese	½ can (7 oz)	230	1	–
Tortellini Meat	½ can (7 oz)	260	4	2
Franco-American				
Beef Raviolios	1 can (7.7 oz)	250	5	2
Beefy Mac	1 can (7.5 oz)	228	8	3
Elbow Macaroni & Cheese	1 can (7.5 oz)	187	6	3
Spaghetti 'N Beef	1 can (7.5 oz)	226	8	4
Spaghetti w/ Meatballs	1 can (7.2 oz)	249	9	4
Kid's Kitchen				
Microwave Meals Cheezy Mac & Beef	1 cup (7.5 oz)	260	7	3
Microwave Meals Noodle Rings & Chicken	1 cup (7.5 oz)	150	4	2
Microwave Meals Spaghetti Rings & Franks	1 cup (7.5 oz)	240	9	4

FOOD	PORTION	CALS	FAT	SAT FAT
Progresso				
Beef Ravioli	1 cup (9.1 oz)	260	5	2
Cheese Ravioli	1 cup (9.1 oz)	220	2	1
FROZEN				
Amy's				
Bowl Stuffed Pasta Shells	1 pkg (10 oz)	300	12	7
Cannelloni w/ Vegetables	1 pkg (9 oz)	330	12	8
Lasagna Cheese	1 pkg (10.25 oz)	330	12	7
Lasagna Garden Vegetable	1 pkg (10.25 oz)	290	9	4
Macaroni & Cheese	1 pkg (9 oz)	410	16	10
Macaroni & Soy Cheese	1 pkg (9 oz)	370	15	2
Pasta & Vegetable Alfredo	1 cup	220	8	4
Pasta Primavera	1 pkg (9 oz)	300	11	6
Ravioli w/ Sauce	1 pkg (8 oz)	340	12	5
Rice Mac & Cheese	1 pkg (9 oz)	140	16	10
Skillet Meals	1 cup	250	11	3
Tofu Vegetable Lasagna	1 pkg (9.5 oz)	300	10	2
Vegetable Lasagna	1 pkg (9.5 oz)	280	12	5
Banquet				
Chicken Pasta Primavera	1 meal (9.5 oz)	320	12	6
Family Size Egg Noodles w/ Beef & Brown Gravy	1 serv	150	5	3
Family Size Lasagna w/ Meat Sauce	1 cup	270	10	6
Family Size Macaroni & Cheese	1 cup	230	7	3
Fettuccine Alfredo	1 meal (9.5 oz)	350	16	7
Homestyle Noodles & Chicken	1 meal (12 oz)	390	19	7
Lasagna w/ Meat Sauce	1 meal (9.5 oz)	260	8	3
Macaroni & Cheese	1 meal (12 oz)	420	14	8
Birds Eye				
Easy Recipe Creations Basil Herb Primavera	2¼ cups	260	11	7
Easy Recipe Creations Tortellini Parmigiana	2¼ cups	240	12	7
Pasta Secrets Italian Pesto	2⅓ cups	240	9	2
Pasta Secrets Primavera	2⅓ cups	230	10	3
Pasta Secrets Ranch	2⅓ cups	300	15	6
Pasta Secrets Three Cheese	2 cups	230	8	3
Pasta Secrets White Cheddar	2 cups	240	10	3
Pasta Secrets Zesty Garlic	2 cups	240	10	3

FOOD	PORTION	CALS	FAT	SAT FAT
Green Giant				
Create A Meal Creamy Alfredo as prep	1¼ cups (10 oz)	380	12	5
Create A Meal Creamy Cheddar as prep	1½ cups (10 oz)	290	10	6
Create A Meal Creamy Chicken Noodle as prep	1¼ cups (10 oz)	350	11	5
Pasta Accents Alfredo	2 cups (5.6 oz)	210	5	3
Pasta Accents Creamy Cheddar	2⅓ cups (6.7 oz)	250	8	3
Pasta Accents Florentine	2 cups (7.3 oz)	310	9	3
Pasta Accents Garden Herb Seasoning	2 cups (6.8 oz)	230	7	4
Pasta Accents Garlic Seasoning	2 cups (6.6 oz)	260	10	5
Pasta Accents Primavera	2¼ cups (7 oz)	320	12	5
Pasta Accents White Cheddar Sauce	1¾ cups (5.6 oz)	300	12	4
Healthy Choice				
Beef Macaroni	1 meal (8.5 oz)	220	4	2
Bowls Cheese & Chicken Tortellini	1 meal (8.7 oz)	250	5	2
Breaded Chicken Breast Strips w/ Macaroni & Cheese	1 meal (8 oz)	270	5	3
Cheese Ravioli Parmigiana	1 meal (9 oz)	260	5	3
Chicken Fettuccine Alfredo	1 meal (8.5 oz)	280	7	3
Fettuccine Alfredo	1 meal (8 oz)	240	5	3
Lasagna Roma	1 meal (13.5 oz)	420	9	3
Macaroni & Cheese	1 meal (9 oz)	240	5	3
Manicotti w/ Three Cheeses	1 meal (11 oz)	300	9	3
Spaghetti & Sauce w/ Seasoned Beef	1 meal (10 oz)	260	8	2
Stuffed Pasta Shells	1 meal (10.35 oz)	370	6	3
Joseph's Pasta				
Grilled Chicken Ravioli w/ Roasted Red Pepper Sauce	1 pkg (14 oz)	540	15	8
Kid Cuisine				
Magical Macaroni & Cheese	1 meal (10.6 oz)	440	13	5
Lean Cuisine				
Cafe Classics Bow Tie Pasta & Chicken	1 pkg (9.5 oz)	220	4	1
Cafe Classics Cheese Lasagna w/ Chicken Scaloppini	1 pkg (10 oz)	270	8	3
Cafe Classics Shrimp & Angel Hair Pasta	1 pkg (10 oz)	240	5	1
Everyday Favorites Alfredo Pasta Primavera	1 pkg (10 oz)	290	7	3

FOOD	PORTION	CALS	FAT	SAT FAT
Everyday Favorites Angel Hair Pasta	1 pkg (10 oz)	240	4	1
Everyday Favorites Cheese Cannelloni	1 pkg (9.1 oz)	230	4	2
Everyday Favorites Cheese Lasagna Casserole	1 pkg (10 oz)	270	6	3
Everyday Favorites Cheese Ravioli	1 pkg (8.5 oz)	260	7	4
Everyday Favorites Chicken Lasagna	1 pkg (10 oz)	280	7	3
Everyday Favorites Classic Cheese Lasagna	1 pkg (11.5 oz)	290	6	4
Everyday Favorites Fettucini Alfredo	1 pkg (9.25 oz)	280	7	3
Everyday Favorites Fettucini Primavera	1 pkg (10 oz)	270	7	3
Everyday Favorites Lasagna w/ Meat Sauce	1 pkg (10.5 oz)	300	8	5
Everyday Favorites Macaroni & Cheese	1 pkg (10 oz)	290	7	4
Everyday Favorites Macaroni & Beef	1 pkg (10 oz)	270	4	2
Everyday Favorites Penne Pasta	1 pkg (10 oz)	260	4	1
Everyday Favorites Spaghetti w/ Meat Sauce	1 pkg (11.5 oz)	290	5	2
Everyday Favorites Spaghetti w/ Meatballs	1 pkg (9.5 oz)	270	6	3
Family Style Favorites Five Cheese Lasagna	1 serv (8 oz)	210	5	3
Skillet Sensations Chicken Alfredo	1 serv	280	6	4
Luigino's				
Cheese Ravioli & Alfredo With Broccoli Sauce	1 pkg (8.5 oz)	420	25	13
Cheese Tortellini & Alfredo Sauce With Broccoli	1 pkg (8 oz)	390	24	12
Fettuccine Alfredo	1 cup (7.5 oz)	330	11	4
Fettuccine Alfredo	1 pkg (9.4 oz)	390	14	5
Fettuccine Alfredo With Broccoli	1 pkg (9.2 oz)	360	16	8
Fettuccine Carbonara	1 pkg (9 oz)	360	13	4
Lasagna Alfredo	1 cup (6.3 oz)	300	17	5
Lasagna Alfredo	1 pkg (9 oz)	360	20	6
Lasagna Pollo	1 pkg (9 oz)	320	14	5
Lasagna With Meat Sauce	1 pkg (9 oz)	290	10	4
Lasagna With Meat Sauce	1 cup (7.2 oz)	240	8	3
Lasagna With Vegetables	1 pkg (9 oz)	290	10	3
Linguini With Clams & Sauce	1 pkg (9 oz)	270	6	2
Linguini With Red Sauce	1 pkg (9 oz)	260	6	1
Linguini With Seafood	1 pkg (9 oz)	290	8	2

FOOD	PORTION	CALS	FAT	SAT FAT
Macaroni & Cheese	1 pkg (9 oz)	370	15	6
Macaroni & Cheese	1 cup (7.2 oz)	310	12	7
Marinara Sauce Penne Pasta Italian Sausage & Peppers	1 cup (7.4 oz)	290	14	3
Marinara Sauce Penne Pasta Italian Sausage & Peppers	1 pkg (9 oz)	350	17	4
Meat Ravioli & Pomodoro Sauce	1 pkg (8.5 oz)	320	13	5
Minestrone With Penne Pasta	1 cup (6.3 oz)	180	6	1
Penne Pollo	1 pkg (9 oz)	330	14	5
Penne Primavera	1 pkg (9 oz)	350	10	4
Rigatoni Pomodoro Italiano	1 pkg (9 oz)	290	8	2
Shells & Cheese With Jalapenos	1 pkg (8.5 oz)	360	15	6
Spaghetti Bolognese	1 pkg (9 oz)	270	8	3
Spaghetti Marinara	1 pkg (10 oz)	250	2	1
Spinach Ravioli & Primavera Sauce	1 pkg (8.5 oz)	360	17	8
Marie Callender's				
Cheese Ravioli In Marinara Sauce w/ Spirals & Garlic Bread	1 meal (16 oz)	750	29	9
Extra Cheese Lasagna	1 meal (15 oz)	590	27	13
Fettuccine Alfredo & Garlic Bread	1 meal (14 oz)	920	55	23
Fettuccine Alfredo Supreme	1 meal (13 oz)	450	27	12
Fettuccine Primavera w/ Tortellini	1 meal (14 oz)	750	49	21
Fettuccine w/ Broccoli & Chicken	1 meal (13 oz)	710	43	17
Lasagna w/ Meat Sauce	1 meal (15 oz)	630	31	15
Macaroni & Cheese	1 meal (12 oz)	540	24	15
Skillet Meal Chicken Alfredo	½ pkg	490	29	14
Skillet Meal Penne Pasta & Meatballs	½ pkg	600	31	11
Skillet Meal Rigatoni Vegetables In Cheese Sauce	1 cup	290	12	7
Spaghetti w/ Meat Sauce & Garlic Bread	1 meal (17 oz)	670	25	11
Stuffed Pasta Trio	1 meal (10.5 oz)	380	16	9
Morton				
Macaroni & Cheese	1 serv (8 oz)	240	8	4
Spaghetti w/ Meat Sauce	1 meal (8.5 oz)	200	6	3
Quorn				
Fettuccine Alfredo	1 pkg (10.5 oz)	360	16	9
Lasagna	1 pkg (10.5 oz)	360	12	4
Seeds Of Change				
Organic Lasagna Creamy Spinach	1 pkg (11 oz)	370	16	11

FOOD	PORTION	CALS	FAT	SAT FAT
Senor Felix's				
Lasagna Southwestern	1 serv (6 oz)	160	7	4
Slim-Fast				
Fettuccine Alfredo	1 pkg	240	6	3
Rotini w/ Tomato & Italian Herb	1 pkg	240	2	1
Shells & Creamy Cheese Sauce	1 pkg	240	6	3
Stouffer's				
Cheddar Pasta w/ Beef & Tomatoes	1 pkg (11 oz)	450	19	10
Cheese Manicotti	1 pkg (9 oz)	380	17	9
Cheese Ravioli	1 pkg (10.6 oz)	380	13	6
Chicken Lasagna	1 serv (7.8 oz)	320	17	5
Fettucini Alfredo	1 pkg (10 oz)	520	28	16
Fettucini Primavera	1 pkg (10 oz)	430	20	12
Five Cheese Lasagna	1 pkg (10.75 oz)	360	13	7
Grilled Chicken & Angel Hair Pasta	1 pkg (10.9 oz)	380	13	4
Homestyle Chicken Fettucini	1 pkg (10.5 oz)	390	15	4
Homestyle Chicken Parmigiana w/ Spaghetti	1 pkg (12 oz)	460	16	4
Homestyle Veal Parmigiana w/ Spaghetti	1 pkg (11.9 oz)	430	17	5
Lasagna Bake	1 pkg (10.25 oz)	370	12	5
Lasagna w/ Meat Sauce	1 pkg (10.5 oz)	370	14	7
Macaroni & Cheese	1 cup (6 oz)	320	16	7
Macaroni & Cheese w/ Broccoli	1 pkg (10.5 oz)	360	17	8
Macaroni & Beef	1 pkg (11.5 oz)	420	20	8
Noodles Romanoff	1 pkg (12 oz)	490	25	6
Pasta Shells w/ American Cheese	1 cup (6 oz)	260	10	4
Salisbury Steak w/ Macaroni & Cheese	1 serv (11.3 oz)	410	19	8
Spaghetti w/ Meat Sauce	1 pkg (10 oz)	350	12	4
Spaghetti w/ Meatballs	1 pkg (12.6 oz)	440	15	5
Tuna Noodle Casserole	1 pkg (10 oz)	320	10	4
Turkey Tettrazini	1 pkg (10 oz)	360	17	7
Vegetable Lasagna	1 pkg (10.5 oz)	440	20	8
Tabatchnick				
Macaroni & Cheese	7.5 oz	280	12	6
Weight Watchers				
Garden Lasagna	1 pkg (11 oz)	270	7	4
Homestyle Macaroni & Cheese	1 pkg (9 oz)	290	7	3
Smart Ones Angel Hair Pasta	1 pkg (9 oz)	180	2	0

FOOD	PORTION	CALS	FAT	SAT FAT
Smart Ones Bowtie Pasta & Mushrooms Marsala	1 pkg (9.65 oz)	270	7	4
Smart Ones Chicken Fettucini	1 pkg (10 oz)	300	7	2
Smart Ones Creamy Rigatoni w/ Broccoli & Chicken	1 pkg (9 oz)	230	2	1
Smart Ones Fettucini Alfredo w/ Broccoli	1 pkg (8.5 oz)	230	6	4
Smart Ones Lasagna Florentine	1 pkg (10 oz)	200	2	0
Smart Ones Lasagna Alfredo	1 pkg (9 oz)	300	7	4
Smart Ones Lasagna w/ Meat Sauce	1 pkg (9 oz)	240	2	1
Smart Ones Lasagna w/ Meat Sauce	1 pkg (10.25 oz)	270	6	4
Smart Ones Macaroni & Cheese	1 pkg (9 oz)	220	2	1
Smart Ones Pasta & Spinach Romano	1 pkg (10.4 oz)	260	8	3
Smart Ones Pasta w/ Tomato Basil Sauce	1 pkg (9.6 oz)	260	7	3
Smart Ones Penne Pasta w/ Sun-Dried Tomatoes	1 pkg (10 oz)	280	8	5
Smart Ones Penne Pollo	1 pkg (10 oz)	290	6	3
Smart Ones Ravioli Florentine	1 pkg (8.5 oz)	220	2	1
Smart Ones Spaghetti Marinara	1 pkg (9 oz)	280	7	2
Smart Ones Spaghetti w/ Meat Sauce	1 pkg (10 oz)	280	6	2
Smart Ones Spicy Penne & Ricotta	1 pkg (10.2 oz)	280	6	2
Smart Ones Tuna Noodle Casserole	1 pkg (9.5 oz)	270	7	3
Smart Ones Zita Mozzarella	1 pkg (9 oz)	290	7	2
Yves				
Veggie Lasagna	1 pkg (10.5 oz)	300	3	0
Veggie Macaroni	1 pkg (10.5 oz)	230	2	0
Veggie Penne	1 pkg (10.5 oz)	220	2	0
MIX				
Annie's Homegrown				
Mac & Cheese Meals	1 pkg	230	5	3
Aramana				
Cheddar Cheeseburger as prep	1 cup	260	17	10
Creamy Chicken Alfredo as prep	1 cup	260	16	10
Mild Mexican as prep	1 cup	260	16	10
Atkins				
Quick Quisine Elbows & Cheese as prep	1 cup	250	7	2
Quick Quisine Fettuccine Alfredo as prep	1 cup	210	7	3

FOOD	PORTION	CALS	FAT	SAT FAT
Quick Quisine Pesto Cream as prep	1 cup	240	6	2
Casbah				
Pasta Fasul	1 pkg (1.6 oz)	150	1	0
Hamburger Helper				
Ravioli as prep	1 cup	280	10	4
Ravioli w/ White Cheese Topping as prep	1 cup	310	10	4
Hodgson Mill				
Macaroni & Cheese Whole Wheat	1 serv	250	1	1
Keto				
Macaroni & Cheese not prep	1 serv	112	10	—
Kraft				
Deluxe Macaroni & Cheese Four Cheese Blend as prep	1 cup (6.2 oz)	320	10	7
Deluxe Macaroni & Cheese Original as prep	1 cup (6.1 oz)	320	10	6
Light Deluxe Macaroni & Cheese as prep	1 cup (6.5 oz)	290	5	3
Macaroni & Cheese All Shapes as prep	1 cup (6.9 oz)	410	18	5
Macaroni & Cheese Original as prep	1 cup (6.9 oz)	410	18	5
Macaroni & Cheese Original as prep light recipe	1 cup (6.4 oz)	290	6	2
Premium Macaroni & Cheese Cheesy Alfredo as prep	1 cup (6.9 oz)	410	19	5
Premium Macaroni & Cheese Mild White Cheddar as prep	1 cup (6.8 oz)	410	19	4
Premium Macaroni & Cheese Thick 'N Creamy as prep	1 cup (7.6 oz)	420	19	5
Premium Macaroni & Cheese Three Cheese as prep	1 cup (6.9 oz)	410	18	4
Spaghetti Classics Mild Italian as prep	1 cup (9.1 oz)	240	3	1
Spaghetti Classics Tangy Italian as prep	1 cup (8.9 oz)	240	2	1
Spaghetti Classics Zesty Cheese as prep	1 cup (8.6 oz)	240	2	1
Spaghetti Classics w/ Meat Sauce as prep	1 cup (8.2 oz)	330	10	4
Lipton				
Pasta & Sauce Angel Hair Chicken Broccoli as prep	1 cup	260	8	1

FOOD	PORTION	CALS	FAT	SAT FAT
Pasta & Sauce Angel Hair Parmesan as prep	1 cup	280	11	3
Pasta & Sauce Bow Tie Chicken Primavera as prep	1 cup	290	10	4
Pasta & Sauce Bow Tie Italian Cheese as prep	1 cup	300	12	5
Pasta & Sauce Butter & Herbs as prep	1 cup	270	10	3
Pasta & Sauce Cheddar Broccoli as prep	1 cup	340	11	4
Pasta & Sauce Chicken Herb Parmesan as prep	1 cup	80	9	2
Pasta & Sauce Chicken Stir-Fry as prep	1 cup	270	8	1
Pasta & Sauce Creamy Garlic as prep	1 cup	350	13	5
Pasta & Sauce Creamy Mushroom as prep	1 cup	320	11	4
Pasta & Sauce Garlic & Butter Linguine as prep	1 cup	260	9	2
Pasta & Sauce Mild Cheddar Cheese as prep	1 cup	290	10	4
Pasta & Sauce Roasted Garlic Chicken as prep	1 cup	290	10	3
Pasta & Sauce Roasted Garlic & Olive Oil w/ Tomato as prep	1 cup	270	9	2
Pasta & Sauce Rotini Primavera as prep	1 cup	320	12	5
Pasta & Sauce Savory Herb w/ Garlic as prep	1 cup	280	9	3
Pasta & Sauce Three Cheese Rotini as prep	1 cup	320	12	5
Melting Pot				
Terrazza Black Beans & Penne	1 cup	180	1	0
Terrazza Florentine Red Beans & Fusilli	1 cup	220	1	0
Terrazza Red Lentils & Bow Ties	1 cup	240	2	1
Terrazza Tuscan White Beans & Gemell	1 cup	220	1	0
Velveeta				
Rotini & Cheese w/ Broccoli as prep	1 cup (7.2 oz)	400	16	10
Shells & Cheese Bacon as prep	1 cup (6.8 oz)	360	14	8
Shells & Cheese Original as prep	1 cup (6.6 oz)	360	13	8
Shells & Cheese Salsa as prep	1 cup (7.5 oz)	380	14	9

FOOD	PORTION	CALS	FAT	SAT FAT
Whey Cool				
High Protein Macaroni & Cheese as prep	1 serv	260	5	2
READY-TO-EAT				
Tyson				
Rosemary Penne	1 pkg (12.5 oz)	330	5	2
SHELF-STABLE				
Hormel				
Microcup Meals Lasagna	1 cup (7.5 oz)	250	14	7
Microcup Meals Macaroni & Cheese	1 cup (7.5 oz)	260	11	6
Microcup Meals Ravioli w/ Tomato Sauce	1 cup (7.5 oz)	220	6	2
Microcup Meals Spaghetti & Meatballs	1 cup (7.5 oz)	220	7	4
It's Pasta Anytime				
Penne With Tomato Italian Sausage Sauce	1 pkg (15.25 oz)	540	8	1
Kid's Kitchen				
Microwave Meals Beefy Macaroni	1 cup (7.5 oz)	190	6	3
Microwave Meals Macaroni & Cheese	1 cup (7.5 oz)	260	11	6
Microwave Meals Mini Ravioli	1 cup (7.5 oz)	240	7	3
Microwave Meals Spaghetti & Meatballs	1 cup (7.5 oz)	220	7	4
Microwave Meals Spaghetti Rings & Meatballs	1 cup (7.5 oz)	250	7	3
Lunch Bucket				
Beef Ravioli In Tomato Sauce	1 pkg (7.5 oz)	180	4	2
Italian Pasta w/ Chicken	1 pkg (7.5 oz)	130	2	1
Lasagna 'n Meatsauce	1 pkg (7.5 oz)	160	3	2
Light 'n Healthy Pasta 'n Garden Vegetables	1 pkg (7.5 oz)	150	1	—
Macaroni 'n Beef in Meatsauce	1 pkg (7.5 oz)	180	5	2
Macaroni 'n Cheese	1 pkg (7.5 oz)	190	7	5
Pasta 'n Chicken	1 pkg (7.5 oz)	150	5	2
Spaghetti 'n Meatsauce	1 pkg (7.5 oz)	160	3	2
My Own Meal				
Cheese Tortellini	1 pkg (10 oz)	340	10	3
TAKE-OUT				
fettuccini alfredo	1 cup	715	170	36
lasagna	1 piece (2.5 in x 2.5 in)	374	21	11

FOOD	PORTION	CALS	FAT	SAT FAT
lasagna vegetarian	2 cups	720	130	24
macaroni & cheese	1 cup	230	10	5
manicotti	¾ cup (6.4 oz)	273	12	6
ravioli cheese w/ tomato sauce	2 cups	530	0	1
rigatoni w/ sausage sauce	¾ cup	260	12	4
spaghetti w/ clam sauce	1 serv	395	65	9
spaghetti w/ marinara sauce	1 cup	260	0	2
spaghetti w/ meatballs & cheese	1 cup	407	19	6
tortellini cheese w/ tomato sauce	1 cup	470	15	7

PASTA MACHINE MIX
Wanda's

FOOD	PORTION	CALS	FAT	SAT FAT
Dried Tomato	⅓ cup mix per serv (1.9 oz)	202	1	0
Durum & Semolina	⅓ cup mix per serv (1.9 oz)	199	1	0
Semolina Blend	⅓ cup mix per serv (1.9 oz)	202	1	0
Spinach	⅓ cup mix per serv (1.9 oz)	202	1	0
Whole Wheat & Semolina	⅓ cup mix per serv (1.9 oz)	198	1	0

PASTA SALAD
MIX
Kraft

FOOD	PORTION	CALS	FAT	SAT FAT
Herb & Garlic as prep	¾ cup (4.9 oz)	280	14	2
Pasta Salad Classic Ranch w/ Bacon as prep	¾ cup (4.7 oz)	350	22	4
Pasta Salad Creamy Caesar as prep	¾ cup (4.8 oz)	340	21	4
Pasta Salad Garden Primavera as prep	¾ cup (5 oz)	240	8	2
Pasta Salad Italian 97% Fat Free as prep	¾ cup (4.9 oz)	190	2	1
Pasta Salad Parmesan Peppercorn as prep	¾ cup (4.9 oz)	360	23	4

Suddenly Salad

FOOD	PORTION	CALS	FAT	SAT FAT
Classic Pasta	¾ cup	250	8	1
Classic Pasta Reduced Fat Recipe	¾ cup	210	4	1
Garden Italian 98% Fat Free	¾ cup	140	1	0

TAKE-OUT

FOOD	PORTION	CALS	FAT	SAT FAT
elbow macaroni salad	3.5 oz	160	5	2

FOOD	PORTION	CALS	FAT	SAT FAT
italian style pasta salad	3.5 oz	140	7	1
mustard macaroni salad	3.5 oz	190	10	1
pasta salad w/ vegetables	3.5 oz	140	4	3

PATE

antipasto pate	1 can (2.25 oz)	110	9	2
chicken liver canned	1 tbsp (13 g)	109	2	–
duck pate	1 oz	96	8	–
fish pate	1 oz	76	7	–
goose liver smoked canned	1 tbsp (13 g)	60	6	–
liver canned	1 tbsp (13 g)	41	4	–
mushroom anchovy pate	1 can (2.25 oz)	130	11	2
pate foie gras	1 oz	127	13	3
pork pate	1 oz	107	10	4
pork pate en croute	1 oz	91	7	3
rabbit pate	1 oz	66	5	3
salmon pate	1 can (2.25 oz)	140	10	2
shrimp	1 can (2.25 oz)	140	10	2
smoked turkey	1 can (2.25 oz)	170	13	3

PEACH
CANNED

halves in heavy syrup	1 half	60	tr	tr
halves in light syrup	1 half	44	tr	tr
halves juice pack	1 half	34	tr	tr
halves water pack	1 half	18	tr	tr
peachsauce	½ cup	120	0	0
spiced in heavy syrup	1 fruit	66	tr	tr
spiced in heavy syrup	1 cup	180	tr	tr

Del Monte

Fruit Cup Diced Extra Light Syrup	1 pkg (4 oz)	50	0	0
Fruit Cup Diced In Heavy Syrup	1 serv (4 oz)	80	0	0
Fruit Cup Fruit Naturals Diced	1 pkg (4 oz)	50	0	0
Fruit Pleasures Raspberry Flavor	½ cup (4.5 oz)	80	0	0
Fruit To Go Banana Berry Peaches	1 pkg (4 oz)	70	0	0
Fruitrageous Peachy Pie	1 pkg (4 oz)	80	0	0
Fruitrageous Wild Raspberry Flavor	1 pkg (4 oz)	80	0	0
Halves Ginger Flavor	½ cup (4.5 oz)	90	0	0
Halves In Extra Light Syrup	½ cup (4.4 oz)	60	0	0
Halves In Heavy Syrup	½ cup (4.5 oz)	100	0	0
Halves Melba In Heavy Syrup	½ cup (4.5 oz)	100	0	0

FOOD	PORTION	CALS	FAT	SAT FAT
Orchard Select Sliced Cling	½ cup	80	0	0
Slice Fruit Natural	½ cup (4.4 oz)	60	0	0
Sliced In Extra Light Syrup	½ cup (4.4 oz)	60	0	0
Sliced Natural Raspberry Flavor	½ cup (4.4 oz)	80	0	0
Sliced Natural Harvest Spice Flavor	½ cup (4.5 oz)	80	0	0
Whole Spiced In Heavy Syrup	½ cup (4.2 oz)	100	0	0
Dole				
All Natural Yellow Cling Sliced	½ cup	80	0	0
DRIED				
halves	1 cup	383	1	tr
halves	10	311	1	tr
halves cooked w/ sugar	½ cup	139	tr	tr
halves cooked w/o sugar	½ cup	99	tr	tr
Del Monte				
Sun Dried	⅓ cup (1.4 oz)	90	0	0
Sonoma				
Pieces	3-5 pieces (1.4 oz)	120	0	0
FRESH				
peach	1	37	tr	tr
sliced	1 cup	73	tr	tr
Chiquita				
Peach	1 med (3.4 oz)	40	0	0
FROZEN				
slices sweetened	1 cup	235	tr	tr
PEACH JUICE				
nectar	1 cup	134	tr	tr
After The Fall				
Peach Vanilla	1 can (12 oz)	170	0	0
Nantucket Nectars				
The Original	8 oz	120	0	0
Snapple				
Dixie Peach	10 fl oz	140	0	0
PEANUT BUTTER				
chunky	1 cup	1520	129	25
chunky	2 tbsp	188	16	3
chunky w/o salt	2 tbsp	188	16	3
chunky w/o salt	1 cup	1520	129	25

FOOD	PORTION	CALS	FAT	SAT FAT
smooth	1 cup	1517	128	25
smooth	2 tbsp	188	16	3
smooth w/o salt	1 cup	1517	129	25
smooth w/o salt	2 tbsp	188	16	3
Carb Options				
Creamy	2 tbsp	190	17	4
Crazy Richard's				
Natural Creamy	2 tbsp (1.1 oz)	190	16	2
Estee				
Creamy Low Sodium	2 tbsp (1 oz)	190	15	3
Jif				
Apple Cinnamon	2 tbsp (1.3 oz)	200	16	3
Berry Blend	2 tbsp (1.2 oz)	200	17	4
Chocolate Silk	2 tbsp (1.3 oz)	190	15	3
Creamy	2 tbsp (1.1 oz)	190	16	3
Extra Crunchy	2 tbsp (1.1 oz)	190	16	3
Reduced Fat Creamy	2 tbsp (1.3 oz)	190	12	3
Reduced Fat Crunchy	2 tbsp (1.3 oz)	190	12	3
Simply	2 tbsp (1.1 oz)	190	16	3
Maranatha				
Crunchy	2 tbsp	190	16	–
Salted	2 tbsp	190	16	3
P.B.				
Slices	1 slice (1 oz)	170	14	3
Peanut Wonder				
Low Sodium	2 tbsp	100	3	0
Regular	2 tbsp	100	3	0
Red Wing				
Creamy	2 tbsp (1.1 oz)	200	16	3
Crunchy	2 tbsp (1.1 oz)	200	16	3
Reese's				
Peanut Butter Chips	1 tbsp (0.5 oz)	80	4	4
Skippy				
Creamy	2 tbsp	190	16	3
Creamy w/ 2 slices white bread	1 sandwich	340	19	3
Reduced Fat Creamy	2 tbsp	190	12	3
Tropical Source				
Chips Dairy Free	13 pieces (1.5 oz)	80	5	3

FOOD	PORTION	CALS	FAT	SAT FAT
PEANUTS				
chocolate coated	10 (1.4 oz)	208	13	6
chocolate coated	1 cup (5.2 oz)	773	50	22
cooked	½ cup	102	7	1
dry roasted	1 cup	855	73	10
dry roasted w/ salt	30 nuts (1 oz)	170	14	2
At Last!				
Chocolate Covered	1 pkg (0.9 oz)	150	11	5
Estee				
Candy Coated	¼ cup	200	9	4
Frito Lay				
Honey Roasted	1 serv (1.5 oz)	270	21	4
Hot	1 serv (1.1 oz)	190	16	3
Salted	1 oz	200	16	4
Judy's				
Sugar Free Coconut Peanut Brittle	¼ piece (1 oz)	90	5	2
Lance				
Honey Toasted	1 pkg (1⅜ oz)	220	15	3
Roasted	1 pkg (1¼ oz)	190	14	3
Salted	1 pkg (1⅛ oz)	200	15	3
Salted Long Tube	¼ cup (1 oz)	180	14	3
Little Debbie				
Salted	¼ cup (1 oz)	160	14	2
Low Carb Creations				
Soft Peanut Brittle	2 pieces (1 oz)	140	10	2
Pennant				
Oil Roasted	1 oz	170	14	2
Planters				
Cocktail Lightly Salted Oil Roasted	1 oz	170	15	2
Cocktail Oil Roasted	1 oz	170	14	2
Cocktail Unsalted Oil Roasted	1 oz	170	14	2
Dry Roasted	1 oz	160	13	2
Fun Size! Oil Roasted	2 pkg (1 oz)	170	15	2
Heat Hot Spicy Oil Roasted	1 pkg (1.7 oz)	290	25	4
Heat Hot Spicy Oil Roasted	1 pkg (2 oz)	330	29	4
Heat Hot Spicy Oil Roasted	1 oz	160	14	2
Heat Mild Spicy Oil Roasted	1 oz	160	14	2
Honey Roasted	1 oz	160	13	2
Honey Roasted Dry Roasted	1 pkg (1.7 oz)	260	19	3

FOOD	PORTION	CALS	FAT	SAT FAT
Lightly Salted Dry Roasted	1 oz	160	14	2
Lightly Salted Dry Roasted	1 pkg (1.75 oz)	290	25	3
Lightly Salted Oil Roasted	1 pkg (1.8 oz)	300	27	4
Munch'N Go Singles Heat Hot Spicy Oil Roasted	1 pkg (2.5 oz)	410	36	5
Reduced Fat Honey Roasted	⅓ cup (1 oz)	130	7	1
Salted Oil Roasted	1 pkg (1 oz)	170	15	2
Spanish Oil Roasted	1 oz	170	14	3
Spanish Raw	1 oz	150	13	3
Sweet N Crunchy	1 oz	140	7	1
Unsalted Dry Roasted	1 oz	160	14	2
Sweet Delight				
Peanut Roasters	⅓ pkg (1 oz)	160	12	–
Tom's				
Double Coated	1 pkg (1.35 oz)	220	15	6
Toasted	1 pkg (1.4 oz)	240	19	4
Weight Watchers				
Honey Roasted	1 pkg (0.7 oz)	100	5	1
PEAR				
CANNED				
halves in heavy syrup	1 cup	188	tr	tr
halves in heavy syrup	1 half	68	tr	tr
halves in light syrup	1 half	45	tr	tr
halves juice pack	1 cup	123	tr	tr
halves water pack	1 half	22	tr	tr
Del Monte				
Fruit Cup Diced In Heavy Syrup	1 pkg (4 oz)	80	0	0
Fruit Cup Diced Extra Light Syrup	1 pkg (4 oz)	50	0	0
Fruit To Go Peachy Peaches	1 pkg (4 oz)	70	0	0
Halves Fruit Naturals	½ cup (4.4 oz)	60	0	0
Halves In Extra Light Syrup	½ cup (4.4 oz)	60	0	0
Halves In Heavy Syrup	½ cup (4.5 oz)	100	0	0
Orchard Select Sliced Bartlett	½ cup	80	0	0
Sliced In Extra Light Syrup	½ cup (4.5 oz)	60	0	0
DRIED				
halves	10	459	1	tr
halves	1 cup	472	1	tr
halves cooked w/ sugar	½ cup	196	tr	tr
halves cooked w/o sugar	½ cup	163	tr	tr

FOOD	PORTION	CALS	FAT	SAT FAT
Sonoma				
Pieces	3-4 pieces (1.4 oz)	120	0	0
FRESH				
asian	1 (4.3 oz)	51	tr	tr
pear	1	98	1	tr
sliced w/ skin	1 cup	97	1	tr
Chiquita				
Pear	1 med (5.8 oz)	100	1	0
PEAR JUICE				
nectar	1 cup	149	tr	tr
PEAS				
CANNED				
green	½ cup	59	tr	tr
green low sodium	½ cup	59	tr	tr
Del Monte				
Sweet	½ cup (4.4 oz)	60	0	0
Sweet No Salt Added	½ cup (4.4 oz)	60	0	0
Sweet Very Young Small	½ cup (4.4 oz)	60	0	0
Green Giant				
Sweet	½ cup (4.3 oz)	60	0	0
Sweet 50% Less Sodium	½ cup (4.3 oz)	60	0	0
LeSueur				
Early Peas	½ cup (4.2 oz)	60	0	0
Early Peas 50% Less Sodium	½ cup (4.2 oz)	60	0	0
Sweet	½ cup (4.2 oz)	60	0	0
Sweet 50% Less Sodium	½ cup (4.2 oz)	60	0	0
S&W				
Petite	½ cup (4.4 oz)	70	0	0
Small	½ cup (4.4 oz)	70	0	0
Veg-All				
Tender Sweet	½ cup	60	1	0
DRIED				
split cooked	1 cup	231	1	tr
Bascom's				
Yellow Split as prep	½ cup	110	0	0
Hurst				
HamBeens Green Split Peas w/ Ham	1 serv	120	1	0

FOOD	PORTION	CALS	FAT	SAT FAT
FRESH				
green cooked	½ cup	67	tr	tr
green raw	½ cup	58	tr	tr
snap peas cooked	½ cup	34	tr	tr
snap peas raw	½ cup	30	tr	tr
FROZEN				
green cooked	½ cup	63	tr	tr
snap peas cooked	1 pkg (10 oz)	132	1	tr
snap peas cooked	½ cup	42	tr	tr
Birds Eye				
Butter Peas	½ cup	110	1	0
Crowder	½ cup	120	1	0
Field Peas w/ Snaps	⅔ cup	130	1	0
Green	½ cup	70	0	0
Purple Hull Peas	½ cup	110	1	0
Sugar Snap	½ cup	40	0	0
Tiny Tender	¾ cup	40	0	0
Fresh Like				
Garden	3.5 oz	85	1	–
Green Giant				
Butter Sauce	¾ cup (4 oz)	100	2	2
Butter Sauce LeSueur Baby Peas	¾ cup (4 oz)	100	2	2
Harvest Fresh LeSueur Baby Peas	⅔ cup (3.2 oz)	70	0	0
Harvest Fresh Sugar Snap	⅔ cup (3.2 oz)	50	0	0
Harvest Fresh Sweet	⅔ cup (3.3 oz)	60	0	0
LaSueur Baby Sweet	⅔ cup (2.8 oz)	60	0	0
LaSueur Early June	⅔ cup (2.8 oz)	80	0	0
LaSueur Early June w/ Mushrooms	¾ cup (3 oz)	60	0	0
Select Sugar Snap	¾ cup (2.8 oz)	35	0	0
Sweet	⅔ cup (3.1 oz)	70	0	0
La Choy				
Snow Pea Pods	½ pkg (3 oz)	35	2	0
Tree Of Life				
Peas	⅔ cup (3.1 oz)	70	0	0
SHELF-STABLE				
TastyBite				
Agra Peas & Greens	½ pkg (5 oz)	260	14	5
TAKE-OUT				
pea & potato curry	1 serv (7 oz)	284	22	–
pea curry	1 serv (4.4 oz)	438	42	–

FOOD	PORTION	CALS	FAT	SAT FAT
PECANS				
dry roasted	1 oz	187	18	1
dry roasted salted	1 oz	187	18	1
halves dry roasted w/ salt	20 (1 oz)	200	21	2
halves dried	1 cup	721	73	6
oil roasted	1 oz	195	20	2
oil roasted salted	1 oz	195	20	2
Keto				
Chocolate Covered	1 oz	207	19	4
Planters				
Chips	1 pkg (2 oz)	390	40	3
Gold Measure Halves	1 pkg (2 oz)	390	40	3
Halves	1 oz	190	20	2
Honey Roasted	1 oz	180	16	2
Pieces	1 oz	190	20	2
Pieces	1 pkg (2 oz)	390	40	3
Sweet Delights				
Pecan Roasters	⅓ pkg (1 oz)	210	21	2
PECTIN				
powder	¼ pkg (0.4 oz)	39	0	0
powder	1 pkg (1.75 oz)	163	tr	–
Slim Set				
Packet	1 pkg	208	0	0
Powder	1 tbsp	3	0	0
Sure Jell				
For Lower Sugar Recipes	1 tsp (2.8 g)	20	0	0
Fruit Pectin	1 tsp (3.6 g)	20	0	0
PEPEAO				
dried	½ cup	36	tr	–
raw sliced	1 cup	25	tr	–
PEPPER				
black	1 tsp	5	tr	tr
cayenne	1 tsp	6	tr	tr
red	1 tsp	6	tr	tr
white	1 tsp	7	tr	–
McCormick				
Lemon & Pepper Seasoning Salt	¼ tsp	0	0	0

FOOD	PORTION	CALS	FAT	SAT FAT
Watkins				
Black	¼ tbsp (0.5 g)	0	0	0
Cajun	¼ tbsp (0.5 g)	0	0	0
Cracked Black	¼ tbsp (0.5 g)	0	0	0
Dijon	¼ tbsp (0.5 g)	0	0	0
Garlic Peppercorn Blend	¼ tbsp (1 g)	0	0	0
Herb	¼ tbsp (0.5 g)	0	0	0
Italian	¼ tbsp (0.5 g)	0	0	0
Lemon	¼ tbsp (1 g)	0	0	0
Mexican	¼ tbsp (0.5 g)	0	0	0
Red Pepper Flakes	¼ tsp (0.5 oz)	0	0	0
Royal Pepper Blend	¼ tbsp (0.5 g)	0	0	0
PEPPERS				
CANNED				
chili green	1 cup (5.5 oz)	29	tr	tr
chili green hot chopped	½ cup	17	tr	tr
chili red hot	1 (2.6 oz)	18	tr	tr
chili red hot chopped	½ cup	17	tr	tr
green halves	½ cup	13	tr	tr
jalapeno chopped	½ cup	17	tr	tr
red halves	½ cup	13	tr	tr
Chi-Chi's				
Chilies Diced Green	2 tbsp (1.2 oz)	10	0	0
Chilies Green Whole	¾ pepper (1 oz)	10	0	0
Old El Paso				
Green Chiles Chopped	2 tbsp (1 oz)	5	0	0
Green Chilies Chopped	2 tbsp (1 oz)	5	0	0
Green Chilies Whole	1 (1.2 oz)	10	0	0
Jalapenos Pickled	2 (0.9 oz)	5	0	0
Jalapenos Slices	2 tbsp (1.1 oz)	15	0	0
Progresso				
Cherry Sliced & So Hot	2 tbsp (1 oz)	25	2	0
Hot Cherry	1 (1 oz)	10	0	0
Pepper Salad (drained)	2 tbsp (1 oz)	15	1	0
Roasted	1 piece (1 oz)	10	0	0
Sweet Fried w/ Onions	2 tbsp (0.9 oz)	20	2	0
Tuscan	3 (1 oz)	10	0	0
Rosarita				
Chilies Diced Green	2 tbsp (1 oz)	6	tr	0

FOOD	PORTION	CALS	FAT	SAT FAT
Chilies Green Strips	¼ cup (1.2 oz)	5	tr	0
Chilies Whole Green	2 tbsp (1.2 oz)	5	tr	0
Jalapeno Whole w/ Escabeche	¼ cup (1.2 oz)	8	tr	0
Jalapenos Diced	2 tbsp (1 oz)	5	tr	0
Jalapenos Nacho Sliced	2 tbsp (1 oz)	2	tr	0
Vlasic				
Hot Sliced Cherry	1 oz	5	0	0
Jalapeno Sliced	1 oz	10	0	0
Mild Cherry	1 oz	5	0	0
Pepper Rings Hot	1 oz	5	0	0
Pepper Rings Mild	1 oz	5	0	0
DRIED				
ancho	1 (0.6 oz)	48	1	tr
green	1 tbsp	1	tr	tr
pasilla	1 (7 g)	24	1	—
red	1 tbsp	1	tr	tr
FRESH				
banana	1 cup (4.4 oz)	33	1	tr
banana	1 (4 in) (1.2 oz)	9	tr	tr
chili green hot	1	18	tr	tr
chili green hot chopped	½ cup	30	tr	tr
chili red chopped	½ cup	30	tr	tr
chili red hot	1 (1.6 oz)	18	tr	tr
green	1 (2.6 oz)	20	tr	tr
green chopped	½ cup	13	tr	tr
green chopped cooked	½ cup	19	tr	tr
green cooked	1 (2.6 oz)	20	tr	tr
habanero chile	1 tsp	9	tr	—
hungarian	1 (0.9 oz)	8	tr	tr
jalapeno	1 (0.5 oz)	4	tr	tr
jalapeno sliced	1 cup (3.2 oz)	27	1	tr
red	1 (2.6 oz)	20	tr	tr
red chopped	½ cup	13	tr	tr
red chopped cooked	½ cup	19	tr	tr
red cooked	1 (2.6 oz)	20	tr	tr
serrano	1 (6 g)	2	tr	0
serrano chopped	1 cup (3.7 oz)	34	tr	tr
yellow	10 strips	14	tr	—
yellow	1 (6.5 oz)	50	tr	—

FOOD	PORTION	CALS	FAT	SAT FAT
Chiquita				
Pepper	1 med (5.2 oz)	30	0	0
FROZEN				
green chopped	1 oz	6	tr	tr
red chopped	1 oz	6	tr	tr
Birds Eye				
Diced Green	¾ cup	20	0	0
PERCH				
FRESH				
cooked	1 fillet (1.6 oz)	54	1	tr
cooked	3 oz	99	1	tr
ocean perch atlantic cooked	3 oz	103	2	tr
ocean perch atlantic cooked	1 fillet (1.8 oz)	60	1	tr
ocean perch atlantic raw	3 oz	80	1	tr
raw	3 oz	77	1	tr
red raw	3.5 oz	114	4	—
FROZEN				
Van De Kamp's				
Battered Fillets	2 (4 oz)	300	20	3
PERSIMMONS				
dried japanese	1	93	tr	—
fresh	1	32	tr	—
fresh japanese	1	118	tr	—
Sonoma				
Dried	6-8 pieces (1.4 oz)	140	0	0
PHEASANT				
breast w/o skin raw	½ breast (6.4 oz)	243	6	2
leg w/o skin raw	1 (3.6 oz)	143	5	2
roasted	3.5 oz	215	9	3
w/ skin raw	½ pheasant (14 oz)	723	37	11
w/o skin raw	½ pheasant (12.4 oz)	470	13	4
PHYLLO				
phyllo dough	1 oz	85	2	tr
sheet	1	57	1	tr
Ekizian				
Sheets	¼ lb	433	9	4

FOOD	PORTION	CALS	FAT	SAT FAT
Fillo Factory				
Fillo Dough Spelt Vegan	3 sheets (2 oz)	180	1	0
Fillo Dough Vegan	3 sheets (2 oz)	170	1	0
Fillo Dough Whole Wheat Vegan	3 sheets (2 oz)	190	1	0
Pastry Shells Vegan	3 (0.4 oz)	45	2	2
PICANTE (see SALSA)				
PICKLES				
dill	1 (2.3 oz)	12	tr	tr
dill low sodium	1 (2.3 oz)	12	tr	tr
dill low sodium sliced	1 slice	1	tr	tr
dill sliced	1 slice	1	tr	tr
gerkins	1 oz	6	tr	—
kosher dill	1 (2.3 oz)	12	tr	tr
polish dill	1 (2.3 oz)	12	tr	tr
quick sour	1 (1.2 oz)	4	tr	tr
quick sour low sodium	1 (1.2 oz)	4	tr	tr
quick sour sliced	1 slice	1	tr	tr
sweet	1 (1.2 oz)	41	tr	tr
sweet gherkin	1 sm (½ oz)	20	tr	tr
sweet low sodium	1 (1.2 oz)	41	tr	tr
sweet sliced	1 slice	7	tr	tr
Claussen				
Bread 'N Butter Chips	4 slices (1 oz)	20	0	0
Deli Style Hearty Garlic Whole	½ (1 oz)	5	0	0
Kosher Dills Spears	1 spear (1.2 oz)	5	0	0
Kosher Dills Halves	1 half (1 oz)	5	0	0
Kosher Dills Mini	1 (0.8 oz)	5	0	0
Kosher Dills Whole	½ (1 oz)	5	0	0
New York Deli Style Half Sours Whole	½ (1 oz)	5	0	0
Sandwich Slices Bread 'N Butter	2 (1.2 oz)	25	0	0
Sandwich Slices Deli Style Hearty Garlic	2 (1.2 oz)	5	0	0
Sandwich Slices Kosher Dills	2 (1.2 oz)	5	0	0
Super Slices For Burgers	1 (0.8 oz)	5	0	0
Mt Olive				
Bread & Butter No Sugar Added	1 oz	0	0	0
Vlasic				
Hamburger Dill Chips	1 oz	5	0	0
Kosher Cross Cuts	1 oz	5	0	0

FOOD	PORTION	CALS	FAT	SAT FAT
Kosher Spears	1 oz	5	0	0
Kosher Whole	1 oz	5	0	0
Sweet Butter Chips	1 oz	30	0	0
Sweet Gerkins	1 oz	35	0	0
Whole Dills	1 oz	5	0	0
PIE				
FROZEN				
apple	⅛ of 9 in pie (4.4 oz)	297	14	3
blueberry	⅛ of 9 in pie (4.4 oz)	289	13	2
cherry	⅛ of 9 in pie (4.4 oz)	325	14	3
chocolate creme	⅙ of 8 in pie (4 oz)	344	22	6
coconut creme	⅙ of 7 in pie (2.2 oz)	191	11	5
lemon meringue	⅙ of 8 in pie (4.5 oz)	303	10	2
peach	⅙ of 8 in pie (4.1 oz)	261	12	2
Amy's				
Apple	1 serv (4 oz)	240	8	5
Kineret				
Apple Homestyle	⅙ pie (4 oz)	313	16	4
Mrs. Smith's				
Apple	1 slice (4.3 oz)	350	19	4
Blueberry	1 slice (4.6 oz)	330	17	4
Cappuccino	1 slice (4.2 oz)	300	13	8
Cherry	1 slice (4.3 oz)	320	17	4
Cherry Crumb	1 slice (4.2 oz)	320	12	3
Chocolate Cream	1 slice (4.6 oz)	340	18	8
Chocolate Mint Cream	1 slice (4.3 oz)	360	15	8
Coconut Custard	1 slice (4.4 oz)	260	14	5
Cookies 'N Cream	1 slice (4.3 oz)	360	16	8
Dutch Apple	1 slice (4.4 oz)	330	13	3
French Silk	1 slice (4.4 oz)	560	40	20
Key West Lime	1 slice (4.3 oz)	430	18	11
Lemon Cream	1 slice (5 oz)	440	26	17

FOOD	PORTION	CALS	FAT	SAT FAT
Lemonade	1 slice (4.3 oz)	340	15	10
Mince	1 slice (4.6 oz)	380	17	4
Mixed Berry	1 slice (4.2 oz)	300	13	3
Peach	1 slice (4.6 oz)	320	17	4
Peach Lattice	1 slice (4.2 oz)	290	13	3
Peanut Butter Silk	1 slice (4.6 oz)	600	41	19
Pecan	1 slice (4.8 oz)	560	27	5
Pumpkin Custard	1 slice (4.6 oz)	270	13	3
Raspberry	1 slice (4.6 oz)	330	17	4
S'Mores Cream	1 slice (4.3 oz)	360	16	8
Strawberry Banana	1 slice (4.3 oz)	330	15	9
Sweet Potato Custard	1 slice (4.6 oz)	340	17	4
Sara Lee				
Apple 45% Reduced Fat	⅙ pie (4.5 oz)	290	8	2
Chocolate Silk	⅕ pie (4.8 oz)	500	32	16
Coconut Cream	⅕ pie (4.8 oz)	480	31	14
Homestyle Apple	⅛ pie (4.6 oz)	340	16	4
Homestyle Blueberry	⅛ pie (4.6 oz)	360	15	4
Homestyle Cherry	⅛ pie (4.6 oz)	320	16	4
Homestyle Dutch Apple	⅛ pie (4.6 oz)	350	15	3
Homestyle Mince	⅛ pie (4.6 oz)	390	17	4
Homestyle Peach	⅛ pie (4.6 oz)	320	14	3
Homestyle Pecan	⅛ pie (4.2 oz)	520	24	5
Homestyle Pumpkin	⅛ pie (4.6 oz)	260	11	3
Homestyle Raspberry	⅛ pie (4.6 oz)	380	19	5
Lemon Meringue	⅙ pie (5 oz)	350	11	3
Weight Watchers				
Mississippi Mud	1 piece (2.45 oz)	160	5	2
MIX				
Jell-O				
No Bake Chocolate Silk as prep	⅙ pie (4.4 oz)	320	16	6
SNACK				
apple	1 (3 oz)	266	14	7
cherry	1 (3 oz)	266	14	7
lemon	1 (3 oz)	266	14	7
Dolly Madison				
Apple	1 (4.5 oz)	480	22	9
Blueberry	1 (4.5 oz)	480	21	10
Cherry	1 (4.5 oz)	470	22	11
Chocolate Pudding	1 (4.5 oz)	530	25	11

FOOD	PORTION	CALS	FAT	SAT FAT
Lemon	1 (4.5 oz)	500	24	11
Peach	1 (4.5 oz)	480	21	10
Pecan	1 (3 oz)	360	19	8
Pecan Fried	1 (4.5 oz)	530	21	9
Pineapple	1 (4.5 oz)	460	21	10
Hostess				
Apple	1 (4.5 oz)	480	22	9
Blackberry	1 (4.5 oz)	520	21	11
Blueberry	1 (4.5 oz)	480	21	10
Cherry	1 (4.5 oz)	470	22	11
French Apple	1 (4.5 oz)	480	22	9
Lemon	1 (4.5 oz)	500	24	11
Peach	1 (4.5 oz)	480	21	10
Pineapple	1 (4.5 oz)	460	21	10
Strawberry	1 (4.5 oz)	510	23	9
Lance				
Pecan	1 (3 oz)	350	17	4
Tastykake				
Apple	1 (4 oz)	270	11	1
Blueberry	1 (4 oz)	300	11	1
Cherry	1 (4 oz)	290	11	1
Coconut Creme	1 (4 oz)	370	21	4
French Apple	1 (4.2 oz)	310	11	1
Lemon	1 (4 oz)	300	13	2
Peach	1 (4 oz)	280	11	1
Pineapple	1 (4 oz)	290	12	1
Pineapple Cheese	1 (4 oz)	320	12	3
Pumpkin	1 (4 oz)	340	14	2
Strawberry	1 (3.5 oz)	320	12	1
Tastyklair	1 (4 oz)	400	20	3
Tom's				
Apple	1 pkg (3 oz)	330	17	8
Banana Marshmallow	1 pkg (2.75 oz)	320	11	7
Cherry	1 pkg (3 oz)	320	18	8
Chocolate Marshmallow	1 pkg (2.75 oz)	320	11	6
TAKE-OUT				
apple	⅛ of 9 in pie (5.4 oz)	411	19	5
banana cream	⅛ of 9 in pie (5.2 oz)	398	20	6

FOOD	PORTION	CALS	FAT	SAT FAT
blueberry	⅛ of 9 in pie (5.2 oz)	360	18	4
butterscotch	⅛ of 9 in pie (4.5 oz)	355	18	5
cherry	⅛ of 9 in pie (6.3 oz)	486	22	5
coconut creme	⅛ of 9 in pie (4.7 oz)	396	21	8
coconut custard	⅙ of 8 in pie (3.6 oz)	271	14	6
custard	⅛ of 9 in pie (4.5 oz)	262	11	4
lemon meringue	⅛ of 9 in pie (4.5 oz)	362	16	4
mince	⅛ of 9 in pie (5.8 oz)	477	18	4
pecan	⅙ of 8 in pie (4 oz)	452	21	4
pumpkin	⅙ of 8 in pie (3.8 oz)	229	10	2
vanilla cream	⅛ of 9 in pie (4.4 oz)	350	18	5
PIE CRUST				
FROZEN				
baked	⅛ of 9 in pie (0.6 oz)	82	5	2
baked	9 in shell (4.4 oz)	647	41	13
puff pastry baked	1 shell (1.4 oz)	223	15	2
Pepperidge Farm				
Puff Pastry Sheets	⅙ sheet (1.4 oz)	170	11	3
Puff Pastry Shell	1 (1.6 oz)	190	13	4
Puff Pastry Squares	1 sq (2 oz)	240	16	5
Pet-Ritz				
Deep Dish	⅛ pie (0.7 oz)	90	5	2
Regular	⅛ pie (0.6 oz)	80	5	2
Tart Shells	1 (1 oz)	130	8	2

FOOD	PORTION	CALS	FAT	SAT FAT
MIX				
as prep	9 in crust (5.6 oz)	801	49	12
as prep	⅛ of 9 in pie (0.7 oz)	100	6	2
Betty Crocker				
Pie Crust as prep	⅛ crust	110	8	2
Flako				
Mix	¼ cup (0.9 oz)	130	8	3
MiniCarb				
Pie Crust Mix	1 slice	105	7	4
READY-TO-EAT				
chocolate cookie crumb	⅛ of 9 in pie (1 oz)	139	9	2
chocolate cookie crumb	9 in crust (7.7 oz)	1130	69	15
graham cracker	9 in crust (8.4 oz)	1181	60	12
graham cracker	⅛ of 9 in pie (1 oz)	148	8	2
vanilla wafer cracker crumbs	9 in crust (6.1 oz)	937	64	13
vanilla wafer cracker crumbs	⅛ of 9 in pie (0.8 oz)	119	8	2
Honey Maid				
Graham	⅛ crust (1 oz)	140	7	2
Keebler				
Graham Single Serve	1 (0.8 oz)	120	6	1
Reduced Fat Graham	⅛ pie (0.7 oz)	90	4	0
Nabisco				
Nilla	⅛ crust (1 oz)	140	8	2
Oreo				
Crumb Crust	⅛ crust (1 oz)	140	11	2
REFRIGERATED				
All Ready				
Crust	⅛ pie (0.9 oz)	120	7	3
PIE FILLING				
apple	1 can (21 oz)	599	1	tr
apple	⅛ can (2.6 oz)	74	tr	tr

FOOD	PORTION	CALS	FAT	SAT FAT
cherry	1 can (21 oz)	683	1	tr
cherry	⅛ can (2.6 oz)	85	tr	tr
pumpkin pie mix	1 cup	282	tr	tr
Colac				
All Flavors	1 tbsp	19	0	0
Comstock				
MoreFruit Light Cherry	⅓ cup (2.9 oz)	60	0	0
Red Ruby Cherry	⅓ cup (3.1 oz)	90	0	0
Libby				
Pumpkin Pie Mix	⅓ cup	90	1	0
Smucker's				
Pie Glaze Strawberry	2 oz	80	0	0

PIEROGI

pierogi	¾ cup (4.4 oz)	307	19	7
Health Is Wealth				
Potato & Cheddar	2 (2.8 oz)	140	2	0
Potato & Onion	2 (2.8 oz)	140	2	0
Mrs. T's				
Broccoli & Cheddar	3 (4.2 oz)	200	5	1
Jalapeno & Cheddar	3 (4.2 oz)	190	3	1
Potato & American Cheese	3 (4.2 oz)	220	4	2
Potato & Roasted Garlic	3 (4.2 oz)	190	4	1
Potato & Cheddar	3 (4.2 oz)	190	3	1
Potato & Onion	3 (4.2 oz)	180	2	0
Rogies Cheddar & Bacon	7 (3 oz)	140	3	1
Rogies Jalapeno & Cheddar	7 (3 oz)	120	2	1
Rogies Potato & Cheddar	7 (3 oz)	130	2	1

PIG'S EARS AND FEET

ear simmered	1	184	12	4
feet pickled	1 lb	921	73	25
feet pickled	1 oz	58	5	2
feet simmered	3 oz	165	11	4
Hormel				
Pickled Feet	2 oz	80	6	2
Pickled Hocks	2 oz	110	8	3

PIGEON

| w/ skin & bone | 3.5 oz | 169 | 10 | — |

FOOD	PORTION	CALS	FAT	SAT FAT
PIGEON PEAS				
dried cooked	½ cup	102	tr	tr
dried cooked	1 cup	204	1	tr
PIGNOLIA (see PINE NUTS)				
PIKE				
northern cooked	3 oz	96	1	tr
northern cooked	½ fillet (5.4 oz)	176	1	tr
northern raw	3 oz	75	1	tr
roe raw	1 oz	37	tr	–
walleye baked	3 oz	101	1	tr
walleye fillet baked	4.4 oz	147	2	tr
PILLNUTS				
canarytree dried	1 oz	204	23	9
PIMIENTOS				
canned	1 slice	0	0	0
canned	1 tbsp	3	tr	tr
Dromedary				
Peeled	½ tsp (4 g)	0	0	0
Unpeeled	½ tsp (4 g)	0	0	0
PINE NUTS				
pignolia dried	1 oz	146	14	2
pignolia dried	1 tbsp	51	5	1
pinyon dried	1 oz	161	17	3
Progresso				
Pignoli	1 jar (1 oz)	170	13	1
PINEAPPLE				
CANNED				
chunks in heavy syrup	1 cup	199	tr	tr
chunks juice pack	1 cup	150	tr	tr
crushed in heavy syrup	1 cup	199	tr	tr
slices in heavy syrup	1 slice	45	tr	tr
slices in light syrup	1 slice	30	tr	tr
slices juice pack	1 slice	35	tr	tr
slices water pack	1 slice	19	tr	tr
tidbits in heavy syrup	1 cup	199	tr	tr
tidbits in juice	1 cup	150	tr	tr
tidbits in water	1 cup	79	tr	tr

FOOD	PORTION	CALS	FAT	SAT FAT
Del Monte				
Chunks In Heavy Syrup	½ cup (4.3 oz)	90	0	0
Chunks In Its Own Juice	½ cup (4.3 oz)	70	0	0
Crushed In Heavy Syrup	½ cup (4.3 oz)	90	0	0
Crushed In Its Own Juice	½ cup (4.3 oz)	70	0	0
Fruit Cup Tidbits	1 pkg (4 oz)	50	0	0
Sliced In Heavy Syrup	2 slices (4.1 oz)	90	0	0
Sliced In Its Own Juice	½ cup (4 oz)	60	0	0
Spears In Its Own Juice	½ cup (4.3 oz)	70	0	0
Tidbits In Its Own Juice	½ cup (4.3 oz)	70	0	0
Wedges In Its Own Juice	½ cup (4.3 oz)	70	0	0
Dole				
All Natural Chunks	½ cup	60	0	0
Chunks Juice Pack	½ cup	60	0	0
SunFresh				
In Lightly Sweetened Juice	½ cup	70	0	0
DRIED				
Sonoma				
Pieces	2 pieces (1.4 oz)	140	2	0
FRESH				
diced	1 cup	77	tr	tr
slice	1 slice	42	tr	tr
Bonita Hill				
Golden Extra Sweet	2 slices (3.9 oz)	60	0	0
Frosty Fresh				
Peeled & Cored	½ cup	60	0	0
FROZEN				
chunks sweetened	½ cup	104	tr	tr
PINEAPPLE JUICE				
canned	1 cup	139	tr	tr
frzn as prep	1 cup	129	tr	tr
frzn not prep	6 oz	387	tr	tr
After The Fall				
Mandarin Pineapple	1 can (12 oz)	150	0	0
Del Monte				
Juice	6 fl oz	80	0	0
Dole				
Chilled	8 oz	130	0	0

FOOD	PORTION	CALS	FAT	SAT FAT
PINK BEANS				
dried cooked	1 cup	252	1	tr
PINTO BEANS				
CANNED				
pinto	1 cup	186	1	tr
Chi-Chi's				
Pinto Beans	½ cup (4.3 oz)	100	1	0
Eden				
Organic Spicy	½ cup (4.6 oz)	125	0	0
Green Giant				
Pinto Beans	½ cup (4.4 oz)	110	1	0
Old El Paso				
Pinto Beans	½ cup (4.6 oz)	110	1	0
Progresso				
Pinto Beans	½ cup (4.6 oz)	110	1	0
DRIED				
cooked	1 cup	235	1	tr
Hurst				
HamBeens w/ Ham	3 tbsp (1.2 oz)	120	1	0
FROZEN				
cooked	3 oz	152	tr	tr
PISTACHIOS				
dried	1 cup	739	62	8
dry roasted	1 oz	172	15	2
dry roasted salted	1 oz	172	15	2
dry roasted salted	1 cup	776	68	9
dry roasted w/ salt	47 nuts (1 oz)	160	13	2
with shells dry roasted unsalted	½ cup	180	14	2
Lance				
Pistachios	1 pkg (1⅛ oz)	90	7	1
Planters				
Munch'N Go Singles Shelled Dry Roasted	1 pkg (2 oz)	330	29	4
Red Salted Dry Roasted	1 pkg	160	14	2
Uncolored Dry Roasted	½ cup	160	14	2
Sonoma				
Salted Shelled	¼ cup (1 oz)	190	14	2
Sweet Delights				
Pistachio Roasters	⅓ pkg (1 oz)	190	14	—

FOOD	PORTION	CALS	FAT	SAT FAT
PITANGA				
fresh	1	2	tr	—
fresh	1 cup	57	1	—
PIZZA (see also PIZZA DOUGH, PIZZA SAUCE)				
Amy's				
Cheese	⅓ pie	300	13	4
Mushroom & Olive	⅓ pie	250	9	3
Pesto	⅓ pie	310	12	4
Pocket Sandwich Cheese Pizza	1 (4.5 oz)	300	9	4
Pocket Sandwich Vegetarian Pizza	1 (4.5 oz)	250	6	3
Roasted Vegetable	⅓ pie	260	8	2
Snacks Cheese	5-6 pieces	180	6	3
Soy Cheese	⅓ pie	290	11	1
Spinach	⅓ pie	300	12	4
Veggie Combo	⅓ pie	280	9	3
Appian Way				
Pizza Mix Thick Crust	⅓ pie (4.2 oz)	290	5	2
Pizza Mix Thin Crust	⅓ pie (4.1 oz)	250	3	1
Banquet				
Pepperoni	1 pie (6.75 oz)	490	23	7
Pizza Snack Cheese	6 pieces (7.5 oz)	200	8	4
Pizza Snack Pepperoni	6 pieces (7.5 oz)	230	11	5
Pizza Snack Pepperoni & Sausage	6 pieces (7.5 oz)	210	9	4
Celeste				
Italian Bread Deluxe	1 (5.1 oz)	290	11	3
Italian Bread Garlic & Herb Zesty Chicken	1 (5 oz)	260	8	2
Italian Bread Pepperoni	1 (5 oz)	320	13	4
Italian Bread Zesty Four Cheese	1 (4.6 oz)	300	12	6
Large Cheese	¼ pie (4.4 oz)	320	16	8
Large Deluxe	¼ pie (5.5 oz)	350	18	6
Large Pepperoni	¼ pie (4.7 oz)	350	20	7
Large Suprema With Meat	⅕ pie (4.6 oz)	290	16	5
Large Zesty Four Cheese	¼ pie (4.4 oz)	330	16	8
Small Cheese	1 (7.5 oz)	540	25	13
Small Deluxe	1 (8.2 oz)	540	29	10
Small Hot & Zesty Four Cheese	1 (7 oz)	530	27	13
Small Original Four Cheese	1 (7 oz)	540	30	12
Small Pepperoni	1 (6.7 oz)	520	27	10

FOOD	PORTION	CALS	FAT	SAT FAT
Small Sausage	1 (7.5 oz)	530	27	9
Small Suprema Vegetable	1 (7.5 oz)	480	23	8
Small Suprema With Meat	1 (9 oz)	580	31	10
Small Zesty Four Cheese	1 (7 oz)	530	27	13
Croissant Pocket				
Stuffed Sandwich Pepperoni Pizza	1 piece (4.5 oz)	350	15	5
Di Giorno				
Rising Crust 12 inch Four Cheese	⅙ pie (4.9 oz)	320	11	6
Rising Crust 12 inch Italian Sausage	⅙ pie (5.3 oz)	360	14	7
Rising Crust 12 inch Pepperoni	⅙ pie (5.2 oz)	370	16	8
Rising Crust 12 inch Supreme	⅙ pie (5.8 oz)	380	17	8
Rising Crust 12 inch Three Meat	⅙ pie (5.4 oz)	380	16	8
Rising Crust 12 inch Vegetable	⅙ pie (5.6 oz)	310	10	5
Rising Crust 8 inch Chicken Supreme	⅓ pie (4.8 oz)	270	9	5
Rising Crust 8 inch Four Cheese	⅓ pie (4 oz)	260	9	5
Rising Crust 8 inch Italian Sausage	⅓ pie (4.4 oz)	300	12	6
Rising Crust 8 inch Pepperoni	⅓ pie (4.2 oz)	300	13	6
Rising Crust 8 inch Spinach	⅓ pie (4.3 oz)	250	8	4
Rising Crust 8 inch Supreme	⅓ pie (4.7 oz)	310	14	6
Rising Crust 8 inch Three Meat	⅓ pie (4.4 oz)	310	13	6
Rising Crust 8 inch Vegetable	⅓ pie (4.6 oz)	250	8	4
Health Is Wealth				
Pizza Munchees	6 (3 oz)	190	5	0
Healthy Choice				
French Bread Cheese	1 piece (6 oz)	340	5	2
French Bread Pepperoni	1 piece (6 oz)	340	5	2
French Bread Sausage	1 piece (6 oz)	320	5	2
French Bread Supreme	1 piece (6.35 oz)	330	5	2
French Bread Vegetable	1 piece (6 oz)	280	4	2
Hot Pocket				
Stuffed Sandwich Pepperoni & Sausage Pizza	1 (4.5 oz)	340	16	6
Stuffed Sandwich Pepperoni Pizza	1 (4.5 oz)	350	17	8
Jack's				
Great Combinations 12 inch Bacon Cheeseburger	¼ pie (4.7 oz)	360	18	9
Great Combinations 12 inch Double Cheese	¼ pie (4.9 oz)	380	19	11
Great Combinations 12 inch Pepperoni	¼ pie (5.2 oz)	410	19	9

FOOD	PORTION	CALS	FAT	SAT FAT
Great Combinations 12 inch Pepperoni & Mushrooms	¼ pie (4.8 oz)	340	16	7
Great Combinations 12 inch Sausage	¼ pie (5.4 oz)	390	18	8
Great Combinations 12 inch Sausage & Mushroom	¼ pie (4.9 oz)	310	15	7
Great Combinations 12 inch Sausage & Pepperoni	¼ pie (4.8 oz)	350	19	8
Great Combinations 12 inch Supreme	¼ pie (5.2 oz)	350	18	8
Great Combinations 9 inch Double Cheese	½ pie (5.5 oz)	430	21	12
Great Combinations 9 inch Pepperoni & Sausage	½ pie (5.1 oz)	380	18	8
Naturally Rising 12 inch Bacon Cheeseburger	⅙ pie (5 oz)	350	15	7
Naturally Rising 12 inch Canadian Bacon	⅙ pie (4.9 oz)	280	9	5
Naturally Rising 12 inch Cheese	⅙ pie (4.5 oz)	290	10	6
Naturally Rising 12 inch Combination w/ Sausage & Pepperoni	⅙ pie (5.2 oz)	360	17	8
Naturally Rising 12 inch Pepperoni	⅙ pie (4.9 oz)	350	16	8
Naturally Rising 12 inch Pepperoni Supreme	⅙ pie (5.1 oz)	340	16	8
Naturally Rising 12 inch Sausage	⅙ pie (5.1 oz)	340	15	7
Naturally Rising 12 inch Spicy Italian Sausage	⅙ pie (5.1 oz)	330	14	7
Naturally Rising 12 inch The Works	⅙ pie (5.3 oz)	330	14	7
Naturally Rising 9 inch Cheese	⅓ pie (4.7 oz)	300	10	6
Naturally Rising 9 inch Combination w/ Sausage & Pepperoni	¼ pie (4.2 oz)	300	14	7
Naturally Rising 9 inch Pepperoni	⅓ pie (5.2 oz)	360	16	8
Naturally Rising 9 inch Sausage	⅓ pie (5.4 oz)	360	16	7
Naturally Rising 9 inch The Works	¼ pie (4.5 oz)	280	12	6
Original 12 inch Canadian Bacon	¼ pie (4.4 oz)	280	10	5
Original 12 inch Cheese	⅓ pie (5 oz)	360	13	7
Original 12 inch Hamburger	¼ pie (4.4 oz)	300	14	7
Original 12 inch Pepperoni	¼ pie (4.3 oz)	330	15	7
Original 12 inch Sausage	¼ pie (4.3 oz)	300	14	7
Original 12 inch Spicy Italian Sausage	¼ pie (4.3 oz)	290	13	6
Original 9 inch Pepperoni	½ pie (5 oz)	380	18	8
Original 9 inch Sausage	½ pie (5.1 oz)	360	16	7

FOOD	PORTION	CALS	FAT	SAT FAT
Pizza Bursts Combination Sausage & Pepperoni	6 pieces (3 oz)	250	12	4
Pizza Bursts Pepperoni	6 pieces (3 oz)	260	14	5
Pizza Bursts Sausage	6 pieces (3 oz)	250	12	4
Pizza Bursts Supercheese	6 pieces (3 oz)	250	12	5
Pizza Bursts Supreme	6 pieces (3 oz)	250	13	4
Kid Cuisine				
Backpacking Pizza Snack	6 pieces	230	11	5
Big League Hamburger	1 meal (8.3 oz)	400	11	4
Fire Chief Cheese	1 pie (5.2 oz)	340	10	5
Pirate Pizza w/ Cheese	1 meal (8 oz)	430	11	5
Poolside Pepperoni	1 (5.2 oz)	380	14	7
Kineret				
Bagel Pizza	2 (4 oz)	300	10	6
Slice	1 (4.9 oz)	490	9	4
Lean Cuisine				
Everyday Favorites French Bread Cheese	1 pkg (6 oz)	320	7	4
Everyday Favorites French Bread Deluxe	1 pkg (6.1 oz)	290	6	3
Everyday Favorites French Bread Pepperoni	1 pkg (5.25 oz)	300	8	4
Everyday Favorites French Bread Sun Dried Tomatoes	1 serv (6 oz)	340	8	5
Lean Pockets				
Stuffed Sandwich Pizza Deluxe	1 (4.5 oz)	270	8	3
Marie Callender's				
French Bread Cheese	1 (7.2 oz)	530	24	14
French Bread Pepperoni	1 (7.5 oz)	570	28	14
French Bread Supreme	1 (7.5 oz)	510	23	11
Old El Paso				
Pizza Burrito Cheese	1 (3.5 oz)	320	9	4
Pizza Burrito Pepperoni	1 (3.5 oz)	260	10	5
Pizza Burrito Sausage	1 (3.5 oz)	260	9	4
Pepperidge Farm				
Gourmet Crust Cheese	1 (4.4 oz)	390	20	7
Gourmet Crust Pepperoni	1 (4.5 oz)	420	23	9
Stouffer's				
French Bread Bacon Cheddar	1 piece (5.7 oz)	430	21	7
French Bread Cheese	1 piece (5.2 oz)	370	16	6

FOOD	PORTION	CALS	FAT	SAT FAT
French Bread Cheeseburger	1 piece (6 oz)	420	20	6
French Bread Deluxe	1 piece (6.2 oz)	430	21	7
French Bread Double Cheese	1 piece (5.9 oz)	400	16	7
French Bread Pepperoni	1 piece (5.6 oz)	430	20	8
French Bread Pepperoni & Mushroom	1 piece (6.1 oz)	440	20	7
French Bread Sausage	1 piece (6 oz)	420	18	7
French Bread Sausage & Pepperoni	1 piece (6.25 oz)	470	23	8
French Bread Three Meat	1 piece (6.25 oz)	460	21	8
French Bread Vegetable Deluxe	1 piece (6.4 oz)	380	16	6
French Bread White Pizza	1 piece (5.1 oz)	460	23	7
Tombstone				
Double Top Pepperoni	⅙ pie (4.5 oz)	340	19	9
Double Top Sausage	⅙ pie (4.6 oz)	320	17	9
Double Top Sausage & Pepperoni	⅙ pie (4.6 oz)	340	19	9
Double Top Supreme	⅙ pie (4.7 oz)	330	18	9
Double Top Two Cheese	⅙ pie (5.2 oz)	380	19	11
For One ½ Less Fat Cheese	1 pie (6.5 oz)	460	10	5
For One ½ Less Fat Vegetable	1 pie (7.2 oz)	360	9	4
For One Extra Cheese	1 pie (6.9 oz)	520	28	13
For One Pepperoni	1 pie (6.9 oz)	550	32	14
For One Supreme	1 pie (7.5 oz)	550	32	14
Light Supreme	⅕ pie (4.8 oz)	270	9	4
Light Vegetable	⅕ pie (4.6 oz)	240	7	3
Original 12 inch Canadian Bacon	¼ pie (5.5 oz)	350	14	7
Original 12 inch Deluxe	⅕ pie (4.8 oz)	310	14	6
Original 12 inch Extra Cheese	¼ pie (5.1 oz)	350	15	8
Original 12 inch Hamburger	⅕ pie (4.4 oz)	310	15	7
Original 12 inch Pepperoni	¼ pie (5.3 oz)	400	21	9
Original 12 inch Sausage	⅕ pie (4.4 oz)	300	14	6
Original 12 inch Sausage & Mushroom	⅕ pie (4.6 oz)	300	14	6
Original 12 inch Sausage & Pepperoni	⅕ pie (4.4 oz)	320	16	7
Original 12 inch Supreme	⅕ pie (5.1 oz)	320	16	7
Original 9 inch Deluxe	⅓ pie (4.4 oz)	280	13	6
Original 9 inch Extra Cheese	½ pie (5.6 oz)	380	19	8
Original 9 inch Hamburger	⅓ pie (4 oz)	280	13	6
Original 9 inch Pepperoni	⅓ pie (4 oz)	300	15	7
Original 9 inch Pepperoni & Sausage	⅓ pie (4.1 oz)	300	15	7
Original 9 inch Sausage	⅓ pie (4 oz)	280	13	6
Original 9 inch Supreme	⅓ pie (4.4 oz)	310	16	7
Oven Rising Italian Sausage	⅙ pie (5.1 oz)	320	13	6

FOOD	PORTION	CALS	FAT	SAT FAT
Oven Rising Pepperoni	1/6 pie (4.9 oz)	340	15	7
Oven Rising Supreme	1/6 pie (5.1 oz)	320	14	6
Oven Rising Three Cheese	1/6 pie (4.8 oz)	320	13	8
Oven Rising Three Meat	1/6 pie (5.1 oz)	340	15	7
Thin Crust Four Meat Combo	1/4 pie (5 oz)	380	23	10
Thin Crust Italian Sausage	1/4 pie (5 oz)	370	22	10
Thin Crust Pepperoni	1/4 pie (4.8 oz)	400	25	11
Thin Crust Supreme	1/4 pie (5 oz)	380	22	10
Thin Crust Supreme Taco	1/4 pie (5.1 oz)	370	23	11
Thin Crust Three Cheese	1/4 pie (4.7 oz)	360	21	11
Weight Watchers				
Smart Ones Deluxe Combo	1 (6.57 oz)	380	11	6
Smart Ones Pepperoni	1 (5.56 oz)	390	12	4
TAKE-OUT				
cheese	12 in pie	1121	26	12
cheese	1/8 of 12 in pie	140	3	2
cheese deep dish individual	1 (5.5 oz)	460	24	9
cheese meat & vegetables	1/8 of 12 in pie	184	5	2
cheese meat & vegetables	12 in pie	1472	43	12
pepperoni	12 in pie	1445	56	18
pepperoni	1/8 of 12 in pie	181	7	2
PIZZA DOUGH				
crust	1 slice (1.7 oz)	130	2	0
Betty Crocker				
Italian Herb Crust Mix	1/4 crust (1.6 oz)	180	2	1
Boboli				
Shell + Sauce	1/6 sm shell (2.6 oz)	170	3	1
Shell + Sauce	1/8 lg shell (2.6 oz)	170	3	1
Thin Crust	1/5 crust (2 oz)	160	4	1
Carbsense				
Garlic & Herb as prep	1 slice	100	1	1
Keto				
Dough Mix as prep	1 slice	79	1	–
MiniCarb				
Parmesan Herb Mix as prep	1 slice	130	5	1
Pillsbury				
Crust	1/5 crust (2 oz)	150	2	0

FOOD	PORTION	CALS	FAT	SAT FAT
Robin Hood				
Crust	¼ crust	160	2	1
Sassafras				
Cornmeal Pizza Crust	1 slice (1.4 oz)	140	0	0
Italian Pizza Crust Mix	1 slice (1.4 oz)	140	0	0
Wanda's				
Crust Mix Oregano & Basil	⅒ pie (1.4 oz)	149	0	0
Crust Mix Oregano & Basil Whole Wheat	⅒ pie (1.4 oz)	141	1	0
Watkins				
Crust Mix	⅛ pkg (1.8 oz)	180	1	0
PIZZA SAUCE				
Boboli				
Sauce	¼ cup (2.5 oz)	40	0	0
Sauce	1 pkg (1.2 oz)	20	0	0
Hunt's				
Fully Prepared	¼ cup (2.2 oz)	21	1	0
Pizza Sauce	¼ cup (2.2 oz)	27	1	0
Prima Choice Supper Heavy	¼ cup (2.2 oz)	28	1	0
Muir Glen				
Organic	¼ cup (2.2 oz)	40	0	0
Progresso				
Pizza Sauce	¼ cup (2.1 oz)	20	0	0
PLANTAINS				
fresh uncooked	1 (6.3 oz)	218	1	—
sliced cooked	½ cup	89	tr	—
Chifles				
Plantain Chips	1 pkg (2 oz)	170	11	2
TAKE-OUT				
ripe fried	2.8 oz	214	7	—
PLUMS				
CANNED				
purple in heavy syrup	3	119	tr	tr
purple in heavy syrup	1 cup	320	tr	tr
purple in light syrup	1 cup	158	tr	tr
purple in light syrup	3	83	tr	tr
purple juice pack	3	55	tr	tr
purple juice pack	1 cup	146	tr	tr

FOOD	PORTION	CALS	FAT	SAT FAT
purple water pack	1 cup	102	tr	tr
purple water pack	3	39	tr	tr
Eden				
Umeboshi Paste	1 tsp	5	0	0
Umeboshi Plums	1	5	0	0
FRESH				
plum	1	36	tr	tr
sliced	1 cup	91	1	tr
Chiquita				
Purple	2 med (4.6 oz)	80	1	0

POI
poi	½ cup	134	tr	tr

POKEBERRY SHOOTS
cooked	½ cup	16	tr	–
fresh	½ cup	18	tr	–

POLENTA
Frieda's				
Dried Tomato	4 oz	80	0	0
Italian Herb	4 oz	80	0	0
Mexicana	4 oz	80	0	0
Original	4 oz	80	0	0
Wild Mushroom	4 oz	80	0	0
Melissa's				
Original	4 oz	80	0	0

POLLACK
altantic fillet baked	5.3 oz	178	2	tr
atlantic baked	3 oz	100	1	tr

POMEGRANATE
fresh	1	104	tr	–

POMEGRANATE JUICE
Cortas				
Concentrated Juice	1 tbsp (0.6 oz)	40	0	0
POM Wonderful				
Pomegranate Blueberry	8 oz	140	0	0
Pomegranate Cherry	8 oz	140	0	0
Pomegranate Tangerine	8 oz	150	0	0
Pomegrante Juice	8 oz	140	0	0

FOOD	PORTION	CALS	FAT	SAT FAT
POMPANO				
florida cooked	3 oz	179	10	4
florida raw	3 oz	140	8	3
POPCORN (see also POPCORN CAKES)				
air-popped	1 cup (0.3 oz)	31	tr	tr
caramel coated	1 cup (1.2 oz)	152	5	1
caramel coated w/ peanuts	⅔ cup (1 oz)	114	2	tr
cheese	1 cup (0.4 oz)	58	4	1
oil popped	1 cup (0.4 oz)	55	3	1
Chester's				
Butter	3 cups	160	12	2
Caramel Craze	¾ cup	130	2	0
Cheddar Cheese	3 cups	190	13	3
Microwave Butter	5 cups	200	12	2
Cracker Jack				
Fat Free Butter Toffee	¾ cup	110	0	0
Fat Free Caramel	¾ cup	110	0	0
Original	½ cup (1 oz)	120	2	0
Estee				
Caramel	1 cup	120	2	0
Herr's				
Regular	3 cups (1 oz)	140	11	2
Husman's				
Cheese Corn	2¼ cups (1 oz)	160	10	2
Jolly Time				
America's Best 94% Fat Free	1 cup	20	0	0
Blast O Butter	1 cup	45	3	1
Blast O Butter Light	1 cup	30	2	0
Butter Licious	1 cup	35	2	0
Butter Licious Light	1 cup	30	2	0
Crispy & White	1 cup	40	3	1
Crispy & White Light	1 cup	25	1	0
Healthy Pop 94% Fat Free	1 cup	20	0	0
White Air Popped	5 cups	100	1	0
Yellow Air Popped	5 cups	100	1	0
Judy's				
Sugar Free Popcorn Nut Brittle	¼ piece (1 oz)	100	5	1
Lance				
Cheese	1 pkg (0.6 oz)	90	5	2

FOOD	PORTION	CALS	FAT	SAT FAT
Plain	1 pkg (0.5 oz)	70	3	1
White Cheddar	1 pkg (0.6 oz)	100	8	2
White Cheddar	1 pkg (0.9 oz)	150	11	3
Louise's				
Fat-Free Apple Cinnamon	1 oz	100	0	0
Fat-Free Buttery Toffee	1 oz	100	0	0
Fat-Free Caramel	1 oz	100	0	0
Newman's Own				
Microwave Butter Flavor	3½ cups	170	11	2
Microwave Light Butter	3½ cups	110	3	1
Microwave Light Natural	3½ cups	110	3	1
Microwave Natural	3½ cups	170	11	2
Popcorn unpopped	3 tbsp	110	2	0
Orville Redenbacher's				
Gourmet Original	3 cups	92	1	tr
Hot Air	3 cups	92	1	tr
Microwave Butter	3 cups	168	13	3
Microwave Butter No Salt Added	3 cups	176	12	3
Microwave Butter Light	3 cups	122	6	1
Microwave Caramel	1 serv	179	10	2
Microwave Golden Cheddar	1 serv	169	13	3
Microwave Natural	3 cups	164	11	2
Microwave Natural No Salt Added	3 cups	174	12	3
Microwave Natural Light	3 cups	118	5	1
Microwave Smartpop	1 serv	96	3	1
Microwave Smartpop Butter Snack Size	1 bag	155	4	1
Microwave Snack Size Butter	1 bag	287	22	5
Microwave Snack Size Butter Light	1 bag	183	8	2
Microwave White Cheddar	1 serv	169	13	3
Redenbudders Microwave Herb & Garlic	1 serv	176	13	3
Redenbudders Microwave Zesty Butter	1 serv	177	13	3
Redenbudders Movie Theater Butter Light	1 serv	113	5	1
Redenbudders Movie Theater Microwave Butter	1 serv	176	13	3
Smart Pop Movie Theater Butter	1 serv	92	2	tr
White	3 cups	92	1	tr

FOOD	PORTION	CALS	FAT	SAT FAT
Planters				
Fiddle Faddle Caramel Fat Free	1 cup (1 oz)	110	0	0
Pop Secret				
94% Fat Free Butter	1 cup (5 g)	20	0	0
94% Fat Free Natural	1 cup (5 g)	20	0	0
Butter	1 cup (7 g)	35	3	1
Cheddar Cheese	1 cup (6 g)	30	2	1
Jumbo Pop Butter	1 cup (7 g)	40	3	1
Jumbo Pop Movie Theater Butter	1 cup (7 g)	40	3	1
Light Butter	1 cup (5 g)	20	1	0
Light Movie Theater Butter	1 cup (5 g)	25	1	0
Light Natural	1 cup (5 g)	25	1	0
Movie Theater Butter	1 cup (7 g)	40	3	1
Nacho Cheese	1 cup (6 g)	30	2	1
Natural	1 cup (7 g)	35	3	1
Real Butter	1 cup (7 g)	35	3	1
Smartfood				
Butter	3 cups	150	9	2
Low Fat Toffee Crunch	¾ cup	110	1	0
Reduced Fat Golden Butter	3½ cups	130	4	1
Reduced Fat White Cheddar	3 cups	140	6	2
White Cheddar	2 cups	190	12	3
Snyder's Of Hanover				
Butter	⅝ oz	110	10	0
Tom's				
Caramel Corn	1 pkg (1.6 oz)	180	3	1
Utz				
Au Natural	3 cups (1 oz)	120	1	0
Butter	2 cups (1 oz)	170	12	2
Cheese	2 cups (1 oz)	150	10	2
Hulless Puff'N Corn	2 cups (1 oz)	180	15	3
Hulless Puff'N Corn Hot Cheese	1 pkg (1.75 oz)	290	22	3
Hulless Puff'N Corn Cheese	2 cups (1 oz)	170	12	2
White Cheddar	2 cups (1 oz)	150	9	2
Weight Watchers				
Butter	1 pkg (0.66 oz)	90	3	0
Butter Toffee	1 pkg (0.9 oz)	110	3	1
Caramel	1 pkg (0.9 oz)	100	1	0
Microwave	1 pkg (1 oz)	100	1	0
White Cheddar Cheese	1 pkg (0.66 oz)	90	4	1

FOOD	PORTION	CALS	FAT	SAT FAT
POPCORN CAKES				
Mother's				
Butter Flavor	1 (0.3 oz)	35	0	0
Unsalted	1 (0.3 oz)	35	0	0
Orville Redenbacher's				
BBQ Mini	8 (0.5 oz)	55	1	tr
Butter	2 (0.6 oz)	134	1	tr
Butter Mini	8 (0.5 oz)	56	1	tr
Caramel	1 (0.4 oz)	34	tr	0
Caramel Mini	7 (0.5 oz)	50	tr	tr
Nacho Cheese Mini	8 (0.5 oz)	56	1	tr
Peanut Crunch Mini	7 (0.5 oz)	55	1	tr
White Cheddar	2 (0.6 oz)	63	1	tr
White Cheddar Mini	8 (0.5 oz)	56	1	tr
Quaker				
Blueberry Crunch	1 (0.5 oz)	50	0	0
Butter Mini	6 (0.5 oz)	50	1	–
Butter Popped	1 (0.3 oz)	35	0	0
Caramel	1 (0.5 oz)	50	0	0
Caramel Mini	5 (0.5 oz)	50	1	–
Cheddar Cheese Mini	6 (0.5 oz)	50	1	–
Lightly Salted Mini	7 (0.5 oz)	50	1	–
Monterey Jack	1 (0.4 oz)	40	0	0
Strawberry Crunch	1 (0.5 oz)	50	0	0
White Cheddar	1 (0.4 oz)	40	0	0
POPOVER				
home recipe as prep w/ 2% milk	1 (1.4 oz)	87	3	1
home recipe as prep w/ whole milk	1 (1.4 oz)	90	3	1
mix as prep	1 (1.2 oz)	67	2	tr
POPPY SEEDS				
poppy seeds	1 tsp	15	1	tr
PORGY				
fresh	3 oz	77	tr	–
PORK (see also HAM, PORK DISHES)				
CANNED				
Hormel				
Pickled Tidbits	2 oz	100	8	3

FOOD	PORTION	CALS	FAT	SAT FAT
FRESH				
boston blade roast lean & fat cooked	3 oz	229	16	6
boston blade steak lean & fat cooked	3 oz	220	14	5
center loin roast lean bone in cooked	3 oz	169	8	3
center loin chop lean bone in cooked	3 oz	172	7	3
center rib chop lean & fat bone in cooked	3 oz	213	13	5
center rib roast lean & fat bone in cooked	3 oz	217	13	5
fresh ham rump lean roasted	3 oz	175	7	2
fresh ham rump lean & fat roasted	3 oz	214	12	4
fresh ham shank lean roasted	3 oz	183	9	3
fresh ham shank lean & fat roasted	3 oz	246	17	6
fresh ham whole lean roasted	3 oz	179	8	3
fresh ham whole lean roasted diced	1 cup	285	13	4
fresh ham whole lean & fat roasted	3 oz	232	15	6
fresh ham whole lean & fat roasted diced	1 cup	369	24	9
ground 97% fat free	4 oz	130	3	1
ground cooked	3 oz	252	18	7
leg loin & shoulder lean only roasted	3 oz	198	11	—
loin chop lean bone in braised	3 oz	191	11	4
loin chop lean bone in broiled	3 oz	199	12	4
loin roast lean bone in roasted	3 oz	210	13	5
loin whole lean & fat braised	3 oz	203	12	4
loin whole lean & fat broiled	3 oz	206	12	4
loin whole lean & fat roasted	3 oz	211	12	5
lungs braised	3 oz	84	3	1
pancreas cooked	3 oz	186	9	3
ribs country style lean & fat braised	3 oz	252	18	7
shoulder arm picnic lean & fat roasted	3 oz	269	20	7
shoulder whole lean & fat roasted	3 oz	248	18	7
shoulder whole lean & fat roasted diced	1 cup	394	29	11
shoulder whole lean roasted	3 oz	196	12	4
shoulder whole lean roasted diced	1 cup	311	18	6
sirloin chop lean & fat bone in braised	3 oz	208	13	5
sirloin roast lean & fat bone in cooked	3 oz	222	14	5
spareribs braised	3 oz	338	26	10
spleen braised	3 oz	127	3	1

FOOD	PORTION	CALS	FAT	SAT FAT
tail simmered	3 oz	336	30	11
tenderloin lean roasted	3 oz	139	4	1
top loin chop boneless lean & fat cooked	3 oz	198	11	4
top loin roast boneless lean & fat cooked	3 oz	192	10	4
Freirich				
Porkette	4 oz	220	18	7
Oscar Mayer				
Sweet Morsel Smoked Boneless Pork Shoulder Butt	3 oz	180	15	5
READY-TO-EAT				
Tyson				
Pork Pattie	1 (3.8 oz)	200	11	4
TAKE-OUT				
chicharrones pork cracklings fried	1 cup	844	72	–

PORK DISHES
Hormel

FOOD	PORTION	CALS	FAT	SAT FAT
Extra Lean Teriyaki	4 oz	140	4	2
Extra Lean Loin Lemon Garlic	1 serv (4 oz)	130	5	2
Pork Roast Au Jus	1 serv (5 oz)	180	7	3
Jimmy Dean				
BBQ Pork Rib Sandwich	1 (5.4 oz)	440	23	7
Smithfield				
Pulled Pork w/ Barbecue Sauce	2 oz	90	4	2
Tenderloin Garlic & Herb	3 oz	100	3	1
Tyson				
Lemon Pepper Pork Roast	1 serv (3 oz)	110	3	1
TAKE-OUT				
chinese spareribs	1 serv	776	166	21
pork roast	2 oz	70	3	1
tourtiere	1 piece (4.9 oz)	451	34	10

PORK RINDS (see SNACKS)

POT PIE
Amy's

FOOD	PORTION	CALS	FAT	SAT FAT
Broccoli	1 (7.5 oz)	430	22	10
Country Vegetable	1 (7.5 oz)	370	16	9
Shepard's	1 (8 oz)	160	4	0

FOOD	PORTION	CALS	FAT	SAT FAT
Vegetable	1 (7.5 oz)	420	19	12
Vegetable Non-Dairy	1 (7.5 oz)	320	9	1
Banquet				
Beef	1 (7 oz)	400	23	11
Cheesy Potato & Broccoli w/ Ham	1 (7 oz)	410	23	10
Chicken	1 (7 oz)	380	22	9
Chicken & Broccoli	1 (7 oz)	350	20	9
Family Size Hearty Chicken	1 cup	460	29	11
Macaroni & Cheese	1 pkg (6.5 oz)	210	5	3
Turkey	1 (7 oz)	370	20	8
Vegetable Cheese	1 (7 oz)	340	17	7
Healthy Choice				
Colonial Chicken	1 (9.5 oz)	310	7	3
Lean Cuisine				
Everyday Favorites Chicken Pie	1 pkg (9.5 oz)	300	8	3
Everyday Favorites Vegetable Eggroll	1 pkg (9 oz)	300	5	1
Marie Callender's				
Beef	1 (9.5 oz)	680	42	21
Chicken	1 (9.5 oz)	680	48	21
Chicken & Broccoli	1 (9.5 oz)	670	43	12
Chicken Au Gratin	1 (9.5 oz)	690	46	21
Turkey	1 (9.5 oz)	680	46	19
Morton				
Macaroni & Cheese	1 (6.5 oz)	210	5	3
Vegetable w/ Beef	1 (7 oz)	340	21	9
Vegetable w/ Chicken	1 (7 oz)	320	18	7
Vegetable w/ Turkey	1 (7 oz)	310	18	9
Mrs. Paterson's				
Aussie Pie Chicken	1 (5.5 oz)	460	25	8
Aussie Pie Chicken Low Fat	1 (5.5 oz)	380	17	6
Aussie Pie Philly Steak	1 (5.5 oz)	420	24	8
Stouffer's				
Beef Pie	1 pkg (10 oz)	450	26	9
Chicken Pie	1 pkg (10 oz)	540	33	10
Turkey	1 pkg (10 oz)	530	33	9
Swanson				
Beef	1 (7 oz)	376	19	8
Chicken	1 (7 oz)	416	22	8
Turkey	1 (7 oz)	440	24	9

FOOD	PORTION	CALS	FAT	SAT FAT
TAKE-OUT				
beef	⅓ of 9 in pie (7.4 oz)	515	30	8
chicken	⅓ of 9 in pie (8.1 oz)	545	31	10
POTATO (see also CHIPS, KNISH, PANCAKES)				
CANNED				
potatoes	½ cup	54	tr	tr
Del Monte				
New Sliced	⅔ cup (5.4 oz)	60	0	0
New Whole	2 med (5.5 oz)	60	0	0
Hormel				
Au Gratin & Bacon	1 can (7.5 oz)	250	14	5
S&W				
Whole Small	2 (5.5 oz)	60	0	0
FRESH				
baked skin only	1 skin (2 oz)	115	tr	tr
baked w/ skin	1 (6.5 oz)	220	tr	tr
baked w/o skin	1 (5 oz)	145	tr	tr
baked w/o skin	½ cup	57	tr	tr
boiled	½ cup	68	tr	tr
microwaved	1 (7 oz)	212	tr	tr
microwaved w/o skin	½ cup	78	tr	tr
raw w/o skin	1 (3.9 oz)	88	tr	tr
PurelyIdaho				
Oven Roasts	1 serv (3 oz)	70	0	0
Yukon Gold				
Fresh	1 (5.3 oz)	110	0	0
FROZEN				
french fries	10 strips	111	4	2
french fries thick cut	10 strips	109	4	2
hashed brown	½ cup	170	9	4
potato puffs	½ cup	138	7	3
potato puffs as prep	1	16	1	tr
Birds Eye				
Baby Gourmet	7 (4 oz)	100	0	0
Whole	3	50	0	0
Fillo Factory				
Petite Fillo Puffs Potato & Herb	7 (4.6 oz)	280	8	4

FOOD	PORTION	CALS	FAT	SAT FAT
Healthy Choice				
Cheddar Broccoli Potatoes	1 meal (10.5 oz)	330	7	3
Kineret				
Crinkle Cut	18 pieces (3 oz)	120	4	1
Kugel	1 piece (2.5 oz)	150	10	2
Latkes	1 (1.5 oz)	90	5	–
Latkes Mini	10 (3 oz)	160	9	1
Lean Cuisine				
Everyday Favorites Deluxe Cheddar Potato	1 pkg (10.4 oz)	250	6	3
Everyday Favorites Roasted Potatoes w/ Broccoli	1 pkg (10.25 oz)	260	6	4
MicroMagic				
French Fries Low Fat	1 pkg (3 oz)	130	3	1
Oh Boy!				
Stuffed With Cheddar Cheese	1 (5 oz)	130	4	1
Stouffer's				
Au Gratin	½ cup (5.75 oz)	130	6	3
Scalloped	½ cup (5.75 oz)	140	6	1
Tree Of Life				
Organic French Fries	20 pieces (3 oz)	110	3	0
Weight Watchers				
Smart Ones Baked Broccoli & Cheese	1 pkg (10 oz)	250	6	4
MIX				
au gratin as prep	½ cup	160	9	6
instant mashed flakes as prep w/ whole milk & butter	½ cup	118	6	4
instant mashed flakes not prep	½ cup	78	tr	tr
instant mashed granules as prep w/ whole milk & butter	½ cup	114	5	3
instant mashed granules not prep	½ cup	372	1	tr
scalloped	½ cup	105	5	3
Betty Crocker				
Au Gratin Low Fat Recipe	½ cup	110	1	1
Au Gratin as prep	½ cup	150	6	2
Cheddar & Bacon	½ cup	150	6	2
Cheddar & Bacon Low Fat Recipe	½ cup	120	3	1
Cheddar & Sour Cream	½ cup	130	3	1
Chicken & Vegetable	⅔ cup	140	4	1
Chicken & Vegetable Low Fat Recipe	⅔ cup	120	3	1

FOOD	PORTION	CALS	FAT	SAT FAT
Hash Browns	½ cup	190	8	2
Homestyle Broccoli Au Gratin	½ cup	140	6	2
Homestyle Broccoli Au Gratin Low Fat Recipe	½ cup	110	3	1
Homestyle Cheddar Cheese	½ cup	120	3	1
Homestyle Cheddar Cheese Stove Top Recipe	½ cup	140	5	2
Homestyle Cheesy Scalloped	½ cup	140	6	2
Homestyle Cheesy Scalloped Low Fat Recipe	½ cup	110	3	1
Julienne	½ cup	150	6	2
Mashed Butter & Herb	½ cup	160	8	3
Mashed Butter & Herb Reduced Fat Recipe	½ cup	130	5	2
Mashed Chicken & Herb	½ cup	150	7	2
Mashed Chicken & Herb Reduced Fat Recipe	½ cup	120	4	1
Mashed Four Cheese	½ cup	150	7	2
Mashed Four Cheese Reduced Fat Recipe	½ cup	120	4	1
Mashed Potato Buds	⅔ cup	160	8	2
Mashed Potato Buds Reduced Fat Recipe	⅔ cup	120	4	1
Mashed Roasted Garlic	½ cup	150	8	2
Mashed Roasted Garlic Reduced Fat Recipe	½ cup	130	5	1
Mashed Sour Cream & Chives	½ cup	150	7	2
Mashed Sour Cream & Chives Reduced Fat Recipe	½ cup	120	4	1
Potato Shakers Original	⅔ cup	140	4	1
Potato Shakers Original Low Fat Recipe	⅔ cup	120	2	0
Ranch	½ cup	160	6	2
Scalloped	½ cup	150	6	2
Scalloped Low Fat Recipe	⅔ cup	110	1	0
Sour Cream'n Chive	½ cup	160	7	2
Three Cheese	½ cup	150	6	2
Twice Baked Cheddar & Bacon Low Fat Recipe	⅔ cup	130	3	1

FOOD	PORTION	CALS	FAT	SAT FAT
Twice Baked Cheddar & Bacon as prep	⅔ cup	210	11	3
Hungry Jack				
Au Gratin as prep	½ cup	150	5	3
Cheddar & Bacon as prep	½ cup	150	5	3
Chessy Scalloped as prep	½ cup	150	5	3
Creamy Scalloped as prep	½ cup	150	5	3
Mashed Butter Flavored as prep	½ cup	150	7	2
Mashed Garlic Flavored as prep	½ cup	150	7	2
Mashed Parsley Butter as prep	½ cup	150	7	2
Mashed Sour Cream 'n Chives as prep	½ cup	150	7	2
Mashed Potato Flakes as prep	½ cup	160	7	2
Sour Cream & Chives as prep	½ cup	160	6	4
Idaho				
Mashed Potato Granules as prep	½ cup	160	7	2
Shake 'N Bake				
Perfect Potatoes Crispy Cheddar	⅙ pkg (7 g)	30	2	2
Perfect Potatoes Herb & Garlic	⅙ pkg (7 g)	20	0	0
Perfect Potatoes Home Fries	⅙ pkg (7 g)	20	0	0
Perfect Potatoes Parmesan Peppercorn	⅙ pkg (7 g)	25	1	1
Perfect Potatoes Savory Onion	⅙ pkg (7 g)	20	0	0
REFRIGERATED				
Purely Idaho				
Cheddar Crusted	¾ cup	120	1	0
SHELF-STABLE				
Lunch Bucket				
Scalloped w/ Ham Chunks	1 pkg (7.5 oz)	170	7	3
Micro Cup Meals				
Microcup Meals Scalloped Potatoes w/ Ham	1 cup (7.5 oz)	240	14	6
TastyBite				
Bombay Potatoes	½ pkg (5 oz)	190	8	2
Mumbai Pav Bhaji	½ pkg (5 oz)	229	6	4
Simla Potatoes	½ pkg (5 oz)	180	8	2
TAKE-OUT				
au gratin w/ cheese	½ cup	178	10	4
baked topped w/ cheese sauce	1	475	29	11

FOOD	PORTION	CALS	FAT	SAT FAT
baked topped w/ cheese sauce & bacon	1	451	26	10
baked topped w/ cheese sauce & broccoli	1	402	14	9
baked topped w/ cheese sauce & chili	1	481	22	13
baked topped w/ sour cream & chives	1	394	22	10
curry	1 serv (6 oz)	292	16	–
french fries	1 reg	235	12	4
french fries	1 lg	355	19	6
hash brown	½ cup (2.5 oz)	151	9	4
indian yogurt potatoes	1 serv	315	9	4
mashed	½ cup	111	4	1
mustard potato salad	3.5 oz	120	6	0
o'brien	1 cup	157	3	2
potato dumpling	3.5 oz	334	1	–
potato pancakes	1 (1.3 oz)	101	7	1
potato salad	½ cup	179	10	2
potato salad w/ vegetables	3.5 oz	120	3	1
red new boiled	5 sm (5 oz)	120	0	0
scalloped	½ cup	127	5	–
twice backed w/ cheese	1 half (10 oz)	392	18	10

POTATO STARCH

potato starch	1 oz	96	tr	–

POUT

ocean baked	3 oz	86	1	tr
ocean fillet baked	4.8 oz	139	2	1

PRETZELS

chocolate covered	1 oz	130	5	2
dutch twist	4 (2.1 oz)	229	2	tr
milk chocolate covered twists	4 (1 oz)	140	7	4
pretzels	1 oz	108	1	tr
rods	4 (2 oz)	229	2	tr
sticks	10	10	tr	tr
twists	1 (½ oz)	65	1	tr
twists	10 (2.1 oz)	229	2	tr
whole wheat	2 sm (1 oz)	103	1	tr

FOOD	PORTION	CALS	FAT	SAT FAT
whole wheat	2 med (2 oz)	205	2	tr
Aramana				
Soy Pretzels	15 (1 oz)	100	3	2
Bachman				
Thin'n Right	12 (1 oz)	120	1	0
Estee				
Chocolate Covered	7	130	6	4
Dutch	2 (1.1 oz)	130	1	0
Unsalted	23 (1 oz)	120	1	0
Gardetto's				
Mustard	1 pkg (0.5 oz)	50	1	0
Herr's				
Hard Sourdough	1 (1 oz)	100	0	0
Lance				
Pretzels	1 pkg (1.25 oz)	140	1	0
Landies Candies				
Sugar Free Chocolate	4 (1.5 oz)	220	12	7
Little Debbie				
Mini Twists	1 pkg (1.2 oz)	140	1	0
Manischewitz				
Bagel Pretzels Original	4 (1 oz)	110	0	0
Mister Salty				
Chips	16 (1 oz)	110	3	0
Dutch	2 (1.1 oz)	120	1	0
Fat Free Chips	16 (1 oz)	100	0	0
Mini	22 (1 oz)	110	1	0
Sticks Fat Free	47 (1 oz)	110	0	0
Mr. Phipps				
Chips Lower Sodium	16 (1 oz)	120	3	0
Chips Original	16 (1 oz)	120	3	0
Chips Original Fat Free	16 (1 oz)	100	0	0
Nabisco				
Air Crisps Fat Free	23 pieces (1 oz)	110	0	0
Nestle				
Flipz Milk Chocolate Covered	9 pieces (1 oz)	130	5	4
Flipz White Fudge Covered	9 pieces (1 oz)	130	6	5
Newman's Own				
Salted Rounds Organic	1 pkg (1.4 oz)	150	2	0
Planters				
Twists	1 oz	100	1	0

FOOD	PORTION	CALS	FAT	SAT FAT
Twists	1 pkg (1.5 oz)	160	1	0
Rold Gold				
Crispy's Thins	4 (1 oz)	110	2	0
Fat Free Honey Mustard	17 (1 oz)	110	0	0
Fat Free Sticks	48 (1 oz)	110	0	0
Fat Free Thins	12 pieces (1 oz)	110	0	0
Fat Free Tiny Twists	18 pieces (1 oz)	110	0	0
Honey Mustard	16 (1 oz)	110	1	0
Rods	3 (1 oz)	110	1	0
Sharp Cheddar	22 (1 oz)	110	1	0
Sour Dough Nuggets	11 (1 oz)	110	0	0
Snyder's Of Hanover				
Dips White Fudge	1 oz	130	6	4
Hard Sourdough	1 oz	100	0	0
Hard Sourdough Unsalted	1 oz	100	0	0
Logs	1 oz	110	1	0
Mini	1 oz	120	0	0
Mini Unsalted	1 oz	110	0	0
Nibblers	1 oz	120	0	0
Nibblers Honey Mustard & Onions	1 oz	130	3	0
Nibblers Oat Bran	1 oz	130	3	0
Nibblers Unsalted	1 oz	120	0	0
Oat Bran	1 oz	100	3	0
Old Fashioned Dipping Stix	1 oz	100	0	0
Old Tyme Unsalted	1 oz	120	1	0
Olde Tyme	1 oz	120	1	0
Olde Tyme Stix	1 oz	120	1	0
Pieces Buttermilk Ranch	1 oz	130	5	1
Pieces Cheddar Cheese	1 oz	190	6	1
Pieces Honey Mustard & Onions	1 oz	140	7	1
Pieces Peppered Pizza	1 oz	150	8	2
Rods	1 oz	120	2	0
Snaps	24 (1 oz)	120	1	0
Thin	1 oz	130	0	0
Whole Wheat Honey	1 oz	120	1	0
Spinzels				
Braided	1 pkg (0.5 oz)	55	1	0
Utz				
Country Store Stix	5 (1 oz)	110	1	0
Fat Free Hard	1 (0.8 oz)	90	0	0

FOOD	PORTION	CALS	FAT	SAT FAT
Fat Free Hard No Salt Added	1 (0.8 oz)	90	0	0
Fat Free Sour Dough Nuggets	10 (1 oz)	100	0	0
Fat Free Stix	14 (1 oz)	100	0	0
Fat Free Thin	10 (1 oz)	100	0	0
Honey Mustard & Onion	⅓ cup (1 oz)	130	6	1
Rods	3 (1 oz)	120	1	0
Specials	5 (1 oz)	110	1	0
Specials Extra Dark	5 (1 oz)	110	1	0
Specials Unsalted	5 (1 oz)	110	1	0
Wheels	20 (1 oz)	100	0	0
Wege				
Honey Wheat	1 (0.8 oz)	120	2	0
Weight Watchers				
Oat Bran Nuggets	1 pkg (1.5 oz)	170	3	0

PRUNE JUICE

canned	1 cup	181	tr	tr

PRUNES

canned in heavy syrup	5	90	tr	tr
canned in heavy syrup	1 cup	245	tr	tr
dried	10	201	tr	tr
dried	1 cup	385	1	tr
dried cooked w/ sugar	½ cup	147	tr	tr
dried cooked w/o sugar	½ cup	113	tr	tr
Del Monte				
Pitted	¼ cup (1.4 oz)	120	0	0
Unpitted	⅓ cup (1.4 oz)	110	0	0
Sonoma				
Pitted	¼ cup (1.4 oz)	120	0	0

PUDDING

MIX

banana as prep w/ 2% milk	½ cup (4.9 oz)	142	2	1
banana as prep w/ whole milk	½ cup (4.9 oz)	157	4	3
chocolate	½ cup (5 oz)	150	3	2
chocolate as prep w/ whole milk	½ cup (5 oz)	158	5	3
coconut cream	½ cup (4.9 oz)	148	4	3
instant banana as prep w/ 2% milk	½ cup (5.2 oz)	152	3	1
instant banana as prep w/ whole milk	½ cup (5.2 oz)	167	4	3
instant chocolate	½ cup (5.2 oz)	149	3	2

FOOD	PORTION	CALS	FAT	SAT FAT
instant chocolate as prep w/ whole milk	½ cup (5.2 oz)	164	5	3
instant lemon	½ cup (5.2 oz)	155	4	1
instant vanilla	½ cup (5 oz)	147	2	1
lemon	½ cup (5.1 oz)	163	2	1
rice as prep w/ whole milk	½ cup (5.1 oz)	175	4	3
tapioca	½ cup (5 oz)	147	2	1
tapioca as prep w/ whole milk	½ cup (5 oz)	161	4	3
vanilla as prep w/ 2% milk	½ cup (4.9 oz)	141	2	1
vanilla as prep w/ whole milk	½ cup (4.9 oz)	155	4	3
Betty Crocker				
Rice as prep	1 serv	200	3	tr
Jell-O				
Americana Rice as prep w/ skim milk	½ cup (5.2 oz)	140	0	0
Americana Tapioca as prep w/ skim milk	½ cup (5.1 oz)	130	0	0
Banana Cream as prep w/ 2% milk	½ cup (5.1 oz)	140	3	2
Butterscotch as prep w/ 2% milk	½ cup (5.2 oz)	160	3	2
Chocolate as prep w/ 2% milk	½ cup (5.2 oz)	150	3	2
Chocolate Fudge as prep w/ 2% milk	½ cup (5.2 oz)	150	3	2
Coconut Cream as prep w/ 2% milk	½ cup (5.1 oz)	150	5	4
Fat Free Chocolate as prep w/ skim milk	½ cup (5.2 oz)	130	0	0
Fat Free Vanilla as prep w/ skim milk	½ cup (5.1 oz)	130	0	0
Instant Banana Cream as prep w/ 2% milk	½ cup (5.2 oz)	150	3	2
Instant Butterscotch as prep w/ 2% milk	½ cup (5.2 oz)	150	3	2
Instant Chocolate as prep w/ 2% milk	½ cup (5.2 oz)	160	3	2
Instant Chocolate Fudge as prep w/ 2% milk	½ cup (4.2 oz)	160	3	2
Instant Coconut Cream as prep w/ 2% milk	½ cup (4.2 oz)	160	5	4
Instant French Vanilla as prep w/ 2% milk	½ cup (4.2 oz)	150	3	2
Instant Lemon as prep w/ 2% milk	½ cup (4.2 oz)	150	3	2
Instant Pistachio as prep w/ 2% milk	½ cup (4.2 oz)	160	3	2
Instant Vanilla as prep w/ 2% milk	½ cup (4.2 oz)	150	3	2
Instant Fat Free Chocolate as prep w/ skim milk	½ cup (5.3 oz)	140	0	0

FOOD	PORTION	CALS	FAT	SAT FAT
Instant Fat Free Devil's Food as prep w/ skim milk	½ cup (5.3 oz)	140	0	0
Instant Fat Free Sugar Free Banana as prep w/ skim milk	½ cup (4.6 oz)	70	0	0
Instant Fat Free Sugar Free Butterscotch as prep w/ skim milk	½ cup (4.6 oz)	70	0	0
Instant Fat Free Sugar Free Chocolate Fudge as prep w/ skim milk	½ cup (4.7 oz)	80	0	0
Instant Fat Free Sugar Free Chocolate as prep w/ skim milk	½ cup (4.6 oz)	80	0	0
Instant Fat Free Sugar Free Vanilla as prep w/ skim milk	½ cup (4.6 oz)	70	0	0
Instant Fat Free Sugar Free White Chocolate as prep w/ skim milk	½ cup (4.6 oz)	70	0	0
Instant Fat Free Vanilla as prep w/ skim milk	½ cup (5.2 oz)	140	0	0
Instant Fat Free White Chocolate as prep w/ skim milk	½ cup (5.2 oz)	140	0	0
Lemon as prep	½ cup (4.4 oz)	140	2	1
Milk Chocolate as prep w/ 2% milk	½ cup (5.2 oz)	150	3	2
Sugar Free Chocolate as prep w/ 2% milk	½ cup (4.6 oz)	90	3	2
Sugar Free Vanilla as prep w/ 2% milk	½ cup (4.5 oz)	80	3	2
Vanilla as prep w/ 2% milk	½ cup (5.1 oz)	150	3	2
Keto				
Banana not prep	½ scoop	62	3	–
Chocolate not prep	½ scoop	66	3	–
French Vanilla not prep	½ scoop	62	3	–
Louisiana Purchase				
Bread	1 serv (1.3 oz)	150	3	3
Lundberg				
Elegant Rice Cinnamon Raisin	½ cup (3.9 oz)	70	0	0
Elegant Rice Coconut	½ cup (3.9 oz)	70	2	2
Elegant Rice Honey Almond	½ cup (3.9 oz)	70	1	0
Uncle Ben's				
Rice Pudding Cinnamon & Raisins as prep	½ cup (1.5 oz)	160	1	0
READY-TO-EAT				
banana	1 pkg (5 oz)	180	5	1

FOOD	PORTION	CALS	FAT	SAT FAT
chocolate	1 pkg (5 oz)	189	6	1
lemon	1 pkg (5 oz)	177	4	1
rice	1 pkg (5 oz)	231	11	2
tapioca	1 pkg (5 oz)	169	5	1
vanilla	1 pkg (4 oz)	146	4	1
Boost				
Vanilla	1 pkg (5 oz)	240	9	1
Handi-Snacks				
Banana	1 serv (3.5 oz)	120	4	1
Butterscotch	1 serv (3.5 oz)	120	4	1
Chocolate	1 serv (3.5 oz)	130	4	1
Chocolate Fudge	1 serv (3.5 oz)	130	4	1
Fat Free Chocolate	1 serv (3.5 oz)	90	0	0
Fat Free Vanilla	1 serv (3.5 oz)	90	0	0
Tapioca	1 serv (3.5 oz)	120	4	1
Vanilla	1 serv (3.5 oz)	120	4	1
Healthy Choice				
Low Fat Chocolate Raspberry	½ cup (3.5 oz)	102	2	1
Low Fat Chocolate Almond	½ cup (3.5 oz)	109	2	1
Low Fat Double Chocolate Fudge	½ cup (3.5 oz)	101	1	tr
Low Fat French Vanilla	½ cup (3.5 oz)	98	1	1
Low Fat Tapioca	½ cup (3.5 oz)	101	1	1
Hunt's				
Snack Pack Banana	1 serv (3.5 oz)	119	4	2
Snack Pack Butterscotch	1 serv (3.5 oz)	130	4	1
Snack Pack Chocolate	1 serv (3.5 oz)	143	5	1
Snack Pack Chocolate Fudge	1 serv (3.5 oz)	147	5	2
Snack Pack Chocolate Marshmallow	1 serv (3.5 oz)	134	5	1
Snack Pack Fat Free Chocolate	1 serv (3.5 oz)	86	tr	tr
Snack Pack Fat Free Tapioca	1 serv (3.5 oz)	82	tr	0
Snack Pack Fat Free Vanilla	1 serv (3.5 oz)	81	tr	0
Snack Pack Lemon	1 serv (3.5 oz)	124	3	1
Snack Pack Milk Chocolate Variety	1 serv (3.5 oz)	143	5	1
Snack Pack Swirl Chocolate Caramel	1 serv (3.5 oz)	143	5	2
Snack Pack Swirl Chocolate Peanut Butter	1 serv (3.5 oz)	146	6	1
Snack Pack Swirl Smores	1 serv (3.5 oz)	136	5	1
Snack Pack Tapioca	1 serv (3.5 oz)	125	4	2
Snack Pack Toppers Chocolate Fudge w/ Rainbow Sprinkles	1 serv (4 oz)	164	6	2

FOOD	PORTION	CALS	FAT	SAT FAT
Snack Pack Toppers Chocolate w/ Dinosaurs	1 serv (4 oz)	161	6	1
Snack Pack Toppers Chocolate w/ Fun Chips	1 serv (4 oz)	176	6	2
Snack Pack Toppers Vanilla w/ Chocolate Sprinkles	1 serv (4 oz)	164	6	2
Snack Pack Vanilla	1 serv (3.5 oz)	135	5	1
Imagine				
Banana	1 pkg (4 oz)	150	3	0
Butterscotch	1 pkg (4 oz)	150	3	0
Chocolate	1 pkg (4 oz)	170	3	0
Lemon	1 pkg (4 oz)	150	3	0
Jell-O				
Chocolate	1 serv (4 oz)	160	5	2
Chocolate Vanilla Swirls	1 serv (4 oz)	160	5	2
Fat Free Chocolate	1 serv (4 oz)	100	0	0
Fat Free Chocolate Vanilla Swirl	1 serv (4 oz)	100	0	0
Fat Free Chocolate Fudge & Caramel	1 serv (4 oz)	100	0	0
Fat Free Devil's Food	1 serv (4 oz)	100	0	0
Fat Free Rocky Road	1 serv (4 oz)	100	0	0
Fat Free Tapioca	1 serv (4 oz)	100	0	0
Fat Free Vanilla	1 serv (4 oz)	100	0	0
Fat Free Vanilla Caramel	1 serv (4 oz)	100	0	0
Vanilla	1 serv (4 oz)	160	5	2
Kozy Shack				
Banana	1 pkg (4 oz)	130	3	2
Chocolate	1 pkg (4 oz)	140	4	2
Light Chocolate	1 pkg (4 oz)	110	1	1
Light Vanilla	1 pkg (4 oz)	110	1	0
Rice	1 pkg (4 oz)	130	3	2
Tapioca	1 pkg (4 oz)	140	3	2
Vanilla	1 pkg (4 oz)	130	3	2
Matthew Walker				
Plum	3.5 oz	290	7	–
NutraBalance				
Low Lactose All Flavors	1 serv (4 oz)	225	8	–
Swiss Miss				
Butterscotch	1 pkg (4 oz)	156	6	1
Chocolate	1 pkg (4 oz)	166	6	2
Chocolate Fudge	1 pkg (4 oz)	175	6	2

FOOD	PORTION	CALS	FAT	SAT FAT
Fat Free Chocolate	1 pkg (4 oz)	98	tr	0
Fat Free Chocolate Fudge	1 pkg (4 oz)	101	tr	0
Fat Free Tapioca	1 pkg (4 oz)	98	tr	0
Fat Free Vanilla	1 pkg (4 oz)	93	tr	0
Fat Free Parfait Vanilla Chocolate	1 pkg (4 oz)	96	tr	0
Lemon Meringue Pie	1 pkg (4 oz)	150	3	1
Low Fat Vanilla	1 serv (4 oz)	120	2	1
Milk Chocolate	1 pkg (4 oz)	166	6	2
Parfait Vanilla Chocolate	1 pkg (4 oz)	164	6	2
Swirl Chocolate Caramel	1 pkg (4 oz)	169	6	2
Swirl Chocolate Vanilla	1 pkg (4 oz)	169	6	1
Swirl Chocolate Vanilla Chocolate	1 pkg (4 oz)	169	6	2
Tapioca	1 pkg (4 oz)	138	4	1
Vanilla	1 pkg (4 oz)	156	6	1
TAKE-OUT				
blancmange	1 serv (4.7 oz)	154	5	—
bread pudding	½ cup (4.4 oz)	212	7	3
bread w/ raisins	½ cup	180	5	2
chocolate	½ cup (5.5 oz)	221	6	3
corn	⅔ cup	181	9	4
queen of puddings	1 serv (4.4 oz)	266	10	—
rice pudding	1 serv (6 oz)	220	8	—
rice w/ raisins	½ cup	246	6	3
tapioca	½ cup (5.3 oz)	189	7	—
vanilla	½ cup (4.3 oz)	130	4	3
yorkshire	1 serv (3 oz)	177	8	—
PUDDING POPS				
chocolate	1 (1.6 oz)	72	2	—
vanilla	1 (1.6 oz)	75	2	—
PUFFERFISH				
raw	3 oz	72	0	0
PUMMELO				
fresh	1	228	tr	—
sections	1 cup	71	tr	—
PUMPKIN				
butter	1 tbsp	32	0	0
canned	½ cup	41	tr	tr
cooked mashed	½ cup	24	tr	tr

FOOD	PORTION	CALS	FAT	SAT FAT
flowers cooked	½ cup	10	tr	tr
flowers raw	1	0	0	0
leaves cooked	½ cup	7	tr	tr
leaves raw	½ cup	4	tr	tr
raw cubed	½ cup	15	tr	tr
Libby				
Puree	½ cup	40	1	0
PUMPKIN SEEDS				
dried	1 oz	154	13	2
roasted	¼ cup	296	24	5
salted & roasted	¼ cup	296	24	5
whole roasted	1 oz	127	6	1
whole roasted	¼ cup	71	3	1
whole salted roasted	¼ cup	71	3	1
PURSLANE				
cooked	1 cup	21	tr	–
fresh	1 cup	7	tr	–
QUAIL				
breast w/o skin raw	1 (2 oz)	69	2	tr
w/ skin raw	1 quail (3.8 oz)	210	13	4
w/o skin raw	1 quail (3.2 oz)	123	4	1
QUICHE				
Atkins				
Crustless Bacon & Onion	1 serv	320	27	14
Crustless Four Cheese	1 serv	290	24	15
Crustless Smoked Ham & Cheese	1 serv	290	24	13
TAKE-OUT				
cheese	1 slice (3 oz)	283	20	–
lorraine	⅛ of 8 in pie	600	48	23
mushroom	1 slice (3 oz)	256	18	–
QUINCE				
fresh	1	53	tr	tr
QUINOA				
quinoa not prep	1 cup (6 oz)	636	10	1
RABBIT				
domestic w/o bone roasted	3 oz	167	7	2

FOOD	PORTION	CALS	FAT	SAT FAT
wild w/o bone stewed	3 oz	147	3	1

RACCOON
| roasted | 3 oz | 217 | 12 | – |

RADICCHIO
| raw shredded | ½ cup | 5 | tr | – |

RADISHES
chinese dried	½ cup	157	tr	tr
chinese raw	1 (12 oz)	62	tr	tr
chinese raw sliced	½ cup	8	tr	tr
chinese sliced cooked	½ cup	13	tr	tr
daikon dried	½ cup	157	tr	tr
daikon raw	1 (12 oz)	62	tr	tr
daikon raw sliced	½ cup	8	tr	tr
daikon sliced cooked	½ cup	13	tr	tr
red raw	10	7	tr	tr
red sliced	½ cup	10	tr	tr
white icicle raw	1 (½ oz)	2	tr	tr
white icicle raw sliced	½ cup	7	tr	tr
Eden				
Daikon Dried Shredded	2 tbsp	45	0	0
Daikon Pickled	2 slices	5	0	0
TAKE-OUT				
korean kimchee	½ cup	31	1	–
moo namul saengche korean salad	1 serv (3.7 oz)	34	tr	tr

RAISINS
chocolate coated	1 cup (6.7 oz)	741	28	17
chocolate coated	10 (0.4 oz)	39	2	1
golden seedless	1 cup	437	1	tr
jumbo golden	¼ cup	130	0	0
seedless	1 cup	434	1	tr
seedless	1 tbsp	27	tr	tr
sultanas	1 oz	88	0	–
Del Monte				
Golden	¼ cup (1.4 oz)	130	0	0
Raisins	1 box (0.5 oz)	45	0	0
Raisins	1 box (1 oz)	90	0	0
Raisins	¼ cup (1.4 oz)	130	0	0
Raisins	1 box (1.5 oz)	140	0	0

FOOD	PORTION	CALS	FAT	SAT FAT
Yogurt Raisins Strawberry	1 pkg (0.9 oz)	110	3	3
Yogurt Raisins Vanilla	1 pkg (0.9 oz)	110	3	3
Yogurt Raisins Vanilla	3 tbsp (1 oz)	130	3	3
Yogurt Raisins Vanilla	1 pkg (1 oz)	120	3	3
Dole				
CinnaRaisins	1 pkg (1 oz)	95	0	0
Estee				
Chocolate Covered	¼ cup	180	6	5
Mariana				
Fruitn Yogurt Milk Chocolate Covered Raisins	32 pieces (1 oz)	130	5	3
Nestle				
Chocolate Covered	1⅓ tbsp	70	3	2
Sonoma				
Monukka Thompson	¼ cup (1.4 oz)	130	0	0
Tree Of Life				
Organic	¼ cup (1.4 oz)	130	0	0
RASPBERRIES				
canned in heavy syrup	½ cup	117	tr	tr
fresh	1 cup	61	1	tr
fresh	1 pint	154	2	tr
frozen sweetened	1 cup	256	tr	tr
frozen sweetened	1 pkg (10 oz)	291	tr	tr
Birds Eye				
Red	5 oz	90	0	0
Tree Of Life				
Organic	⅔ cup (5 oz)	50	0	0
RASPBERRY JUICE				
Crystal Light				
Raspberry Ice Drink	1 serv (8 oz)	5	0	0
Raspberry Ice Drink Mix as prep	1 serv (8 oz)	5	0	0
Dole				
Country Raspberry	8 fl oz	140	0	0
Fresh Samantha				
Raspberry Dream	1 cup (8 oz)	120	1	0
Kool-Aid				
Drink Mix as prep	1 serv (8 oz)	60	0	0
Raspberry Drink as prep w/ sugar	1 serv (8 oz)	100	0	0
Splash Blue Raspberry Drink	1 serv (8 oz)	120	0	0

FOOD	PORTION	CALS	FAT	SAT FAT
Squeezit				
Blue Raspberry	1 bottle (7 oz)	110	0	0
RED BEANS				
CANNED				
Green Giant				
Red Beans	½ cup (4.5 oz)	100	1	0
Hunt's				
Small	½ cup (4.5 oz)	89	1	0
Van Camp				
Red Beans	½ cup (4.6 oz)	90	0	0
DRIED				
Hurst				
HamBeens w/ Ham	1 serv	120	1	0
MIX				
Bean Cuisine				
Pasta & Beans Barcelona Red With Radiatore	1 serv	210	1	0
RELISH				
cranberry orange	½ cup	246	tr	—
hamburger	1 tbsp	19	tr	tr
hamburger	½ cup	158	1	tr
hot dog	½ cup	111	1	tr
hot dog	1 tbsp	14	tr	tr
piccalilli	1.4 oz	13	tr	—
sweet	1 tbsp	19	tr	tr
sweet	½ cup	159	1	tr
Claussen				
Sweet Pickle	1 tbsp (0.5 oz)	15	0	0
Green Giant				
Corn	1 tbsp (0.6 oz)	20	0	0
Matouk's				
Hot Chow	2 tbsp	20	0	0
Kuchela	1 tsp	9	1	0
Old El Paso				
Jalapeno	1 tbsp (0.5 oz)	5	0	0
Vlasic				
Fancy Sweet	1 tbsp	15	0	0

FOOD	PORTION	CALS	FAT	SAT FAT
RENNIN				
tablet	1 (0.9 g)	1	0	–
RHUBARB				
fresh	½ cup	13	tr	–
frozen	½ cup	60	tr	–
frzn as prep w/ sugar	½ cup	139	tr	–
RICE (see also RICE CAKES, WILD RICE)				
arborio	½ cup	100	0	–
brown long grain cooked	1 cup (6.8 oz)	216	2	tr
brown medium grain cooked	1 cup (6.8 oz)	218	2	tr
glutinous cooked	1 cup (6.1 oz)	169	tr	tr
starch	1 oz	98	0	0
white long grain cooked	1 cup (5.5 oz)	205	tr	tr
white long grain instant cooked	1 cup (5.8 oz)	162	tr	tr
white medium grain cooked	1 cup (6.5 oz)	242	tr	tr
white short grain cooked	1 cup (6.5 oz)	242	tr	tr
Amy's				
Bowls Brown Rice & Vegetables	1 pkg (10 oz)	240	8	1
Birds Eye				
Rice & Broccoli In Cheese Sauce	1 pkg	290	9	3
White & Wild w/ Green Beans	1 cup (6.6 oz)	180	4	2
Carolina				
Black Beans & Rice Mix as prep	1 serv	200	2	0
Gold as prep	1 cup	160	0	0
Spanish Rice Mix as prep	1 serv	180	1	0
Casbah				
Basmati as prep	1 cup	158	tr	–
Jambalaya	1 pkg (1.4 oz)	130	0	0
La Fiesta	1 pkg (1.59 oz)	170	1	0
Nutted Pilaf as prep	1 cup	220	3	0
Pilaf as prep	1 cup	200	tr	0
Spanish Pilaf as prep	1 cup	200	1	0
Thai Yum	1 pkg (1.7 oz)	180	3	0
Chun King				
Fried Rice Mix	½ cup (1.4 oz)	126	tr	0
Gourmet House				
Brown & White not prep	¼ cup	160	10	0
Goya				
Arroz Amarillo	¼ cup (1.6 oz)	170	0	0

FOOD	PORTION	CALS	FAT	SAT FAT
Green Giant				
Rice & Broccoli	1 pkg (10 oz)	320	12	4
Rice Medley	1 pkg (10 oz)	240	3	2
Rice Pilaf	1 pkg (10 oz)	230	3	2
White & Wild	1 pkg (10 oz)	250	5	1
Kitchen Del Sol				
Mediterranean Paella Costa Brave as prep	½ cup (1.2 oz)	130	2	tr
Mediterranean Sunny Lemon Pilaf as prep	½ cup (1.2 oz)	110	1	0
Mediterranean Tomato & Basil With Pine Nuts	½ cup (1 oz)	110	4	1
La Choy				
Fried Rice	1 cup (4.9 oz)	236	1	tr
Lipton				
Golden Saute Onion Mushroom	½ cup (2.1 oz)	240	4	2
Oriental Stir Fry as prep	1 cup	270	8	1
Rice & Sauce Alfredo Broccoli as prep	1 cup	320	12	5
Rice & Sauce Beef as prep	1 cup	270	8	1
Rice & Sauce Cajun Style as prep	1 cup	270	7	1
Rice & Sauce Cajun Style w/ Beans as prep	1 cup	310	8	1
Rice & Sauce Cheddar Broccoli as prep	1 cup	280	9	3
Rice & Sauce Chicken & Parmesan Risotto as prep	1 cup	270	9	2
Rice & Sauce Chicken Broccoli as prep	1 cup	280	9	2
Rice & Sauce Chicken Flavor as prep	1 cup	280	9	2
Rice & Sauce Creamy Chicken as prep	1 cup	290	11	3
Rice & Sauce Herb & Butter as prep	1 cup	280	11	4
Rice & Sauce Medley as prep	1 cup	270	9	2
Rice & Sauce Mushroom as prep	1 cup	270	8	1
Rice & Sauce Mushroom & Herb as prep	1 cup	290	8	2
Rice & Sauce Oriental as prep	1 cup	280	8	1
Rice & Sauce Pilaf as prep	1 cup	260	11	1
Rice & Sauce Scampi Style as prep	1 cup	270	9	2
Rice & Sauce Spanish as prep	1 cup	270	8	1
Rice & Sauce Teriyaki as prep	1 cup	270	8	1
Roasted Chicken as prep	1 cup	260	8	1
Salsa Style as prep	1 cup	220	7	1

FOOD	PORTION	CALS	FAT	SAT FAT
Southwestern Chicken Flavor as prep	1 cup	260	11	1
Luigino's				
Fried Rice Chicken	1 pkg (8 oz)	250	5	2
Fried Rice Pork	1 pkg (8 oz)	250	7	3
Fried Rice Pork & Shrimp	1 pkg (8 oz)	250	5	2
Fried Rice Shrimp	1 pkg (8 oz)	220	4	2
Risotto Parmesano	1 pkg (8 oz)	360	20	6
Lundberg				
One-Step Curry	1 cup (7.4 oz)	160	1	0
Quick Brown Rice Savory Vegetarian Chicken	1 cup (2.5 oz)	260	3	1
Risotto Tomato Basil	1 serv	140	1	0
Mahatma				
Jambalaya as prep	1 cup	190	1	0
Nacho Cheese Mix as prep	1 serv	250	3	2
Thai Jasmine as prep	¾ cup	160	0	0
Melting Pot				
Risotto Melanese w/ Saffron	1 cup	210	0	0
Risotto Primavera	1 cup	200	1	0
Risotto Sun-Dried Tomatoes & Peas	1 cup	200	1	0
Risotto Three Cheese	1 cup	200	2	1
Risotto Wild Mushroom	1 cup	200	1	0
Minute				
Boil-In-Bag White as prep	1 cup (5.7 oz)	190	0	0
Instant Brown as prep	⅔ cup	170	2	0
Instant White as prep	1 cup (5.7 oz)	160	0	0
Long Grain & Wild Seasoned w/ Herbs as prep	1 cup (7.8 oz)	230	1	0
Near East				
Barley Pilaf as prep	1 cup	220	4	1
Beef Pilaf as prep	1 cup	220	5	1
Curry Rice as prep	1 cup	220	4	1
Lentil Pilaf as prep	1 cup	210	4	1
Long Grain & Wild as prep	1 cup	220	5	1
Pilaf Brown Rice as prep	1 cup	220	5	1
Pilaf Chicken as prep	1 cup	220	5	1
Pilaf Kosher as prep	1 cup	220	5	1
Spanish Pilaf as prep	1 cup	230	6	1

FOOD	PORTION	CALS	FAT	SAT FAT
Old El Paso				
Mexican	½ cup (4 oz)	410	2	1
Spanish	1 cup (8.6 oz)	130	1	–
Pritikin				
Mexican	⅓ cup (2 oz)	200	2	0
Oriental	⅓ cup (2 oz)	190	2	0
River Rice				
Brown Long Grain not prep	¼ cup	150	1	0
S&W				
Arborio as prep	¾ cup	150	0	0
Basmati Mix as prep	¾ cup	160	0	0
Brown Long Grain not prep	¼ cup	150	1	0
Long Grain Organic not prep	¼ cup	150	0	0
Success				
Beef Mix as prep	1 cup	240	7	1
Broccoli & Cheese	½ cup	130	4	2
Brown	1 cup	150	1	0
Brown & Wild Mix	½ cup	120	3	1
Classic Chicken	½ cup	90	1	1
Grilled Chicken & Broccoli Mix as prep	1 cup	240	6	1
Long Grain & Wild	½ cup	120	3	1
Pilaf	½ cup	120	3	1
Red Beans & Rice Mix as prep	1 cup	300	7	2
Spanish	½ cup	120	3	1
White as prep	1 cup	190	0	0
Yellow Mix as prep	1 cup	170	3	1
TastyBite				
Pilaf Curried Vegetable	½ pkg (4.5 oz)	180	6	3
Pilaf Green Peas	½ pkg (4.5 oz)	208	4	1
Pilaf Vegetable Kofta	½ pkg (4.5 oz)	229	5	2
Uncle Ben's				
White Converted as prep	1 cup	170	0	0
Van Camp				
Spanish	½ cup (4.5 oz)	90	2	tr
Water Maid				
White Medium Grain not prep	¼ cup	160	0	0
Watkins				
Brown & Wild	¼ cup (1.6 oz)	160	0	0
Calico Medley	¼ cup (1.6 oz)	160	0	0

FOOD	PORTION	CALS	FAT	SAT FAT
East/West Medley	¼ cup (1.6 oz)	160	0	0
Heartland Medley	¼ cup (1.6 oz)	160	0	0
Minnesota Medley	¼ cup (1.6 oz)	160	0	0
White & Wild	¼ cup (1.6 oz)	160	0	0
Zatarain's				
Dirty Rice Mix as prep w/o meat and oil	½ cup	130	0	0
Red Beans & Rice as prep w/o oil	½ cup	100	0	0
TAKE-OUT				
coconut rice	1 serv	500	42	–
nasi goreng (fried rice)	1 serv	206	4	–
nasi goreng indonesian rice & vegetables	1 cup (4.9 oz)	130	0	0
paella	1 serv (7 oz)	308	16	3
pilaf	½ cup	84	3	1
risotto	6.6 oz	426	18	–
spanish	¾ cup	363	27	10

RICE CAKES *(see also POPCORN CAKES)*

FOOD	PORTION	CALS	FAT	SAT FAT
Estee				
Banana Nut	5	60	1	0
Cinnamon Spice	5	60	0	0
Granny Smith Apple	5	60	0	0
Mixed Berry	5	60	0	0
Peanut Butter Crunch	5	60	0	0
Lundberg				
Nutra Farmed Brown Rice	1 (0.7 oz)	70	0	0
Nutra Farmed Sesame Tamari	1 (0.7 oz)	70	1	0
Organic Koku Sesame	1 (0.7 oz)	80	0	0
Mother's				
Mini Apple	5 (0.5 oz)	50	0	0
Mini Caramel	5 (0.5 oz)	50	0	0
Mini Cinnamon	5 (0.5 oz)	50	0	0
Mini Plain Unsalted	7 (0.5 oz)	60	0	0
Multigrain Lightly Salted	1 (0.3 oz)	35	0	0
Rye Unsalted	1 (0.3 oz)	35	0	0
Wheat Unsalted	1 (0.3 oz)	35	0	0
Pritikin				
Mini Apple Crisp	5 (0.5 oz)	50	0	0
Multigrain	1 (0.3 oz)	35	0	0

FOOD	PORTION	CALS	FAT	SAT FAT
Multigrain Unsalted	1 (0.3 oz)	35	0	0
Plain	1 (0.3 oz)	35	0	0
Plain Unsalted	1 (0.3 oz)	35	0	0
Sesame Low Sodium	1 (0.3 oz)	35	0	0
Sesame Unsalted	1 (0.3 oz)	35	0	0
Quaker				
Apple Cinnamon	1 (0.5 oz)	50	0	0
Banana Crunch	1 (0.5 oz)	50	0	0
Cinnamon Crunch	1 (0.5 oz)	50	0	0
Mini Apple Cinnamon	5 (0.5 oz)	50	0	0
Mini Banana Nut	5 (0.5 oz)	50	0	0
Mini Butter Popped Corn	6 (0.5 oz)	50	0	0
Mini Caramel Corn	5 (0.5 oz)	50	0	0
Mini Chocolate Crunch	5 (0.5 oz)	50	0	0
Mini Cinnamon Crunch	5 (0.5 oz)	50	0	0
Mini Honey Nut	5 (0.5 oz)	50	0	0
Mini Monterey Jack	6 (0.5 oz)	50	0	0
Mini White Cheddar	6 (0.5 oz)	50	0	0
Salt-Free	1 (0.3 oz)	35	0	0
Salted	1 (0.3 oz)	35	0	0
Weight Watchers				
Apple Cinnamon	1 oz	110	1	0
Butter	1 oz	110	2	0
Caramel	1 oz	110	1	0
White Cheddar	1 oz	100	1	0
ROCKFISH				
pacific cooked	3 oz	103	2	tr
pacific cooked	1 fillet (5.2 oz)	180	3	1
pacific raw	3 oz	80	1	tr
ROE (see also individual fish names)				
fish	1 oz	11	tr	tr
fresh baked	1 oz	58	2	1
fresh baked	3 oz	173	7	2
ROLL				
FROZEN				
New York				
Garlic	1 (2 oz)	210	10	2

FOOD	PORTION	CALS	FAT	SAT FAT
Pillsbury				
Dinner Rolls Crusty French	1	110	2	0
Sara Lee				
Deluxe Cinnamon Rolls w/o Icing	1 (2.7 oz)	370	15	9
READY-TO-EAT				
bialy	1 (2.2 oz)	138	0	0
brioche sweet roll	1 (3.5 oz)	410	23	14
brown & serve	1 (1 oz)	85	2	tr
cheese	1 (2.3 oz)	238	12	4
cinnamon raisin	1 (2¾ in)	223	10	3
dinner	1 (1 oz)	85	2	tr
egg	1 (2½ in)	107	2	1
french	1 (1.3 oz)	105	2	tr
hamburger	1 (1½ oz)	123	2	1
hamburger multi-grain	1 (1½ oz)	113	2	1
hamburger reduced calorie	1 (1½ oz)	84	1	tr
hard	1 (3½ in)	167	2	tr
hot cross bun	1	202	4	—
hotdog	1 (1½ oz)	123	2	1
hotdog reduced calorie	1 (1½ oz)	84	1	tr
hotdog whole wheat	1 (1.5 oz)	110	2	0
kaiser	1 (3½ in)	167	2	tr
oat bran	1 (1.2 oz)	78	2	tr
rye	1 (1 oz)	81	1	tr
submarine	1 (4.7 oz)	155	2	tr
wheat	1 (1 oz)	77	2	tr
whole wheat	1 (1 oz)	75	1	tr
Alvarado St. Bakery				
Burger Buns	1 (2.2 oz)	140	2	0
Hot Dog Buns	1 (2.2 oz)	140	2	0
Bread Du Jour				
Cracked Wheat	1 (1.2 oz)	100	1	0
Italian	1 (1.2 oz)	90	1	0
Sourdough	1 (1.2 oz)	90	1	0
Country Kitchen				
Wheat Light	1	80	2	0
Freihofer's				
Brown 'N Serve	1 (1 oz)	80	2	0
Pepperidge Farm				
Brown & Serve Club	1 (1.6 oz)	120	1	0

FOOD	PORTION	CALS	FAT	SAT FAT
Dinner Rolls Finger Poppy	1 (0.9 oz)	80	2	1
Parker House	1 (0.9 oz)	80	2	1
San Francisco				
Sourdough	1 (1.8 oz)	180	0	0
Stroehmann				
Hamburger	1 (1.4 oz)	100	2	0
Hamburger Potato	1 (1.9 oz)	140	2	0
Hot Dog	1 (1.4 oz)	100	2	0
Hot Dog Potato	1 (1.9 oz)	140	2	0
The Baker				
Honey Cinnamon Raisin	1 (2 oz)	150	2	0
Wonder				
Brown & Serve	1 (1 oz)	80	2	1
Brown & Serve Sourdough	1 (1 oz)	70	2	0
Brown & Serve Wheat	1 (1 oz)	80	2	0
Bun	1 (3 oz)	220	3	1
Club French	1 (1.6 oz)	120	2	0
Club Grain	1 (1.6 oz)	120	2	0
Club Sourdough	1 (1.6 oz)	120	2	0
Dinner	2 (1.6 oz)	130	1	0
Dinner Honey Rich	1 (1.3 oz)	100	2	0
Dinner Wheat	2 (1.6 oz)	140	3	0
Hamburger	1 (2 oz)	150	2	0
Hamburger	1 (2.5 oz)	180	3	0
Hamburger	1 (1.5 oz)	110	2	0
Hamburger Wheat	1 (1.9 oz)	140	2	0
Hamburger Wheat	1 (1.5 oz)	120	2	1
Hoagie French	1 (3 oz)	220	3	1
Hoagie Grain	1 (3 oz)	220	3	1
Hoagie Sourdough	1 (3 oz)	220	3	1
Hot Dog	1 (2 oz)	160	3	1
Kaiser	1 (2.2 oz)	180	3	1
Kaiser Hoagie	1 (3 oz)	220	3	1
Multigrain	1 (1.8 oz)	140	2	1
Potato Bun	1 (1.5 oz)	110	1	0
Steak	1 (2.5 oz)	190	3	1
REFRIGERATED				
cinnamon w/ frosting	1	109	4	1
crescent	1 (1 oz)	98	4	1

FOOD	PORTION	CALS	FAT	SAT FAT
Pillsbury				
Apple Cinnamon	1 (1.5 oz)	150	6	2
Caramel	1 (1.7 oz)	170	7	2
Cinnamon w/ Icing	1 (1.5 oz)	150	6	2
Cinnamon w/ Icing Reduced Fat	1 (1.5 oz)	140	4	1
Cinnamon Raisin w/ Icing	1 (1.7 oz)	170	6	2
Cornbread Twists	1 (1.4 oz)	140	6	2
Crecents Reduced Fat	1 (1 oz)	100	5	1
Crescent	1 (1 oz)	110	6	2
Dinner	1 (1.4 oz)	110	2	0
Dinner Wheat	1 (1.4 oz)	110	2	0
Orange Sweet Roll w/ Icing	1 (1.7 oz)	150	7	2
ROSE APPLE				
fresh	3.5 oz	32	tr	–
ROSE HIP				
fresh	1 oz	26	0	0
ROSELLE				
fresh	1 cup	28	tr	–
ROSEMARY				
dried	1 tsp	4	tr	–
ROUGHY				
orange baked	3 oz	75	1	tr
RUTABAGA				
cooked mashed	½ cup	41	tr	tr
raw cubed	½ cup	25	tr	tr
SABLEFISH				
baked	3 oz	213	17	3
fillet baked	5.3 oz	378	30	6
smoked	1 oz	72	6	1
smoked	3 oz	218	17	4
SAFFLOWER				
seeds dried	1 oz	147	11	1
SAFFRON				
saffron	1 tsp	2	tr	–

FOOD	PORTION	CALS	FAT	SAT FAT
SAGE				
ground	1 tsp	2	tr	tr
Watkins				
Sage	¼ tsp (0.5 g)	0	0	0
SALAD				
MIX				
Dole				
All American Toss	2 cups (3.5 oz)	50	1	0
American Blend	1½ cups (3 oz)	15	0	0
Classic	1½ cups (3 oz)	15	0	0
Classic Romaine Blend	1½ cups (3 oz)	15	0	0
Coleslaw	1½ cups (3 oz)	25	0	0
European Special Blend	2 cups (3 oz)	15	0	0
Garlic Caesar Complete w/ Dressing	1½ cups (3.5 oz)	180	15	3
Greek Marinade	1½ cups (3.5 oz)	100	8	2
Greener Selection	1½ cups (3 oz)	15	0	0
Light Caesar Complete w/ Dressing	1½ cups (3.5 oz)	60	1	0
Light Herb Ranch Complete w/ Dressing	1½ cups (3.5 oz)	50	1	1
Light Roasted Garlic Caesar Complete w/ Dressing	1½ cups (3.5 oz)	60	1	0
Light Zesty Italian Complete w/ Dressing	1½ cups (3.5 oz)	50	1	0
Mediterranean Marinade	2 cups (3.5 oz)	90	8	1
Oriental Complete w/ Dressing	1½ cups (3.5 oz)	120	6	1
Romano Complete w/ Dressing	1½ cups (3.5 oz)	150	12	2
Sunflower Ranch Complete w/ Dressing	1½ cups (3.5 oz)	160	16	2
Tomato & Mozzarella Medley	2 cups (3.5 oz)	60	2	1
Triple Cheese Toss	2 cups (3.5 oz)	80	5	3
Earthbound Farm				
Baby Caesar Mix	1 pkg (5 oz)	25	0	0
Baby Greens w/ Low Fat Honey Dijon Vinaigrette & Tomato Croutons	1 serv (3.5 oz)	90	3	0
Caesar w/ Garlic Croutons	1 serv (3.5 oz)	170	15	2
Italian Salad Organic	1⅔ cups (2.9 oz)	15	0	0
Mixed Baby Greens Organic	1 pkg (4 oz)	30	0	0
Organic Baby Greens w/ Vinaigrette & Garlic Croutons	1 serv (3.5 oz)	230	20	3

FOOD	PORTION	CALS	FAT	SAT FAT
Organic Baby Spinach w/ Sesame Soy Vinaigrette & Peanuts	1 serv (3.5 oz)	150	11	2
Organic Italian Salad w/ Blue Cheese Dressing & Walnuts	1 serv (3.5 oz)	190	17	3
Romaine Blend Organic	1⅔ cups (2.9 oz)	15	0	0
Fresh Express				
Baby Spinach Trio	4 cups (3 oz)	20	0	0
Fancy Field Greens	1½ cups (3 oz)	15	0	0
Original Iceberg Garden w/ Zip	1½ cups (3 oz)	15	0	0
Veggie Lover's	1½ cups (3 oz)	20	0	0
Suddenly Salad				
Caesar	¾ cup	220	9	2
Caesar Low Fat Recipe	¾ cup	170	3	0
Italian Pepperoni	1 cup	190	4	1
Italian Pepperoni Low Fat Recipe	1 cup	180	2	0
Ranch & Bacon	¾ cup	330	20	3
Ranch & Bacon Low Fat Recipe	¾ cup	180	2	0
Weight Watchers				
Caesar Salad	1 serv (3.5 oz)	60	0	0
Caesar Salad w/ Cookies	1 pkg (4.3 oz)	160	3	1
European Salad	1 serv (3.5 oz)	60	0	0
European Salad w/ Cookies	1 pkg (4.3 oz)	160	3	1
Garden Salad	1 serv (3.5 oz)	60	0	0
Garden Salad w/ Cookies	1 pkg (4 oz)	120	2	1
TAKE-OUT				
caesar	2 cups (5 oz)	235	20	2
chef w/o dressing	1½ cups	386	28	13
tossed w/o dressing	¾ cup	16	0	0
tossed w/o dressing	1½ cups	32	tr	0
tossed w/o dressing w/ cheese & egg	1½ cups	102	6	3
tossed w/o dressing w/ chicken	1½ cups	105	2	tr
tossed w/o dressing w/ pasta & seafood	1½ cups (14.6 oz)	380	21	3
tossed w/o dressing w/ shrimp	1½ cups	107	2	tr
waldorf	½ cup	79	6	2

SALAD DRESSING
MIX
Et Tu

FOOD	PORTION	CALS	FAT	SAT FAT
Caesar Salad Kit	1 serv	140	12	1

FOOD	PORTION	CALS	FAT	SAT FAT
Good Seasons				
Cheese Garlic as prep	2 tbsp (1 oz)	140	16	3
Fat Free Honey Mustard as prep	2 tbsp (1.2 oz)	20	0	0
Fat Free Italian as prep	2 tbsp (1.1 oz)	10	0	0
Fat Free Ranch as prep	2 tbsp (1.2 oz)	20	0	0
Fat Free Zesty Herb as prep	2 tbsp (1.1 oz)	10	0	0
Garlic & Herbs as prep	2 tbsp (1 oz)	140	15	2
Gourmet Parmesan Italian as prep	2 tbsp (1.1 oz)	150	16	3
Honey French as prep	2 tbsp (1.2 oz)	160	15	2
Honey Mustard as prep	2 tbsp (1.1 oz)	150	15	2
Italian as prep	2 tbsp	130	14	2
Italian not prep	⅛ pkg (3 g)	5	0	0
Mexican Spice as prep	2 tbsp (1.1 oz)	140	15	3
Mild Italian as prep	2 tbsp (1.1 oz)	150	15	3
Oriental Sesame as prep	2 tbsp (1.1 oz)	150	16	3
Reduced Calorie Italian as prep	2 tbsp (1 oz)	50	5	1
Reduced Calorie Zesty Italian as prep	2 tbsp (1 oz)	50	5	1
Roasted Garlic as prep	2 tbsp (1.1 oz)	150	15	2
Zesty Italian as prep	2 tbsp (1 oz)	140	15	2
McCormick				
Mediterranean Potato Salad	1 tbsp	25	0	0
Pasta Salad Vinaigrette	1 tsp (5 g)	15	0	0
READY-TO-EAT				
blue cheese	1 tbsp	77	8	2
french	1 tbsp	67	6	2
french reduced calorie	1 tbsp	22	1	tr
italian	1 tbsp	69	7	1
italian reduced calorie	1 tbsp	16	2	tr
russian	1 tbsp	76	8	1
russian reduced calorie	1 tbsp	23	1	tr
sesame seed	1 tbsp	68	7	1
thousand island	1 tbsp	59	6	1
thousand island reduced calorie	1 tbsp	24	2	tr
Annie Chun				
Lemongrass	2 tbsp	60	3	0
Sesame Cilantro	1 tbsp	4	0	–
Carb Options				
Italian	2 tbsp	70	8	1
Ranch	2 tbsp	150	17	3

FOOD	PORTION	CALS	FAT	SAT FAT
Drew's				
Low Carb Garlic Italian	1 tbsp	80	9	1
Low Carb Lemon Tahini Goddess	1 tbsp	80	9	1
Low Carb Sesame Orange	1 tbsp	80	9	1
Estee				
Creamy French	2 tbsp (1 oz)	10	0	0
Italian	2 tbsp	5	0	0
Hellmann's				
Citrus Splash Ruby Red Ginger	2 tbsp (1 oz)	90	7	1
Kraft				
⅓ Less Fat Catalina	2 tbsp (1.2 oz)	80	5	1
⅓ Less Fat Cucumber Ranch	2 tbsp (1.1 oz)	60	5	1
⅓ Less Fat Italian	2 tbsp (1.1 oz)	70	7	1
⅓ Less Fat Ranch	2 tbsp (1.1)	110	11	2
⅓ Less Fat Thousand Island	2 tbsp (1.2 oz)	70	5	1
Bacon & Tomato	2 tbsp (1.1 oz)	140	14	3
Buttermilk Ranch	2 tbsp (1.1 oz)	150	16	3
Caesar Italian	2 tbsp (1.1 oz)	100	10	2
Caesar Ranch	2 tbsp (1.1 oz)	110	11	2
Catalina	2 tbsp (1.1 oz)	120	10	2
Catalina With Honey	2 tbsp (1.1 oz)	130	11	2
Classic Caesar	2 tbsp (1.1 oz)	110	11	2
Coleslaw	2 tbsp (1.1 oz)	130	11	2
Creamy French	2 tbsp (1.1 oz)	160	15	3
Creamy Garlic	2 tbsp (1.1 oz)	110	11	2
Creamy Italian	2 tbsp (1.1 oz)	110	11	2
Cucumber Ranch	2 tbsp (1.1 oz)	140	15	2
Free Blue Cheese	2 tbsp (1.2 oz)	45	0	0
Free Caesar Italian	2 tbsp (1.2 oz)	25	0	0
Free Catalina	2 tbsp (1.2 oz)	35	0	0
Free Classic Caesar	2 tbsp (1.2 oz)	45	0	0
Free Creamy Italian	2 tbsp (1.2 oz)	50	0	0
Free French	2 tbsp (1.2 oz)	45	0	0
Free Garlic Ranch	2 tbsp (1.2 oz)	45	0	0
Free Honey Dijon	2 tbsp (1.2 oz)	45	0	0
Free Italian	2 tbsp (1.2 oz)	20	0	0
Free Peppercorn Ranch	2 tbsp (1.2 oz)	45	0	0
Free Ranch	1 tbsp (1.2 oz)	50	0	0
Free Red Wine Vinegar	2 tbsp (1.1 oz)	15	0	0
Free Thousand Island	2 tbsp (1.2 oz)	40	0	0

FOOD	PORTION	CALS	FAT	SAT FAT
Garlic Ranch	2 tbsp (1.1 oz)	180	19	3
Herb Vinaigrette	2 tbsp (1.1 oz)	140	15	2
Honey Dijon	2 tbsp (1.1 oz)	110	10	2
Honey Mustard	2 tbsp (1.1 oz)	110	10	2
House Italian w/ Olive Oil Blend	2 tbsp (1.1 oz)	120	12	2
Peppercorn Ranch	2 tbsp (1 oz)	170	18	3
Pesto Italian	2 tbsp (1.1 oz)	90	9	2
Ranch	2 tbsp (1 oz)	170	18	3
Roka Blue Cheese	2 tbsp (1.1 oz)	130	13	3
Russian	2 tbsp (1.2 oz)	130	10	2
Sour Cream & Onion Ranch	2 tbsp (1 oz)	170	18	3
Thousand Island	2 tbsp (1.1 oz)	110	10	2
Thousand Island With Bacon	2 tbsp (1.1 oz)	130	12	2
Tomato & Herb Italian	2 tbsp (1.1 oz)	100	9	1
Zesty Italian	2 tbsp (1.1 oz)	110	11	1
LaMartinique				
Blue Cheese Vinaigrette	2 tbsp	160	17	6
Poppy Seed	2 tbsp	170	15	4
Marzetti				
Bacon Spinach Salad	2 tbsp	80	15	2
Blue Cheese	2 tbsp	160	17	3
Buttermilk & Herb	2 tbsp	180	20	3
Buttermilk Bacon Ranch	2 tbsp	180	19	3
Buttermilk Blue Cheese	2 tbsp	160	18	3
Buttermilk Parmesan Pepper	2 tbsp	170	18	3
Buttermilk Parmesan Ranch	2 tbsp	160	17	3
Buttermilk Ranch	2 tbsp	180	20	3
Buttermilk Veggie Dip	2 tbsp	170	18	3
Caesar	2 tbsp	150	16	3
Caesar Ranch	2 tbsp	190	20	3
California French	2 tbsp	160	13	2
Celery Seed	2 tbsp	160	13	2
Chunky Blue Cheese	2 tbsp	150	16	3
Classic Caesar Ranch	2 tbsp	190	20	3
Country French	2 tbsp	150	13	2
Cracked Peppercorn	2 tbsp	140	14	3
Creamy Garlic Italian	2 tbsp	160	17	3
Creamy Italian	2 tbsp	150	16	3
Crispy Celery Seed	2 tbsp	160	13	2
Dijon Honey Mustard	2 tbsp	140	13	2

FOOD	PORTION	CALS	FAT	SAT FAT
Dijon Ranch	2 tbsp	170	18	3
Dutch Sweet'N Sour	2 tbsp	160	13	2
Fat Free California French	2 tbsp	45	0	0
Fat Free Honey Dijon	2 tbsp	60	0	0
Fat Free Honey French	2 tbsp	45	0	0
Fat Free Italian	2 tbsp	15	0	0
Fat Free Peppercorn Ranch	2 tbsp	30	0	0
Fat Free Ranch	2 tbsp	30	0	0
Fat Free Raspberry	2 tbsp	70	0	0
Fat Free Slaw	2 tbsp	45	0	0
Fat Free Sweet & Sour	2 tbsp	45	0	0
Fat Free Thousand Island	2 tbsp	35	0	0
Garden Ranch	2 tbsp	180	19	3
Gusto Italian	2 tbsp	120	13	2
Honey Dijon	2 tbsp	140	13	2
Honey Dijon Ranch	2 tbsp	150	15	3
Honey French	2 tbsp	160	14	2
Honey French Blue Cheese	2 tbsp	160	13	2
House Caesar	2 tbsp	150	16	3
Italian With Olive Oil	2 tbsp	120	13	2
Light Blue Cheese	2 tbsp	60	6	2
Light Buttermilk Ranch	2 tbsp	90	9	2
Light California French	2 tbsp	80	6	1
Light Chunky Blue Cheese	2 tbsp	80	7	2
Light French	2 tbsp	40	2	0
Light Honey French	2 tbsp	80	4	1
Light Italian	2 tbsp	60	5	1
Light Ranch	2 tbsp	90	8	2
Light Red Wine Vinegar & Oil	2 tbsp	20	1	0
Light Slaw	2 tbsp	60	7	1
Light Sweet & Sour	2 tbsp	100	6	1
Light Thousand Island	2 tbsp	70	5	1
Old Fashioned Poppyseed	2 tbsp	140	11	2
Olde Venice Italian	2 tbsp	130	13	2
Olde World Caesar	2 tbsp	150	16	3
Parmesan Pepper	2 tbsp	160	17	3
Peppercorn Ranch	2 tbsp	180	19	3
Poppyseed	2 tbsp	160	13	2
Potato Salad Dressing	2 tbsp	120	13	2
Ranch	2 tbsp	180	20	3

FOOD	PORTION	CALS	FAT	SAT FAT
Red Wine Vinegar & Oil	2 tbsp	130	14	2
Romano Cheese Caesar	2 tbsp	150	16	3
Romano Italian	2 tbsp	160	17	3
Savory Italian	2 tbsp	110	12	2
Slaw	2 tbsp	170	16	3
Southern Slaw	2 tbsp	100	11	2
Sweet & Saucy	2 tbsp	140	12	2
Sweet & Sour	2 tbsp	160	13	2
Thousand Island	2 tbsp	150	15	2
Vintage Champagne	2 tbsp	150	16	2
Wilde Raspberry	2 tbsp	150	12	2
Nasoya				
Creamy Dill	2 tbsp	70	7	1
Creamy Italian	2 tbsp	60	6	1
Garden Herb	2 tbsp	70	7	1
Sesame Garlic	2 tbsp	60	6	1
Thousand Island	2 tbsp	70	6	1
Newman's Own				
Balsamic Vinaigrette	2 tbsp (1.1 oz)	90	9	1
Caesar	2 tbsp (1.1 oz)	150	16	2
Light Italian	2 tbsp (1.1 oz)	20	1	0
Olive Oil & Vinegar	2 tbsp (1 oz)	150	16	3
Ranch	2 tbsp (1 oz)	180	19	3
Old Dutch				
Sweet & Sour	2 tbsp	50	0	0
Paul's				
No-Fat Raspberry & Balsamic	2 tbsp	20	0	0
No-Oil Orange & Basil	2 tbsp	15	0	0
Pfeiffer				
1000 Island	2 tbsp	140	14	2
California French	2 tbsp	140	12	2
French	2 tbsp	150	13	2
Honey Dijon	2 tbsp	140	13	2
Lite Italian	2 tbsp	50	5	1
Ranch	2 tbsp	180	20	3
Savory Italian	2 tbsp	110	12	2
Pritikin				
Dijon Balsamic Vinaigrette	2 tbsp (1 oz)	3	0	0
French	2 tbsp (1 oz)	35	0	0
Honey Dijon	2 tbsp (1 oz)	45	0	0

FOOD	PORTION	CALS	FAT	SAT FAT
Honey French	2 tbsp (1 oz)	40	0	0
Italian	2 tbsp (1 oz)	20	0	0
Raspberry Vinaigrette	2 tbsp (1 oz)	45	0	0
Red Wing				
"K" Dressing	1 tbsp (0.5 oz)	70	7	1
Chunky Blue Cheese	2 tbsp (1 oz)	130	13	2
Creamy Ranch	2 tbsp (1 oz)	150	15	2
French Traditional	2 tbsp (1 oz)	130	11	2
Italian Traditional	2 tbsp (1 oz)	100	9	2
Spicy Sweet French	2 tbsp (1 oz)	130	11	2
Thousand Island Thick & Rich	2 tbsp (1 oz)	110	9	2
Seven Seas				
⅓ Less Fat Creamy Italian	2 tbsp (1.1 oz)	60	5	1
⅓ Less Fat Italian w/ Olive Oil Blend	2 tbsp (1.1 oz)	45	4	0
⅓ Less Fat Ranch	2 tbsp (1.1 oz)	100	9	2
⅓ Less Fat Red Wine Vinegar & Oil	2 tbsp (1.1 oz)	45	4	0
⅓ Less Fat Viva Italian	2 tbsp (1.1 oz)	45	4	0
2 Cheese Italian	2 tbsp (1.1 oz)	70	7	1
Chunky Blue Cheese	2 tbsp (1.1 oz)	130	13	3
Classic Caesar	2 tbsp (1.1 oz)	100	10	2
Creamy Italian	2 tbsp (1.1 oz)	120	12	2
Free Ranch	2 tbsp (1.2 oz)	45	0	0
Free Red Wine Vinegar	2 tbsp (1.1 oz)	15	0	0
Free Sour Cream & Onion Ranch	2 tbsp (1.2 oz)	50	0	0
Free Viva Italian	2 tbsp (1.1 oz)	10	0	0
Green Goddess	2 tbsp (1.1 oz)	130	13	2
Herbs & Spices	2 tbsp (1.1 oz)	90	9	1
Ranch	2 tbsp (1.1 oz)	160	17	3
Red Wine Vinegar & Oil	2 tbsp (1.1 oz)	90	9	1
Viva Italian	2 tbsp (1.1 oz)	90	9	1
Viva Russian	2 tbsp (1.1 oz)	150	16	3
Steel's				
Honey Mustard	1 tbsp	90	7	1
Sweet Ginger Lime	1 tbsp	68	7	0
Walden Farms				
Fat Free Balsamic Vinaigrette	2 tbsp (1 oz)	15	0	0
Fat Free Caesar	2 tbsp (1 oz)	25	0	0
Fat Free Italian	2 tbsp (1 oz)	10	0	0
Fat Free Ranch	2 tbsp (1 oz)	25	0	0
Fat Free Raspberry Vinaigrette	2 tbsp (1 oz)	20	0	0

FOOD	PORTION	CALS	FAT	SAT FAT
Fat Free Russian	2 tbsp (1 oz)	30	0	0
Fat Free Sodium Free Italian	2 tbsp (1 oz)	10	0	0
Fat Free Sugar Free Italian	2 tbsp (1 oz)	0	0	0
Italian With Sun Dried Tomato	2 tbsp (1 oz)	15	0	0
Ranch With Sun Dried Tomato	2 tbsp (1 oz)	25	0	0
Weight Watchers				
Fat Free Caesar	2 tbsp	10	0	0
Fat Free Caesar	1 pkg (0.75 oz)	5	0	0
Fat Free Creamy Italian	2 tbsp	30	0	0
Fat Free French Style	2 tbsp	40	0	0
Fat Free Honey Dijon	2 tbsp	45	0	0
Fat Free Italian	2 tbsp	10	0	0
Fat Free Ranch	2 tbsp	35	0	0
Fat Free Ranch	1 pkg (0.75 oz)	25	0	0
Wishbone				
Caesar	2 tbsp (1 oz)	90	10	2
Chunky Blue Cheese	2 tbsp (1 oz)	150	17	3
Classic House Italian	2 tbsp (1 oz)	140	14	2
Classic Olive Oil Italian	2 tbsp (1 oz)	60	5	1
Creamy Caesar	2 tbsp (1 oz)	180	18	3
Creamy Italian	2 tbsp (1 oz)	110	10	2
Creamy Roasted Garlic	2 tbsp (1 oz)	110	10	2
Deluxe French	2 tbsp (1 oz)	120	11	2
Fat Free Chunky Blue Cheese	2 tbsp (1 oz)	35	0	0
Fat Free Creamy Italian	2 tbsp (1 oz)	35	0	0
Fat Free Creamy Roasted Garlic	2 tbsp (1 oz)	40	0	0
Fat Free Deluxe French	2 tbsp (1 oz)	30	0	0
Fat Free Honey Dijon	2 tbsp (1 oz)	45	0	0
Fat Free Italian	2 tbsp (1 oz)	10	0	0
Fat Free Parmesan & Onion	2 tbsp (1 oz)	45	0	0
Fat Free Ranch	2 tbsp (1 oz)	40	0	0
Fat Free Red Wine Vinaigrette	2 tbsp (1 oz)	35	0	0
Fat Free Sweet N' Spicy French	2 tbsp (1 oz)	30	0	0
Fat Free Thousand Island	2 tbsp (1 oz)	35	0	0
Italian	2 tbsp (1 oz)	80	8	1
Lite French	2 tbsp (1 oz)	50	2	1
Lite Italian	2 tbsp (1 oz)	15	1	0
Lite Ranch	2 tbsp (1 oz)	100	8	1
Olive Oil Vinaigrette	2 tbsp (1 oz)	60	5	1
Oriental	2 tbsp (1 oz)	70	5	1

FOOD	PORTION	CALS	FAT	SAT FAT
Parmesan & Onion	2 tbsp (1 oz)	110	10	2
Ranch	2 tbsp (1 oz)	160	17	3
Red Wine Vinaigrette	2 tbsp (1 oz)	80	5	1
Robusto Italian	2 tbsp (1 oz)	90	8	1
Russian	2 tbsp (1 oz)	110	6	1
Sweet N' Spicy French	2 tbsp (1 oz)	140	12	2
Thousand Island	2 tbsp (1 oz)	140	12	2
TAKE-OUT				
vinegar & oil	1 tbsp	72	8	2
SALMON				
CANNED				
chum w/ bone	1 can (13.9 oz)	521	20	5
chum w/ bone	3 oz	120	5	1
pink w/ bone	1 can (15.9 oz)	631	27	7
pink w/ bone	3 oz	118	5	1
sockeye w/ bone	3 oz	130	6	1
sockeye w/ bone	1 can (12.9 oz)	566	27	6
Bumble Bee				
Keta	½ cup (3.5 oz)	160	8	–
Red	½ cup (3.5 oz)	180	10	–
Libby				
Keta	½ can (3.8 oz)	140	6	–
Pink	½ can (3.8 oz)	150	7	–
FRESH				
atlantic baked	3 oz	155	7	1
chinook baked	3 oz	196	11	3
chum baked	3 oz	131	4	1
coho cooked	½ fillet (5.4 oz)	286	12	2
coho cooked	3 oz	157	6	1
coho raw	3 oz	124	5	1
pink baked	3 oz	127	4	1
roe raw	1 oz	59	3	–
sockeye cooked	½ fillet (5.4 oz)	334	17	3
sockeye cooked	3 oz	183	9	2
sockeye raw	3 oz	143	7	1
SMOKED				
chinook	1 oz	33	1	tr
chinook	3 oz	99	4	1

FOOD	PORTION	CALS	FAT	SAT FAT
Lascco				
Nova Sliced	2 oz	60	1	0
Nathan's				
Nova	2 oz	80	3	1
TAKE-OUT				
roulette w/ spinach stuffing	1 serv (4 oz)	160	6	2
salmon cake	1 (3 oz)	241	15	7
SALSA				
black bean & corn	2 tbsp (1 oz)	15	0	0
citrus	2 tbsp (1 oz)	10	0	0
peach	2 tbsp	15	0	0
Chi-Chi's				
Con Queso	2 tbsp (1.1 oz)	90	7	3
Hot	2 tbsp (1 oz)	10	0	0
Medium	2 tbsp (1 oz)	10	0	0
Mild	2 tbsp (1 oz)	10	0	0
Picante Hot	2 tbsp (1 oz)	10	0	0
Picante Medium	2 tbsp (1 oz)	10	0	0
Picante Mild	2 tbsp (1 oz)	10	0	0
Verde Medium	2 tbsp (1.2 oz)	15	0	0
Verde Mild	2 tbsp (1.2 oz)	15	0	0
Del Salsa				
Fire Roasted All Flavors	2 tbsp	8	0	0
Gringo Billy's				
Salsa Mix	1 tsp	5	1	0
Guiltless Gourmet				
Roasted Red Pepper	2 tbsp (1 oz)	10	0	0
Southwestern Grill	2 tbsp (1 oz)	10	0	0
Hunt's				
Alfresco All Varieties	2 tbsp (1.1 oz)	10	tr	tr
Hot	2 tbsp (1.1 oz)	27	tr	0
Medium	2 tbsp (1.1 oz)	27	tr	0
Mild	2 tbsp (1.1 oz)	27	tr	0
Picante All Varieties	2 tbsp (1.1 oz)	11	tr	0
Squeeze Mild & Medium	2 tbsp (1.1 oz)	27	tr	0
Louise's				
Fat Free BBQ Black Bean	1 oz	10	0	0
Fat Free Black Bean	1 oz	10	0	0
Fat Free Medium	1 oz	10	0	0

FOOD	PORTION	CALS	FAT	SAT FAT
Fat Free Mild	1 oz	10	0	0
Fat Free Nacho Queso	1 oz	15	0	0
Muir Glen				
Black Bean & Corn Medium	2 tbsp (1.1 oz)	15	0	0
Chipotle Medium	2 tbsp (1.1 oz)	10	0	0
Fire Roasted Tomato Medium	2 tbsp (1.1 oz)	10	0	0
Garlic Cilantro Medium	2 tbsp (1.1 oz)	10	0	0
Habanero Hot	2 tbsp (1.1 oz)	10	0	0
Organic Medium	2 tbsp (1.1 oz)	10	0	0
Organic Mild	2 tbsp (1.1 oz)	10	0	0
Roasted Garlic Medium	2 tbsp (1.1 oz)	10	0	0
Newman's Own				
Bandito Hot	2 tbsp (1.1 oz)	10	0	0
Bandito Medium	2 tbsp (1.1 oz)	10	0	0
Bandito Mild	2 tbsp (1.1 oz)	10	0	0
Peach	2 tbsp (1.1 oz)	25	0	0
Pineapple	2 tbsp (1.1 oz)	15	0	0
Roasted Garlic	2 tbsp (1.1 oz)	10	0	0
Old El Paso				
Green Chili Medium	2 tbsp (1 oz)	10	0	0
Homestyle	2 tbsp (1 oz)	5	0	0
Homestyle Mild	2 tbsp (1 oz)	5	0	0
Picante Hot	2 tbsp (1 oz)	10	0	0
Picante Medium	2 tbsp (1 oz)	10	0	0
Picante Mild	2 tbsp (1 oz)	10	0	0
Picante Thick'n Chunky Hot	2 tbsp (1 oz)	10	0	0
Picante Thick'n Chunky Medium	2 tbsp (1 oz)	10	0	0
Picante Thick'n Chunky Mild	2 tbsp (1 oz)	10	0	0
Pico De Gallo Hot	2 tbsp (1 oz)	5	0	0
Pico De Gallo Medium	1 tbsp (1 oz)	5	0	0
Salsa Verde	2 tbsp (1 oz)	10	0	0
Thick'n Chunky Hot	2 tbsp (1 oz)	10	0	0
Thick'n Chunky Medium	2 tbsp (1 oz)	10	0	0
Thick'n Chunky Mild	2 tbsp (1 oz)	10	0	0
Pace				
Picante Mild or Medium	2 tbsp	10	0	0
Thick & Chunky Mild or Medium	2 tbsp	10	0	0
Rosarita				
Extra Chunky Medium	2 tbsp (1 oz)	7	tr	0
Green Tomatillo Medium	2 tbsp (1 oz)	8	tr	0

FOOD	PORTION	CALS	FAT	SAT FAT
Picante Zesty Jalapeno Hot	2 tbsp (1 oz)	8	tr	0
Picante Zesty Jalapeno Medium	2 tbsp (1 oz)	9	tr	0
Picante Zesty Jalapeno Mild	2 tbsp (1 oz)	8	tr	0
Roasted Mild	2 tbsp (1 oz)	10	tr	0
Traditional Medium	2 tbsp (1 oz)	7	tr	0
Traditional Mild	2 tbsp (1 oz)	7	tr	0
Snyder's Of Hanover				
Mild	2 tbsp	10	0	0
Taco Bell				
Smooth 'N Zesty Picante Medium	2 tbsp (1.1 oz)	15	0	0
Smooth 'N Zesty Picante Mild	2 tbsp (1.1 oz)	15	0	0
Thick 'N Chunky Salsa Hot	2 tbsp (1.1 oz)	15	0	0
Thick 'N Chunky Salsa Medium	2 tbsp (1.1 oz)	15	0	0
Thick 'N Chunky Salsa Mild	2 tbsp (1.1 oz)	15	0	0
Tostitos				
Con Queso	2.3 oz	80	5	2
Hot	2.3 oz	30	0	0
Low Fat Con Queso	2.5 oz	80	3	2
Medium	2.3 oz	30	0	0
Mild	2.3 oz	30	0	0
Restaurant Style	2.2 oz	30	0	0
Ultimate Garden	2.4 oz	30	0	0
Tree Of Life				
Medium	2 tbsp (1 oz)	10	0	0
Mild	2 tbsp (1 oz)	10	0	0
Utz				
Chunky	2 tbsp (1 fl oz)	60	0	0
Watkins				
Salsa Seasoning Blend	⅛ tsp (0.5 g)	0	0	0
Tropical	2 tbsp (1 oz)	60	0	0
SALSIFY				
fresh sliced cooked	½ cup	46	tr	–
raw sliced	½ cup	55	tr	–
SALT SUBSTITUTES				
Cardia				
Salt Alternative	1 pkg (0.6 g)	0	0	0
Eden				
Shiso Leaf Powder	1 tsp	0	0	0

FOOD	PORTION	CALS	FAT	SAT FAT
Estee				
Salt-It	¼ tsp	0	0	0
Halsosalt				
All Flavors	¼ tsp (7 g)	1	0	0
Molly McButter				
Lite Sodium	1 tsp	5	0	0
Morton				
Salt Substitute	¼ tsp (1.2 g)	tr	0	0
Mrs. Dash				
Onion & Herb	¼ tsp	0	0	0
NoSalt				
Salt Alternative	1 pkg (0.75 g)	0	0	0
SALT/SEASONED SALT				
salt	1 tbsp (18 g)	0	0	0
salt	1 tsp (6 g)	0	0	0
Eden				
Atlantic Sea Salt	¼ tsp	0	0	0
Brittany Sea Salt	¼ tsp	0	0	0
Morton				
Garlic	1 tsp	3	tr	—
Iodized	1 tsp	tr	0	—
Kosher	1 tsp	0	0	—
Lite	¼ tsp (1.4 g)	tr	0	0
Nature's Season Seasoning Blend	1 tsp	3	tr	—
Non-Iodized	1 tsp	0	0	—
Seasoned	1 tsp	4	tr	—
Watkins				
Bacon Cheese Salt	¼ tbsp (1 g)	0	0	0
Butter Salt	¼ tbsp (1 g)	0	0	0
Cheese Salt	¼ tbsp (1 g)	0	0	0
Garlic Salt	¼ tsp (1 g)	0	0	0
Salt & Vinegar Seasoning	¼ tsp (1 g)	0	0	0
Seasoning Salt	¼ tsp (1 g)	0	0	0
Sour Cream & Onion Salt	¼ tbsp (1 g)	0	0	0
SANDWICHES				
Amy's				
Pocket Sandwich Broccoli & Cheese	1 (4.5 oz)	270	10	4
Pocket Sandwich Roasted Vegetables	1 (4.5 oz)	220	8	2

FOOD	PORTION	CALS	FAT	SAT FAT
Pocket Sandwich Spinach Feta	1 (4.5 oz)	250	9	5
Pocket Sandwich Tofu Scramble	1 (4 oz)	160	6	0
Pocket Sandwich Vegetable Pie	1 (5 oz)	300	9	2
Toaster Pops Grilled Cheese	1	180	8	4
Croissant Pocket				
Stuffed Sandwich Chicken Broccoli & Cheddar	1 piece (4.5 oz)	300	11	4
Stuffed Sandwich Ham & Cheddar	1 piece (4.5 oz)	360	17	7
Healthy Choice				
Bread Stuffs Chicken & Broccoli	1 (6.1 oz)	310	4	2
Bread Stuffs Ham & Cheese w/ Broccoli	1 (6.1 oz)	320	5	2
Bread Stuffs Italian Style Meatball	1 (6.1 oz)	330	5	2
Bread Stuffs Philly Beef Steak	1 (6.1 oz)	310	5	2
Hot Pocket				
Stuffed Sandwich Barbecue	1 (4.5 oz)	340	12	5
Stuffed Sandwich Beef & Cheddar	1 (4.5 oz)	360	18	9
Stuffed Sandwich Beef Fajita	1 (4.5 oz)	360	17	8
Stuffed Sandwich Chicken & Cheddar With Broccoli	1 (4.5 oz)	300	12	5
Stuffed Sandwich Ham & Cheese	1 (4.5 ox)	340	15	7
Stuffed Sandwich Turkey & Ham With Cheese	1 (4.5 oz)	320	13	6
Lean Pockets				
Stuffed Sandwich Beef & Broccoli	1 (4.5 oz)	250	7	3
Stuffed Sandwich Chicken Fajita	1 (4.5 oz)	260	8	3
Stuffed Sandwich Chicken Parmesan	1 (4.5 oz)	260	8	3
Stuffed Sandwich Glazed Chicken Supreme	1 (4.5 oz)	240	7	3
Stuffed Sandwich Turkey & Ham With Cheddar	1 (4.5 oz)	260	7	3
Stuffed Sandwich Turkey Broccoli & Cheese	1 (4.5 oz)	260	8	3
Smucker's				
Uncrustables Grape	1 (2 oz)	200	8	2
TAKE-OUT				
chicken fillet plain	1	515	29	9
chicken fillet w/ cheese lettuce mayonnaise & tomato	1	632	39	12

FOOD	PORTION	CALS	FAT	SAT FAT
croque monsieur	1 (12.4 oz)	765	46	26
fish fillet w/ tartar sauce	1	431	55	5
fish fillet w/ tartar sauce & cheese	1	524	29	8
fried egg w/ cheese	1	340	19	7
fried egg w/ cheese & ham	1	348	16	7
ham w/ cheese	1	353	15	6
roast beef submarine sandwich w/ tomato lettuce & mayonnaise	1	411	13	7
roast beef w/ cheese	1	402	18	9
roast beef plain	1	346	14	4
steak w/ tomato lettuce salt & mayonnaise	1	459	14	4
submarine w/ salami ham cheese lettuce tomato onion & oil	1	456	19	7
tuna salad submarine sandwich w/ lettuce & oil	1	584	28	5

SAPODILLA

fresh	1	140	2	–
fresh cut up	1 cup	199	3	–

SAPOTES

fresh	1	301	1	–

SARDINES
CANNED

atlantic in oil w/ bone	2	50	3	tr
atlantic in oil w/ bone	1 can (3.2 oz)	192	11	1
pacific in tomato sauce w/ bone	1 can (13 oz)	658	44	11
pacific in tomato sauce w/ bone	1	68	5	1
Bumble Bee				
In Hot Sauce	½ can (2 oz)	109	8	2
In Mustard	½ can (2 oz)	88	5	2
In Oil	½ can (2 oz)	125	7	2
In Water	½ can (2 oz)	83	3	1
King Oscar				
In Olive Oil	1 can (3.75 oz)	150	11	3
Skinless Boneless In Soya Oil	3 pieces (1.9 oz)	120	7	2
Season				
Brisling In Water	1 can (3.75 oz)	145	10	4

FOOD	PORTION	CALS	FAT	SAT FAT
FRESH				
raw	3.5 oz	135	5	–

SAUCE (see also BARBECUE SAUCE, GRAVY, PIZZA SAUCE, SPAGHETTI SAUCE)

FOOD	PORTION	CALS	FAT	SAT FAT
JARRED				
fish sauce chinese	1 tbsp	9	0	0
fish sauce vietnamese nuoc mam	1 tbsp	6	0	0
hoisin	1 tbsp	35	1	–
morroccan tagine	½ cup (4 oz)	70	3	0
oyster	1 tbsp	8	0	0
teriyaki	1 oz	30	0	0
teriyaki	1 tbsp	15	0	0
A1				
Bold Steak Sauce	1 tbsp	20	0	0
Annie Chun				
Shiitake Mushroom	1 tbsp	15	0	0
Thai Peanut	2 tbsp	120	7	1
Armour				
Chili Hot Dog	¼ cup (2.2 oz)	120	9	4
Meatless Sloppy Joe Sauce	¼ cup (2.2 oz)	30	0	0
Atkins				
Steak Sauce	1 tbsp	5	0	0
Teriyaki	1 tbsp	10	1	0
Boar's Head				
Ham Glaze Brown Sugar & Spice	2 tbsp (1.4 oz)	120	0	0
Carb Options				
Alfredo	¼ cup	110	10	4
Asian Teriyaki Marinade	1 tbsp	5	1	–
Cheese	¼ cup	90	8	3
Garden Style	½ cup	80	5	1
Steak Sauce	1 tbsp	5	0	0
Cheez Whiz				
Cheese	2 tbsp (1.2 oz)	90	7	5
Cheese Jalapeno Pepper	2 tbsp (1.2 oz)	90	7	5
Cheese Mild Salsa	2 tbsp (1.2 oz)	100	7	5
Chi-Chi's				
Enchilada	¼ cup (2.1 oz)	30	2	1
Taco	1 tbsp (0.5 oz)	10	0	0
Chun King				
Sweet And Sour	2 tbsp (1.2 oz)	58	tr	0

FOOD	PORTION	CALS	FAT	SAT FAT
Teriyaki	1 tbsp (0.6 oz)	17	tr	0
Teriyaki Hot	1 tbsp (0.6 oz)	17	tr	0
Del Monte				
Seafood Cocktail	¼ cup (2.7 oz)	100	0	0
Sloppy Joe Hickory Flavor	¼ cup (2.4 oz)	70	0	0
Sloppy Joe Hickory Flavor	¼ cup (2.4 oz)	70	0	0
Sloppy Joe Original	¼ cup (2.4 oz)	70	0	0
Fritos				
Texas-Style Chili Hearty Topping	2.3 oz	50	2	1
Utimate Taco Hearty Topping	2.3 oz	50	2	1
Gebhardt				
Enchilada Sauce	¼ cup (2.2 oz)	35	2	1
Hot Dog Chili Sauce	¼ cup (2.2 oz)	60	3	1
Hot Sauce	1 tsp (5 g)	1	tr	0
Green Giant				
Sloppy Joe	¼ cup (2.6 oz)	50	0	0
Sloppy Joe as prep w/ meat	1 serv (4.4 oz)	200	11	4
Gringo Billy's				
Chipotle Dipping & Grilling Sauce	1 tsp	5	0	0
Hormel				
Not-So-Sloppy-Joe Sauce	¼ cup (2.2 oz)	70	0	0
House Of Tsang				
Bangkok Padang	1 tbsp (0.6 oz)	45	3	1
Hoisin	1 tsp (6 g)	15	0	0
Mandarin Marinade	1 tbsp (0.6 oz)	25	0	0
Saigon Sizzle	1 tbsp (0.6 oz)	40	1	0
Spicy Brown Bean	1 tsp (6 g)	15	0	0
Stir Fry Classic	1 tbsp (0.6 oz)	25	1	0
Stir Fry Sweet & Sour	1 tbsp (0.6 oz)	30	0	0
Stir Fry Szechuan Spicy	1 tbsp (0.6 oz)	20	1	0
Sweet & Sour Concentrate	1 tsp (6 g)	10	0	0
Teriyaki Korean	1 tbsp (0.6 oz)	30	1	0
Hunt's				
Light w/ Mushrooms	½ cup (4.4 oz)	42	tr	tr
Steak	1 tbsp (0.6 oz)	10	tr	0
Jok'n'Al				
Cocktail	¼ cup	29	0	0
Plum	1 tbsp	10	0	0
Just Rite				
Hot Dog	¼ cup (2.2 oz)	50	3	1

FOOD	PORTION	CALS	FAT	SAT FAT
Kikkoman				
Teriyaki	1 tbsp	15	0	0
Kraft				
Cocktail	¼ cup (2.3 oz)	60	1	0
Fat Free Tartar Sauce	2 tbsp (1.1 oz)	25	0	0
Lemon & Herb Tartar Sauce	2 tbsp (1 oz)	150	16	3
Reduced Fat Sandwich Spread	1 tbsp (0.5 oz)	35	3	0
Sandwich Spread	1 tbsp (0.5 oz)	50	4	1
Sweet'n Sour	2 tbsp (1.2 oz)	60	0	0
Tartar	2 tbsp (1.1 oz)	90	9	2
La Choy				
Duck Sauce Sweet & Sour	2 tbsp (1.3 oz)	61	tr	0
Sweet & Sour	2 tbsp (1.2 oz)	58	tr	0
Teriyaki	1 tbsp (0.6 oz)	17	tr	0
Lawry's				
Marinade Lemon Pepper	1 tbsp (0.5 oz)	10	1	–
Lea & Perrins				
Worcestershire	1 tsp	5	0	0
Manwich				
BBQ Sloppy Joe	¼ cup (2.2 oz)	57	tr	tr
Bold	¼ cup (2.2 oz)	62	1	0
Mexican	¼ cup (2.2 oz)	27	tr	0
Original	¼ cup (2.2 oz)	32	tr	0
Taco Season	¼ cup (2.2 oz)	27	tr	tr
Thick & Chunky	¼ cup (2.3 oz)	44	tr	0
Marzetti				
Teriyaki Stir-Fry	2 tbsp	80	2	0
Matouk's				
Flambeau Sauce	1 tsp	0	0	0
McCormick				
Flavor Medleys Garlic & Herb	2 tbsp	50	5	–
Flavor Medleys Italian Herb	2 tbsp	50	4	–
Flavor Medleys Lemon Pepper	2 tbsp	50	4	–
Flavor Medleys Tomato & Basil	2 tbsp	50	3	–
Newman's Own				
Spicy Simmer Sauce Diavolo	½ cup (4.4 oz)	70	3	0
Old El Paso				
Enchilada Hot	¼ cup (2 oz)	30	2	–
Enchilada Mild	¼ cup	20	1	0
Green Chili Enchilada Sauce	¼ cup (2.1 oz)	30	2	–

FOOD	PORTION	CALS	FAT	SAT FAT
Taco Hot	1 tbsp (0.5 oz)	5	0	0
Taco Medium	1 tbsp (0.5 oz)	5	0	0
Taco Mild	1 tbsp (0.5 oz)	5	0	0
Taco Sauce	1 tbsp (0.5 oz)	5	0	0
Taco Sauce Extra Chunky Medium	1 tbsp (0.5 oz)	5	0	0
Taco Sauce Extra Chunky Mild	1 tbsp (0.5 oz)	5	0	0
Open Range				
Hot Dog Chili	¼ cup (2.2 oz)	61	3	2
Pace				
Enchilada Sauce	¼ cup	36	0	0
Taco Sauce	¼ cup	32	2	0
Progresso				
Alfredo	½ cup (4.4 oz)	200	15	10
Red Wing				
Chili Sauce	1 tbsp (0.6 oz)	20	0	0
Seafood Cocktail	¼ cup (2 oz)	90	1	0
Sauce Arturo				
Original	¼ cup (2.2 fl oz)	50	1	0
Steel's				
Sugar Free Cocktail w/ Dill & Lemon	¼ cup	36	0	0
Sugar Free Hoisin	2 tbsp	15	0	0
Sugar Free Peanut Sauce	1 tbsp	34	2	–
Sugar Free Sweet & Sour	2 tbsp	10	0	0
Tabasco				
Caribbean Steak Sauce	1 tbsp (0.6 oz)	15	0	0
Garlic Basting Sauce	1 tbsp (0.6 oz)	20	0	0
Habanero Sauce	1 tsp (0.2 oz)	5	0	0
Hot Sauce w/ Garlic	1 tsp (0.2 oz)	0	0	0
Jalepeno Pepper Sauce	1 tbsp	15	0	0
New Orleans Steak Sauce	1 tbsp (0.6 oz)	15	0	0
Pepper Sauce	1 tsp (0.2 oz)	0	0	0
Taco Bell				
Taco Sauce Medium	2 tbsp (1.1 oz)	15	0	0
Taco Sauce Mild	2 tbsp (1.1 oz)	15	0	0
The Restaurant Hot Sauce	1 tsp (5 g)	0	0	0
Tostitos				
Beef Fiesta Nacho	2.4 oz	120	8	3
Chicken Quesadilla Topping	2.5 oz	90	6	2
Walden Farms				
Calorie Free Seafood Sauce	1 tbsp	0	0	0

FOOD	PORTION	CALS	FAT	SAT FAT
Scampi Sauce Calorie Free	2 tbsp	0	0	0
Watkins				
Inferno Hot Pepper Sauce	2 tbsp (1 oz)	35	0	0
Steak Sauce	1 tbsp (0.5 oz)	20	0	0
Wild Thyme Farms				
Chili Ginger Honey	1 tbsp	30	0	0
MIX				
cheese as prep w/ milk	1 cup	307	17	9
curry as prep w/ milk	1 cup	270	15	6
mushroom as prep w/ milk	1 cup	228	10	5
sour cream as prep w/ milk	1 cup	509	30	16
stroganoff as prep	1 cup	271	11	7
sweet & sour as prep	1 cup	294	tr	tr
teriyaki as prep	1 cup	131	1	tr
white as prep w/ milk	1 cup	241	13	6
Durkee				
A La King as prep	1 cup	60	4	1
Cheese as prep	¼ cup	25	2	1
Hollandaise as prep	2 tbsp	10	0	0
White as prep	¼ cup	20	1	0
French's				
Cheese as prep	¼ cup	25	1	0
Hollandaise as prep	2 tbsp	10	0	0
Manwich				
Mix	¼ oz	22	tr	0
McCormick				
Bernaise Blend	1 tsp (3 g)	10	0	0
Chicken Dijon Blend	1⅓ tbsp (10 g)	40	2	–
Green Peppercorn Blend as prep	¼ cup	20	0	0
Grill Mates Mesquite Marinade as prep	1 tbsp	15	0	0
Grill Mates Southwest Marinade	2 tsp (5 g)	15	0	0
Hollandaise Blend	2 tsp (4 g)	15	0	–
Hunter Blend as prep	¼ cup	25	0	0
Meat Marinade	1 tsp (4 g)	15	0	0
Pepper Medley Blend as prep	¼ cup	30	2	–
White Blend	2 tsp (6 g)	20	1	–
Watkins				
Beef Marinade	¼ tbsp (2 g)	5	0	0
Calypso Hot Pepper Sauce	1 tsp (5 g)	10	0	0

FOOD	PORTION	CALS	FAT	SAT FAT
Caribbean Red Pepper Sauce	1 tsp (5 g)	10	0	0
Chicken & Pork Marinade	¼ tbsp (2 g)	5	0	0
Fish & Seafood Marinade	¼ tbsp (2 g)	10	0	0
Meat Magic	1 tsp (6 g)	10	0	0
SHELF-STABLE				
Cheez Whiz				
Cheese Sqeezable	2 tbsp (1.2 oz)	100	8	4
Fresh Gourmet				
Stir 'n Sauce Italian	1 tbsp (0.5 oz)	30	1	—
TAKE-OUT				
bearnaise	1 oz	177	19	12
SAUERKRAUT				
canned	½ cup	22	tr	tr
B&G				
Sauerkraut	2 tbsp (1 oz)	6	0	0
Boar's Head				
Sauerkraut	2 tbsp (1 oz)	5	0	0
Claussen				
Sauerkraut	¼ cup (1.1 oz)	5	0	0
Del Monte				
Bavarian Style	2 tbsp (1 oz)	15	0	0
Sauerkraut	2 tbsp (1 oz)	0	0	0
Eden				
Organic	½ cup	25	0	0
S&W				
Canned	2 tbsp (1 oz)	5	0	0
Red Cabbage	2 tbsp (1 oz)	15	0	0
SAUSAGE				
bierschinken	3.5 oz	174	11	—
bierwurst	3.5 oz	258	21	—
blutwurst uncooked	3.5 oz	424	39	—
bockwurst	3.5 oz	276	25	—
bratwurst pork cooked	1 link (3 oz)	256	22	8
brotwurst pork & beef	1 link (2.5 oz)	226	19	7
chipolata	3.5 oz	342	32	12
chorizo	3.5 oz	499	45	17
fleischwurst	3.5 oz	305	29	—
free range chicken breakfast	2 links (2.7 oz)	110	6	1
gelbwurst uncooked	3.5 oz	363	33	—

FOOD	PORTION	CALS	FAT	SAT FAT
italian pork cooked	1 (3 oz)	268	21	8
jagdwurst	3.5 oz	211	16	—
kielbasa pork	1 oz	88	8	3
knockwurst pork & beef	1 (2.4 oz)	209	19	7
mettwurst uncooked	3.5 oz	483	45	—
plockwurst uncooked	3.5 oz	312	45	—
polish pork	1 (8 oz)	739	65	23
pork cooked	1 link (½ oz)	48	4	1
regensburger uncooked	3.5 oz	354	31	—
vienna canned	7 (4 oz)	315	28	10
vienna canned	1 (½ oz)	45	4	1
weisswurst uncooked	3.5 oz	305	27	—
zungenwurst (tongue)	3.5 oz	285	24	—
Aidells				
Andouille Cajun Cooked	1 (3.5 oz)	220	17	8
Burmese Curry Cooked	1 (3.5 oz)	220	15	5
Chicken & Apple Fresh	1 (1.9 oz)	110	8	2
Chicken & Apple Smoked	1 (3.5 oz)	220	16	5
Chicken & Turkey New Mexico Smoked	1 (3.5 oz)	220	16	5
Chicken & Turkey Thai Fresh	1 (3.5 oz)	200	16	5
Chicken & Turkey Thai Smoked	1 (3.5 oz)	220	16	5
Chicken & Turkey With Sun-Dried Tomatoes & Basil Fresh	1 (3.5 oz)	200	15	6
Chicken & Turkey With Sun-Dried Tomatoes & Basil Smoked	1 (3.5 oz)	200	14	5
Creole Hot Cooked	1 (3.5 oz)	220	16	7
Duck & Turkey Smoked	1 (3.5 oz)	220	16	4
Hunter's Cooked	1 (3.5 oz)	240	19	5
Italian Hot Fresh	1 (3.5 oz)	230	18	6
Italian Mild Fresh	1 (3.5 oz)	230	18	6
Lamb & Beef With Rosemary Fresh	1 (3.5 oz)	220	16	6
Lemon Chicken Cooked	1 (3.5 oz)	220	16	5
Mexican Chorizo Beef Fresh	1 (3.5 oz)	400	37	14
Whiskey Fennel Cooked	1 (3.5 oz)	230	18	7
Armour				
Vienna Sausage 25% Less Fat	3 (1.9 oz)	130	11	4
Vienna Sausage 50% Less Fat	3 (1.9 oz)	90	7	3
Vienna Sausage Chicken & Beef	3 (1.9 oz)	120	10	4
Vienna Sausage Hot'n Spicy	3 (2.1 oz)	150	13	5

FOOD	PORTION	CALS	FAT	SAT FAT
Vienna Sausage In BBQ Sauce	3 (2.1 oz)	150	13	5
Vienna Sausage In Beef Stock	3 (1.9 oz)	150	14	6
Vienna Sausage Jalapeno In Beef Stock	3 (1.9 oz)	170	16	6
Banner				
Sausage Stomachs	2 oz	90	5	3
Sausage Tripe	2 oz	90	5	3
Bilinski's				
Chicken & Vegetable	1 (3 oz)	80	2	1
Chicken Italian With Peppers & Onions	1 (3 oz)	120	4	1
Boar's Head				
Bratwurst	1 (4 oz)	300	25	11
Hot Smoked	1 (3.2 oz)	280	25	10
Kielbasa	2 oz	120	10	4
Knockwurst	1 (4 oz)	310	27	11
Brown'N Serve				
Turkey	3 (2.1 oz)	120	8	3
Healthy Choice				
Low Fat Smoked	2 oz	70	2	1
Low Fat Smoked Polska Kielbasa	2 oz	70	2	1
Hormel				
Kielbasa	2 oz	150	13	5
Light & Lean 97 Dinner Smoked	2 oz	60	2	1
Pickled Hot	6 (2 oz)	140	11	5
Pickled Smoked	6 (2 oz)	140	11	5
Smoked Summer	2 oz	200	18	8
Vienna	2 oz	140	14	5
Vienna Chicken	2 oz	110	9	3
Jimmy Dean				
Brick Sausage	2.5 oz	270	25	9
Bulk	2.5 oz	300	28	10
Hickory Smoked Dinner Sausage	2 oz	170	14	5
Pattie Pre-Cooked	1 (1.9 oz)	230	22	8
Polska Kielbasa	2 oz	170	15	5
Sage Pattie	1 (2 oz)	200	19	7
Sausage Pattie Raw	1 (2 oz)	200	19	6
Skinless Link	2 (2 oz)	200	19	7
Skinless Link	4 (2 oz)	200	19	7

FOOD	PORTION	CALS	FAT	SAT FAT
Jones				
Light 50% Less Fat	2 (1.6 oz)	100	8	3
Little Sizzlers				
Brown & Serve	2 patties (1.8 oz)	190	18	6
Brown & Serve	3 links (2.1 oz)	190	22	8
Cooked	3 links (1.8 oz)	230	22	8
Cooked	2 patties (1.8 oz)	230	22	8
Heat & Serve Pork cooked	3 links (1.8 oz)	230	22	8
Louis Rich				
Polska Kielbasa	2 oz	90	5	2
Turkey Hot	2.5 oz	120	8	3
Turkey Original	2.5 oz	120	8	3
Turkey Smoked	2 oz	90	5	2
Mr. Turkey				
Breakfast	2.5 oz	130	9	—
Hearty Blend Polish Kielbasa	1 oz	70	6	—
Hearty Blend Smoked	1 oz	70	6	—
Hot Smoked	1 oz	45	3	—
Italian Smoked	1 oz	45	3	—
Polish Kielbasa	1 oz	45	3	—
Smoked	1 oz	45	3	—
Old Smokehouse				
Summer Sausage	2 oz	200	18	8
Oscar Mayer				
Pork cooked	2 links (1.7 oz)	170	15	5
Smokies Beef	1 (1.5 oz)	120	11	5
Smokies Cheese	1 (1.5 oz)	130	12	5
Smokies Link	1 (1.5 oz)	130	12	4
Smokies Little	6 (2 oz)	170	15	6
Smokies Little Cheese	6 (2 oz)	180	16	6
Perdue				
Hot Italian Turkey Cooked	1 link (2.4 oz)	150	9	3
Sweet Italian Turkey Cooked	1 link (2.4 oz)	150	9	3
Rudy's Farm				
Italian Hot	2.5 oz	240	22	7
Italian Mild	2.5 oz	240	22	7
Italian Mild Natural Casing	1 (2 oz)	190	17	6
Morning Right Link	3 (2.9 oz)	150	10	4
Morning Right Pattie	2 (2.9 oz)	150	10	4
Pattie Pre-Cooked	1 (1.4 oz)	100	6	2

FOOD	PORTION	CALS	FAT	SAT FAT
Smoked	4 (2.1 oz)	200	18	6
Sweet Link	1 (3.9 oz)	380	35	12
Shady Brook				
Turkey Breakfast	2 oz	80	4	2
Turkey Hot Italian	2 oz	100	5	2
Turkey Old World Style	4 oz	190	11	3
Turkey Sweet Italian	2 oz	100	5	2
Turkey Store				
Breakfast	2 links (2 oz)	140	11	3
Wampler				
Breakfast Turkey	2 (2.4 oz)	110	6	2
Italian Turkey	1 (2.7 oz)	120	6	2
TAKE-OUT				
pork	1 patty (1 oz)	100	8	3
pork	1 link (0.5 oz)	48	4	1

SAUSAGE DISHES
Jimmy Dean

Italian Sausage & Mozzarella Sandwich	1 (4.5 oz)	380	22	9
TAKE-OUT				
italian sausage w/ peppers & onions	1 cup	210	11	–
sausage roll	1 (2.3 oz)	311	24	–

SAUSAGE SUBSTITUTES

nonmeat sausage	1 link (25 g)	64	5	1
nonmeat sausage	1 patty (38 g)	97	7	1
Boca Burgers				
Breakfast Patties	1 (1.3 oz)	70	3	0
GardenSausage				
Patty	1 (2.5 oz)	140	3	2
Lightlife				
Gimme Lean	2 oz	70	0	0
Lean Links Breakfast	1 (1.2 oz)	60	3	1
Lean Links Italian	1 (1.4 oz)	60	2	1
Light	2 patties (2.3 oz)	80	0	0
Loma Linda				
Linketts	1 (1.2 oz)	70	5	1
Little Links	2 (1.6 oz)	90	6	1
Morningstar Farms				
Breakfast Links	2 (1.6 oz)	60	2	1

FOOD	PORTION	CALS	FAT	SAT FAT
Breakfast Patties	1 (1.3 oz)	80	3	1
Grillers	1 patty (2.2 oz)	140	7	2
Sausage Style Recipe Crumbles	⅔ cup (1.9 oz)	90	3	0
Natural Touch				
Vegan Sausage Crumbles	½ cup (1.9 oz)	60	0	0
Quron				
Meat-Free Links	2 (1.6 oz)	70	3	0
Worthington				
Leanies	1 link (1.4 oz)	100	7	1
Prosage Links	2 (1.6 oz)	60	3	1
Saucettes	1 link (1.3 oz)	90	6	1
Super Links	1 (1.7 oz)	110	8	1
Veja Links	1 (1.1 oz)	50	3	1
Yves				
Veggie Breakfast Links	1 (1.6 oz)	60	0	0
Veggie Breakfast Patties	1 (2 oz)	70	2	0
SAVORY				
ground	1 tsp	4	tr	–
SCALLOP				
raw	3 oz	75	1	tr
TAKE-OUT				
breaded & fried	2 lg	67	3	1
SCONE				
Finnegan's				
Cranberry	1 (2.7 oz)	90	2	0
Irish Raisin	1 (2.7 oz)	90	2	0
Health Valley				
Apple Kiwi	1	180	0	0
Cinnamon Raisin	1	180	0	0
Cranberry Orange	1	180	0	0
Mountain Blueberry	1	180	0	0
Pineapple Banana	1	180	0	0
TAKE-OUT				
apricot	1	232	7	–
blueberry	1 (3 oz)	270	9	4
cheese	1 (3.5 oz)	364	18	–
orange poppy	1 (3 oz)	260	6	4
plain	1 (3.5 oz)	362	14	–

FOOD	PORTION	CALS	FAT	SAT FAT
raisin	1 (3 oz)	270	8	3
SCUP				
fresh baked	3 oz	115	3	–
SEA BASS (see BASS)				
SEA CUCUMBER				
dried	1 oz	74	1	–
fresh	1 oz	20	tr	–
SEA TROUT (see TROUT)				
SEA URCHIN				
canned	1 oz	39	1	–
fresh	1 oz	36	1	–
roe paste	1 tbsp	19	tr	–
SEAWEED				
agar dried	1 oz	87	tr	tr
agar fresh	1 oz	tr	tr	tr
hijiki dried	1 tbsp	9	0	0
irishmoss fresh	1 oz	14	tr	tr
kelp fresh	1 oz	12	tr	tr
kombu fresh	1 oz	12	tr	tr
laver fresh	1 oz	10	tr	tr
nori fresh	1 oz	10	tr	tr
nori sheet dried	1 (8 x 8 in)	5	0	0
seahair dried	1 tbsp	13	0	0
spirulina dried	1 oz	83	2	1
spirulina fresh	1 oz	7	tr	tr
tangle fresh	1 oz	12	tr	tr
wakame fresh	1 oz	13	tr	tr
Maine Coast				
Alaria	⅓ cup (7 g)	18	0	0
Dulse	⅓ cup (7 g)	18	0	0
Dulse Flakes	1 oz	75	1	–
Kelp	⅓ cup (7 g)	17	0	0
Kelp Crunch	1 bar (1 oz)	129	6	1
Kelp Crunch Peanut-Raisin	1 bar (1 oz)	129	6	1
Laver	⅓ cup (7 g)	22	0	0
Sea Seasoning Dulse	1 g	3	0	0
Sea Seasoning Dulse With Celery	1 g	3	0	0

FOOD	PORTION	CALS	FAT	SAT FAT
Sea Seasoning Dulse With Garlic	1 g	3	0	0
Sea Seasoning Dulse With Sesame	1 g	3	0	0
Sea Seasoning Kelp	1 g	3	0	0
Sea Seasoning Kelp With Cayenne	1 g	3	0	0
Sea Seasoning Nori	1 g	3	0	0
Sea Seasoning Nori With Ginger	1 g	3	0	0

SEITAN (see WHEAT)

SEMOLINA
dry	1 cup (5.9 oz)	601	2	tr

SESAME
seeds	1 tsp	16	2	–
sesame butter	1 tbsp	95	8	1
sesame crunch candy	20 pieces (1.2 oz)	181	12	2
sesame crunch candy	1 oz	146	9	1
tahini from roasted & toasted kernels	1 tbsp	89	8	1
tahini from stone ground kernels	1 tbsp	86	7	1
tahini from unroasted kernels	1 tbsp	85	8	1
Casbah				
Tahini Sauce Mix as prep	¼ cup	160	13	0
Eden				
Organic Seaweed Gomasio	1 serv (1.5 oz)	10	1	0
Organic Gomasio	½ tsp	10	1	0
Organic Gomasio Garlic	½ tsp	10	1	0
Joyva				
Tahini	2 tbsp (1 oz)	200	18	3
Maranatha				
Raw Tahini	2 tbsp	190	16	2
Roasted Tahini	2 tbsp	210	16	2
Planters				
Nut Mix	1 oz	150	12	2
Stone-Buhr				
Seeds Raw	4 tsp (1 oz)	180	16	3

SESBANIA
flower	1	1	0	0
flowers	1 cup	5	tr	–
flowers cooked	1 cup	23	tr	–

FOOD	PORTION	CALS	FAT	SAT FAT
SHAD				
american baked	3 oz	214	15	—
roe baked w/ butter & lemon	1 oz	36	1	—
roe raw	1 oz	37	tr	—
SHARK				
batter-dipped & fried	3 oz	194	12	3
fin dried	1 oz	32	tr	—
raw	3 oz	111	4	1
SHEEPSHEAD FISH				
cooked	3 oz	107	1	tr
cooked	1 fillet (6.5 oz)	234	3	1
raw	3 oz	92	2	1
SHELLFISH (see individual names, SHELLFISH SUBSTITUTES)				
SHELLFISH SUBSTITUTES				
crab imitation	3 oz	87	1	—
scallop imitation	3 oz	84	tr	—
shrimp imitation	3 oz	86	1	—
surimi	3 oz	84	1	—
surimi	1 oz	28	tr	—
Louis Kemp				
Crab Delights	½ cup (3 oz)	90	0	0
Lobster Delights	½ cup (3 oz)	80	0	0
Scallop Delights	13 pieces (3 oz)	80	0	0
Ocean Magic				
Imitation King Crab	3 oz	80	tr	—
SHELLIE BEANS				
canned	½ cup	37	tr	tr
SHERBET				
orange	½ cup (4 fl oz)	132	2	1
orange	½ gal	2158	31	19
orange	1 bar (2.75 fl oz)	91	1	1
orange home recipe	½ cup	120	2	—
Breyers				
Orange	½ cup	120	2	1
Rainbow	½ cup	120	2	1
Hood				
Lime Orange Lemon	½ cup (3.1 oz)	120	1	1

FOOD	PORTION	CALS	FAT	SAT FAT
Orange	½ cup (3.1 oz)	120	1	1
Rainbow Swirl	½ cup (3.1 oz)	120	1	1
Raspberry Orange Lime	½ cup (3.1 oz)	120	1	1
Turkey Hill				
Fruit Rainbow	½ cup	120	1	—
Orange Grove	½ cup	120	1	—
SHRIMP				
canned	3 oz	102	2	tr
canned	1 cup	154	3	tr
chinese shrimp paste	1 tbsp	15	tr	—
cooked	3 oz	84	1	tr
cooked	4 large	22	tr	tr
raw	3 oz	90	1	tr
raw	4 large	30	tr	tr
Bumble Bee				
Medium	⅓ can (2 oz)	45	tr	0
Orleans Tiny Cocktail	½ can (3 oz)	44	0	—
Gorton's				
Popcorn Garlic & Herb	22 pieces (3.6 oz)	270	14	3
Popcorn Original	20 pieces (3.2 oz)	240	13	3
Van De Kamp's				
Breaded Butterfly	7 (4 oz)	280	14	3
Breaded Popcorn	20 (4 oz)	270	13	2
Breaded Whole	7 (4 oz)	240	10	2
TAKE-OUT				
breaded & fried	3 oz	206	10	2
gingered	4	80	tr	tr
jambalaya	¾ cup	188	5	2
scampi	2 cups	438	480	10
SMELT				
rainbow cooked	3 oz	106	3	tr
rainbow raw	3 oz	83	2	tr
SMOOTHIE (see FRUIT DRINKS)				
SNACKS				
cheese puffs	1 oz	157	10	2
corn puffs cheese	1 bag (8 oz)	1256	78	15

FOOD	PORTION	CALS	FAT	SAT FAT
corn twists cheese	1 oz	157	10	2
corn twists cheese	1 bag (8 oz)	1256	78	15
oriental mix	1 oz	155	12	–
pork skins	1 oz	154	9	3
pork skins barbecue	1 oz	152	9	3
trail mix	1 oz	131	8	2
trail mix	1 cup (5.3 oz)	693	44	8
trail mix tropical	1 oz	115	5	2
trail mix w/ chocolate chips	1 cup (5.1 oz)	707	47	9
trail mix w/ chocolate chips	1 oz	137	9	2
Baken-ets				
BBQ	9 (0.5 oz)	70	5	2
Hot N'Spicy	7 (0.5 oz)	70	5	2
Hot N'Spicy Cracklins	8 (0.5 oz)	80	5	2
Regular	9 (0.5 oz)	80	5	3
Regular Cracklins	8 (0.5 oz)	40	6	2
Barbara's Bakery				
Cheese Puffs Bakes	1½ cups (1 oz)	160	11	2
Cheese Puffs Jalapeno	¾ cup (1 oz)	150	10	2
Cheese Puffs Original	¾ cup (1 oz)	150	10	2
Big Dipper				
Bagel Chips Lowfat Barbeque	12 (1 oz)	110	2	0
Bagel Chips Lowfat Garlic	12 (1 oz)	120	2	0
Bagel Chips Lowfat Original	12 (1 oz)	110	2	0
Bowlby's				
Bits Almond	½ cup	100	19	3
Bits Pecan	½ cup	200	19	3
Bits Ranch	½ cup	170	16	2
Bits Salsa	½ cup	170	16	2
Bits Sour Cream Onion & Dill	½ cup	170	16	2
Bits'N'Pops	¾ cup	130	7	3
Mix-Ups Country Mix	½ cup	170	14	2
Mix-Ups Nuttyest-Of-All	½ cup	160	13	2
Mix-Ups Trail Mix	½ cup	165	12	2
Bugles				
Baked Original	1⅓ cup	130	4	1
Chile Con Queso	1⅓ cups	160	9	7
Nacho	1⅓ cups	160	9	7
Original	1⅓ cups	160	9	8
Smokin' BBQ	1⅓ cups	150	8	7

FOOD	PORTION	CALS	FAT	SAT FAT
Cheetos				
Crunchy	21 pieces (1 oz)	160	10	3
Curls	15 pieces (1 oz)	150	10	3
Flamin' Hot	21 pieces (1 oz)	160	10	2
Nacho Cheese	23 pieces (1 oz)	160	10	3
Puffed Balls	38 pieces (1 oz)	150	10	3
Puffs	29 pieces (1 oz)	160	10	3
Zig Zags	17 pieces (1 oz)	170	11	3
Chex Mix				
Cheddar	⅔ cup	140	5	1
Hot'N Spicy	⅔ cup	130	5	1
Nacho Fiesta	⅔ cup	120	4	1
Party Blend Bold	⅔ cup	140	6	1
Peanut Lovers	⅔ cup	140	6	1
Traditional	⅔ cup	130	4	1
Combos				
Cheddar Cheese Cracker	1 pkg (1.7 oz)	250	13	3
Cheddar Cheese Cracker	1 oz	140	8	2
Cheddar Cheese Pretzel	1 pkg (1.8 oz)	240	9	2
Cheddar Cheese Pretzel	1 oz	130	5	1
Chili Cheese w/ Corn Shell	1 oz	140	6	1
Chili Cheese w/ Corn Shell	1 pkg (1.7 oz)	230	11	2
Mustard Pretzel	1 pkg (1.8 oz)	230	8	1
Mustard Pretzel	1 oz	130	4	1
Nacho Cheese Pretzel	1 pkg (1.7 oz)	230	8	2
Nacho Cheese Pretzel	1 oz	130	5	1
Nacho Cheese w/ Tortilla Shell	1 oz	140	6	1
Nacho Cheese w/ Tortilla Shell	1 pkg (1.7 oz)	230	11	2
Peanut Butter Cracker	1 oz	140	8	2
Pepperoni & Cheese Pizza	1 oz	140	7	1
Pepperoni & Cheese Pizza	1 pkg (1.7 oz)	240	11	2
Pizzeria Pretzel	1 pkg (1.8 oz)	230	8	2
Pizzeria Pretzel	1 oz	130	5	1
Tortilla Ranch	1 oz	140	7	2
Tortilla Ranch	1 bag (1.7 oz)	240	12	3
Dakota Gourmet				
Amazing Corn Classic	1 pkg (1 oz)	360	7	1
Amazing Corn Cool Ranch	1 pkg (1 oz)	367	9	1
Amazing Corn Mesquite BBQ	1 pkg (1 oz)	369	8	1
Heart Smart Toasted Corn	⅓ cup (1 oz)	110	2	0

FOOD	PORTION	CALS	FAT	SAT FAT
Toasted Corn Heart Smart	1 pkg (1.75 oz)	177	3	tr
Trail Mix Heart Smart	1 pkg (1.75 oz)	172	0	0
Eden				
Rice Puffs Five Flavor Arare	1 oz	110	0	0
Energy Food Factory				
Poprice Cheddar Cheese	½ oz	60	3	—
Poprice Herb & Garlic	½ oz	50	2	—
Poprice Lite	½ oz	50	2	—
Poprice Original No Salt	½ oz	45	0	0
Frito Lay				
Funyuns	13 (1 oz)	140	7	2
Munchos	16 (1 oz)	160	10	2
Munchos BBQ	14 (1 oz)	160	10	2
Glenny's				
Soy Crisps All Flavors	5	60	4	3
Gram's Gourmet				
Crunchies Pork Rinds	⅛ pkg (0.5 oz)	70	5	2
Hapi				
Chili Bits	½ cup (1 oz)	110	0	0
Health Valley				
Cheddar Lites Green Onion	1¾ cups	120	3	—
Cheddar Lites Original	1¾ cups	120	3	—
Corn Puffs Caramel	2 cups	120	2	—
Low Fat Potato Puffs Cheddar Cheese	1½ cups	110	3	—
Low Fat Potato Puffs Garlic w/ Cheese	1½ cups	260	3	—
Low Fat Potato Puffs Zesty Ranch	1½ cups	110	3	—
Innovative Foods				
Roasted Sweet Corn	1 pkg (0.8 oz)	76	0	0
J&J				
Microwave Pork Rinds All Flavors	1 oz	130	4	2
Lance				
Cheese Balls	1 pkg (1 oz)	150	8	2
Crunchy Cheese Twists	1 pkg (1.25 oz)	190	4	—
Gold-N-Chees	1 pkg (1 oz)	130	5	2
Onion Rings	1 pkg (0.9 oz)	100	8	2
Pork Skins	1 pkg (0.4 oz)	65	4	2
Pork Skins BBQ	1 pkg (0.4 oz)	60	4	2
Maranatha				
High Energy Mix	¼ cup	120	7	1
Organic Harvest Mix	¼ cup	150	9	1

FOOD	PORTION	CALS	FAT	SAT FAT
Organic Nature Mix	¼ cup	150	9	2
Snack Attack Mix	¼ cup	140	8	3
Trail Mix Organic Raw	¼ cup	140	9	2
Trail Mix Deluxe	¼ cup	150	11	1
Trail Mix Navajo	¼ cup	140	9	1
Trail Mix Olympic w/ Chocolate	¼ cup	140	8	2
Trail Mix Organic Delight	¼ cup	150	10	2
Mr. Peanut				
Peanut Butter Crisps Graham	12 pieces (1.1 oz)	150	8	2
Old Dutch Foods				
Baked Cheese Curls	2 cups (1.1 oz)	180	12	3
Cheese Puffcorn Curls	2 cups (1.1 oz)	170	12	1
Pita Puffs				
Barbeque	35 (1 oz)	120	3	0
Lowfat Garlic	35 (1 oz)	110	1	0
Lowfat Original	35 (1 oz)	110	1	0
Lowfat Salsa	35 (1 oz)	110	1	0
Pizza	35 (1 oz)	120	2	0
Ranch	35 (1 oz)	120	2	0
Planters				
Cheez Balls	1 pkg (1 oz)	150	10	2
Cheez Balls	1 oz	150	10	2
Cheez Curls	1 pkg (1.2 oz)	190	12	3
Cheez Mania Original	42 pieces (1 oz)	150	10	2
Heat Snack Mix	1 oz	140	8	1
Pumpkorn				
Caramel	⅓ cup	150	11	2
Chili	⅓ cup	150	11	2
Curry	⅓ cup	150	11	2
Maple Vanilla	⅓ cup	150	11	2
Mesquite	⅓ cup	150	11	2
Original	⅓ cup	150	11	2
Robert's American Gourmet				
Pirate's Booty Puffed Rice & Corn w/ Cheddar	1 oz	120	3	0
Rold Gold				
Snack Mix Colossal Cheddar	1 pkg (1 oz)	140	7	2
Snyder's Of Hanover				
Cheese Twists	1 oz	230	14	2

FOOD	PORTION	CALS	FAT	SAT FAT
Fried Pork Skins	1 oz	80	4	2
Fried Pork Skins Barbecue	1 oz	80	4	2
Kruncheez	1.25 oz	200	10	1
Onion Toasters	1 oz	188	10	1
Utz				
Caramel Corn Clusters	1⅛ cups (1 oz)	120	2	0
Cheese Balls	50 (1 oz)	150	9	3
Cheese Curls	18 (1 oz)	150	9	3
Cheese Curls Crunchy	30 (1 oz)	160	10	2
Cheese Curls Reduced Fat	32 (1 oz)	140	6	1
Onion Rings	41 (1 oz)	140	7	1
Party Mix	¾ cup (1 oz)	140	6	1
Pork Cracklins	0.5 oz	90	7	3
Pork Cracklins Hot & Spicy	0.5 oz	80	5	2
Pork Rinds	0.5 oz	80	5	2
Pork Rinds BBQ	0.5 oz	80	5	2
Weight Watchers				
Cheese Curls	1 pkg (0.5 oz)	70	3	1
SNAIL				
cooked	3 oz	233	1	tr
raw	3 oz	117	tr	tr
TAKE-OUT				
escargot cooked	5	25	0	0
SNAKE				
fresh	3 oz	78	tr	—
SNAPPER				
cooked	1 fillet (6 oz)	217	3	1
cooked	3 oz	109	1	tr
raw	3 oz	85	1	tr
SODA				
Orange	1 can (12 oz)	160	0	0
club	12 oz	0	0	0
cola	12 oz	151	tr	—
cream	12 oz	191	0	0
diet cola	12 oz	2	0	0
diet cola w/ equal	12 oz	2	0	0
diet cola w/ saccharin	12 oz	2	0	0

FOOD	PORTION	CALS	FAT	SAT FAT
ginger ale	12 oz can	124	0	–
grape	12 oz	161	0	0
lemon lime	12 oz	149	0	0
orange	12 oz	177	0	0
pepper type	12 oz	151	tr	–
quinine	12 oz	125	0	0
root beer	12 oz	152	0	0
shirley temple	1 serv	159	0	0
tonic water	12 oz	125	0	0
7 Up				
Diet	8 oz	0	0	0
Original	1 can	140	0	0
A & W				
Root Beer	1 can (12 oz)	170	0	0
After The Fall				
Raspberry Ginger Ale	1 can (12 oz)	150	0	0
Barq's				
Root Beer	1 can (12 oz)	160	0	0
Barritts				
Ginger Beer	1 bottle (12 oz)	200	0	0
Best Health				
Root Beer	1 bottle (12 oz)	165	0	0
Vanilla Cream	1 bottle (12 oz)	170	0	0
Canada Dry				
Ginger Ale	1 can (12 oz)	140	0	0
Tonic Water	8 fl oz	90	0	0
Coca-Cola				
Classic	1 can (12 oz)	140	0	0
Diet	1 can (12 oz)	0	0	0
Crush				
Tropical Fruit Punch	1 can (11.5 fl oz)	200	0	0
Dr Pepper				
Diet	1 oz	tr	0	–
Original	1 can (12 oz)	150	0	0
Fanta				
Orange	1 can (12 oz)	160	0	0
Hansen's				
Black Cherry	8 fl oz	110	0	0
Diet All Flavors	1 can	0	0	0

FOOD	PORTION	CALS	FAT	SAT FAT
Ginger Beer	8 fl oz	100	0	0
Natural Black Cherry	1 can	160	0	0
Natural Cherry Vanilla	1 can	140	0	0
Natural Creamy Rootbeer	1 can	160	0	0
Natural Ginger Ale	1 can	140	0	0
Natural Grapefruit	1 can	130	0	0
Natural Key Lime	1 can	130	0	0
Natural Kiwi Strawberry	1 can	130	0	0
Natural Mandarin Lime	1 can	130	0	0
Natural Orange Mango	1 can	170	0	0
Natural Raspberry	1 can	130	0	0
Natural Tangerine	1 can	160	0	0
Natural Tropical Passion	1 can	160	0	0
Natural Vanilla Cola	1 can	140	0	0
Orange Creme	8 fl oz	110	0	0
Sangria	8 fl oz	110	0	0
Sarsaparilla	8 fl oz	110	0	0
Sparkling Orangeade	8 fl oz	100	0	0
Vanilla Creme	8 fl oz	110	0	0
Health Valley				
Ginger Ale	1 bottle	160	0	0
Rootbeer Old Fashioned	1 bottle	160	0	0
Sarsaparilla Rootbeer	1 bottle	160	0	0
IBC				
Root Beer	1 can	160	0	0
Jones Soda				
Sugar Free All Flavors	1 bottle (12 oz)	0	0	0
Like				
Cola	1 oz	13	0	—
Lucozade				
Soda	7 oz	136	0	0
Olde Brooklyn				
Flatbush Orange	8 oz	130	0	0
Williamsburg Root Beer	8 oz	120	0	0
Olde Philadelphia				
Black Cherry	1 bottle (12 oz)	180	0	0
Cream	1 bottle (12 oz)	190	0	0
Cream Diet	1 bottle (12 oz)	0	0	0
Grape	1 bottle (12 oz)	180	0	0
Orange Cream	1 bottle (12 oz)	190	0	0

FOOD	PORTION	CALS	FAT	SAT FAT
Pineapple	1 bottle	190	0	0
Root Beer	1 bottle (12 oz)	180	0	0
Pennsylvania Dutch				
Birch Beer	8 fl oz	110	0	0
Pepsi				
Blue Berry Cola Fusion	8 fl oz	100	0	0
Diet	1 can (12 oz)	0	0	0
Regular	1 can (12 oz)	150	0	0
Vanilla	1 can	160	0	0
Vanilla Diet	1 can	0	0	0
Prism				
Green Tea Soda Cola	8 oz	105	0	0
Lemon Lime	8 oz	117	0	0
Qibla				
Cola	1 bottle (18 oz)	185	tr	–
Diet Cola	1 bottle (18 oz)	1	0	0
Saranac				
Diet Root Beer	1 bottle (12 oz)	35	0	0
Ginger Beer	1 bottle (12 oz)	160	0	0
Root Beer	1 bottle (12 oz)	180	0	0
Seagram's				
Ginger Ale	1 can (12 oz)	130	0	0
Sex Cola				
All Flavors	1 bottle (12 oz)	0	0	0
Shasta				
Black Cherry	1 can (12 oz)	170	0	0
Caffeine Free Cola	1 can (12 oz)	160	0	0
Cherry Cola	1 can (12 oz)	160	0	0
Club Soda	1 can (12 oz)	0	0	0
Cola	1 can (12 oz)	170	0	0
Creme	1 can (12 oz)	190	0	0
Diet Black Cherry	1 can (12 oz)	0	0	0
Diet Caffeine Free Cola	1 can (12 oz)	0	0	0
Diet Cherry Cola	1 can (12 oz)	0	0	0
Diet Cola	1 can (12 oz)	0	0	0
Diet Creme	1 can (12 oz)	0	0	0
Diet Doc Shasta	1 can (12 oz)	0	0	0
Diet Ginger Ale	1 can (12 oz)	0	0	0
Diet Grape	1 can (12 oz)	0	0	0
Diet Grapefruit	1 can (12 oz)	0	0	0

FOOD	PORTION	CALS	FAT	SAT FAT
Diet Grapefruit	1 can (12 oz)	0	0	0
Diet Kiwi-Strawberry	1 can (12 oz)	0	0	0
Diet Lemon-Lime Twist	1 can (12 oz)	0	0	0
Diet Orange	1 can (12 oz)	0	0	0
Diet Pineapple-Orange	1 can (12 oz)	0	0	0
Diet Raspberry Creme	1 can (12 oz)	0	0	0
Diet Red Pop	1 can (12 oz)	0	0	0
Diet Root Beer	1 can (12 oz)	0	0	0
Diet Strawberry	1 can (12 oz)	0	0	0
Diet Strawberry-Peach	1 can (12 oz)	0	0	0
Doc Shasta	1 can (12 oz)	160	0	0
Fruit Punch	1 can (12 oz)	200	0	0
Ginger Ale	1 can (12 oz)	130	0	0
Grape	1 can (12 oz)	190	0	0
Kiwi-Strawberry	1 can (12 oz)	170	0	0
Lemon-Lime Twist	1 can (12 oz)	150	0	0
Moon Mist	1 can (12 oz)	180	0	0
Orange	1 can (12 oz)	200	0	0
Peach	1 can (12 oz)	170	0	0
Pineapple	1 can (12 oz)	200	0	0
Pineapple-Orange	1 can (12 oz)	180	0	0
Quinine/Tonic	1 can (12 oz)	130	0	0
Raspberry Creme	1 can (12 oz)	170	0	0
Red Pop	1 can (12 oz)	170	0	0
Root Beer	1 can (12 oz)	170	0	0
Strawberry	1 can (12 oz)	190	0	0
Strawberry-Peach	1 can (12 oz)	170	0	0
Ski				
Citrus	1 bottle (10 oz)	150	0	0
Snapple				
Amazin' Grape	8 fl oz	120	0	0
Cherry Lime Ricky	8 fl oz	110	0	0
Creme D'Vanilla	8 fl oz	130	0	0
French Cherry	8 fl oz	120	0	0
Kiwi Peach	8 fl oz	120	0	0
Kiwi Strawberry	8 fl oz	130	0	0
Mango Madness	8 fl oz	130	0	0
Passion Supreme	8 fl oz	120	0	0
Peach Melba	8 fl oz	120	0	0
Raspberry	8 fl oz	120	0	0

FOOD	PORTION	CALS	FAT	SAT FAT
Seltzer Black Cherry	8 fl oz	0	0	0
Seltzer Lemon Lime	8 fl oz	0	0	0
Seltzer Original	8 fl oz	0	0	0
Seltzer Tangerine	8 fl oz	0	0	0
Tru Root Beer	8 fl oz	110	0	0
Steap				
Green Tea Soda Root Beer	8 oz	90	0	0
Organic Green Tea Soda Raspberry	8 oz	90	0	0
Stewart's				
Root Beer	1 bottle (12 oz)	160	0	0
Sunkist				
Orange	1 can	190	0	0
Vermont Sweetwater				
Country Apple Jack	1 bottle	180	0	0
Kickin' Cow Cola	1 bottle	129	0	0
Mango Moonshine	1 bottle	180	0	0
Maple	1 bottle	101	0	0
Raspberry Rhubarb Ramble	1 bottle	180	0	0
Tangerine Cream Twister	1 bottle	180	0	0
Vermont Maple Seltzer	1 bottle	53	0	0
White T				
All Flavors	1 bottle (12 oz)	128	0	0
Diet All Flavors	1 bottle (12 oz)	0	0	0
Yoo-Hoo				
Original	9 fl oz	150	tr	tr
SOLE				
cooked	3 oz	99	1	tr
cooked	1 fillet (4.5 oz)	148	2	tr
lemon raw	3.5 oz	85	1	—
raw	3.5 oz	90	1	—
Van De Kamp's				
Lightly Breaded Fillets	1 (4 oz)	220	11	2
Natural Fillets	1 (4 oz)	110	2	0
TAKE-OUT				
battered & fried	3.2 oz	211	11	3
breaded & fried	3.2 oz	211	11	3
SORGHUM				
sorghum	1 cup (6.7 oz)	651	6	1

FOOD	PORTION	CALS	FAT	SAT FAT
SOUFFLE				
lemon chilled	1 cup	176	tr	—
raspberry chilled	1 cup	173	tr	—
spinach	1 cup	218	18	7
SOUP				
CANNED				
asparagus cream of as prep w/ milk	1 cup	161	8	3
asparagus cream of as prep w/ water	1 cup	87	4	1
beef broth ready-to-serve	1 can (14 oz)	27	1	tr
beef broth ready-to-serve	1 cup	16	1	tr
beef noodle as prep w/water	1 cup	84	3	1
black bean turtle soup	1 cup	218	1	tr
black bean as prep w/water	1 cup	116	2	tr
celery cream of as prep w/ milk	1 cup	165	10	4
celery cream of as prep w/ water	1 cup	90	6	1
celery cream of not prep	1 can (10¾ oz)	219	14	3
cheese as prep w/ milk	1 cup	230	15	9
cheese as prep w/ water	1 cup	155	10	7
cheese not prep	1 can (11 oz)	377	25	16
chicken broth as prep w/ water	1 cup	39	1	tr
chicken cream of as prep w/ milk	1 cup	191	11	5
chicken cream of as prep w/ water	1 cup	116	7	2
chicken gumbo as prep w/ water	1 cup	56	1	tr
chicken noodle as prep w/ water	1 cup	75	2	1
chicken rice as prep w/ water	1 cup	251	2	tr
clam chowder manhattan as prep w/ water	1 cup	77	2	tr
clam chowder new england as prep w/ water	1 cup	95	3	tr
clam chowder new england as prep w/ milk	1 cup	163	7	3
consomme w/ gelatin not prep	1 can (10½ oz)	71	0	0
consomme w/ gelatin as prep w/ water	1 cup	29	0	0
escarole ready-to-serve	1 cup	27	2	1
french onion as prep w/ water	1 cup	57	2	tr
gazpacho ready-to-serve	1 cup	57	2	tr
minestrone as prep w/water	1 cup	83	3	1

FOOD	PORTION	CALS	FAT	SAT FAT
mushroom cream of as prep w/ milk	1 cup	203	14	5
mushroom cream of as prep w/ water	1 cup	129	9	2
oyster stew as prep w/ milk	1 cup	134	8	5
oyster stew as prep w/ water	1 cup	59	4	3
pepperpot as prep w/ water	1 cup	103	5	2
potato cream of as prep w/ milk	1 cup	148	6	4
potato cream of as prep w/ water	1 cup	73	2	1
scotch broth as prep w/ water	1 cup	80	3	1
split pea w/ ham as prep w/ water	1 cup	189	4	2
tomato as prep w/ milk	1 cup	160	6	3
tomato as prep w/ water	1 cup	86	2	tr
vegetarian vegetable as prep w/ water	1 cup	72	2	tr
vichyssoise	1 cup	148	6	4
Amy's				
Organic Barley	1 cup	50	1	0
Organic Black Bean Vegetable	1 cup	110	1	0
Organic Cream Of Mushroom	1 cup	120	9	2
Organic Cream Of Tomato	1 cup	100	2	2
Organic Lentil	1 cup	130	4	1
Organic Minestrone	1 cup	90	2	0
Organic No Chicken Noodle Soup	1 cup	90	3	0
Organic Vegetable	1 cup	35	0	0
Boston Market				
Chicken Broth Reduced Sodium	1 cup	15	1	0
Butterball				
Chicken Broth Reduced Sodium 99% Fat Free	1 cup	10	0	0
Campbell's				
98% Fat Free Cream Of Chicken as prep	1 cup	70	2	1
Bean With Bacon as prep	1 cup	168	4	2
Beef Barley as prep	1 cup	81	2	1
Cheddar Cheese	1 cup	110	5	3
Cheddar Cheese as prep	1 cup	134	8	4
Chicken Vegetable as prep	1 cup	74	3	1
Chicken & Pasta With Garden Vegetables	1 cup (8.4 oz)	90	1	0
Chicken Gumbo as prep	1 cup	55	1	1

FOOD	PORTION	CALS	FAT	SAT FAT
Chunky Savory Chicken w/ White & Wild Rice	1 cup	140	3	1
Chunky Classic Chicken Noodle	1 cup (8.4 oz)	130	4	1
Clam Chowder New England as prep	1 cup	89	3	1
Classics Chicken Rice	1 cup (8.4 oz)	80	2	1
Classics Beef Noodle	1 cup	70	3	1
Consomme as prep	1 cup	24	tr	0
Cream Of Asparagus as prep	1 cup	72	4	1
Cream Of Mushroom as prep	1 cup	108	7	2
Cream Of Celery as prep	1 cup	107	7	2
Cream Of Chicken as prep	1 cup	120	8	3
Cream Of Potato as prep	1 cup	102	4	2
Cream of Chicken w/ Herbs	1 cup	90	4	2
Fiesta Tomato as prep	1 cup	72	tr	tr
Garden Vegetable as prep	1 cup	69	2	1
Green Pea as prep	1 cup	173	3	1
Healthy Request Chicken Noodle as prep	1 cup	70	2	1
Healthy Request Chicken Rice as prep	1 cup	60	2	1
Healthy Request Cream Of Mushroom as prep	1 cup	66	2	1
Healthy Request Cream Of Chicken & Broccoli as prep	1 cup	78	3	1
Healthy Request Cream Of Chicken as prep	1 cup	70	3	1
Healthy Request Hearty Pasta w/ Vegetables	1 cup	87	1	tr
Healthy Request Tomato as prep	1 cup	91	2	tr
Healthy Request Vegetable as prep	1 cup	84	1	tr
Home Cookin' Chicken Vegetable	1 cup (8.4 oz)	130	4	1
Home Cookin' Chicken Rice	1 cup	110	1	1
Home Cookin' Chicken With Egg Noodles	1 cup (8.4 oz)	90	2	1
Home Cookin' Oriental Noodles w/ Vegetables	1 cup (8.4 oz)	100	1	1
Italian Tomato as prep	1 cup	105	tr	tr
Kitchen Classics Chicken Noodle	1 cup	980	1	1
Kitchen Classics Lentil	1 cup	120	1	1
Low Sodium Chicken Broth	1 can (10.75 oz)	27	1	1
Low Sodium Chicken W/ Noodles	1 can (10.75 oz)	162	5	2

FOOD	PORTION	CALS	FAT	SAT FAT
Low Sodium Chunky Vegetable Beef	1 can (10.75 oz)	159	4	1
Low Sodium Cream of Mushroom	1 can (10.75 oz)	200	13	4
Low Sodium Green Pea	1 can (10.75 oz)	235	4	2
Low Sodium Tomato w/ Pieces	1 can (10.75 oz)	170	5	2
Minestrone as prep	1 cup	81	2	1
Ready To Serve Bean w/ Bacon 'N Ham	1 can (10.5 oz)	274	7	2
Ready To Serve Chicken Noodle	1 cup	80	2	1
Ready To Serve Chicken w/ Rice	1 can (10.5 oz)	122	2	1
Ready-To-Serve Vegetable Beef	1 can (10.5 oz)	143	1	tr
Savory Tomato & Dill as prep	1 cup	99	2	tr
Select Chicken & Pasta With Roasted Garlic	1 cup (8.4 oz)	100	1	1
Select Chicken Rice	1 cup	100	1	1
Select Fiesta Vegetable	1 cup (8.4 oz)	120	1	0
Select Herbed Chicken w/ Roasted Vegetables	1 cup	90	1	1
Select Italian Style Wedding	1 cup	120	3	2
Select Mushroom w/ White & Wild Rice	1 cup	90	1	0
Select Roasted Chicken w/ Rotini & Penne Pasta	1 cup	90	1	1
Select Rosemary Chicken w/ Roasted Potatoes	1 cup	110	1	0
Select Split Pea w/ Ham	1 cup (8.4 oz)	170	2	1
Select Tuscany-Style Minestrone	1 cup (8.4 oz)	190	9	2
Simply Home Chicken Noodle	1 cup (8.4 oz)	80	1	1
Simply Home Chicken With Rice	1 cup (8.4 oz)	100	1	0
Soup At Hand Blended Vegetable Medley	1 pkg (10.75 oz)	110	2	2
Tomato as prep	1 cup	80	0	0
Vegetable Beef as prep	1 cup	68	2	1
Vegetarian Vegetable as prep	1 cup	79	2	2
College Inn				
Beef Broth 99% Fat Free	1 cup	20	1	0
Chicken Broth Fat Free 50% Less Sodium	1 cup	5	0	0
Gold's				
Russian Borscht	8 oz	70	0	0

FOOD	PORTION	CALS	FAT	SAT FAT
Health Valley				
5 Bean Vegetable	1 cup	250	0	0
Beef Broth Fat Free	1 cup	20	0	0
Beef Broth Fat Free No Salt	1 cup	20	0	0
Black Bean & Vegetable	1 cup	110	0	0
Chicken Broth	1 cup	45	2	—
Chicken Broth Fat Free	1 cup	30	0	0
Chicken Broth No Salt	1 cup	45	2	—
Country Corn & Vegetable	1 cup	70	0	0
Garden Vegetable	1 cup	80	0	0
Italian Plus Carotene	1 cup	80	0	0
Lentil & Carrot	1 cup	100	0	0
Organic Black Bean	1 cup	110	0	0
Organic Lentil No Salt	1 cup	90	0	0
Organic Minestrone	1 cup	100	0	0
Organic Mushroom Barley No Salt	1 cup	60	0	0
Organic Potato Leek	1 cup	70	0	0
Organic Potato Leek No Salt	1 cup	70	0	0
Organic Split Pea	1 cup	110	0	0
Organic Split Pea No Salt	1 cup	110	0	0
Organic Tomato	1 cup	90	0	0
Organic Vegetable No Salt	1 cup	80	0	0
Pasta Bolognese	1 cup	100	0	0
Pasta Cacciatore	1 cup	100	0	0
Pasta Romano	1 cup	100	0	0
Real Italian Minestrone	1 cup	90	0	0
Rotini & Vegetable	1 cup	100	0	0
Split Pea & Carrots	1 cup	110	0	0
Super Broccoli Carotene	1 cup	70	0	0
Tomato Vegetable	1 cup	80	0	0
Vegetable Barley	1 cup	90	0	0
Vegetable Power Carotene	1 cup	70	0	0
Healthy Choice				
Bean & Ham	1 cup (8.7 oz)	166	1	tr
Beef & Potato	1 cup (8.5 oz)	116	1	1
Broccoli Cheddar	1 cup (8.4 oz)	116	2	1
Chicken Corn Chowder	1 cup (8.8 oz)	176	3	1
Chicken Pasta	1 cup (8.6 oz)	119	3	1
Chicken Rice	1 cup (8.4 oz)	119	2	1
Chili Beef	1 cup (9.1 oz)	189	2	1

FOOD	PORTION	CALS	FAT	SAT FAT
Clam Chowder	1 cup (8.8 oz)	123	1	1
Classic Italian Bean and Pasta	1 cup (8 oz)	100	2	1
Country Vegetable	1 cup (8.6 oz)	112	1	tr
Cream Of Mushroom	1 cup (8.8 oz)	77	1	tr
Cream Of Celery as prep	1 cup	73	2	1
Cream Of Chicken Vegetable	1 cup (8.9 oz)	127	2	1
Cream Of Roasted Chicken as prep	1 cup	80	3	1
Cream Of Roasted Garlic as prep	1 cup	57	1	tr
Garden Tomato Herbs as prep	1 cup	80	1	tr
Garden Vegetable	1 cup (8.6 oz)	108	1	1
Hearty Chicken	1 cup (8.7 oz)	136	3	1
Lentil	1 cup (8.7 oz)	135	1	tr
Minestrone	1 cup (8.6 oz)	107	1	tr
Old Fashion Chicken Noodle	1 cup (8.8 oz)	137	3	1
Split Pea & Ham	1 cup (8.8 oz)	164	2	1
Tomato Garden	1 cup (8.6 oz)	101	1	1
Turkey Wild Rice	1 cup (8.4 oz)	72	1	tr
Vegetable Beef	1 cup (8.8 oz)	96	1	tr
Herb-Ox				
Beef Liquid	2 tsp (0.4 oz)	20	0	0
Chicken Liquid	2 tsp (0.4 oz)	15	0	0
Imagine				
Creamy Broccoli	1 serv (8 oz)	70	2	0
Creamy Butternut Squash	1 serv (8 oz)	120	2	2
Creamy Mushroom	1 serv (8 oz)	80	3	1
Creamy Potato Leek	1 serv (8 oz)	90	3	0
Creamy Sweet Corn	1 serv (8 oz)	100	3	1
Creamy Tomato	1 serv (8 oz)	90	2	0
Vegetable Broth	1 serv (8 oz)	45	1	0
Zesty Gazpacho	1 serv (8 oz)	80	0	0
Manischewitz				
Clear Chicken Condensed	½ cup	15	1	0
Natural Choice				
Orangic Vegan Classic Tomato	1 cup	100	1	0
Organic Vegan Classic Mushroom	1 cup	50	2	0
Organic Vegan Country Corn	1 cup	100	1	0
Organic Vegan Kabocha Squash	1 cup	60	1	0
Organic Vegan Southern Greens	1 cup	80	3	0
Organic Vegan Split Pea	1 cup	120	1	0
Organic Vegan Vegetable Curry	1 cup	110	4	1

FOOD	PORTION	CALS	FAT	SAT FAT
Old El Paso				
Black Bean With Bacon	1 cup (8.6 oz)	160	2	1
Chicken Vegetable	1 cup (8.4 oz)	110	3	1
Chicken With Rice	1 cup (8.4 oz)	90	3	1
Garden Vegetable	1 cup (8.4 oz)	110	3	1
Hearty Beef	1 cup (8.4 oz)	120	3	2
Hearty Chicken Noodle	1 cup (8.4 oz)	110	3	1
Pacific				
Free Range Organic Chicken Broth	1 cup	5	0	0
Pritikin				
Chicken & Rice	1 cup (8.8 oz)	80	1	0
Chicken Broth	1 cup (8.5 oz)	15	0	0
Chicken Pasta	1 cup (8.6 oz)	100	1	0
Hearty Vegetable	1 cup (8.8 oz)	90	1	0
Lentil	1 cup (8.4 oz)	130	1	0
Minestrone	1 cup (8.8 oz)	90	1	0
Split Pea	1 cup (9.2 oz)	140	1	0
Three Bean Chili	½ cup (4.5 oz)	90	1	0
Vegetable Broth	1 cup (8.3 oz)	20	0	0
Vegetarian Vegetables	1 cup (9 oz)	100	0	0
Progresso				
99% Fat Free Beef Barley	1 cup (8.5 oz)	140	2	1
99% Fat Free Beef Vegetable	1 cup (8.5 oz)	160	2	1
99% Fat Free Chicken Noodle	1 cup	90	2	0
99% Fat Free Chicken Rice w/ Vegetables	1 cup (8.4 oz)	110	2	0
99% Fat Free Creamy Mushroom Chicken	1 cup (8.3 oz)	90	2	1
99% Fat Free Lentil	1 cup (8.5 oz)	130	2	0
99% Fat Free Minestrone	1 cup (8.5 oz)	130	2	0
99% Fat Free Roasted Chicken w/ Italian Style Vegetable	1 cup (8 oz)	90	2	0
99% Fat Free Split Pea	1 cup (8.9 oz)	170	2	0
99% Fat Free Tomato Garden Vegetable	1 cup (8.6 oz)	100	2	0
99% Fat Free Vegetable	1 cup (8.4 oz)	70	1	0
99% Fat Free White Cheddar Potato	1 cup (8.6 oz)	140	3	2
Basil Rotini Tomato	1 cup (8.9 oz)	120	2	0
Bean & Ham	1 cup (8.4 oz)	160	2	1
Beef & Vegetable	1 cup	130	3	2

FOOD	PORTION	CALS	FAT	SAT FAT
Beef Barley	1 cup (8.5 oz)	130	4	2
Beef Minestrone	1 cup (8.5 oz)	140	3	1
Beef Noodle	1 cup (8.5 oz)	140	4	2
Cheese & Herb Tortellini Tomato	1 cup (8.6 oz)	140	3	1
Chickarina	1 cup (8.3 oz)	130	5	2
Chicken Minestrone	1 cup (8.4 oz)	110	2	0
Chicken Vegetable	1 cup (8.4 oz)	90	2	0
Chicken & Wild Rice	1 cup (8.4 oz)	100	2	1
Chicken Barley	1 cup (8.5 oz)	110	2	0
Chicken Broth	1 cup (8.2 oz)	20	2	0
Chicken Noodle	1 cup (8.4 oz)	90	2	0
Chicken Rice w/ Vegetable	1 cup (8.4 oz)	90	2	0
Clam & Rotini Chowder	1 cup (8.8 oz)	190	9	2
Escarole In Chicken Broth	1 cup (8.1 oz)	25	1	0
Green Split Pea	1 cup (8.6 oz)	170	3	1
Hearty Black Bean	1 cup (8.5 oz)	170	2	0
Hearty Penne In Chicken Broth	1 cup (8.4 oz)	80	1	0
Hearty Tomato	1 cup (8.7 oz)	100	2	0
Herb Rotini Vegetable	1 cup (9.1 oz)	120	2	0
Homestyle Chicken w/ Vegetable	1 cup (8.4 oz)	90	2	0
Italian Herb Shells Minestrone	1 cup (9.1 oz)	120	2	0
Lentil	1 cup (8.5 oz)	140	2	0
Macaroni & Bean	1 cup (8.6 oz)	160	4	1
Manhattan Clam Chowder	1 cup (8.4 oz)	110	2	0
Meatballs & Pasta Pearls	1 cup (8.3 oz)	140	7	3
Minestrone	1 cup (8.4 oz)	120	2	0
Minestrone Parmesan	1 cup (8.3 oz)	100	3	1
New England Clam Chowder	1 cup (8.4 oz)	190	10	3
Oregano Penne Italian Style Vegetable	1 cup (8.7 oz)	90	2	0
Peppercorn Penne Vegetable	1 cup (9.1 oz)	100	1	0
Potato Broccoli & Cheese	1 cup (8.8 oz)	160	6	2
Potato Ham & Cheese	1 cup (8.6 oz)	170	7	2
Rich & Hearty Beef Pot Roast	1 cup	130	2	1
Roasted Garlic Pasta Lentil	1 cup (9.3 oz)	120	2	0
Rotisserie Seasoned Chicken	1 cup (8.5 oz)	100	2	0
Spicy Chicken & Penne	1 cup (8.5 oz)	110	2	0
Split Pea w/ Ham	1 cup (8.4 oz)	150	4	2
Tomato	1 cup (8.5 oz)	100	2	0
Tomato Basil	1 cup (8.8 oz)	100	2	0

FOOD	PORTION	CALS	FAT	SAT FAT
Tomato Vegetable	1 cup (8.5 oz)	90	2	0
Tortellini In Chicken Broth	1 cup (8.3 oz)	70	2	1
Turkey Noodle	1 cup (8.4 oz)	90	2	0
Turkey Rice w/ Vegetables	1 cup (8.5 oz)	110	1	0
Vegetable	1 cup (8.4 oz)	90	2	1
White Meat Roasted Chicken Rotini	1 cup (8.1 oz)	80	2	0
Streit's				
Hearty Vegetarian Vegetable	1 cup	90	0	0
Mushroom Barley	1 cup	100	2	0
Swanson				
Beef Broth 100% Fat Free Lower Sodium	1 cup	15	0	–
Beef Broth 99% Fat Free	1 cup	10	1	–
Beef Broth Onion Seasoned	1 cup (8.4 oz)	20	0	0
Chicken Broth 100% Fat Free 33% Less Sodium	1 cup	15	0	0
Chicken Broth Seasoned Italian Herbs	1 cup (8.4 oz)	20	1	0
Vegetable Broth	1 cup	19	1	0
Walnut Acres				
Organic Country Corn Chowder	1 cup (8.8 oz)	150	3	2
Weight Watchers				
Chicken & Rice	1 can (10.5 oz)	110	2	0
Chicken Noodle	1 can (10.5 oz)	150	2	1
Minestrone	1 can (10.5 oz)	130	2	1
Vegetable	1 can (10.5 oz)	130	1	0
FROZEN				
Birds Eye				
Hearty Spoonfuls Pasta & Chicken	1 bowl (11.2 oz)	140	2	0
Nature's Entree				
Chowder	1 pkg (12 oz)	230	6	3
Tortellini Minestone	1 pkg (12 oz)	360	9	1
Tabatchnick				
Barley Mushroom No Salt Added	1 serv (7.5 oz)	70	0	0
Broccoli Cream Of	1 serv (7.5 oz)	90	4	2
Cabbage	1 serv (7.5 oz)	60	0	0
Chicken With Dumplings	1 serv (7.5 oz)	70	2	0
Corn Chowder	1 serv (7.5 oz)	150	6	2
Minestrone	1 serv (7.5 oz)	150	1	0
New England Potato	1 serv (7.5 oz)	150	6	3

FOOD	PORTION	CALS	FAT	SAT FAT
Old Fashion Potato	1 serv (7.5 oz)	70	0	0
Pea	1 serv (7.5 oz)	180	2	0
Pea No Salt Added	1 serv (7.5 oz)	180	2	0
Spinach Cream Of	1 serv (7.5 oz)	90	4	2
Vegetable	1 serv (7.5 oz)	110	1	0
Vegetable No Salt Added	1 serv (7.5 oz)	110	1	0
Wisconsin Cheddar Vegetable	1 serv (7.5 oz)	140	9	3
Yankee Bean	1 serv (7.5 oz)	160	2	0
MIX				
asparagus cream of as prep w/ water	1 cup	59	2	tr
beef broth	1 pkg (0.2 oz)	14	1	tr
beef broth as prep w/ water	1 cup	19	1	tr
beef broth cube	1 cube (3.6 g)	6	tr	tr
beef broth cube as prep w/ water	1 cup	8	tr	tr
celery cream of as prep w/ water	1 cup	63	2	tr
chicken broth	1 pkg (0.2 oz)	16	1	tr
chicken broth as prep w/ water	1 cup	21	1	tr
chicken broth cube	1 cube (4.8 g)	9	tr	tr
chicken broth cube, as prep w/ water	1 cup	13	tr	tr
chicken cream of as prep w/ water	1 cup	107	5	3
chicken noodle as prep w/ water	1 cup	53	1	tr
french onion not prep	1 pkg (1.4 oz)	115	2	1
leek as prep w/ water	1 cup	71	2	1
onion as prep w/ water	1 cup	28	1	tr
tomato as prep w/ water	1 cup	102	2	1
Alpine Aire				
Low Carb Bay Shrimp Bisque	1 pkg	150	11	6
Low Carb Beefy Vegetable	1 pkg	100	4	2
Low Carb Broccoli Cheddar	1 pkg	140	10	6
Low Carb Mushroom & Chicken w/ Roasted Garlic	1 pkg	130	8	5
Armour				
Bouillon Cubes Beef	1 (4 g)	5	0	0
Bouillon Cubes Chicken	1 (4 g)	5	0	0
Azumaya				
Thin Cut Noodle	1 cup	120	0	0
Wide Cut Noodle	1 cup	120	0	0
Bean Cuisine				
13 Bean Bouillabaisse	1 cup	220	0	0

FOOD	PORTION	CALS	FAT	SAT FAT
Island Black Bean	1 cup	210	0	0
Lots of Lentil	1 cup	230	0	0
Mesa Maize	1 cup	160	0	0
White Bean Provencal	1 cup	250	1	0
Casbah				
Black Bean	1 pkg (1.7 oz)	170	2	0
Split Pea	1 pkg (2.3 oz)	230	1	0
Sweet Corn Chowder	1 pkg (1.2 oz)	125	1	0
Vegetarian Chili	1 pkg (1.8 oz)	170	2	0
Cup-a-Soup				
Broccoli & Cheese as prep	1 serv (6 oz)	70	3	1
Chicken Vegetable as prep	1 serv (6 oz)	50	1	0
Chicken Broth as prep	1 serv (6 oz)	20	0	0
Chicken Broth w/ Pasta Fat Free as prep	1 serv (6 oz)	45	0	0
Chicken Noodle as prep	1 serv (6 oz)	50	1	0
Cream Of Chicken as prep	1 serv (6 oz)	70	2	0
Creamy Chicken Vegetable as prep	1 serv (6 oz)	80	5	2
Creamy Mushroom as prep	1 serv (6 oz)	60	2	0
Green Pea as prep	1 serv (6 oz)	80	1	0
Hearty Chicken Noodle as prep	1 serv (6 oz)	60	1	0
Ring Noodle as prep	1 serv (6 oz)	50	1	0
Spring Vegetable as prep	1 serv (6 oz)	45	1	0
Tomato as prep	1 serv (6 oz)	100	1	0
George Washington				
Broth & Brown Seasoning	1 serv	6	0	–
Broth & Golden Seasoning	1 serv	6	0	–
Broth & Onion Seasoning	1 serv	12	0	–
Broth & Vegetable Seasoning	1 serv	12	0	–
Health Valley				
Chicken Noodles w/ Vegetables	1 serv	110	0	0
Corn Chowder w/ Tomatoes	1 serv	100	0	0
Creamy Potato w/ Broccoli	1 serv	70	0	0
Garden Split Pea w/ Carrots	1 serv	130	0	0
Lentil w/ Couscous	1 serv	130	0	0
Pasta Italiano	1 serv	140	0	0
Pasta Marinara	1 serv	100	0	0
Pasta Parmesan	1 serv	100	0	0
Spicy Black Bean w/ Couscous	1 serv	130	0	0
Zesty Black Bean w/ Rice	1 serv	100	0	0

FOOD	PORTION	CALS	FAT	SAT FAT
Herb-Ox				
Beef Bouillon	1 cube (3.5 g)	5	0	0
Beef Instant Bouillon Powder	1 tsp (4 g)	5	0	0
Beef Instant Broth & Seasoning Pack	1 pkg (4.5 g)	5	0	0
Beef Instant Broth & Seasoning Pack Low Sodium	1 pkg (4 g)	10	0	0
Chicken Bouillon	1 cube (4 g)	5	0	0
Chicken Instant Bouillon Powder	1 tsp (4 g)	5	0	0
Chicken Instant Broth & Seasoning Pack	1 pkg (4 g)	5	0	0
Chicken Instant Broth & Seasoning Pack Low Sodium	1 pkg (4 g)	10	0	0
Vegetable Bouillon	1 cube (4 g)	5	0	0
Hodgson Mill				
Choice Bean not prep	¼ cup (1.5 oz)	150	0	0
Hurst				
15 Bean Soup Beef	1 serv (6 oz)	120	1	0
15 Bean Soup Cajun	1 serv	120	1	0
15 Bean Soup Chicken	1 serv (6 oz)	120	1	0
15 Bean Soup Chili	1 serv (6 oz)	120	1	0
15 Bean Soup Ham	1 serv	120	1	0
HamBeens Great Northern Bean	1 serv	120	1	0
HamBeens Navy Bean	1 serv	120	1	0
Pasta Fagioli	1 serv	120	1	0
Spanish American Pinto Bean	1 serv	120	1	0
Spanish American Black Bean	1 serv	120	1	0
Kojel				
Hearty Potato With Vegetables Instant	1 serv (6 fl oz)	60	0	0
Noodle Soup Chicken Flavor Instant	1 serv (6 fl oz)	70	1	0
Split Pea Instant	1 serv (6 fl oz)	60	tr	0
Tomato Instant	1 serv (6 fl oz)	50	0	0
Vegetable Chicken Couscous Instant	1 serv (6 fl oz)	80	1	tr
Lipton				
Chicken Noodle w/ White Chicken Meat as prep	1 cup	80	2	1
Extra Noodle w/ Chicken Broth as prep	1 cup	90	2	1
Giggle Noodle w/ Chicken Broth as prep	1 cup	70	2	1

FOOD	PORTION	CALS	FAT	SAT FAT
Recipe Secrets Beefy Mushroom	1½ tbsp (0.4 oz)	35	0	0
Recipe Secrets Beefy Onion	1 tbsp (0.3 oz)	25	1	0
Recipe Secrets Fiesta Herb w/ Red Pepper as prep	1 cup	30	0	0
Recipe Secrets Golden Herb w/ Lemon as prep	1 cup	35	1	0
Recipe Secrets Golden Onion	1⅔ tbsp (0.5 oz)	50	1	0
Recipe Secrets Italian Herb w/ Tomato as prep	1 cup	40	1	0
Recipe Secrets Onion as prep	1 cup	20	0	0
Recipe Secrets Onion Mushroom as prep	1 cup	30	1	0
Recipe Secrets Savory Herb With Garlic as prep	1 cup	30	0	0
Recipe Secrets Vegetable as prep	1 cup	30	0	0
Ring-O-Noodle w/ Chicken Broth as prep	1 cup	70	2	1
Soup Secrets Chicken 'N Onion as prep	1 cup	120	2	0
Soup Secrets Chicken w/ Pasta & Beans as prep	1 cup	110	2	0
Soup Secrets Country Chicken w/ Pasta & Herbs as prep	1 cup	100	2	0
Soup Secrets Homestyle Lentil w/ Bow Tie Pasta as prep	1 cup	130	1	0
Soup Secrets Minestrone as prep	1 cup	110	1	0
Spiral Pasta w/ Chicken Broth as prep	1 cup	60	1	0
MiniCarb				
Miso w/ Tofu & Shitake	1 pkg	33	1	0
Szechuan Beef	1 pkg	24	1	0
Thai Coconut Cream	1 pkg	100	6	4
Miso-Cup				
Golden Vegetable as prep	1 cup	30	1	—
Miso Reduced Sodium as prep	1 cup	25	1	—
Organic Miso as prep	1 cup	35	1	—
Savory Seaweed as prep	1 cup	30	1	—
Morga				
Vegetable Bouillon No Salt Added	½ cube (5 g)	25	2	1
Vegetable Broth Fat Free	1 tsp (4 g)	10	0	0

FOOD	PORTION	CALS	FAT	SAT FAT
Ramen Noodle				
Beef Low Fat as prep	1 pkg (2.2 oz)	216	1	tr
Beef as prep	1 pkg (2.2 oz)	280	11	6
Chicken Low Fat as prep	1 pkg (2.2 oz)	216	1	tr
Chicken as prep	1 pkg (2.2 oz)	279	11	5
Oriental Low Fat as prep	1 pkg (2.2 oz)	217	1	tr
Shrimp Low Fat as prep	1 pkg (2.2 oz)	218	1	tr
Shrimp as prep	1 pkg (2.2 oz)	294	13	4
Tomato as prep	1 pkg (2.2 oz)	295	13	5
Rapunzel				
Cubes Vegetable Bouillon No Salt Added	½ cube	25	2	—
Cubes Vegetable Bouillon w/ Sea Salt	½ cube	15	1	—
Cubes Vegetable Bouillon w/ Sea Salt & Herbs	½ cube	15	2	—
Slim-Fast				
Creamy Broccoli	1 pkg	210	5	2
Creamy Chicken	1 pkg	220	5	2
Creamy Potato Cheddar & Chive	1 pkg	220	5	2
Steero				
Beef Bouillon Cube	1 (3.5 g)	5	0	0
Beef Bouillon Cube Reduced Sodium	1 cube (3.5 oz)	5	0	0
Beef Bouillon Instant	1 tsp (3.5 oz)	5	0	0
Beef Bouillon Instant Reduced Sodium	1 tsp (3.5 oz)	5	0	0
Chicken Bouillon Cube	1 (3.5 g)	5	0	0
Chicken Bouillon Cube Reduced Sodium	1 (3.5 g)	5	0	0
Chicken Bouillon Cube Reduced Sodium	1 (3.5 g)	5	0	0
Chicken Bouillon Instant	1 tsp (3.5 g)	5	0	0
Chicken Bouillon Instant Reduced Sodium	1 tsp (3.5 g)	5	0	0
Thai Kitchen				
Instant Rice Noodle Bangkok Curry	1 pkg	192	5	0
Rice Noodle Bowl Roasted Garlic	1 bowl	170	2	0
Rice Noodle Bowl Spring Onion	1 bowl	170	2	0
Weight Watchers				
Instant Beef Broth	1 pkg (0.16 oz)	10	0	0
Instant Chicken Broth	1 pkg (0.16 oz)	10	0	0

FOOD	PORTION	CALS	FAT	SAT FAT
Wyler's				
Beef Bouillon Cube	1 (3.5 g)	5	0	0
Beef Bouillon Cube Reduced Sodium	1 (3.5 g)	5	0	0
Beef Bouillon Instant	1 tsp (3.5 g)	5	0	0
Beef Bouillon Instant Reduced Sodium	1 tsp (3.5 g)	5	0	0
Chicken Bouillon Cube	1 (3.5 g)	5	0	0
Chicken Bouillon Cube Reduced Sodium	1 (3.5 g)	5	0	0
Chicken Bouillon Instant	1 tsp (3.5)	5	0	0
Chicken Bouillon Instant Reduced Sodium	1 tsp (3.5 g)	5	0	0
SHELF-STABLE				
Annie Chun				
Ginger Chicken	1 cup	30	0	0
Shiitake Mushroom	1 cup	25	0	0
Traditional Miso	1 cup	35	1.	0
Campbell's				
Soup At Hand Blended Vegetable Medley	1 pkg (10.75 oz)	110	2	2
Hormel				
Micro Cup Bean & Ham	1 cup (7.5 oz)	190	4	1
Micro Cup Beef Vegetable	1 cup (7.5 oz)	90	1	0
Micro Cup Broccoli Cheese w/ Ham	1 cup (7.5 oz)	170	13	5
Micro Cup Chicken & Rice	1 cup (7.5 oz)	110	3	1
Micro Cup Chicken Noodle	1 cup (7.5 oz)	110	3	2
Micro Cup New England Clam Chowder	1 cup (7.5 oz)	130	5	3
Micro Cup Potato Cheese w/ Ham	1 cup (7.5 oz)	190	13	5
Lunch Bucket				
Chicken Noodle	1 pkg (7.25 oz)	80	2	1
Country Vegetable	1 pkg (7.25 oz)	60	1	0
TastyBite				
Tom Yum	½ pkg (5.3 oz)	92	7	5
TAKE-OUT				
albondigas meatball soup	1 bowl	318	17	7
beef stew soup	1 cup (8.8 oz)	221	5	2
black bean turtle soup	1 cup	241	1	tr
brunswick stew soup	1 cup (8.5 oz)	232	6	2
caldo de res beef soup	1 bowl	327	12	4

FOOD	PORTION	CALS	FAT	SAT FAT
chinese velvet corn	1¼ cup	135	0	0
corn & cheese chowder	¾ cup	215	12	7
egg drop	1 cup	73	103	1
gazpacho	1 cup	46	tr	—
greek lemon	¾ cup	63	2	1
hot & sour	1 serv (14 oz)	173	8	2
middle eastern chilled fruit	1 cup	99	0	0
middle eastern chilled yogurt & cucumber	1 bowl	85	3	—
minestrone	1 cup	154	0	tr
miso w/ tofu	1 bowl	36	0	0
onion soup gratinee	1 serv	492	27	16
oxtail	5 oz	64	3	—
pasta e fagioli	1 cup (8.8 oz)	194	5	1
ratatouille	1 cup (7.5 oz)	266	25	3
thai lemon grass	1 bowl	100	4	—
vietnamese pho beef noodle	1 serv (7.8 oz)	480	12	5
wonton soup	1 cup	205	3	1
zupa koprowa polish dill soup	1 bowl	54	2	—
zuppa toscana	1 bowl	543	123	18

SOUR CREAM

FOOD	PORTION	CALS	FAT	SAT FAT
sour cream	1 cup (8 oz)	493	48	30
sour cream	1 tbsp (0.4 oz)	26	3	2
Breakstone's				
Free	2 tbsp (1.1 oz)	35	0	0
Reduced Fat	2 tbsp (1.1 oz)	45	4	3
Sour Cream	2 tbsp (1 oz)	60	5	4
Cabot				
Light	2 tbsp	35	3	2
No Fat	2 tbsp	20	0	0
Sour Cream	2 tbsp	50	5	3
Hood				
Fat Free	2 tbsp (1 oz)	20	0	0
Light	2 tbsp (1 oz)	40	3	2
Sour Cream	2 tbsp (1 oz)	60	5	4
Knudsen				
Free	2 tbsp (1.1 oz)	35	0	0
Hampshire	2 tbsp (1 oz)	60	6	4
Light	2 tbsp (1.1 oz)	50	3	2

FOOD	PORTION	CALS	FAT	SAT FAT
Land O Lakes				
Fat Free	2 tbsp (1.1 oz)	25	0	0
Light	2 tbsp (1 oz)	40	3	2
Sour Cream	2 tbsp (1 oz)	60	6	4
SOUR CREAM SUBSTITUTES				
nondairy	1 cup	479	45	41
nondairy	1 oz	59	6	5
SOURSOP				
fresh	1	416	2	—
fresh cut up	1 cup	150	1	—
SOY *(see also* CHEESE SUBSTITUTES, ICE CREAM, FROZEN DESSERTS, MILK SUBSTITUTES, MISO, SOY SAUCE, SOYBEANS, TEMPEH, TOFU, YOGURT FROZEN*)*				
lecithin	1 tbsp	104	14	2
soy milk	1 cup	79	5	1
soya cheese	1.4 oz	128	11	—
Bob's Red Mill				
Flour	⅓ cup	130	6	—
Dakota Gourmet				
Soy Nuts	1 oz	129	7	1
Fearn				
Granules	¼ cup	110	1	—
Powder	¼ cup	100	5	—
GeniSoy				
Soy Nuts Deep Sea Salted	1 oz	120	4	1
Soy Nuts Old Hickory Smoked	1 oz	120	4	1
Soy Nuts Praline	55 pieces (1 oz)	120	3	0
Soy Nuts Unsalted	1 oz	120	4	0
Soy Nuts Zesty Barbeque	1 oz	120	4	1
Health Trip				
Soynut Butter Honey Sweet	2 tbsp	170	13	2
Soynut Butter Original	2 tbsp	180	13	2
Soynut Butter Unsalted	2 tbsp	180	13	2
I.M. Healthy				
SoyNut Butter Chocolate	2 tbsp (1.1 oz)	190	14	2
SoyNut Butter Honey Creamy	2 tbsp (1.1 oz)	170	11	2
SoyNut Butter Original Creamy	2 tbsp (1.1 oz)	170	11	2
SoyNut Butter Unsweetened Chunky	2 tbsp (1.1 oz)	160	13	2
SoyNut Butter Unsweetened Creamy	2 tbsp (1.1 oz)	160	13	2

FOOD	PORTION	CALS	FAT	SAT FAT
Loma Linda				
Soyagen All Purpose	¼ cup (1 oz)	130	6	1
Soyagen Carob	¼ cup (1 oz)	130	6	1
Soyagen No Sucrose	¼ cup (1 oz)	130	6	1
Natural Touch				
Roasted Soy Butter	2 tbsp (1.1 oz)	170	11	2
Revival				
Shake Chocolate Daydream Fructose	1 pkg	240	3	1
Shake Strawberry Smile Unsweetened	1 pkg	130	2	1
Shake Strawberry Smile Fructose	1 pkg	225	2	1
Shake Strawberry Smile Splenda	1 pkg	130	2	1
Soy Shake Plain	1 pkg	110	2	1
Soy Shake Vanilla Pleasure	1 pkg	220	2	1
Soy Shake Vanilla Pleasure Splenda	1 pkg	120	2	1
Soy Shake Vanilla Pleasure Unsweetened	1 pkg	120	2	1
Soynuts Chocolate Covered	⅙ cup	70	4	2
Soynuts Hot Jalapeno & Cheddar	⅙ cup	78	4	1
Soynuts Unsalted	⅙ cup	78	4	1
Soynuts Yogurt Covered	⅙ cup	720	4	3
Soy Juicy				
All Flavors	8 oz	160	3	1
Soy Wonder				
Creamy	2 tbsp	170	11	2
Crunchy	2 tbsp	170	11	2
SOY SAUCE				
shoyu	1 tbsp	9	tr	tr
soy sauce	1 tbsp	7	tr	tr
tamari	1 tbsp	11	tr	tr
Chun King				
Lite	1 tbsp (0.5 oz)	15	tr	0
Soy Sauce	1 tbsp (0.6 oz)	11	tr	0
Eden				
Organic Shoyu Reduced Sodium	1 tbsp	10	0	0
Organic Tamari	1 tbsp	15	0	0
Ponzu Sauce	1 tbsp	5	0	0
Shoyu	1 tbsp	15	0	0
House Of Tsang				
Dark	1 tbsp (0.6 oz)	10	0	0

FOOD	PORTION	CALS	FAT	SAT FAT
Ginger Flavored	1 tbsp (0.6 oz)	20	0	0
Light	1 tbsp (0.6 oz)	5	0	0
Low Sodium	1 tbsp (0.6 oz)	5	0	0
Low Sodium Ginger	1 tbsp (0.6 oz)	10	0	0
Low Sodium Mushroom	1 tbsp (0.6 oz)	10	0	0
Just Rite				
Soy Sauce	1 tbsp (0.5 oz)	11	tr	0
Kikkoman				
Lite	1 tbsp (0.5 oz)	10	0	0
Soy Sauce	1 tbsp (0.5 oz)	10	0	0
La Choy				
Lite	1 tbsp (0.5 oz)	15	tr	0
Soy Sauce	1 tbsp (0.6 oz)	11	tr	0
Tree Of Life				
Shoyu	1 tbsp (0.5 oz)	15	0	0
Tamari Wheat Free	1 tbsp (0.5 oz)	15	0	0
SOYBEANS				
dried cooked	1 cup	298	15	2
dry roasted	½ cup	387	19	3
green cooked	½ cup	127	6	1
honey toasted	¼ cup (1 oz)	130	4	1
roasted	½ cup	405	22	3
roasted & toasted	1 oz	129	7	1
roasted & toasted	1 cup	490	26	3
roasted & toasted salted	1 cup	490	26	3
roasted & toasted salted	1 oz	129	7	1
sprouts raw	½ cup	43	2	tr
sprouts steamed	½ cup	38	2	tr
sprouts stir fried	1 cup	125	7	1
Arrowhead				
Organic not prep	¼ cup	180	8	–
Eden				
Organic Black	½ cup (4.6 oz)	120	6	1
Seapoint Farms				
Edamame Organic	½ cup (2.6 oz)	100	3	0
Edamame In Pods frzn	½ cup (2.6 oz)	100	3	0
Edamame Rice Bowl Kung Pao Vegetable	1 pkg (12 oz)	420	6	1

FOOD	PORTION	CALS	FAT	SAT FAT
Edamame Rice Bowl Szechwan Vegetables	1 pkg (12 oz)	420	4	1
Edamame Rice Bowl Teriyaki Vegetable	1 pkg (12 oz)	430	5	1
Edamame Rice Bowl Vegetable Fried Rice	1 pkg (11 oz)	220	6	1
Edamame Shelled	½ cup (2.6 oz)	100	3	0

SPAGHETTI (see PASTA, PASTA DINNERS, PASTA SALAD, SPAGHETTI SAUCE)

SPAGHETTI SAUCE
JARRED

FOOD	PORTION	CALS	FAT	SAT FAT
marinara sauce	1 cup	171	8	tr
spaghetti sauce	1 cup	272	12	2
Amy's				
Family Marinara	½ cup	50	1	0
Garlic Mushroom	½ cup	120	7	3
Puttanesca	½ cup	40	2	0
Tomato Basil	½ cup	80	3	0
Wild Mushroom	½ cup	60	3	0
Colavita				
Garden Style	½ cup (4.4 oz)	60	3	0
Del Monte				
Chunky Garlic & Herb	½ cup (4.4 oz)	60	2	0
Chunky Italian Herb	½ cup (4.4 oz)	60	1	0
Tomato & Basil	½ cup (4.4 oz)	70	1	0
Traditional	½ cup (4.4 oz)	60	1	0
With Garlic & Onion	½ cup (4.4 oz)	80	1	0
With Green Peppers & Mushrooms	½ cup (4.4 oz)	80	1	0
With Meat	½ cup (4.4 oz)	60	1	0
With Mushrooms	½ cup (4.4 oz)	60	1	0
Eden				
Organic Lightly Seasoned	½ cup (4.4 oz)	80	3	0
Enrico's				
Fat Free Organic Basil	½ cup (4 oz)	50	0	0
Fat Free Organic Garlic	½ cup (4 oz)	50	0	0
Fat Free Organic Hot Pepper	½ cup (4 oz)	50	0	0
Fat Free Organic Mushroom	½ cup (4 oz)	60	0	0
Fat Free Organic Traditional	½ cup (4 oz)	45	0	0
Francesco Rinaldi				
Alfredo	¼ cup (2.1 oz)	70	5	3

FOOD	PORTION	CALS	FAT	SAT FAT
Chunky Garden Mushroom & Onion	½ cup (4.4 oz)	80	2	0
Chunky Garden Tomato Garlic & Onion	½ cup (4.4 oz)	80	2	0
Dolce Sweet & Tasty Tomato	½ cup (4.4 oz)	110	5	1
Dolce Three Cheese	½ cup (4.4 oz)	90	2	1
Dulce Super Mushroom	½ cup (4.4 oz)	110	5	1
Hearty Diavolo	½ cup (4.4 oz)	70	4	1
Hearty Mushroom Pepper & Onion	½ cup (4.4 oz)	80	3	1
Hearty Tomato & Basil	½ cup (4.4 oz)	80	3	0
Puttanesca	½ cup (4.3 oz)	70	4	1
Tomato Alfredo	¼ cup (2.1 oz)	60	4	2
Traditional Meat Flavored	½ cup (4.4 oz)	90	4	1
Traditional Mushroom	1.2 cup (4.4 oz)	90	4	1
Traditional No Salt Added	½ cup (4.4 oz)	70	3	0
Traditional Original	½ cup (4.4 oz)	90	4	1
Vodka Sauce	¼ cup (2.1 oz)	60	4	2
Healthy Choice				
Chunky Italian Vegetable	½ cup (4.4 oz)	40	tr	0
Chunky Mushroom	½ cup (4.4 oz)	42	tr	0
Garlic & Herbs	½ cup (4.4 oz)	49	tr	0
Garlic Lovers Garlic & Mushroom	½ cup (4.4 oz)	44	tr	0
Garlic Lovers Roasted Garlic	½ cup (4.4 oz)	52	tr	0
Garlic Lovers Roasted Garlic & Sun Dried Tomato	½ cup (4.4 oz)	52	tr	0
Super Chunky Mushroom & Sweet Peppers	½ cup (4.4 oz)	43	tr	0
Super Chunky Tomato Mushroom & Garlic	½ cup (4.4 oz)	45	tr	0
Super Chunky Vegetable Primavera	½ cup (4.4 oz)	43	tr	0
Traditional	½ cup (4.4 oz)	48	tr	0
With Mushrooms	½ cup (4.4 oz)	48	tr	0
Hunt's				
Angela Mia Marinara	¼ cup (2.2 oz)	24	1	tr
Chunky	½ cup (4.4 oz)	38	1	tr
Chunky Italian Sausage	½ cup (4.5 oz)	72	3	1
Chunky Italian Style Vegetable	½ cup (4.4 oz)	63	1	tr
Chunky Marinara	½ cup (4.4 oz)	61	1	tr
Chunky Tomato Garlic & Onion	½ cup (4.4 oz)	63	1	tr
Classic Four Cheese	½ cup (4.4 oz)	50	1	0
Classic Garlic & Herb	½ cup (4.4 oz)	53	2	tr

FOOD	PORTION	CALS	FAT	SAT FAT
Classic Parmesan	½ cup (4.4 oz)	49	2	tr
Classic Tomato & Basil	½ cup (4.4 oz)	48	1	tr
Family Favorites Seasoned Diced Tomato Sauce	½ cup (4.3 oz)	50	1	0
Homestyle Meat Flavored	½ cup (4.4 oz)	51	2	tr
Homestyle Mushrooms	½ cup (4.4 oz)	48	1	tr
Homestyle Traditional	½ cup (4.4 oz)	49	1	tr
Light Meat Flavored	½ cup (4.4 oz)	45	1	1
Light w/ Garlic & Herb	½ cup (4.5 oz)	40	1	tr
Original Meat Flavored	½ cup (4.4 oz)	68	2	tr
Original Traditional	½ cup (4.4 oz)	67	2	tr
Original w/ Mushrooms	½ cup (4.4 oz)	62	2	tr
Original w/ Italian Cheese & Garlic	½ cup (4.5 oz)	64	2	1
Tomato Bits	½ cup (4.5 oz)	49	tr	0
Traditional Light	½ cup (4.4 oz)	40	tr	tr
Mama Rizzo's				
Mushroom Onion	½ cup (4.3 oz)	60	2	0
Pepper Mushroom Onion	½ cup (4.3 oz)	60	2	0
Pepper Primavera Vegetable	½ cup (4.2 oz)	50	2	0
Pepper Tomato Basil Garlic	½ cup (4.7 oz)	60	2	0
Primavera Vegetable	½ cup (4.2 oz)	50	2	0
Tomato Basil Garlic	½ cup (4.6 oz)	60	2	0
Muir Glen				
Organic Balsamic Roasted Onion	½ cup (4.4 oz)	50	1	0
Organic Cabernet Marinara	½ cup (4.4 oz)	50	1	0
Organic Chunky Herb	½ cup (4.4 oz)	50	1	0
Organic Garden Vegetable	½ cup (4.4 oz)	50	1	0
Organic Garlic & Onion	½ cup (4.4 oz)	55	1	0
Organic Garlic Roasted Garlic	½ cup (4.4 oz)	50	1	0
Organic Green Olive	½ cup (4.4 oz)	60	2	0
Organic Italian Herb	½ cup (4.4 oz)	55	1	0
Organic Mushroom Marinara	½ cup (4.4 oz)	45	0	0
Organic Portabello Mushroom	½ cup (4.4 oz)	50	0	0
Organic Sun Dried Tomato	½ cup (4.4 oz)	55	1	1
Organic Tomato Basil	½ cup (4.4 oz)	50	1	1
Newman's Own				
Marinara Venetian	½ cup (4.4 oz)	60	2	0
Marinara Venetian w/ Mushrooms	½ cup (4.4 oz)	60	2	0
Pasta Sauce Bambolina	½ cup (4.5 oz)	100	5	1

FOOD	PORTION	CALS	FAT	SAT FAT
Pasta Sauce Roasted Garlic & Red & Green Peppers	½ cup (4.7 oz)	70	3	0
Pasta Sauce Say Cheese	½ cup (4.4 oz)	90	3	2
Sockarooni	½ cup (4.4 oz)	60	2	0
Prego				
Pasta Bake Sauce Tomato Garlic & Basil	1 serv (3.4 oz)	80	4	1
Traditional	½ cup (4.2 oz)	140	5	2
Pritikin				
Chunky Garden	½ cup (4 oz)	50	1	0
Marinara	½ cup (4 oz)	60	0	0
Original	½ cup (4 oz)	60	1	0
Progresso				
Marinara	½ cup (4.3 oz)	80	5	1
Meat Flavored	½ cup (4.4 oz)	100	5	1
Sauce	½ cup (4.4 oz)	100	5	1
Ragu				
Chunky Garden Style Tomato Garlic & Onion	½ cup (4.5 oz)	110	3	0
Sara Lee				
Chunky Garden Mushroom & Peppers	½ cup (4.4 oz)	80	2	0
Tree Of Life				
Pasta Sauce	½ cup (4 oz)	50	2	—
Pasta Sauce Fat Free Classic	½ cup (3.9 oz)	40	0	0
Pasta Sauce Fat Free Mushroom & Basil	½ cup (3.9 oz)	30	0	0
Pasta Sauce Fat Free Onion & Garlic	½ cup (3.9 oz)	30	0	0
Pasta Sauce Fat Free Sweet Pepper	½ cup (3.9 oz)	30	0	0
Pasta Sauce No Salt Added	½ cup (3.9 oz)	50	2	—
Walden Farms				
Alfredo Sauce Calorie Free	¼ cup	0	0	0
Marinara Calorie Free	⅓ cup	0	0	0
MIX				
Durkee				
Spaghetti Sauce as prep	½ cup	15	0	0
With Mushrooms as prep	½ cup	15	0	0
French's				
Italian as prep	½ cup	16	0	0
Mushroom as prep	½ cup	20	1	0
Thick as prep	½ cup	10	0	0

FOOD	PORTION	CALS	FAT	SAT FAT
McCormick				
Alfredo Pasta Blend as prep	½ cup	60	2	–
Pasta Rosa Blend	1 tbsp (10 g)	40	2	1
Pesto Pasta Sauce as prep	2 tsp (4 g)	10	0	0
Primavera Pasta Blend	1 tbsp (7 g)	30	1	–
Spaghetti Sauce	1 tbsp (8 g)	25	0	0
REFRIGERATED				
Di Giorno				
Alfredo	¼ cup (2.2 oz)	180	18	7
Basil Pesto	¼ cup (2.2 oz)	320	31	6
Four Cheese	¼ cup (2.2 oz)	160	15	7
Garlic Pesto	¼ cup (2.1 oz)	340	33	7
Light Alfredo Sauce	¼ cup (2.4 oz)	140	9	6
Marinara	½ cup (4.5 oz)	70	0	0
Plum Tomato Cream Sauce	½ cup (4.4 oz)	160	13	7
Plum Tomato & Mushroom	½ cup (4.4 oz)	60	0	0
Roasted Red Bell Pepper Cream Sauce	¼ cup (2.3 oz)	140	10	6
TAKE-OUT				
bolognese	5 oz	195	15	–
SPANISH FOOD				
CANNED				
Chi-Chi's				
Pico De Gallo	2 tbsp (1.2 oz)	10	0	0
Derby				
Tamales	3 (6.5 oz)	253	17	8
Gebhardt				
Enchiladas	2 (5.7 oz)	258	19	9
Tamales	2 (5.7 oz)	268	21	10
Tamales Jumbo	2 (6.9 oz)	332	25	12
Hormel				
Tamales Beef	3 (7.5 oz)	280	21	8
Tamales Chicken	3 (7.5 oz)	210	11	4
Tamales Hot Spicy Beef	3 (7.5 oz)	280	21	8
Tamales Jumbo Beef	2 (6.9 oz)	270	20	8
Old El Paso				
Tamales	3 (7.2 oz)	330	19	7
Rosarita				
Enchilada Sauce Mild	¼ cup (2.1 oz)	23	1	tr

FOOD	PORTION	CALS	FAT	SAT FAT
Van Camp				
Tamales	2 (5 oz)	210	13	5
FROZEN				
Amy's				
Black Bean Vegetable Enchilada	1 (4.75 oz)	130	4	0
Bowls Santa Fe Enchilada	1 pkg (10 oz)	340	9	2
Burrito Bean & Cheese	1 (6 oz)	280	8	3
Burrito Bean & Rice Non-Dairy	1 (6 oz)	270	6	1
Burrito Black Bean Vegetable	1 (6 oz)	320	8	1
Burrito Breakfast	1 (6 oz)	210	6	tr
Burrito Especial	1 (6 oz)	260	6	2
Cheese Enchilada	1 (4.75 oz)	210	12	6
Mexican Tamale Pie	1 (8 oz)	150	3	0
Banquet				
Chimichanga Meal	1 meal (9.5 oz)	500	24	8
Enchilada Beef	1 pkg (11 oz)	370	12	5
Enchilada Cheese	1 pkg (11 oz)	360	10	4
Enchilada Chicken	1 pkg (11 oz)	350	10	3
Enchilada Beef & Tamale Combo	1 pkg (11 oz)	450	20	6
Mexican Style Enchilada Combo	1 meal (11 oz)	360	11	5
Chi-Chi's				
Burro Beef	1 pkg (15.9 oz)	590	19	8
Burro Chicken	1 pkg (15.9 oz)	540	14	5
Chimichanga Beef	1 pkg (15.9 oz)	630	24	9
Chimichanga Chicken	1 pkg (15.9 oz)	580	19	6
Enchilada Chicken Suprema	1 pkg (15.9 oz)	600	20	9
Enchilida Baja	1 pkg (15.9 oz)	590	20	9
Health Is Wealth				
Burrito Munchees	10 (5 oz)	310	7	2
Mexican Munchees	2 (1 oz)	49	1	0
Healthy Choice				
Chicken Enchiladas Supreme	1 meal (11.3 oz)	300	7	3
Chicken Enchiladas Suiz	1 meal (10 oz)	280	6	3
Chicken Breast Con Queso Burrito	1 meal (10.55 oz)	350	6	3
Jimmy Dean				
Burrito Breakfast Bacon	1 (4 oz)	260	8	3
Burrito Breakfast Sausage	1 (4 oz)	250	8	3

FOOD	PORTION	CALS	FAT	SAT FAT
Lean Cuisine				
Everyday Favorites Chicken Enchilada Suiza	1 pkg (9 oz)	280	5	2
Old El Paso				
Burrito Bean & Cheese	1 (4.9 oz)	290	9	5
Burrito Beef & Bean Hot	1 (5 oz)	320	10	4
Burrito Beef & Bean Medium	1 (5 oz)	320	10	4
Burrito Beef & Bean Mild	1 (5 oz)	330	9	3
Chimichanga Beef	1 (4.5 oz)	370	20	5
Chimichanga Chicken	1 (4.5 oz)	350	16	4
Patio				
Beef & Cheese Enchiladas Chili 'N Beans	1 meal (15.5 oz)	670	30	14
Beef Enchiladas Chili 'N Beans	1 meal (15.5 oz)	540	27	10
Burrito Bean & Cheese	1 (5 oz)	300	9	5
Burrito Beef & Bean Hot	1 (5 oz)	320	12	5
Burrito Beef & Bean Mild	1 (5 oz)	330	12	4
Burrito Chicken	1 (5 oz)	290	6	3
Burrito Beef & Bean Medium	1 (5 oz)	310	10	5
Burrito Beef & Bean Red Chili Pepper Red Hot	1 (5 oz)	320	12	5
Enchilada Beef	1 meal (12 oz)	320	12	5
Enchilada Cheese	1 meal (12 oz)	370	12	5
Enchilada Chicken	1 meal (12 oz)	400	12	4
Fiesta	1 meal (12 oz)	350	11	5
Mexican Style	1 meal (13.25 oz)	470	19	6
Rudy's Farm				
Burrito Beef/Bean	1 (5 oz)	326	12	4
Burrito Hot Beef/Bean	1 (5 oz)	305	9	3
Senor Felix's				
Burrito Black Bean	1 (10 oz)	540	18	9
Burrito Black Bean Soy	1 (5 oz)	240	7	1
Burrito Chicken	1 (10 oz)	520	20	4
Burrito Hot Potato	1 (10 oz)	560	24	9
Burrito Soy Hot	1 (10 oz)	520	20	3
Burrito Charbroiled Chicken	1 + 4 tsp sauce (6.7 oz)	320	11	3
Burrito Sonora Style	1 + 4 tsp sauce (6.7 oz)	280	8	2

FOOD	PORTION	CALS	FAT	SAT FAT
Burrito Yucatan Style	1 + 4 tsp sauce (6.7 oz)	310	9	2
Empanadas Chicken	1 (4.7 oz)	340	15	30
Empanadas Corn & Rice	1 (4.7 oz)	280	13	4
Empanadas Pumpkin & Mushroom	1 (4.7 oz)	260	11	4
Empanadas Spinach & Ricotta	1 (4.7 oz)	260	12	4
Enchilada Red Pepper	1 (10 oz)	420	19	5
Enchilada Soy Verda	1 (10 oz)	430	24	3
Enchilada Supreme Soy Cheese	1 (10 oz)	460	23	4
Enchilada Verde	1 (5 oz)	423	23	5
Tamales Blue Corn & Soy Cheese	2 + 4 tsp sauce (5.7 oz)	240	10	3
Tamales Chicken	2 + 4 tsp sauce (5.7 oz)	240	9	2
Tamales Gourmet Vegetarian	2 + 4 tsp sauce	240	9	2
Taquitos Blue Corn Soy	3 + 4 tsp sauce (5.2 oz)	230	11	2
Taquitos Chicken	2 + 4 tsp sauce (5.7 oz)	240	10	3
Stouffer's				
Chicken Enchilada	1 serv (4.8 oz)	230	11	5
Today's Tamales				
Cheese & Chili	1 pkg (7 oz)	390	21	10
Del Sol	1 pkg (6.5 oz)	310	15	2
Original Bean	1 pkg (7 oz)	330	11	1
Spicy Taco	1 pkg (7 oz)	310	15	1
Tyson				
Beef Fajita	3½ pieces (12.5 oz)	550	16	4
Chicken Fajita	3½ pieces (13.1 oz)	460	11	3
Weight Watchers				
Smart Ones Chicken Enchiladas Suiza	1 pkg (9 oz)	270	9	5
Smart Ones Santa Fe Style Rice & Beans	1 pkg (10 oz)	290	8	4
MIX				
Gebhardt				
Menudo Mix	¼ tsp (0.4 g)	1	tr	0
McCormick				
Burrito Seasoning	1 tbsp (8 g)	25	1	—

FOOD	PORTION	CALS	FAT	SAT FAT
Fajitas Marinade Mix	2 tsp (4 g)	15	0	0
Taco Seasoning Hot	2 tsp (6 g)	20	0	0
Taco Seasoning Mild	2 tsp (7 g)	20	0	0
Old El Paso				
Burrito Seasoning Mix	2 tsp (6 g)	20	0	0
Dinner Kit Burrito as prep	1	280	7	3
Dinner Kit Soft Taco as prep	2	380	10	4
Dinner Kit Taco as prep	2	270	13	5
Enchilada Sauce Mix	2 tsp (4 g)	10	0	0
Taco Mix 40% Less Sodium	2 tsp (6 g)	20	0	0
Taco Seasoning Mix	2 tsp (6 g)	20	0	0
Taco Bell				
Home Originals Chicken Fajita Dinner as prep	2 (6.9 oz)	340	9	2
Home Originals Chicken Fajita Seasoning Mix	1 tbsp (8 g)	25	0	0
Home Originals Soft Taco Dinner as prep	2 (6.3 oz)	410	18	4
Home Originals Taco Dinner as prep	2 (4.4 oz)	280	15	5
Home Originals Taco Seasoning Mix	2 tsp (6 g)	20	0	0
Home Originals Ultimate Bean Burrito Dinner as prep	1 (4.4 oz)	200	5	2
Home Originals Ultimate Nachos as prep	12 pieces (4.6 oz)	240	11	3
READY-TO-EAT				
taco shell baked	1 med (0.5 oz)	61	3	tr
taco shell baked w/o salt	1 med (½ oz)	61	3	tr
Chi-Chi's				
Taco Shells White Corn	2 (1.2 oz)	170	8	2
Taco Shells Yellow Corn	2 shells (1.2 oz)	170	8	0
Gebhardt				
Taco Shells	3 (1.1 oz)	155	8	2
La Mexicana				
Flour Burritos	1 (1.6 oz)	160	5	1
Old El Paso				
Taco Shells Mini	7 (1.1 oz)	160	10	2
Taco Shells Regular	3 (1.1 oz)	170	10	2
Taco Shells Super	2 (1.3 oz)	190	12	2
Taco Shells White Corn	3 (1.1 oz)	170	10	2
Tostaco Shells	1 (0.8 oz)	130	7	1

FOOD	PORTION	CALS	FAT	SAT FAT
Tostada Shells	3 (1.1 oz)	160	10	2
Rosarita				
Taco Shells	3 (1.1 oz)	155	8	2
Tostada Shells	2 (1 oz)	125	5	1
Taco Bell				
Home Originals Taco Shells	3 (1.1 oz)	150	6	1
TAKE-OUT				
burrito w/ apple	1 lg (5.4 oz)	484	20	7
burrito w/ apple	1 sm (2.6 oz)	231	10	5
burrito w/ beans	2 (7.6 oz)	448	14	7
burrito w/ beans & cheese	2 (6.5 oz)	377	12	7
burrito w/ beans & chili peppers	2 (7.2 oz)	413	15	8
burrito w/ beans & meat	2 (8.1 oz)	508	18	8
burrito w/ beans cheese & beef	2 (7.1 oz)	331	13	7
burrito w/ beans cheese & chili peppers	2 (11.8 oz)	663	23	11
burrito w/ beef	2 (7.7 oz)	523	21	10
burrito w/ beef & chili peppers	2 (7.1 oz)	426	17	8
burrito w/ beef cheese & chili peppers	2 (10.7 oz)	634	25	10
burrito w/ cherry	1 sm (2.6 oz)	231	10	5
burrito w/ cherry	1 lg (5.4 oz)	484	20	7
chimichanga w/ beef	1 (6.1 oz)	425	20	9
chimichanga w/ beef & cheese	1 (6.4 oz)	443	23	11
chimichanga w/ beef & red chili peppers	1 (6.7 oz)	424	19	8
chimichanga w/ beef cheese & red chili peppers	1 (6.3 oz)	364	18	8
enchilada eggplant	1	142	5	–
enchilada w/ cheese	1 (5.7 oz)	320	19	11
enchilada w/ cheese & beef	1 (6.7 oz)	324	18	9
enchirito w/ cheese beef & beans	1 (6.8 oz)	344	16	8
frijoles w/ cheese	1 cup (5.9 oz)	226	8	4
nachos w/ cheese	6 to 8 (4 oz)	345	19	8
nachos w/ cheese & jalapeno peppers	6 to 8 (7.2 oz)	607	34	14
nachos w/ cheese beans ground beef & peppers	6 to 8 (8.9 oz)	568	31	12
nachos w/ cinnamon & sugar	6 to 8 (3.8 oz)	592	36	18
quesadilla	1	290	16	8
taco	1 sm (6 oz)	370	21	11

FOOD	PORTION	CALS	FAT	SAT FAT
taco salad	1½ cups	279	15	7
taco salad w/ chili con carne	1½ cups	288	13	6
tostada w/ beans & cheese	1 (5.1 oz)	223	10	5
tostada w/ beans beef & cheese	1 (7.9 oz)	334	17	11
tostada w/ beef & cheese	1 (5.7 oz)	315	16	10
tostada w/ guacamole	2 (9.2 oz)	360	23	10

SPICES *(see individual names,* HERBS/SPICES)

SPINACH
CANNED

spinach	½ cup	25	1	tr
Del Monte				
Chopped	½ cup (4 oz)	30	0	0
No Salt Added	½ cup (4 oz)	30	0	0
Whole Leaf	½ cup (4 oz)	30	0	0
S&W				
Spinach	½ cup (4.5 oz)	30	0	0
FRESH				
baby raw	2 cups	20	0	0
cooked	½ cup	21	tr	tr
malabar cooked	1 cup (1.5 oz)	10	tr	—
mustard chopped cooked	½ cup	14	tr	—
mustard raw chopped	½ cup	17	tr	—
new zealand chopped cooked	½ cup	11	tr	tr
new zealand raw	½ cup	4	tr	tr
raw chopped	½ cup	6	tr	tr
raw chopped	1 pkg (10 oz)	46	1	tr
Dole				
Baby Spinach	3½ cups (3 oz)	35	0	0
Fresh Express				
Baby Spinach	3 cups	20	0	0
Ready Pac				
Baby	½ cup	20	0	0
FROZEN				
cooked	½ cup	27	tr	tr
Birds Eye				
Chopped	⅓ cup	20	0	0
Creamed	½ cup	100	7	3
Cut Leaf	1 cup	20	0	0

FOOD	PORTION	CALS	FAT	SAT FAT
Fresh Like				
Cut Leaf	3.5 oz	21	tr	–
Green Giant				
Butter Sauce	½ cup (3.4 oz)	40	2	1
Creamed	½ cup (3.8 oz)	80	3	2
Cut Leaf	¾ cup (2.6 oz)	25	0	0
Harvest Fresh	½ cup (3.5 oz)	25	0	0
Health Is Wealth				
Spinach Munchees	2 (1 oz)	60	3	0
Spinach Feta Munchees	2 (1 oz)	70	3	1
Stouffer's				
Creamed	1 serv (4.5 oz)	160	12	4
Souffle	1 serv (4 oz)	150	10	2
Tabatchnick				
Creamed	7.5 oz	60	2	1
Tree Of Life				
Organic	1 cup (3 oz)	20	0	0
SHELF-STABLE				
TastyBite				
Kashmir Spinach	½ pkg (5 oz)	170	10	4
TAKE-OUT				
indian saag	1 serv	28	2	tr
spanakopita spinach pie	1 cup (6 oz)	196	3	2
SPINACH JUICE				
juice	7 oz	14	0	0
SPORTS DRINKS (see ENERGY DRINKS)				
SPOT				
baked	3 oz	134	5	2
SPROUTS				
kidney bean	½ cup	27	tr	tr
kidney bean cooked	1 lb	152	3	tr
lentil sprouts	½ cup	40	tr	tr
mung bean	½ cup	16	tr	tr
mung bean canned	½ cup	8	tr	tr
mung bean cooked	½ cup	13	tr	tr
navy bean	½ cup	35	tr	–
navy bean cooked	3½ oz	78	1	–
pea	½ cup	77	tr	tr

FOOD	PORTION	CALS	FAT	SAT FAT
pinto bean	3½ oz	62	1	–
pinto bean cooked	3½ oz	22	tr	–
radish	½ cup	8	tr	tr
Chun King				
Bean Sprouts	1 cup (3 oz)	11	tr	0
Fresh Alternatives				
BroccoSprouts	½ cup (1 oz)	10	0	0
Deli Blend	½ cup (1 oz)	10	0	0
Salad Blend	½ cup (1 oz)	10	0	0
Sandwich Blend	½ cup (1 oz)	5	0	0
La Choy				
Bean Sprouts	1 cup (2.9 oz)	11	tr	0
TAKE-OUT				
mung bean stir fried	½ cup	31	tr	tr
SQUAB				
boneless baked	3.5 oz	175	3	1
breast w/o skin raw	1 (3.5 oz)	135	5	1
w/o skin raw	1 squab (5.9 oz)	239	13	3
SQUASH (see also ZUCCHINI)				
seeds dried	1 oz	154	13	2
seeds whole roasted	1 oz	127	6	1
CANNED				
crookneck sliced	½ cup	14	tr	tr
FRESH				
acorn cooked mashed	½ cup	41	tr	tr
acorn cubed baked	½ cup	57	tr	tr
butternut baked	½ cup	41	tr	tr
crookneck raw sliced	½ cup	12	tr	tr
crookneck sliced cooked	½ cup	18	tr	tr
hubbard baked	½ cup	51	tr	tr
hubbard cooked mashed	½ cup	35	tr	tr
scallop raw sliced	½ cup	12	tr	tr
scallop sliced cooked	½ cup	14	tr	tr
spaghetti cooked	½ cup	23	tr	tr
FROZEN				
butternut cooked mashed	½ cup	47	tr	tr
crookneck sliced cooked	½ cup	24	tr	tr
Birds Eye				
Cooked Squash	½ cup	50	0	0

FOOD	PORTION	CALS	FAT	SAT FAT
Sliced Yellow	⅔ cup	15	0	0
SEEDS				
dried	1 cup	747	63	12
roasted	1 cup	1184	96	18
roasted	1 oz	148	12	2
salted & roasted	1 oz	148	12	2
salted & roasted	1 cup	1184	96	18
whole roasted	1 cup	285	12	2
whole salted roasted	1 cup	285	12	2
SQUID				
fried	3 oz	149	6	2
raw	3 oz	78	1	tr
TAKE-OUT				
calamari deep fried	1 serv	451	423	3
SQUIRREL				
roasted	3 oz	147	4	tr
STARFRUIT				
fresh	1	42	tr	–
Sonoma				
Dried	7-9 pieces (1.4 oz)	140	0	0
STRAWBERRIES				
CANNED				
in heavy syrup	½ cup	117	tr	tr
FRESH				
strawberries	1 cup	45	1	tr
strawberries	1 pint	97	1	tr
FROZEN				
sweetened sliced	1 cup	245	tr	tr
sweetened sliced	1 pkg (10 oz)	273	tr	tr
unsweetened	1 cup	52	tr	tr
whole sweetened	1 cup	200	tr	tr
whole sweetened	1 pkg (10 oz)	223	tr	tr
Birds Eye				
In Syrup	½ cup	120	0	0
Lite Syrup	1 pkg (10 oz)	120	0	0
Whole	½ cup	100	0	0
Tree Of Life				
Organic	¾ cup (5 oz)	50	0	0

FOOD	PORTION	CALS	FAT	SAT FAT
STRAWBERRY JUICE				
After The Fall				
Strawberry Vanilla	1 can (12 oz)	160	0	0
Twist O' Strawberry	1 can (12 oz)	190	0	0
Capri Sun				
Strawberry Cooler Drink	1 pkg (7 oz)	90	0	0
Kool-Aid				
Drink as prep w/ sugar	1 serv (8 oz)	100	0	0
Drink Mix as prep	1 serv (8 oz)	60	0	0
Squeezit				
Strawberry	1 bottle (7 oz)	110	0	0
Veryfine				
Juice-Ups	8 fl oz	140	0	0
STUFFING/DRESSING				
bread as prep w/ water & fat	½ cup	251	15	6
bread as prep w/ water egg & fat	½ cup	107	7	4
bread dry as prep	½ cup	178	9	2
cornbread as prep	½ cup	179	9	2
Kellogg's				
Croutettes Mix	1 cup (1.2 oz)	120	0	0
Pepperidge Farm				
Corn Bread	¾ cup (1.5 oz)	170	2	0
Herb Seasoned	¾ cup (1.5 oz)	170	2	0
Herb Seasoned Cubed	¾ cup (1.3 oz)	140	2	0
One Step Chicken	½ cup (1.2 oz)	140	4	1
One Step Southwestern Corn Bread	½ cup (1.2 oz)	150	5	1
One Step Turkey	½ cup (1.2 oz)	150	5	1
Stove Top				
Chicken as prep w/ margarine	½ cup (3.6 oz)	170	9	2
Cornbread as prep w/ margarine	½ cup (3.6 oz)	170	8	2
Flexible Serve Chicken as prep w/ margarine	½ cup (3.3 oz)	170	8	2
Flexible Serve Cornbread as prep w/ margarine	½ cup (3.3 oz)	160	8	2
Flexible Serve Homestyle Herb as prep w/ margarine	½ cup (3.3 oz)	170	8	2
For Beef as prep w/ margarine	½ cup (3.7 oz)	180	9	2
For Pork as prep w/ margarine	½ cup (3.6 oz)	170	9	2
For Turkey as prep w/ margarine	½ cup (3.6 oz)	170	9	2

FOOD	PORTION	CALS	FAT	SAT FAT
Long Grain & Wild Rice as prep w/ margarine	½ cup (3.7 oz)	180	9	2
Lower Sodium Chicken as prep w/ margarine	½ cup (3.6 oz)	180	9	2
Microwave Chicken as prep w/ margarine	½ cup (3.5 oz)	160	7	2
Microwave Homestyle Cornbread as prep w/ margarine	½ cup (3 oz)	160	7	2
Mushroom & Onion as prep w/ margarine	½ cup (3.6 oz)	180	9	2
San Francisco Style as prep w/ margarine	½ cup (3.6 oz)	170	9	2
Savory Herb as prep w/ margarine	½ cup (3.6 oz)	170	9	2
Traditional Sage as prep w/ margarine	½ cup (3.6 oz)	180	9	2
TAKE-OUT				
bread	½ cup (3½ oz)	195	8	2
sausage	½ cup	292	11	2
STURGEON				
cooked	3 oz	115	4	1
raw	3 oz	90	3	1
roe raw	1 oz	59	3	–
smoked	3 oz	147	4	1
smoked	1 oz	48	1	tr
SUCKER				
white baked	3 oz	101	3	tr
SUGAR				
brown packed	1 cup (7.7 oz)	828	0	0
brown unpacked	1 cup (5.1 oz)	546	0	0
maple	1 piece (1 oz)	100	tr	–
powdered	1 tbsp (0.3 oz)	31	0	0
powdered unsifted	1 cup (4.2 oz)	467	tr	–
sugarcane stem	3 oz	54	0	0
white	1 cup (7 oz)	773	0	0
white	1 tbsp	45	0	0
white	1 packet (6 g)	25	0	0
white	1 tsp (4 g)	15	0	0

FOOD	PORTION	CALS	FAT	SAT FAT
Billington's				
Muscovado Light Brown	1 tsp	15	0	0
Domino				
Dark Brown	1 tsp	15	0	0
Light Brown	1 tsp	15	0	0
White	1 tsp	16	0	0
Maui Brand				
Raw Sugar	1 tsp	15	0	0
Princess Of Yum				
Citrus Lemon	2.5 tsp	40	0	0
French Vanilla	2.5 tsp	40	0	0
SUGAR SUBSTITUTES				
Equal				
Packet	1 pkg	0	0	0
Fran Gare's				
Miracle Sweet	1 tsp	10	0	0
Keto				
Sweet	½ tsp	0	0	0
Lo Han				
Sweet	2 scoops	2	0	0
Mrs. Bateman's				
Sugarlike	1 tsp (4 g)	4	0	0
SomerSweet				
Sweetener	¼ tsp	0	0	0
Splenda				
Sweetener	1 pkg	0	0	0
Steel's				
Brown	1 tsp	10	0	0
Sugar Substitute	1 tsp	10	0	0
Stevita				
Stevia Spoonable	⅓ tsp	0	0	0
Sugar Twin				
Packets	1	0	0	0
Spoonable Brown	1 tsp	0	0	0
Spoonable White	1 tsp	0	0	0
Weight Watchers				
Sweetener	1 serv (1 g)	5	0	0

FOOD	PORTION	CALS	FAT	SAT FAT
SUGAR-APPLE				
fresh	1	146	tr	–
fresh cut up	1 cup	236	1	–
SUNCHOKE				
fresh raw sliced	½ cup	57	tr	0
SUNFISH				
pumpkinseed baked	3 oz	97	1	tr
SUNFLOWER				
seeds dried	1 oz	162	14	7
seeds dried	1 cup	821	71	7
seeds dry roasted	1 oz	165	14	1
seeds dry roasted	1 cup	745	64	7
seeds dry roasted salted	1 oz	165	14	1
seeds dry roasted salted	1 cup	745	64	7
seeds oil roasted	1 cup	830	78	8
seeds oil roasted salted	1 oz	175	16	2
seeds oil roasted salted	1 cup	830	78	8
seeds toasted	1 oz	176	16	2
seeds toasted	1 cup	826	76	8
seeds toasted salted	1 cup	826	76	8
seeds toasted salted	1 oz	176	16	2
sunflower butter	1 tbsp	93	8	1
sunflower butter w/o salt	1 tbsp	93	8	1
Dakota Gourmet				
Honey Roasted Kernels	1 pkg (1 oz)	158	12	1
Lightly Salted Kernels	1 pkg (1 oz)	168	14	1
Frito Lay				
Seeds	1 oz	180	15	2
Lance				
Seeds In Shell	⅔ cup (1.8 oz)	160	13	3
Seeds Roasted & Shelled	1 pkg (1⅛ oz)	190	16	3
Maranatha				
Tamari Seeds	¼ cup	160	14	2
Planters				
Kernels	1 pkg (1.7 oz)	290	25	3
Kernels	1 pkg (2 oz)	340	29	3
Kernels Barbecue	1 pkg (1.7 oz)	290	25	3
Kernels Honey Roasted	1 pkg (1.7 oz)	280	22	3

FOOD	PORTION	CALS	FAT	SAT FAT
Kernels Salted	1 oz	170	14	2
Munch'N Go Singles Dry Roasted	1 pkg	120	11	1
Nuts Dry Roasted	¼ cup (1.1 oz)	190	17	2
Original With Shell Dry Roasted	¾ cup	160	15	2
Stone-Buhr				
Seeds Raw	4 tsp (1 oz)	170	14	2
SunGold				
SunButter	2 tbsp	200	16	2

SUSHI
TAKE-OUT

FOOD	PORTION	CALS	FAT	SAT FAT
california roll	1 piece (0.8 oz)	28	1	tr
sashimi	1 serv (6 oz)	198	7	1
tuna roll	1 piece (0.7 oz)	23	tr	tr
vegetable roll	1 piece (1.2 oz)	27	1	tr
vinegared ginger	⅓ cup (1.6 oz)	48	tr	tr
wasabi	2 tsp (0.3 oz)	5	tr	0
yellowtail roll	1 piece (0.6 oz)	25	1	tr

SWAMP CABBAGE

FOOD	PORTION	CALS	FAT	SAT FAT
chopped cooked	½ cup	10	tr	–
raw chopped	1 cup	11	tr	–

SWEET POTATO *(see also YAM)*

FOOD	PORTION	CALS	FAT	SAT FAT
baked w/ skin	1 (3½ oz)	118	tr	tr
canned in syrup	½ cup	106	tr	tr
canned pieces	1 cup	183	tr	tr
frzn cooked	½ cup	88	tr	tr
leaves cooked	½ cup	11	tr	tr
mashed	½ cup	172	tr	tr

TAKE-OUT

FOOD	PORTION	CALS	FAT	SAT FAT
candied	3½ oz	144	3	1

SWEETBREADS

FOOD	PORTION	CALS	FAT	SAT FAT
beef braised	3 oz	230	15	–
lamb braised	3 oz	199	13	6
veal braised	3 oz	218	12	–

SWISS CHARD

FOOD	PORTION	CALS	FAT	SAT FAT
cooked	½ cup	18	tr	–
raw chopped	½ cup	3	tr	–

FOOD	PORTION	CALS	FAT	SAT FAT
SWORDFISH				
cooked	3 oz	132	4	1
raw	3 oz	103	3	1
SYRUP				
corn	2 tbsp	122	0	0
corn dark	1 cup (11.5 oz)	925	tr	–
corn dark	1 tbsp (0.7 oz)	56	0	–
corn light	1 cup (11.5 oz)	925	tr	–
corn light	1 tbsp (0.7 oz)	56	0	–
date syrup	1 tbsp	63	tr	–
malt	1 cup (13 oz)	1222	tr	–
malt	1 tbsp (0.8 oz)	76	0	–
maple	1 cup (11.1 oz)	824	1	–
maple	1 tbsp (0.8 oz)	52	0	–
raspberry	1 oz	76	0	0
rose hip	1 oz	9	0	0
sorghum	1 cup (11.6 oz)	957	0	0
sorghum	1 tbsp (0.7 oz)	61	0	0
DaVinci Gourmet				
Sugar Free All Flavors	1 tbsp	0	0	0
Eden				
Organic Barley Malt	1 tbsp	60	0	0
Estee				
Blueberry	¼ cup	80	0	0
Hershey				
Strawberry	2 tbsp (1.4 oz)	100	0	0
Karo				
Corn Syrup Light	2 tbsp (1 oz)	120	0	0
Quik				
Strawberry	2 tbsp (1.5 oz)	110	0	0
Red Wing				
Strawberry	2 tbsp (1.4 oz)	110	0	0
Smucker's				
Apricot	¼ cup	210	0	0
Blackberry	¼ cup	210	0	0
Plate Scapers Kiwi Lime	2 tbsp (1.3 oz)	100	0	0
Plate Scapers Mango Orange	2 tbsp	100	0	0
Plate Scapers Raspberry	2 tbsp (1.3 oz)	100	0	0

TAHINI (see SESAME)

FOOD	PORTION	CALS	FAT	SAT FAT
TAMARIND				
fresh	1	5	tr	tr
fresh cut up	1 cup	287	1	tr
TANGERINE				
CANNED				
in light syrup	½ cup	76	tr	tr
juice pack	½ cup	46	tr	tr
FRESH				
sections	1 cup	86	tr	tr
tangerine	1	37	tr	tr
Chiquita				
Tangerine	1 med (3.5 oz)	50	1	0
TANGERINE JUICE				
canned sweetened	1 cup	125	1	tr
fresh	1 cup	106	tr	tr
frzn sweetened as prep	1 cup	110	tr	tr
frzn sweetened not prep	6 oz	344	1	tr
After The Fall				
Juice	1 can (12 oz)	170	0	0
Fresh Samantha				
Fresh Juice	1 cup (8 oz)	110	0	0
Odwalla				
Juice	8 fl oz	110	0	0
TAPIOCA				
pearl dry	½ cup (2.7 oz)	272	tr	tr
starch	1 oz	98	tr	—
Minute				
Minute Tapioca	1½ tsp (6 g)	20	0	0
TARO				
chips	1 oz	141	7	2
chips	10 (0.8 oz)	115	6	1
leaves cooked	½ cup	18	tr	tr
raw sliced	½ cup	56	tr	tr
shoots sliced cooked	½ cup	10	tr	tr
sliced cooked	½ cup (2.3 oz)	94	tr	tr
tahitian sliced cooked	½ cup	30	tr	tr

FOOD	PORTION	CALS	FAT	SAT FAT
TARPON				
fresh	3 oz	87	2	–
TARRAGON				
ground	1 tsp	5	tr	–
TEA/HERBAL TEA (see also ICED TEA)				
HERBAL				
chamomile brewed	1 cup	2	tr	tr
Celestial Seasonings				
Mandarin Orange Spice	1 tea bag	0	0	0
Eden				
Organic Genmaicha Tea	1 cup	0	0	0
Organic Kukicha Tea	1 cup	0	0	0
Guayaki				
Yerba Mate Magical Mint	1 tea bag	5	0	0
Yerba Mate Organic Chai Spice	1 tea bag	5	0	0
Yerba Mate Organic Chocolatte	1 tea bag	5	0	0
Yerba Mate Organic Orange Blossom	1 tea bag	5	0	0
Yerba Mate Organic Rooiboost	1 tea bag	5	0	0
Yerba Mate Organic Traditional	1 tea bag	5	0	0
Lipton				
Bedtime Story	1 tea bag	0	0	0
Cinnamon Apple	1 tea bag	0	0	0
Ginger Twist	1 tea bag	0	0	0
Lemon	1 tea bag	0	0	0
Orange	1 tea bag	0	0	0
Peppermint	1 tea bag	0	0	0
Quietly Chamomile	1 tea bag	0	0	0
Silk				
Chai	1 cup	140	4	0
REGULAR				
brewed tea	6 oz	2	0	0
instant unsweetened as prep w/ water	8 oz	2	0	0
Activitea				
Green Tea	1 cup	36	0	0
Celestial Seasonings				
Green Tea Raspberry Garden as prep	1 cup	0	0	0
Green Tea Honey Lemon Ginseng	1 cup	0	0	0
Honey Darjeeling as prep	1 cup	0	0	0

FOOD	PORTION	CALS	FAT	SAT FAT
DaVinci Gourmet				
Sugar Free Tea Concentrate Green	2 tbsp	0	0	0
Sugar Free Tea Concentrate Lemon	2 tbsp	0	0	0
Sugar Free Tea Concentrate Spiced Chai	1.5 tbsp	0	0	0
General Foods				
International Instant Tea Decaffeinated English Breakfast Creme	1 serv (8 oz)	70	2	1
International Instant Tea Decaffeinated Viennese Cinnamon Creme	1 serv (8 oz)	70	2	1
International Instant Tea English Breakfast Creme as prep	1 serv (8 oz)	70	2	1
International Instant Tea English Raspberry Creme as prep	1 serv (8 oz)	70	2	1
International Instant Tea Island Orange Creme as prep	1 serv (8 oz)	70	2	1
International Instant Tea Viennese Cinnamon Creme as prep	1 serv (8 oz)	70	2	1
Guayaki				
Yerba Mate Organic Greener Green Tea	1 tea bag	5	0	0
Lipton				
Brisk Tea as prep	1 serv	0	0	0
Decaffeinated Brisk Tea as prep	1 serv	0	0	0
English Blend as prep	1 cup	0	0	0
Flavored Decaffeinated Orange & Spice	1 tea bag	0	0	0
Green Tea	1 tea bag	0	0	0
Loose Tea	1 tsp (2 g)	0	0	0
Pacific Chai				
All Flavors as prep	1 serv	93	1	1
Paradise				
Tropical Tea	8 fl oz	1	0	0
Tropical Tea Decafe	8 fl oz	1	0	0
Tropical Tea Passion Fruit	8 fl oz	1	0	0
Salada				
Green Tea	1 cup	0	0	0
Green Tea Decaffeinated	1 tea bag	0	0	0
Tetley				
British Blend Round Teabags	1 cup	0	0	0

FOOD	PORTION	CALS	FAT	SAT FAT
Decaffeinated Tea Bag as prep	1	0	0	0
Tea Bag as prep	1	0	0	0
TAKE-OUT				
chai spiced latte decaf	1 cup	130	3	1
TEMPEH				
tempeh	½ cup	165	6	1
Lightlife				
Garden Vege	4 oz	200	8	1
Quinoa Sesame	4 oz	220	8	1
Smokey Strips	3 slices (2 oz)	80	3	1
Soy	4 oz	210	8	1
Three Grain	4 oz	200	7	1
Wild Rice	4 oz	190	7	1
Turtle Island				
Five Grain	3 oz	190	6	1
Low Fat Millet	3 oz	130	2	1
Soy	3 oz	160	4	1
Wild Rice Rhapsody	3 oz	160	4	1
White Wave				
Five Grain	⅓ block	140	4	1
Organic Original Soy	⅓ block	150	6	1
Organic Sea Veggie	⅓ block	120	3	0
Soy Rice	⅓ block	140	5	1
THYME				
ground	1 tsp	4	tr	tr
Watkins				
Thyme	¼ tsp (0.5 oz)	0	0	0
TILEFISH				
cooked	3 oz	125	4	1
cooked	½ fillet (5.3 oz)	220	7	1
raw	3 oz	81	2	tr
TOFU				
firm	¼ block (3 oz)	118	7	1
firm	½ cup	183	11	2
fresh fried	1 piece (0.5 oz)	35	3	tr
fuyu salted & fermented	1 block (⅓ oz)	13	1	tr
koyadofu dried frozen	1 piece (⅓ oz)	82	5	1
okara	½ cup	47	1	tr

FOOD	PORTION	CALS	FAT	SAT FAT
regular	¼ block (4 oz)	88	6	1
regular	½ cup	94	6	1
Azumaya				
Baked Chili Picante	2 pieces	200	10	2
Baked Mesquite	2 pieces	100	10	2
Baked Spicy Thai Peanut	2 pieces	190	10	2
Baked Teriyaki	2 pieces	200	10	2
Extra Firm	1 serv (2.8 oz)	70	4	1
Firm	1 serv (2.8 oz)	70	4	1
Lite Extra Firm	1 serv (2.8 oz)	60	2	0
Lite Silken	1 serv (3.2 oz)	40	1	0
Silken	1 serv (3.2 oz)	40	2	0
Casbah				
Gyro as prep w/ tofu	1 patty (2 oz)	105	3	0
Galaxy				
Slices Hickory Smoked	1 slice (1 oz)	50	2	0
Slices Italian Garlic Herb	1 slice (1 oz)	50	2	0
Slices Original	1 slice (1 oz)	50	2	0
Slices Savory	1 slice (1 oz)	50	2	0
Hinoichi				
Firm	1 inch slice (3 oz)	60	3	0
Long Life				
Tofu	3 oz	60	3	0
Nasoya				
5 Spice	1 serv (3 oz)	70	4	1
Baked Mesquite Smoke	2 pieces	220	9	2
Baked Teriyaki	2 pieces	230	9	2
Baked TexMex	2 pieces	230	9	2
Baked Thai Peanut	2 pieces	240	10	2
Extra Firm	1 serv (3 oz)	90	5	1
Firm	1 serv (3 oz)	70	4	1
Firm Enriched	1 serv (3 oz)	45	1	0
Garlic & Onion	1 serv (3 oz)	70	4	1
Silken	1 serv (3.2 oz)	45	3	1
Soft	1 serv (3 oz)	60	4	1
TofuMate Breakfast Scramble	¼ pkg	15	0	0
TofuMate Eggless Salad	¼ pkg	15	0	0
TofuMate Mandarin Stirfry	¼ pkg	30	0	0
TofuMate Mediterranean Herb	¼ pkg	15	0	0
TofuMate Szechwan Stirfry	¼ pkg	25	0	0

FOOD	PORTION	CALS	FAT	SAT FAT
TofuMate Texas Taco	¼ pkg	15	0	0
Pete's Tofu				
Dessert Peach Mango	1 serv (6 oz)	120	3	0
Dessert Very Berry	1 serv (6 oz)	120	3	1
Medium Firm	3 oz	70	4	1
Soft	3 oz	56	3	1
Super Firm Italian Herb	3 oz	120	7	1
Super Firm	3 oz	130	8	2
Tofu 2 Go Lemon Pepper	2 pieces + sauce	160	9	1
Tofu 2 Go Santa Fe	2 pieces + sauce	150	9	1
Tofu 2 Go Sesame Ginger	2 pieces + sauce	160	10	2
Tofu 2 Go Thai Tango	2 pieces + sauce	165	10	2
Tree Of Life				
30% Reduced Fat Firm	⅕ block (3.2 oz)	90	4	0
Easymeal Pasta Primavera as prep	1 serv	460	16	3
Easymeal Southwest Medley as prep	1 serv	380	14	2
Easymeal Teriyaki Stir Fry as prep	1 serv	270	14	2
Easymeal Thai Stir Fry as prep	1 serv	270	14	2
Organic Baked	⅓ block (2.7 oz)	150	8	1
Organic Baked Island Spice	⅓ pkg (2.7 oz)	130	7	1
Organic Baked Oriental	⅓ pkg (2.7 oz)	130	7	1
Organic Baked Savory	⅓ block (2.7 oz)	140	7	1
Organic Firm	⅕ block (3.2 oz)	100	5	0
Raw Firm	⅕ block (3.2 oz)	100	5	0
White Wave				
Baked Garlic Herb Italian	1 piece	120	6	1
Baked Hickory Smoke BBQ	1 piece	75	3	1
Baked Roma Italian Basil	1 piece	100	6	1
Baked Teriyaki Oriental	1 piece	120	6	1
Baked Thai Style	1 piece	120	6	1
Baked Zesty Lemon Pepper	1 piece	120	8	1
Extra Firm	¼ block	80	5	1
Organic Extra Firm	⅕ block	90	6	1
Organic Soft	⅕ block	90	6	1
Reduced Fat	⅕ block	90	4	0
TOMATILLO				
fresh	1 (1.2 oz)	11	tr	–
fresh chopped	½ cup	21	1	–

FOOD	PORTION	CALS	FAT	SAT FAT
TOMATO				
CANNED				
paste	½ cup	110	1	tr
puree	1 cup	102	tr	tr
puree w/o salt	1 cup	102	tr	tr
red whole	½ cup	24	tr	tr
sauce	½ cup	37	tr	tr
sauce spanish style	½ cup	40	tr	tr
sauce w/ mushrooms	½ cup	42	tr	tr
sauce w/ onion	½ cup	52	tr	tr
stewed	½ cup	34	tr	tr
w/ green chiles	½ cup	18	tr	tr
wedges in tomato juice	½ cup	34	tr	tr
Amore				
Sun-Dried Tomato Paste	1 tsp (6 g)	15	1	0
Big R				
Cajun Stewed	½ cup (4.2 oz)	25	0	0
Diced w/ Chilies	½ cup (4.2 oz)	25	0	0
Mexican Stewed	½ cups (4.2 oz)	25	0	0
Stewed	½ cup (4.2 oz)	25	0	0
Whole	½ cup (4.2 oz)	25	0	0
Claussen				
Halves	1 serv (1 oz)	5	0	0
Contadina				
Italian Paste	2 tbsp	35	1	—
Italian Paste Roasted Garlic	2 tbsp	35	1	—
Paste	2 tbsp	30	0	0
Puree	¼ cup (2.2 oz)	20	0	0
Recipe Ready Diced Roasted Garlic	½ cup (4.3 oz)	45	0	0
Stewed	½ cup	35	0	0
Stewed w/ Celery & Green Peppers	½ cup	35	0	0
Del Monte				
Chunky Chili Style	½ cup (4.5 oz)	30	0	0
Chunky Pasta Style	½ cup (4.5 oz)	45	0	0
Crushed Italian Recipe	½ cup (4.4 oz)	45	0	0
Crushed Original Recipe	½ cup (4.4 oz)	45	0	0
Crushed w/ Garlic	½ cup (4.4 oz)	50	0	0
Diced	½ cup (4.4 oz)	25	0	0
Diced No Salt Added	½ cup (4.4 oz)	25	0	0
Diced w/ Basil Garlic & Oregano	½ cup	50	0	0

FOOD	PORTION	CALS	FAT	SAT FAT
Diced w/ Garlic & Onion	½ cup (4.4 oz)	40	1	–
Diced w/ Green Pepper & Onion	½ cup (4.4 oz)	40	0	0
Paste	2 tbsp (1.2 oz)	30	0	0
Petite Cut Garlic & Olive Oil	½ cup	45	1	0
Sauce	¼ cup (2.1 oz)	20	0	0
Sauce No Salt Added	¼ cup (2.1 oz)	20	0	0
Stewed Cajun Recipe	½ cup (4.4 oz)	35	0	0
Stewed Italian Recipe	½ cup (4.4 oz)	30	0	0
Stewed Mexican Recipe	½ cup (4.4 oz)	35	0	0
Stewed Original	½ cup (4.4 oz)	35	0	0
Stewed Original No Salt Added	½ cup (4.4 oz)	35	0	0
Wedges	½ cup (4.4 oz)	35	0	0
Zesty Diced w/ Mild Green Chilies	½ cup (4.4 oz)	30	0	0
Eden				
Organic Diced	½ cup	30	0	0
Organic Diced w/ Green Chilies	½ cup	30	0	0
Hunt's				
Angela Mia Puree	¼ cup (2.2 oz)	16	tr	0
Choice Cut	½ cup (4.2 oz)	23	tr	0
Choice Cut Diced Tomatoes & Italian Herb	½ cup (4.2 oz)	24	0	0
Choice Cut Diced Tomatoes & Roasted Garlic	½ cup (4.2 oz)	24	0	0
Choice Cut Diced Tomatoes w/ Red Pepper & Basil	¼ cup (4.2 oz)	27	tr	0
Crushed Pear Tomatoes	½ cup (4.2 oz)	29	tr	0
Diced In Juice	½ cup	20	0	0
Diced In Puree	½ cup (4.3 oz)	23	tr	0
Diced W/ Green Chilies	2 tbsp (0.4 oz)	1	tr	0
Paste	2 tbsp (1.2 oz)	30	tr	0
Paste Italian	2 tbsp (1.2 oz)	27	tr	0
Paste No Salt Added	2 tbsp (1.2 oz)	30	tr	0
Paste With Garlic	2 tbsp (1.2 oz)	28	tr	0
Petite Diced	½ cup	20	0	0
Petite Diced w/ Mushrooms	½ cup	45	2	0
Puree	¼ cup (2.2 oz)	24	tr	0
Ready Sauce Chunky Chili	¼ cup (2.2 oz)	22	tr	0
Ready Sauce Chunky Italian	¼ cup (2.2 oz)	30	1	0
Ready Sauce Chunky Mexican	¼ cup (2.2 oz)	21	tr	0
Ready Sauce Chunky Salsa	¼ cup (2.2 oz)	18	tr	0

FOOD	PORTION	CALS	FAT	SAT FAT
Ready Sauce Chunky Tomato	¼ cup (2.2 oz)	15	tr	0
Ready Sauce Garlic & Herb	¼ cup (2.2 oz)	26	tr	0
Sauce	¼ cup (2.2 oz)	16	tr	0
Sauce Herb	¼ cup (2.2 oz)	32	1	0
Sauce Italian	¼ cup (2.2 oz)	32	1	0
Sauce Meatloaf Fixins	¼ cup (2.2 oz)	23	tr	0
Sauce No Salt Added	¼ cup (2.2 oz)	16	tr	0
Sauce Special	¼ cup (2.2 oz)	21	1	0
Stewed	½ cup (4.2 oz)	33	tr	0
Stewed No Salt Added	½ cup (4.2 oz)	33	tr	0
Whole Peeled	2 (5.2 oz)	24	tr	0
Whole Peeled No Salt Added	2 (4.8 oz)	21	tr	0
Muir Glen				
Diced Fire Roasted	¼ cup	30	0	0
Diced w/ Green Chilies	½ cup (4.5 oz)	25	0	0
Organic Chunky Sauce	¼ cup (2.3 oz)	20	0	0
Organic Crushed Fire Roasted	¼ cup	20	0	0
Organic Diced	½ cup (4.5 oz)	25	0	0
Organic Diced No Salt Added	½ cup (4.5 oz)	25	0	0
Organic Diced w/ Basil & Garlic	½ cup (4.5 oz)	25	0	0
Organic Diced w/ Italian Herbs	½ cup (4.4 oz)	25	0	0
Organic Ground Peeled	¼ cup (2.3 oz)	10	0	0
Organic Paste	2 tbsp (1.2 oz)	30	0	0
Organic Puree	¼ cup (2.2 oz)	20	0	0
Organic Sauce	¼ cup (2.2 oz)	20	0	0
Organic Sauce No Salt Added	¼ cup (2.2 oz)	20	0	0
Organic Stewed	½ cup (4.5 oz)	30	0	0
Organic Whole Peeled	½ cup (4.6 oz)	30	0	0
Whole Peeled w/ Basil	½ cup (4.6 oz)	30	0	0
Old El Paso				
Tomatoes & Jalapenos	¼ cup (2 oz)	15	0	0
Tomatoes & Green Chilies	¼ cup (2 oz)	10	0	–
Progresso				
Crushed w/ Added Puree	¼ cup (2.1 oz)	20	0	0
Italian Style Peeled	½ cup (4.2 oz)	20	0	0
Paste	2 tbsp (1.2 oz)	30	0	0
Puree	¼ cup (2.2 oz)	25	0	0
Puree Thick Style	¼ cup (2.2 oz)	20	0	0
Sauce	¼ cup (2.1 oz)	20	0	0
Whole Peeled	½ cup (4.2 oz)	25	0	0

FOOD	PORTION	CALS	FAT	SAT FAT
Redpack				
Crushed In Puree	¼ cup	20	0	0
Puree	¼ cup (2.2 oz)	25	0	0
Ro-Tel				
Diced Tomatoes & Green Chilies	½ cup (4.4 oz)	20	0	0
Sonoma				
Dried Spice Medley oil drained	1 tbsp (0.5 oz)	50	4	0
Pesto	¼ cup (2 oz)	110	9	2
Tapenade	1 tbsp (0.7 oz)	70	6	1
DRIED				
sun dried	1 piece	5	tr	tr
sun dried	1 cup	140	2	tr
sun dried in oil	1 cup (4 oz)	235	15	2
sun dried in oil	1 piece (3 g)	6	tr	tr
sun dried	5 pieces (0.5 oz)	40	0	0
Sonoma				
Bits	2-3 tsp (5 g)	15	0	0
Dried	2-3 halves (5 g)	15	0	0
Julienne	7-9 pieces (5 g)	15	0	0
Pasta Toss	½ cup (0.7 oz)	70	0	0
Season It	2-3 tsp (5 g)	20	0	0
FRESH				
cooked	½ cup	32	1	tr
grape tomatoes	20	30	0	0
green	1	30	tr	tr
red	1 (4.5 oz)	26	tr	tr
red chopped	1 cup	35	tr	tr
Chiquita				
Tomato	1 med (5.2 oz)	35	1	0
Eurofresh				
Tomatoes On The Vine	1 med (5.2 oz)	35	1	0
TAKE-OUT				
bruschetta on toasted italian bread	1 slice	106	3	0
stewed	1 cup	80	3	1
TOMATO JUICE				
beef broth & tomato	5½ oz	61	tr	tr
clam & tomato	1 can (5½ oz)	77	tr	tr
tomato juice	6 oz	32	tr	tr
tomato juice	½ cup	21	tr	tr

FOOD	PORTION	CALS	FAT	SAT FAT
Campbell's				
Juice	8 oz	51	1	tr
Del Monte				
Juice	8 fl oz	50	0	0
Snap-E-Tom Chile Cocktail	6 fl oz	40	0	0
Dole				
Juice	1 bottle (12 oz)	85	0	0
Hunt's				
Juice	1 can (6 oz)	22	tr	0
No Salt Added	8 fl oz	34	tr	0
Mott's				
Tomato Juice	8 fl oz	40	0	0
Muir Glen				
Organic	5.5 oz	40	0	0
TONGUE				
beef simmered	3 oz	241	18	8
lamb braised	3 oz	234	17	7
pork braised	3 oz	230	16	5
TORTILLA				
corn	1 (6 in diam)	56	1	tr
corn w/o salt	1-6 in diam (.9 oz)	56	1	tr
flour w/o salt	1-8 in diam (1.2 oz)	114	3	tr
Alvarado St. Bakery				
Burrito Size	1 (2.2 oz)	170	4	0
Fajita Size	1 (1.6 oz)	130	3	0
La Mexicana				
Corn	1 (0.8 oz)	50	1	0
Flour	1 (0.8 oz)	80	3	1
Tortillas de Trigo	1 (1 oz)	140	7	1
La Tortilla Factory				
Low Carb Whole Wheat	1 lg	100	3	–
Low Carb Whole Wheat	1 reg	60	2	–
Mariachi				
Tortilla	1	112	3	–
Old El Paso				
Flour	1 (1.4 oz)	130	4	1
Soft Taco Tortilla	2 (1.8 oz)	180	4	1

FOOD	PORTION	CALS	FAT	SAT FAT
Tyson				
Flour	1 (1.7 oz)	150	4	1
Flour Heat Pressed	2 (2 oz)	170	4	1
White Corn	2 (1.8 oz)	100	1	0
Whole Wheat Heat Pressed	1 (1.4 oz)	120	3	1
Yellow Corn	3 (1.9 oz)	140	2	0
TORTILLA CHIPS (see CHIPS)				
TREE FERN				
chopped cooked	½ cup	28	tr	—
TRITICALE				
dry	1 cup (6.7 oz)	645	4	1
triticale not prep	1 oz	94	tr	—
TROUT				
baked	3 oz	162	7	1
rainbow cooked	3 oz	129	4	1
seatrout baked	3 oz	113	4	1
TRUFFLES				
fresh	0.5 oz	4	tr	—
TUNA				
CANNED				
light in oil	1 can (6 oz)	399	14	3
light in oil	3 oz	169	7	1
light in water	3 oz	99	1	tr
light in water	1 can (5.8 oz)	192	1	tr
white in oil	1 can (6.2 oz)	331	14	—
white in oil	3 oz	158	7	—
white in water	1 can (6 oz)	234	4	1
white in water	3 oz	116	2	1
Bumble Bee				
Chunk Light In Water	2 oz	60	1	—
Chunk Light In Water Pouch	2 oz	60	1	0
Chunk Light In Water Touch Of Lemon	2 oz	60	1	0
Solid White Albacore In Water	2 oz	70	1	0
Solid White In Water	2 oz	70	1	0

FOOD	PORTION	CALS	FAT	SAT FAT
Progresso				
In Olive Oil drained	¼ cup (2 oz)	160	12	2
StarKist				
Chunk Light In Water	¼ cup (2 oz)	60	1	0
Chunk Light No Drain Package	¼ cup (2 oz)	60	1	0
Low Sodium Chunk White In Water	2 oz	60	1	0
Solid White Albacore In Water	¼ cup	70	1	0
Tuna Fillet In Spring Water	¼ cup (2 oz)	60	1	0
FRESH				
bluefin cooked	3 oz	157	5	1
bluefin raw	3 oz	122	4	1
skipjack baked	3 oz	112	1	tr
yellowfin baked	3 oz	118	1	tr

TUNA DISHES
MIX
Tuna Helper

FOOD	PORTION	CALS	FAT	SAT FAT
AuGratin 50% Less Fat Recipe as prep	1 cup	240	6	2
AuGratin as prep	1 cup	300	11	3
Cheesy Broccoli 50% Less Fat Recipe as prep	1 cup	240	5	2
Cheesy Broccoli as prep	1 cup	290	9	3
Cheesy Pasta 50% Less Fat Recipe as prep	1 cup	230	5	2
Cheesy Pasta as prep	1 cup	280	11	3
Creamy Broccoli 50% Less Fat Recipe as prep	1 cup	240	5	2
Creamy Broccoli as prep	1 cup	310	12	3
Creamy Pasta 50% Less Fat Recipe as prep	1 cup	230	6	2
Creamy Pasta as prep	1 cup	300	13	4
Fettuccine Alfredo 50% Less Fat Recipe as prep	1 cup	240	6	2
Fettuccine Alfredo as prep	1 cup	310	14	4
Garden Cheddar 50% Less Fat Recipe as prep	1 cup	240	5	2
Garden Cheddar as prep	1 cup	290	11	3
Pasta Salad Low Fat Recipe as prep	⅔ cup	230	2	0
Pasta Salad as prep	⅔ cup	380	27	3

FOOD	PORTION	CALS	FAT	SAT FAT
Tetrazzini 50% Less Fat Recipe as prep	1 cup	230	5	2
Tetrazzini as prep	1 cup	300	12	4
Tuna Melt Reduced Fat Recipe as prep	1 cup	240	6	2
Tuna Melt as prep	1 cup	300	12	4
Tuna Pot Pie as prep	1 cup	440	24	7
Tuna Romanoff 50% Less Fat Recipe as prep	1 cup	240	3	1
Tuna Romanoff as prep	1 cup	280	8	2
READY-TO-EAT				
Bumble Bee				
Tuna Salad Fat Free	1 pkg (3.5 oz)	190	2	0
Tuna Salad Kit	1 pkg (3.8 oz)	250	13	2
StarKist				
Lunch To-Go	1 pkg	310	13	3
Ready-Mixed Tuna Salad Kit	1 pkg (3.5 oz)	190	6	3
Tuna Salad Lunch Kit	1 pkg (4.3 oz)	230	9	2
Wampler				
Salad	⅓ cup	180	12	–
Salad Chunky	⅓ cup	180	13	–
TAKE-OUT				
tuna salad	3 oz	159	8	1
tuna salad	1 cup	383	19	3

TURBOT

FOOD	PORTION	CALS	FAT	SAT FAT
european baked	3 oz	104	3	–

TURKEY (see also TURKEY DISHES, TURKEY SUBSTITUTES)

FOOD	PORTION	CALS	FAT	SAT FAT
CANNED				
w/ broth	½ can (2.5 oz)	116	5	1
w/ broth	1 can (5 oz)	231	10	3
Mary Kitchen				
Roast Turkey Hash	1 can (14.9 oz)	420	11	3
FRESH				
back w/ skin roasted	½ back (9 oz)	637	38	11
breast w/ skin roasted	4 oz	212	8	2
dark meat w/ skin roasted	3.6 oz	230	12	4
dark meat w/o skin roasted	3 oz	170	7	2
dark meat w/o skin roasted	1 cup (5 oz)	262	10	3
ground cooked	3 oz	188	11	3
leg w/ skin roasted	2.5 oz	147	7	2

FOOD	PORTION	CALS	FAT	SAT FAT
leg w/ skin roasted	1 (1.2 lbs)	1133	54	17
light meat w/ skin roasted	4.7 oz	268	11	3
light meat w/ skin roasted	from ½ turkey (2.3 lbs)	2069	87	25
light meat w/o skin roasted	4 oz	183	4	1
neck simmered	1 (5.3 oz)	274	11	4
skin roasted	1 oz	141	13	3
skin roasted	from ½ turkey (9 oz)	1096	98	26
w/ skin roasted	½ turkey (4 lbs)	3857	181	53
w/ skin roasted	8.4 oz	498	23	7
w/ skin neck & giblets roasted	½ turkey (8.8 lbs)	4123	190	56
w/o skin roasted	7.3 oz	354	10	3
w/o skin roasted	1 cup (5 oz)	238	7	2
wing w/ skin roasted	1 (6.5 oz)	426	23	6
Jennie-O				
Ground	4 oz	160	8	3
Louis Rich				
Ground	4 oz	190	12	4
Patties White	1 (4 oz)	170	10	3
Mr. Turkey				
Ground 85% Fat Free	3.5 oz	210	16	–
Ground 91% Fat Free	3.5 oz	170	10	–
Perdue				
Breast Tenderloins Butter Garlic	3 oz	100	1	–
Burger Cooked	1 (4 oz)	160	9	3
Dark Cooked	3 oz	180	11	4
Drumsticks Cooked	1 (2.2 oz)	110	6	2
Ground Cooked	3 oz	160	9	3
Tenderloins Black Pepper Cooked	3 oz	90	1	–
Thighs Cooked	1 (3.2 oz)	240	19	6
White Cooked	3 oz	150	7	2
Shady Brook				
Cutlets	4 oz	130	1	0
Drumstick	4 oz	170	9	3
Ground Breast	4 oz	120	1	0
Ground Lean	4 oz	170	9	3
Ground Turkey 85%	4 oz	220	15	5

FOOD	PORTION	CALS	FAT	SAT FAT
Mesquite Seasoned Tenderloin	4 oz	110	1	0
OnlyOne Boneless Breast Roast	4 oz	130	1	0
Split Breast	4 oz	190	9	3
Tenderloin	4 oz	130	1	0
Teriyaki Seasoned Tenderloin	4 oz	120	1	0
Thigh	4 oz	220	15	5
Turkey Burgers	4 oz	170	9	3
Turkey Meatloaf Lean	4 oz	150	7	2
Whole Breast	4 oz	190	9	3
Whole Turkey	4 oz	180	9	3
Wing	4 oz	220	14	4
Zesty Lemon Seasoned Tenderloin	4 oz	120	1	0
Turkey Store				
Breakfast Sausage Patties Mild	2 patties (2.3 oz)	160	13	4
Lean Ground Italian Style	4 oz	190	10	4
Seasoned Cuts Turkey Breast Roast	4 oz	110	1	0
Wampler				
Boneless Breast Roast	4 oz	160	6	1
Breast Half	4 oz	160	6	1
Breast Steaks	4 oz	120	1	–
Drumsticks	4 oz	180	10	3
Ground	4 oz	210	15	3
Ground Breast	4 oz	130	1	0
Ground Lean	4 oz	160	8	2
Thighs	4 oz	170	10	2
Wings	4 oz	220	14	4
Woodfire Grill Burger	1 (3 oz)	180	9	3
FROZEN				
roast boneless seasoned light & dark meat roasted	1 pkg (1.7 lbs)	1213	45	–
Wampler				
Burger BBQ	1 (4 oz)	240	17	–
Burgers Cracked Peppercorn & Garlic	1 (3 oz)	170	9	3
Seasoned Burgers Cracker Peppercorn & Garlic	1 (3 oz)	170	9	3
READY-TO-EAT				
bologna	1 oz	57	4	–
breast	1 slice (0.75 oz)	23	tr	tr
diced light & dark seasoned	1 oz	39	2	1
diced light & dark seasoned	½ lb	313	14	4

FOOD	PORTION	CALS	FAT	SAT FAT
ham thigh meat	1 pkg (8 oz)	291	12	4
ham thigh meat	2 oz	73	3	1
pastrami	1 pkg (8 oz)	320	14	4
pastrami	2 oz	80	4	1
patties battered & fried	1 (3.3 oz)	266	17	–
patties battered & fried	1 (2.3 oz)	181	12	–
patties breaded & fried	1 (3.3 oz)	266	17	–
patties breaded & fried	1 (2.3 oz)	181	12	–
poultry salad sandwich spread	1 oz	238	4	1
poultry salad sandwich spread	1 tbsp	109	2	tr
prebasted breast w/ skin roasted	½ breast (1.9 lbs)	1087	30	8
prebasted breast w/ skin roasted	1 breast (3.8 lbs)	2175	60	17
prebasted thigh w/ skin roasted	1 thigh (11 oz)	494	27	8
roll light & dark meat	1 oz	42	2	1
roll light meat	1 oz	42	2	1
salami cooked	1 pkg (8 oz)	446	31	–
salami cooked	2 oz	111	8	–
turkey loaf breast meat	2 slices (1.5 oz)	47	1	tr
turkey loaf breast meat	1 pkg (6 oz)	187	3	1
turkey sticks battered & fried	1 stick (2.3 oz)	178	11	–
turkey sticks breaded & fried	1 stick (2.3 oz)	178	11	–
Alpine Lace				
Breast Fat Free	2 oz	45	0	0
Boar's Head				
Breast Cracked Pepper Smoked	2 oz	60	1	0
Breast Golden Skin On	2 oz	60	2	1
Breast Golden Skinless	2 oz	60	1	0
Breast Hickory Smoked	2 oz	70	2	1
Breast Low Sodium Skinless	2 oz	60	1	0
Breast Lower Sodium Skin On	2 oz	60	2	1
Breast Maple Glazed Honey Coat	2 oz	70	1	0
Breast Ovengold Skin On	2 oz	60	2	0
Breast Ovengold Skinless	2 oz	60	1	0
Breast Roasted Mesquite Smoked Skinless	2 oz	60	1	0
Breast Roasted Salsalito	2 oz	60	1	0
Pastrami Seasoned	2 oz	60	1	0

FOOD	PORTION	CALS	FAT	SAT FAT
Carl Buddig				
Honey Roasted Turkey Breast	1 pkg (2.5 oz)	120	7	3
Lean Slices Honey Roasted Breast	1 pkg (2.5 oz)	70	1	1
Lean Slices Oven Roasted Breast	1 pkg (2.5 oz)	70	1	1
Lean Slices Smoked Breast	1 pkg (2.5 oz)	70	1	1
Oven Roasted Breast	1 pkg (2.5 oz)	110	7	3
Smoked Breast	1 pkg (2.5 oz)	110	7	3
Turkey Ham	1 pkg (2.5 oz)	100	5	2
Healthy Choice				
Deli-Thin Roasted Breast	6 slices (2 oz)	60	2	1
Deli-Thin Smoked Breast	6 slices (2 oz)	60	2	1
Deli-Thin Turkey Ham	6 slices (2 oz)	60	2	1
Fresh-Trak Honey Roasted & Smoked Breast	1 slice (1 oz)	35	1	0
Fresh-Trak Oven Roasted Breast	1 slice (1 oz)	35	1	0
Honey Roasted & Smoked	1 slice (1 oz)	35	1	0
Oven Roasted Breast	1 slice (1 oz)	35	1	0
Smoked Breast	1 slice (1 oz)	30	1	0
Variety Pack Regular	3 slices (2.2 oz)	70	2	1
Hormel				
Light & Lean 97 Breast Sliced	1 slice (1 oz)	30	1	0
Light & Lean 97 Mesquite Smoked Breast	1 slice (1 oz)	30	1	0
turkey pepperoni	17 slices (1 oz)	80	4	2
Jennie-O				
Turkey Breast Golden Roast	3 oz	100	3	1
Jordan's				
Healthy Trim Fat Free Oven Roasted Breast	1 slice (1 oz)	20	0	0
Healthy Trim Fat Free Oven Roasted Smoked Breast	1 slice (1 oz)	20	0	0
Louis Rich				
Bologna	1 slice (28 g)	50	4	1
Breaded Nuggets	4 (3.2 oz)	260	16	3
Breaded Patties	1 (3 oz)	220	13	3
Breaded Sticks	3 (3 oz)	230	15	3
Breast Skinless Hickory Smoked	2 oz	50	0	0
Breast Skinless Honey Roasted	2 oz	60	0	0
Breast Skinless Oven Roasted	2 oz	50	0	0
Breast Skinless Rotisserie	2 oz	50	0	0

FOOD	PORTION	CALS	FAT	SAT FAT
Breast Slices Hickory Smoked	1 slice (2 oz)	50	0	0
Breast Slices Honey Roasted	1 slice (2 oz)	60	0	0
Breast Slices Oven Roasted	1 slice (2 oz)	50	0	0
Breast Slices Rotisserie	1 slice (2 oz)	50	0	0
Carving Board Hickory Smoked	2 slices (1.6 oz)	40	1	0
Carving Board Oven Roasted Thin	6 slices (2.1 oz)	60	1	0
Carving Board Oven Roasted Traditional	2 slices (1.6 oz)	40	1	0
Carving Board Rotisserie	2 slices (1.6 oz)	40	1	0
Cotto Salami	1 slice (28 g)	40	3	1
Deli-Thin Oven Roasted	4 slices (1.8 oz)	50	1	0
Deli-Thin Smoked	4 slices (1.8 oz)	50	2	1
Fat Free Hickory Smoked Breast	1 slice (1 oz)	25	0	0
Fat Free Oven Roasted Breast	1 slice (1 oz)	25	0	0
Fat Free Oven Roasted Deli-Thin Breast	4 slices (1.8 oz)	45	0	0
Fat Free Turkey Ham Honey	2 slices (1.7 oz)	35	0	0
Fat Free Turkey Ham Smoked	2 slices (1.7 oz)	35	0	0
Hickory Smoked	1 slice (1 oz)	30	1	0
Oven Roasted	1 slice (1 oz)	30	1	0
Pastrami	1 slice (1 oz)	30	1	0
Salami	1 slice (28 g)	40	3	1
Smoked	1 slice (1 oz)	30	1	0
Turkey Ham	1 slice (1 oz)	30	1	0
Turkey Ham Chopped	1 slice (1 oz)	45	3	1
Turkey Ham Honey Cured	1 slice (1 oz)	30	1	0
Mr. Turkey				
Deli Cuts Hardwood Smoked Breast	3 slices	30	1	–
Deli Cuts Honey Roasted Breast	3 slices	30	1	–
Deli Cuts Oven Roasted Breast	3 slices	30	1	–
Deli Cuts Turkey Ham	3 slices	35	2	–
Deli Cuts Turkey Pastrami	3 slices	35	1	–
Hardwood Smoked Breast	1 slice	30	1	–
Hardwood Smoked Turkey Ham	1 slice	35	2	–
Honey Cured Turkey Ham	1 slice	30	1	–
Oven Roasted Breast	1 slice	30	1	–
Smoked Breakfast Turkey Ham	1 oz	30	1	–
Turkey Bologna	1 slice	70	5	–
Turkey Cotto Salami	1 slice	50	4	–
Turkey Ham	1 slice	35	2	–

FOOD	PORTION	CALS	FAT	SAT FAT
Turkey Pastrami	1 slice	30	1	—
Oscar Mayer				
Free Oven Roasted Breast	4 slices (1.8 oz)	40	0	0
Free Smoked Breast	4 slices (1.8 oz)	40	0	0
Lunchables Turkey Bagels	1 pkg	420	10	4
Oven Roasted White	1 slice (1 oz)	30	1	0
Smoked White	1 slice (1 oz)	30	1	0
Perdue				
Breast Sliced Cajun Style	2 oz	50	1	—
Breast Sliced Honey Smoked	2 oz	50	0	—
Breast Sliced Pan Roasted	2 oz	70	2	1
Ham Hickory Smoked	2 oz	60	3	1
Healthsense Breast Sliced Oven Roasted	2 oz	60	0	—
Pastrami Hickory Smoked	2 oz	70	3	1
Sara Lee				
Hardwood Smoked Breast Of Turkey	2 oz	60	1	0
Hardwood Smoked Turkey Ham	2 oz	60	2	1
Honey Roasted Breast Of Turkey	2 oz	60	0	0
Honey Roasted Turkey Ham	2 oz	70	3	1
Mesquite Smoked Breast Of Turkey	2 oz	60	2	1
Oven Roasted Breast Of Turkey	2 oz	60	2	1
Peppered Breast Of Turkey	2 oz	50	0	0
Seasoned Breast Of Turkey Pastrami	2 oz	60	1	0
Shady Brook				
Black Forest Turkey Ham	2 oz	70	3	1
Browned Homestyle Oven Roasted Breast	2 oz	60	1	0
Browned Slow Roasted Breast	2 oz	60	0	0
Carved Breast Italian Seasoned	2 oz	60	0	0
Carved Breast Natural Roast	2 oz	60	0	0
Carved Breast Peppered	2 oz	60	0	0
Hickory Smoked Breast	2 oz	50	0	0
Honey Roasted Breast	2 oz	60	1	0
Honey Roasted Breast Covered w/ Cracked Pepper	2 oz	60	0	0
Meatballs Italian Style	3 (3 oz)	130	7	3
Smoked Drumstick	3 oz	180	8	3
Smoked Neck	3 oz	150	6	2

FOOD	PORTION	CALS	FAT	SAT FAT
Smoked Whole Turkey	3 oz	150	4	2
Smoked Wing	3 oz	200	10	3
Wampler				
Bologna	2 oz	130	11	–
Dark Cured	2 oz	80	5	–
Deli Roast Breast	2 oz	50	1	–
Deli Roast Classic Spiced Breast	2 oz	70	1	–
Deli Roast Pan Roasted Breast	2 oz	70	2	–
Deli Roast Pan Roasted Skinless Breast	2 oz	50	0	–
Deli Roast Peppered Breast	2 oz	40	0	–
Deli Roast Rotisserie Breast	2 oz	50	2	–
Pastrami	2 oz	90	5	–
Salami	2 oz	90	6	–
Turkey Ham	2 oz	60	3	–
TURKEY DISHES				
gravy & turkey	1 pkg (5 oz)	95	4	1
gravy & turkey	1 cup (8.4 oz)	160	6	2
Banquet				
Sandwich Toppers Gravy & Sliced Turkey	1 pkg (5 oz)	160	11	4
Dinty Moore				
Microwave Cup Stew	1 pkg (7.5 oz)	130	3	1
Stew	1 cup (8.5 oz)	140	3	1
Jennie-O				
Stuffed Turkey Breast Pepper Cheese & Rice	1 piece (6 oz)	250	7	4
Turkey Breast Roast In Homestyle Gravy	1 serv (5 oz)	110	1	0
Luigino's				
Gravy Dressing & Turkey	1 pkg (8 oz)	340	15	4
Mosey's				
Turkey Breast w/ Gravy	1 serv (5 oz)	140	1	0
Shady Brook				
Meatloaf	1 serv (16 oz)	470	17	10
Wampler				
Turkey Ham Salad	⅓ cup	150	10	–
TAKE-OUT				
boneless breast w/ cranberry apple stuffing	1 serv (5 oz)	260	9	2

FOOD	PORTION	CALS	FAT	SAT FAT
TURKEY SUBSTITUTES				
Lightlife				
Smart Deli Turkey	3 slices (1.5 oz)	40	0	0
Soy Is Us				
Turkey Not!	½ cup (1.75 oz)	140	2	1
Tofurkey				
Deli Slices Hickory	1.5 oz	120	2	0
Deli Slices Original	1.5 oz	120	2	0
Deli Slices Peppered	1.5 oz	120	2	0
Drummettes	1 (3 oz)	105	2	1
Giblet Gravy	1 serv (3.5 oz)	42	2	0
Stuffed Tofu Roast	1 serv (4 oz)	193	5	0
Worthington				
Smoked Turkey Meatless	3 slices (2 oz)	140	10	2
Turkee Slices	3 slices (3.3 oz)	130	14	3
Yves				
Veggie Turkey Deli Slices	1 serv (2.2 oz)	85	0	0
TURMERIC				
ground	1 tsp	8	tr	—
TURNIPS				
canned greens	½ cup	17	tr	tr
cooked mashed	½ cup (4.2 oz)	47	tr	tr
cubed cooked	½ cup (3 oz)	33	tr	tr
frzn greens cooked	½ cup	24	tr	tr
greens chopped cooked	½ cup	15	tr	tr
greens raw chopped	½ cup	7	tr	tr
raw cubed	½ cup (2.4 oz)	25	tr	tr
Birds Eye				
Greens w/ Diced Turnip	1 cup	25	0	0
TURTLE				
raw	3.5 oz	85	1	—
TUSK FISH				
raw	3.5 oz	79	tr	—
VANILLA				
Steel's				
Sugar Free	1 tbsp	24	0	0

FOOD	PORTION	CALS	FAT	SAT FAT
Virginia Dare				
Extract	1 tsp	10	0	—
VEAL *(see also VEAL DISHES)*				
cutlet lean only braised	3 oz	172	4	2
cutlet lean only fried	3 oz	156	4	1
ground broiled	3 oz	146	6	3
loin chop w/ bone lean & fat braised	1 chop (2.8 oz)	227	14	5
loin chop w/ bone lean only braised	1 chop (2.4 oz)	155	6	2
shoulder w/ bone lean only braised	3 oz	169	5	1
sirloin w/ bone lean & fat roasted	3 oz	171	9	4
sirloin w/ bone lean only roasted	3 oz	143	5	2
VEAL DISHES				
TAKE-OUT				
parmigiana	4.2 oz	279	18	10
scallopini	1 serv (8 oz)	608	146	13
VEGETABLE JUICE				
vegetable juice cocktail	6 fl oz	34	tr	tr
vegetable juice cocktail	½ cup	22	tr	tr
Dole				
Vegetable Blend	1 bottle (12 oz)	90	0	0
Hunt's				
Cocktail	1 can (6 oz)	20	0	0
Muir Glen				
Organic	5.5 oz	50	0	0
V8				
Lightly Tangy	8 oz	58	1	0
Low Sodium	8 oz	53	tr	tr
Original	8 oz	51	1	0
Picante Vegetable	8 oz	51	tr	0
Spicy Hot	8 oz	49	tr	0
Splash Tropical Blend	8 fl oz	120	0	0
VEGETABLES MIXED				
CANNED				
mixed vegetables	½ cup	39	tr	tr
peas & carrots	½ cup	48	tr	tr
peas & carrots low sodium	½ cup	48	tr	tr
peas & onions	½ cup	30	tr	tr
succotash	½ cup	102	1	tr

FOOD	PORTION	CALS	FAT	SAT FAT
Chi-Chi's				
Diced Tomatoes & Green Chilies	¼ cup (2.5 oz)	20	0	0
Chun King				
Chow Mein Vegetables	⅔ cup (3 oz)	14	tr	0
Del Monte				
Mixed	½ cup (4.4 oz)	40	0	0
Mixed No Salt Added	½ cup (4.4 oz)	40	0	0
Peas And Carrots	½ cup (4.5 oz)	60	0	0
Green Giant				
Garden Medley	½ cup (4.2 oz)	40	0	0
Mixed	½ cup (4.3 oz)	60	0	0
Sweet Peas & Carrots	½ cup (4.3 oz)	50	0	0
Sweet Peas & Tiny Pearl Onion	½ cup (4.4 oz)	60	0	0
House Of Tsang				
Vegetables & Sauce Cantonese Classic	½ cup (4.2 oz)	70	1	0
Vegetables & Sauce Hong Kong Sweet & Sour	½ cup (4.5 oz)	160	0	0
Vegetables & Sauce Szechuan Hot & Spicy	½ cup (4.2 oz)	70	1	0
Vegetables & Sauce Tokyo Teriyaki	½ cup (4.4 oz)	100	0	0
La Choy				
Chop Suey Vegetables	½ cup (2.2 oz)	10	tr	0
LeSueur				
Early Peas w/ Mushrooms & Pearl Onions	½ cup (4.3 oz)	60	0	0
S&W				
Mixed	½ cup (4.4 oz)	35	0	0
Peas & Carrots	½ cup (4.5 oz)	60	0	0
Peas & Onions	½ cup (4.3 oz)	40	0	0
Veg-All				
Cajun Mixed	½ cup	50	0	0
FROZEN				
mixed vegetables cooked	½ cup	54	tr	tr
peas & carrots cooked	½ cup	38	tr	tr
peas & onions cooked	½ cup	40	tr	tr
succotash cooked	½ cup	79	1	tr
Birds Eye				
Baby Sweet Peas & Pearl Onions	⅔ cup	60	1	0
Bavarian Vegetables	1 cup (5.5 oz)	150	8	4

FOOD	PORTION	CALS	FAT	SAT FAT
Broccoli Cauliflower & Carrots	½ cup	25	0	0
Broccoli Cauliflower & Carrots In Cheese Sauce	½ cup	70	4	1
Broccoli Cauliflower & Red Peppers	½ cup	20	0	0
Broccoli & Cauliflower	½ cup	20	0	0
Broccoli Carrots & Water Chestnuts	½ cup	30	0	0
Broccoli Corn & Red Peppers	½ cup	50	0	0
Broccoli Red Peppers Onions & Mushrooms	½ cup	25	0	0
Brussels Sprouts Cauliflower & Carrots	½ cup	30	0	0
California Style Vegetables	½ cup	100	5	2
Cauliflower Nuggets Corn Carrots & Snow Peapods	½ cup	30	0	0
Gumbo Blend	¾ cup	40	0	0
Italian Style Vegetables & Bow Tie Pasta	1 cup	150	9	3
Mixed Vegetables	⅓ cup	50	0	0
New England Style Vegetables & Pasta Shells	1 pkg (9 oz)	260	14	5
Oriental Style Vegetables	½ cup	60	4	2
Peas & Pearl Onions	⅔ cup	90	1	0
Peas & Potatoes In Real Cream Sauce	½ cup	90	3	1
Radiatore Pasta & Vegetables	1 cup	200	8	2
Roasted Potatoes & Broccoli	⅔ cup (3.9 oz)	100	4	1
Roletti Pasta & Vegetables	1 cup (4.4 oz)	190	8	2
Simply Grillin' Garden Herb	1 cup	140	6	1
Stir Fry Asparagus	2 cups	90	1	0
Stir Fry Broccoli	1 cup	30	0	0
Stir Fry Pepper	1 cup	25	0	0
Stir Fry Sugar Snap	¾ cup	35	0	0
Stir Fry Whole Green Bean	1¾ cups	100	1	0
Stir Fry Style Vegetables	½ cup	60	4	2
Vegetables For Soup	⅔ cup	45	0	0
Vegetables For Stew	⅔ cup	40	0	0
Voila! Italian Pesto Chicken	2 cups	240	9	3
Voila! Three Cheese Chicken	1¾ cups	220	8	3
Fresh Like				
California Blend	3.5 oz	31	tr	–
Midwestern Blend	3.5 oz	42	tr	–

FOOD	PORTION	CALS	FAT	SAT FAT
Mixed	3.5 oz	69	tr	—
Oriental Blend	3.5 oz	26	tr	—
Winter Blend	3.5 oz	26	tr	—
Green Giant				
Alfredo Vegetables	¾ cup	70	2	1
American Mixtures Broccoli Carrots Cauliflower	¾ cup (2.6 oz)	25	0	0
American Mixtures Broccoli Carrots Waterchestnuts	¾ cup (3 oz)	30	0	0
American Mixtures Carrots Green Bean Cauliflower	¾ cup (2.7 oz)	25	0	0
American Mixtures Cauliflower Broccoli Sugar Snap & Sweet Pea	¾ cup (2.8 oz)	35	0	0
American Mixtures Corn Broccoli Red Pepper	¾ cup (3.1 oz)	60	0	0
American Mixtures Green Beans Potatoes Onions Red Peppers	¾ cup (2.8 oz)	45	1	0
American Mixtures Sweet Peas Potatoes Carrots	⅔ cup (3 oz)	70	2	0
Butter Sauce Broccoli Cauliflower Carrots Corn Sweet Peas	¾ cup (3.6 oz)	60	2	2
Butter Sauce Broccoli Pasta Sweet Peas Corn Red Peppers	¾ cup (3.5 oz)	70	2	2
Butter Sauce Mixed	¾ cup (3.6 oz)	70	2	1
Cheese Sauce Broccoli Cauliflower Carrots	1 cup (4.1 oz)	60	3	1
Harvest Fresh Broccoli Cauliflower Carrots	1 cup (3.4 oz)	30	0	0
Harvest Fresh Mixed Vegetables	⅔ cup (3.1 oz)	50	0	0
Harvest Fresh Sweet Peas & Pearl Onions	½ cup (2.7 oz)	55	0	0
Mixed	¾ cup (2.9 oz)	50	0	0
Select Sweet Peas & Pearl Onions	⅔ cup (3.1 oz)	60	0	0
Health Is Wealth				
Veggie Munchees	2 (1 oz)	50	1	0
La Choy				
Fancy Chinese Mixed Vegetables	½ cup (2.9 oz)	9	tr	0
McKenzie's				
Gumbo Mixture	1 serv (2.9 oz)	35	0	0

FOOD	PORTION	CALS	FAT	SAT FAT
Soglowek				
Golden Vegetarian Nuggets	4 pieces (2.5 oz)	190	11	2
Tree Of Life				
Mixed	½ cup (3 oz)	65	0	0
SHELF-STABLE				
TastyBite				
Curry Bangkok Red	½ pkg (5.3 oz)	88	6	5
Curry Patong Yellow	½ pkg (5.3 oz)	118	7	6
Curry Siam Green	½ pkg (5.3 oz)	63	3	3
Jaipur Vegetables	½ pkg (5 oz)	220	15	4
Malabar Mixed	½ pkg (5 oz)	67	1	1
TAKE-OUT				
buddha's delight	1 serv (16 oz)	174	5	1
caponata	¼ cup	28	1	—
curry	1 serv (7.7 oz)	398	33	—
gyoza potstickers vegetable	8 (4.9 oz)	210	4	1
pakoras	1 (2 oz)	108	5	—
ratatouille	1 serv (3.5 oz)	96	7	1
samosa	2 (4 oz)	519	46	—
succotash	½ cup	111	1	tr
tapenade grilled vegetables	¼ cup	40	3	0
VENISON				
roasted	3 oz	134	3	1
VINEGAR				
balsamic	1 tbsp (0.5 oz)	5	0	0
cider	1 tbsp	tr	0	0
Eden				
Organic Brown Rice	1 tbsp	2	0	0
Ume Plum	1 tsp	2	0	0
Progresso				
Balsamic	2 tbsp (0.5 oz)	10	0	0
Victoria				
Balsamic	1 tbsp (0.5 oz)	5	0	0
White House				
Apple Cider	1 tbsp (0.5 oz)	0	0	0
White	1 tbsp (0.5 oz)	0	0	0
Wild Thyme Farms				
Balsamic Red Raspberry	1 tbsp	13	0	0

FOOD	PORTION	CALS	FAT	SAT FAT
WAFFLES				
FROZEN				
buttermilk	1 4 in sq (1.2 oz)	88	3	tr
plain	1 4 in sq (1.2 oz)	88	3	tr
Aunt Jemima				
Blueberry	2 (2.5 oz)	190	7	2
Buttermilk	2 (2.5 oz)	170	6	2
Cinnamon	2 (2.5 oz)	180	6	2
Oatmeal	2 (2.5 oz)	170	7	1
Whole Grain	2 (2.5 oz)	170	7	1
Belgian Chef				
Belgian	2 (2.5 oz)	140	3	1
Eggo				
Apple Cinnamon	2 (2.7 oz)	220	8	2
Banana Bread	2 (2.7 oz)	200	7	1
Blueberry	2 (2.7 oz)	220	9	2
Buttermilk	2 (2.7 oz)	220	8	2
Golden Oat	2 (2.7 oz)	150	3	1
Homestyle	2 (2.7 oz)	220	8	2
Minis Cinnamon Toast	12 (3.2 oz)	290	10	2
Minis Cinnamon Toast	12 (3.2 oz)	280	9	2
Minis Homestyle	12 (3.3 oz)	260	9	2
Nut & Honey	2 (2.7 oz)	240	10	2
Nutri-Grain	2 (2.7 oz)	190	6	1
Nutri-Grain Multi-Bran	2 (2.7 oz)	180	6	1
Nutri-Grain Raisin & Bran	2 (2.9 oz)	210	6	1
Special K	2 (2 oz)	120	0	0
Strawberry	2 (2.7 oz)	220	8	2
Kellogg's				
Homestyle Low Fat	2 (2.7 oz)	180	3	1
Nutri-Grain Low Fat	2 (2.7 oz)	160	3	0
Nutri-Grain Low Fat Blueberry	2 (2.7 oz)	160	2	0
Kid Cuisine				
Wave Rider Waffle Sticks	1 meal (6.6 oz)	380	8	2
Van's				
7 Grain Belgian	2	152	4	0
Belgian Original	2	145	4	0
Belgian Original Toaster	2	145	4	0
Blueberry Toaster	2	157	4	0
Blueberry Wheat Free Toaster	2	225	5	1

FOOD	PORTION	CALS	FAT	SAT FAT
Fat Free	2	155	2	0
Mini	4	107	4	0
Multigrain Toaster	2	160	4	0
Organic Whole Wheat	2	190	5	0
Organic Whole Wheat Blueberry	2	190	5	0
Wheat Free Cinnamon Apple Toaster	2	220	5	1
Wheat Free Toaster	2	220	5	1
MIX				
plain as prep	1 7 in diam (2.6 oz)	218	10	2
READY-TO-EAT				
Gol D Lite				
Low Carb Belgian	1 (0.9 oz)	100	5	0
Low Carb Belgian Chocolate Covered	1 (l.1 oz)	130	8	0
Kashi				
GoLean Blueberry	2	170	3	0
GoLean Original	2	170	3	0
Thomas'				
Buttermilk	1 (1.6 oz)	130	5	1
Homestyle	1 (1.6 oz)	140	5	1
TAKE-OUT				
plain	1 (7 in diam)	218	11	2
WALNUTS				
black dried chopped	1 cup	759	71	5
english dried	1 oz	182	18	2
english dried chopped	1 cup	770	74	7
halves	14 (1 oz)	190	19	2
Planters				
Black	1 pkg (2 oz)	340	31	2
Gold Measure Halves	1 pkg (2 oz)	380	38	4
Halves	⅓ cup (1.2 oz)	220	22	3
Pieces	¼ cup (1 oz)	190	20	2
Sweet Delights				
Walnut Roasters	⅓ pkg (1 oz)	210	20	2
WASABI (see HORSERADISH)				
WATER				
ice cubes	3	0	0	0
tap water	8 oz	0	0	0

FOOD	PORTION	CALS	FAT	SAT FAT
Absopure				
Natural Spring	8 fl oz	0	0	0
Aquafina				
Essentials B-Power Wild Berry	8 fl oz	40	0	0
Essentials Calcium + Tangerine Pineapple	8 fl oz	40	0	0
Essentials Daily C Citrus	8 fl oz	40	0	0
Essentials Multi-V Watermelon	8 fl oz	40	0	0
Water	8 fl oz	0	0	0
Aquess				
Purified Water w/ Soluble Fiber	1 bottle (18 oz)	30	0	0
Bong Water				
Chronic Tonic	12 oz	144	0	0
Cottonmouth Quencher	12 oz	165	0	0
Green Dreams	12 oz	165	0	0
Purple Haze	12 oz	165	0	0
Castellina				
Sparking Spring	8 fl oz	0	0	0
Crystal Geyser				
Spring Water	8 fl oz	0	0	0
Dasani				
Purified Water	8 oz	0	0	0
Evamor				
Artesian Water	8 fl oz	0	0	0
Evian				
Spring Water	1 bottle (11.5 oz)	0	0	0
Ferrarelle				
Sparkling	8 fl oz	0	0	0
Gerolsteiner				
Sparkling Mineral	8 fl oz	0	0	0
Glaceau				
Smartwater	8 oz	0	0	0
Vitamin Water Tropical Citrus	1 cup (8 oz)	40	0	0
Glacier Springs				
Drinking Water	8 fl oz	0	0	0
Hansen's				
Energy Water Lemon	8 oz	10	0	0
Iceland Spring				
Spring Water	1 liter	0	0	0

FOOD	PORTION	CALS	FAT	SAT FAT
LaCroix				
Spring	1 bottle (12 oz)	0	0	0
Meridian				
Clear All Flavors	8 oz	100	0	0
Mt Shasta				
Natural Spring	1 bottle (20 oz)	0	0	0
Propel				
Fitness Water Berry	8 fl oz	10	0	0
Fitness Water Black Cherry	8 fl oz	10	0	0
Reebok				
Fitness Water Berry	1 bottle (24 oz)	30	0	0
Fitness Water Natural	1 bottle (24 oz)	0	0	0
Replenish				
Elements Enhanced Water Orange	8 oz	40	0	0
San Pellegrino				
Acqua Panna	8 fl oz	0	0	0
Mineral Water	1 liter (33.8 oz)	0	0	0
Saratoga				
Spring	8 oz	0	0	0
Snapple				
Natural Spring	8 fl oz	0	0	0
Spa				
Mineral Water Reine	1 bottle (17.5 oz)	0	0	0
Ty Nant				
Mineral Water	1 liter	0	0	0
Vasa				
Natural Spring	8 oz	0	0	0
Veryfine				
Fruit$_2$0 Lemon	8 fl oz	0	0	0
Fruit$_2$0 Lemon Lime	8 fl oz	0	0	0
Fruit$_2$0 Orange	8 fl oz	0	0	0
Fruit$_2$0 Raspberry	8 fl oz	0	0	0
Vittel				
Mineral Water	1 bottle (18 oz)	0	0	0
Volvic				
Spring Water	8 oz	0	0	0
Water Joe				
Caffeine Enhanced	8 fl oz	0	0	0

FOOD	PORTION	CALS	FAT	SAT FAT
WATER CHESTNUTS				
chinese sliced canned	½ cup	35	tr	–
fresh sliced	½ cup	66	tr	–
Chun King				
Sliced	2 tbsp (0.8 oz)	11	tr	0
Whole	2 (0.7 oz)	10	tr	0
La Choy				
Chopped	2 tbsp (0.6 oz)	9	tr	0
Sliced	2 tbsp (0.8 oz)	11	tr	0
Whole	2 (0.7 oz)	10	tr	0
WATERCRESS				
fresh chopped	½ cup	2	tr	tr
garden fresh	½ cup	8	tr	tr
garden fresh cooked	½ cup	16	tr	tr
WATERMELON				
cut up	1 cup	50	1	–
seeds dried	1 oz	158	13	3
seeds dried	1 cup	602	51	3
wedge	⅟₁₆	152	2	–
WATERMELON JUICE				
Kool-Aid				
Splash Drink	1 serv (8 oz)	110	0	0
Squeezit				
Watermelon	1 bottle (7 oz)	110	0	0
WAX BEANS				
CANNED				
Del Monte				
Cut Golden	½ cup (4.2 oz)	20	0	0
S&W				
Cut	½ cup (4.2 oz)	20	0	0
WHALE				
raw	3.5 oz	134	3	–
WHEAT				
sprouted	1 cup (3.8 oz)	214	1	tr
starch	3.5 oz	348	tr	–
Bob's Red Mill				
Vital Wheat Gluten	¼ cup	120	1	–

FOOD	PORTION	CALS	FAT	SAT FAT
Lightlife				
Savory Seitan Barbecue	4 oz	160	2	1
Savory Seitan Teriyaki	4 oz	160	2	1
Near East				
Taboule Salad Mix as prep	⅔ cup	120	3	1
Wheat Pilaf as prep	1 cup	220	5	1
Sonoma				
Wheat Nuts Salted	2 tbsp (0.5 oz)	60	3	0
WHEAT GERM				
plain toasted	¼ cup (1 oz)	108	3	1
plain toasted	1 cup	431	12	2
w/ brown sugar & honey toasted	1 oz	107	2	tr
w/ brown sugar & honey toasted	1 cup	426	9	2
Hodgson Mill				
Untoasted	2 tbsp	55	1	0
Kretschmer				
Original Toasted	2 tbsp (0.5 oz)	50	1	0
Stone-Buhr				
Untoasted	2 tbsp (0.5 oz)	58	2	0
WHEY				
acid dry	1 tbsp (3 g)	10	tr	tr
acid fluid	1 cup (8 fl oz)	59	tr	tr
sweet dry	1 tbsp (8 g)	26	tr	tr
sweet fluid	1 cup (8 fl oz)	66	1	1
whey cheese	1 oz	126	8	5
WHIPPED TOPPINGS				
cream pressurized	1 cup (2.1 oz)	154	13	8
cream pressurized	1 tbsp (3 g)	8	tr	tr
nondairy frzn	1 tbsp	13	1	1
nondairy powdered as prep w/ whole milk	1 cup	151	10	9
nondairy powdered as prep w/ whole milk	1 tbsp (4 g)	8	tr	tr
nondairy pressurized	1 tbsp (4 g)	11	1	1
nondairy pressurized	1 cup	184	16	13
Cool Whip				
Extra Creamy	2 tbsp (0.3 oz)	25	2	2
Free	2 tbsp (0.3 oz)	15	0	0

FOOD	PORTION	CALS	FAT	SAT FAT
Lite	2 tbsp (0.3 oz)	20	1	1
Original	2 tbsp (0.3 oz)	25	2	2
Dream Whip				
Mix as prep	2 tbsp (0.3 oz)	20	1	1
Estee				
Whipped Topping	1 serv	10	1	0
Hood				
Instant	2 tbsp	20	2	1
Light Instant	2 tbsp	15	1	0
Kraft				
Dairy Whip Light Cream	2 tbsp (0.2 oz)	10	1	1
Fat Free	1 tbsp (0.3 oz)	15	0	0
Reddiwip				
Lite	2 tbsp (8 g)	15	1	0
Non-Dairy	2 tbsp (8 g)	20	2	1
Real Whipped Heavy Cream	2 tbsp (8 g)	30	3	2
Real Whipped Light Cream	2 tbsp (8 g)	20	2	1
WHITE BEANS				
canned	1 cup	306	1	tr
dried regular cooked	1 cup	249	1	tr
dried small cooked	1 cup	253	1	tr
Progresso				
Cannellini	½ cup (4.6 oz)	100	1	0
WHITEFISH				
baked	3 oz	146	6	1
smoked	1 oz	39	tr	tr
smoked	3 oz	92	1	tr
WHITING				
cooked	3 oz	98	1	tr
raw	3 oz	77	1	tr
WILD RICE				
cooked	1 cup (5.7 oz)	166	1	tr
Gourmet House				
Cracked not prep	¼ cup	170	0	0
Hand Harvested not prep	¼ cup	170	0	0
Quick Cooking not prep	½ cup	170	0	0
White & Wild not prep	¼ cup	170	0	0
Wild & Rice Garden Blend not prep	¼ cup	190	1	0

FOOD	PORTION	CALS	FAT	SAT FAT
Haddon House				
Extra Fancy	¼ cup (1.6 oz)	170	1	0
WINE				
haiku	1 serv	93	0	0
japanese plum	3 oz	139	tr	—
japanese sake	1 oz	33	0	0
kir	1 serv	78	0	0
madeira	3.5 oz	169	0	—
port	3.5 oz	156	0	—
red	1 serv (3.5 oz)	74	0	0
rose	1 serv (3.5 oz)	73	0	0
sake screwdriver	1 serv	175	tr	tr
sangria	1 serv	88	tr	0
sangria blanco	1 serv	155	tr	tr
sherry	2 oz	84	0	0
sweet dessert	1 serv (3.5 oz)	158	0	0
vermouth dry	3½ oz	105	0	0
vermouth sweet	3½ oz	167	0	0
wassail wine	1 serv	142	tr	tr
white	1 serv (3.5 oz)	70	0	0
wine cooler	1 serv	218	tr	tr
wine spritzer	1 serv	60	0	0
Boone's				
Country Kwencher	4 fl oz	96	0	0
Delicious Apple	4 fl oz	84	0	0
Sangria	4 fl oz	88	0	0
Snow Creek Berry	4 fl oz	72	0	0
Strawberry Hill	4 fl oz	88	0	0
Sun Peak Peach	4 fl oz	72	0	0
Wild Island	4 fl oz	72	0	0
Carlo Rossi				
Blush	4 fl oz	84	0	0
Burgundy	4 fl oz	88	0	0
Chablis	4 fl oz	84	0	0
Paisano	4 fl oz	92	0	0
Red Sangria	4 fl oz	92	0	0
Rhine	4 fl oz	84	0	0
Vin Rose'	4 fl oz	84	0	0
White Grenache	4 fl oz	80	0	0

FOOD	PORTION	CALS	FAT	SAT FAT
Eden				
Mirin Rice Cooking Wine	1 tbsp	25	0	0
Fairbanks				
Cream Sherry	4 fl oz	168	0	0
Port	4 fl oz	176	0	0
Sherry	4 fl oz	136	0	0
White Port	4 fl oz	136	0	0
Gallo				
Blush Chablis	4 fl oz	88	0	0
Burgundy	4 fl oz	88	0	0
Cabernet Sauvignon	4 fl oz	88	0	0
Chablis Blanc	4 fl oz	80	0	0
Chardonnay	4 fl oz	92	0	0
Classic Burgundy	4 fl oz	84	0	0
French Colombard	4 fl oz	84	0	0
Hearty Burgundy	4 fl oz	88	0	0
Pink Chablis	4 fl oz	80	0	0
Red Rose'	4 fl oz	92	0	0
Rhine	4 fl oz	88	0	0
Sheffield Cellars				
Sherry	4 fl oz	136	0	0
Tawny Port	4 fl oz	180	0	0
Vermouth Extra Dry	1 fl oz	28	0	0
Vermouth Sweet	1 fl oz	43	0	0
Very Dry Sherry	4 fl oz	128	0	0
WINGED BEANS				
dried cooked	1 cup	252	10	1
WOLFFISH				
atlantic baked	3 oz	105	3	tr
WRAPS (see BREAD)				
XANTHAN GUM				
Bob's Red Mill				
Xanthan Gum	1 tbsp	8	0	0
YAM (see also SWEET POTATO)				
CANNED				
S&W				
Candied	½ cup (4.9 oz)	170	0	0

FOOD	PORTION	CALS	FAT	SAT FAT
FRESH				
mountain yam hawaii cooked	½ cup	59	tr	tr
yam cubed cooked	½ cup	79	tr	tr
YAMBEAN				
cooked	¾ cup	38	tr	–
YARDLONG BEANS				
dried cooked	1 cup	202	1	tr
YAUTIA (TANNIER)				
fresh sliced	1 cup (4.7 oz)	132	1	–
root raw	1 (10.7 oz)	299	1	–
YEAST				
baker's compressed	1 cake (0.6 oz)	18	tr	tr
baker's dry	1 pkg (¼ oz)	21	tr	tr
baker's dry	1 tbsp	35	1	tr
brewer's dry	1 tbsp	25	tr	tr
Fleischmann's				
Active Dry	1 pkg (7 g)	23	3	–
Bread Machine	1 pkg (7 g)	26	2	–
RapidRise	1 pkg (7 g)	26	2	–
Hodgson Mill				
Fast Rise	1 tsp (9 g)	25	0	0
YELLOW BEANS				
canned	½ cup	13	tr	tr
canned low sodium	½ cup	13	tr	tr
dried cooked	1 cup	254	2	tr
fresh cooked	½ cup	22	tr	tr
fresh raw	½ cup	17	tr	tr
frozen cooked	½ cup	18	tr	tr
YELLOWEYE BEANS				
CANNED				
B&M				
Baked	½ cup (4.6 oz)	170	2	1
YELLOWTAIL				
baked	3 oz	159	6	–
YOGURT (see also YOGURT DRINKS, YOGURT FROZEN)				
coffee lowfat	8 oz	194	3	2

FOOD	PORTION	CALS	FAT	SAT FAT
fruit lowfat	4 oz	113	1	1
fruit lowfat	8 oz	225	3	2
plain	8 oz	139	7	5
plain lowfat	8 oz	144	4	2
plain no fat	8 oz	127	tr	tr
vanilla lowfat	8 oz	194	3	2
Breyers				
Blended Blueberry	4.4 oz	130	1	1
Blended Peach	4.4 oz	130	1	1
Blended Strawberry	4.4 oz	130	1	1
Light Nonfat Apple Pie A La Mode	8 oz	120	0	0
Light Nonfat Berry Banana Split	8 oz	120	0	0
Light Nonfat Black Cherry Jubilee	8 oz	120	0	0
Light Nonfat Blueberries N' Cream	8 oz	120	0	0
Light Nonfat Cherry Bon-Bon	8 oz	120	0	0
Light Nonfat Cherry Vanilla Cream	8 oz	120	0	0
Light Nonfat Classic Strawberry	8 oz	120	0	0
Light Nonfat Key Lime Pie	8 oz	120	0	0
Light Nonfat Lemon Chiffon	8 oz	120	0	0
Light Nonfat Peaches N' Cream	8 oz	120	0	0
Light Nonfat Raspberries N' Cream	8 oz	120	0	0
Light Nonfat Strawberry Cheesecake	8 oz	120	0	0
Lowfat Black Cherry	8 oz	240	3	2
Lowfat Blueberry	8 oz	230	3	2
Lowfat Mixed Berry	8 oz	320	3	2
Lowfat Peach	8 oz	240	3	2
Lowfat Pineapple	8 oz	240	3	2
Lowfat Red Raspberry	8 oz	230	3	2
Lowfat Strawberry	8 oz	230	3	2
Lowfat Strawberry Banana	8 oz	240	3	2
Smooth & Creamy Apple Cobbler	8 oz	230	2	1
Smooth & Creamy Black Cherry Parfait	8 oz	240	2	1
Smooth & Creamy Black Cherry Parfait	4.4 oz	130	1	1
Smooth & Creamy Blueberries 'N Cream	8 oz	240	2	1
Smooth & Creamy Blueberries 'N Cream	4.4 oz	130	1	1
Smooth & Creamy Classic Strawberry	8 oz	230	2	1

FOOD	PORTION	CALS	FAT	SAT FAT
Smooth & Creamy Classic Strawberry	4.4 oz	130	1	1
Smooth & Creamy Orange Vanilla Cream	8 oz	230	2	1
Smooth & Creamy Peaches 'N Cream	8 oz	230	2	1
Smooth & Creamy Peaches 'N Cream	4.4 oz	130	1	1
Smooth & Creamy Raspberries 'N Cream	8 oz	230	2	1
Smooth & Creamy Strawberry Banana Split	8 oz	240	2	1
Smooth & Creamy Strawberry Cheesecake	8 oz	240	2	1
Vanilla 98% Fat Free	½ cup	90	2	1
Cabot				
Non Fat	8 oz	100	0	0
Non Fat Berry Banana	8 oz	130	0	0
Non Fat Blueberry	8 oz	130	0	0
Non Fat Lemon	8 oz	130	0	0
Non Fat Raspberry	8 oz	130	0	0
Non Fat Very Berry	8 oz	130	0	0
Colombo				
Fat Free Plain	8 oz	100	0	0
Fat Free Vanilla	8 oz	160	0	0
French Vanilla	8 oz	180	2	2
Fruit On The Bottom Strawberry Banana	8 oz	230	2	2
Lowfat Plain	8 oz	130	3	2
Multipack Blended All Flavors	4 oz	110	1	1
Strawberry	8 oz	190	3	2
Dannon				
Chunky Fruit Nonfat Apple Cinnamon	6 oz	160	0	0
Chunky Fruit Nonfat Blueberry	6 oz	160	0	0
Chunky Fruit Nonfat Cherry Vanilla	6 oz	160	0	0
Chunky Fruit Nonfat Peach	6 oz	160	0	0
Chunky Fruit Nonfat Strawberry	6 oz	160	0	0
Chunky Fruit Nonfat Strawberry Banana	6 oz	160	0	0
Daniamls Lowfat Tropical Punch	4.4 oz	130	1	1
Danimals Lowfat Blueberry	4.4 oz	130	1	1
Danimals Lowfat Grape Lemonade	4.4 oz	120	1	1
Danimals Lowfat Lemon Ice	4.4 oz	120	1	1

FOOD	PORTION	CALS	FAT	SAT FAT
Danimals Lowfat Orange Banana	4.4 oz	130	1	1
Danimals Lowfat Strawberry	4.4 oz	130	1	1
Danimals Lowfat Vanilla	4.4 oz	120	1	1
Danimals Lowfat Wild Raspberry	4.4 oz	120	1	1
Double Delights Banana Creme Strawberry	6 oz	160	1	1
Double Delights Bavarian Creme Raspberry	6 oz	170	1	1
Double Delights Cheesecake Cherry	6 oz	170	1	1
Double Delights Cheesecake Strawberry	6 oz	170	1	1
Double Delights Chocolate Cheesecake	6 oz	220	1	1
Double Delights Chocolate Dipped Strawberry	6 oz	210	1	1
Double Delights Chocolate Eclair	6 oz	220	1	1
Double Delights Vanilla Strawberry	6 oz	170	1	1
Double Delights Vanilla Peach & Apricot	6 oz	170	1	1
Fruit On The Bottom Lowfat Apple Cinnamon	8 oz	240	3	2
Fruit On The Bottom Lowfat Blueberry	8 oz	240	3	2
Fruit On The Bottom Lowfat Boysenberry	8 oz	240	3	2
Fruit On The Bottom Lowfat Cherry	8 oz	240	3	2
Fruit On The Bottom Lowfat Minipack Mixed Berry	4.4 oz	130	2	1
Fruit On The Bottom Lowfat Minipack Strawberry	4.4 oz	130	2	1
Fruit On The Bottom Lowfat Mixed Berries	8 oz	240	3	2
Fruit On The Bottom Lowfat Orange	8 oz	240	3	2
Fruit On The Bottom Lowfat Peach	8 oz	240	3	2
Fruit On The Bottom Lowfat Raspberry	8 oz	240	3	2
Fruit On The Bottom Lowfat Strawberry	8 oz	240	3	2
Fruit On The Bottom Lowfat Strawberry Banana	8 oz	240	3	2

FOOD	PORTION	CALS	FAT	SAT FAT
La Creme Mousse French Vanilla	1 pkg (2.6 oz)	120	5	4
La Creme Vanilla	1 pkg (4.4 oz)	140	5	3
Light 'N Crunchy Mint Chocolate Chip	8 oz	140	0	0
Light 'N Crunchy Nonfat Caramel Apple Crunch	8 oz	140	0	0
Light 'N Crunchy Nonfat Lemon Blueberry Cobbler	8 oz	140	0	0
Light 'N Crunchy Nonfat Mocha Cappuccino	8 oz	140	0	0
Light 'N Crunchy Nonfat Raspberry w/ Granola	8 oz	140	0	0
Light 'N Crunchy Nonfat Vanilla Chocolate Crunch	8 oz	130	0	0
Light Duets Cherry Cheesecake	6 oz	90	0	0
Light Duets Peaches N' Cream	6 oz	90	0	0
Light Duets Raspberry Royale	6 oz	90	0	0
Light Duets Strawberry Cheesecake	6 oz	90	0	0
Light Nonfat Banana Cream Pie	8 oz	100	0	0
Light Nonfat Blueberry	8 oz	100	0	0
Light Nonfat Cappuccino	8 oz	100	0	0
Light Nonfat Cherry Vanilla	8 oz	100	0	0
Light Nonfat Coconut Cream Pie	8 oz	100	0	0
Light Nonfat Creme Caramel	8 oz	100	0	0
Light Nonfat Lemon Chiffon	8 oz	100	0	0
Light Nonfat Mint Chocolate Cream Pie	8 oz	100	0	0
Light Nonfat Peach	8 oz	100	0	0
Light Nonfat Raspberry	8 oz	100	0	0
Light Nonfat Strawberry	8 oz	100	0	0
Light Nonfat Strawberry Banana	8 oz	100	0	0
Light Nonfat Strawberry Kiwi	8 oz	100	0	0
Light Nonfat Tangerine Chiffon	8 oz	100	0	0
Light Nonfat Vanilla	8 oz	100	0	0
Lowfat Coffee	8 oz	210	3	2
Lowfat Cranberry Raspberry	8 oz	210	3	2
Lowfat Lemon	8 oz	210	3	2
Lowfat Vanilla	8 oz	210	3	2
Minipack Blended Nonfat Blueberry	4.4 oz	120	0	0
Minipack Blended Nonfat Cherry	4.4 oz	110	0	0

FOOD	PORTION	CALS	FAT	SAT FAT
Minipack Blended Nonfat Peach	4.4 oz	120	0	0
Minipack Blended Nonfat Raspberry	4.4 oz	120	0	0
Minipack Blended Nonfat Strawberry	4.4 oz	120	0	0
Minipack Blended Nonfat Strawberry Banana	4.4 oz	120	0	0
Sprinkl'ins Cherry Vanilla	1 (4.1 oz)	130	2	1
Sprinkl'ins Strawberry	1 (4.1 oz)	130	2	1
Sprinkl'ins Strawberry Banana	1 (4.1 oz)	130	2	1
Sprinkl'ins Vanilla w/ Cherry Crystals	1 (4.1 oz)	110	1	1
Sprinkl'ins Vanilla w/ Orange Crystals	1 (4.1 oz)	110	1	1
Hood				
Fat Free Blueberry	1 (8 oz)	190	0	0
Fat Free Cherry	1 (8 oz)	190	0	0
Fat Free Peach	1 (8 oz)	190	0	0
Fat Free Plain	1 (8 oz)	130	0	0
Fat Free Raspberry	1 (8 oz)	190	0	0
Fat Free Strawberry	1 (8 oz)	190	0	0
Fat Free Strawberry Banana	1 (8 oz)	190	0	0
Fat Free Vanilla	1 (8 oz)	190	0	0
Fat Free Swiss Blueberry	1 (8 oz)	210	0	0
Fat Free Swiss Lemon	1 (8 oz)	210	0	0
Fat Free Swiss Raspberry	1 (8 oz)	210	0	0
Fat Free Swiss Strawberry	1 (8 oz)	210	0	0
Fat Free Swiss Strawberry Banana	1 (8 oz)	210	0	0
Fat Free Swiss Vanilla	1 (8 oz)	210	0	0
Horizon Organic				
Fat Free Apricot Mango	¾ cup (6 oz)	120	0	0
Fat Free Honey	1 cup (8 oz)	160	0	0
Jell-O				
Lowfat Cherry	4.4 oz	130	1	1
Lowfat Grape	4.4 oz	130	1	1
Lowfat Raspberry	4.4 oz	130	1	1
Lowfat Tropical Berry Twist	4.4 oz	130	1	1
Lowfat Tropical Punch	4.4 oz	130	1	1
Lowfat Watermelon	4.4 oz	130	1	1
Lowfat Wild Berry	4.4 oz	130	1	1
Lowfat Wild Strawberry	4.4 oz	130	1	1
La Yogurt				
French Style Banana	6 oz	180	3	2
French Style Blueberry	6 oz	180	3	2

FOOD	PORTION	CALS	FAT	SAT FAT
French Style Cherry	6 oz	180	3	2
French Style Cherry Vanilla	6 oz	190	3	2
French Style Guava	6 oz	180	3	2
French Style Key Lime	6 oz	180	3	2
French Style Mango	6 oz	180	3	2
French Style Mixed Berry	6 oz	180	3	2
French Style Nonfat Blueberry	6 oz	70	0	0
French Style Nonfat Cherry	6 oz	75	0	0
French Style Nonfat Raspberry	6 oz	70	0	0
French Style Nonfat Strawberry	6 oz	70	0	0
French Style Nonfat Strawberry Banana	6 oz	70	0	0
French Style Peach	6 oz	180	3	2
French Style Pina Colada	6 oz	180	3	2
French Style Raspberry	6 oz	180	3	2
French Style Strawberry	6 oz	180	3	2
French Style Strawberry Banana	6 oz	180	3	2
French Style Strawberry Fruit Cup	6 oz	180	3	2
French Style Tropical Orange	6 oz	180	4	2
French Style Vanilla	6 oz	170	3	2
Latin Style Banana	6 oz	190	3	2
Latin Style Guava	6 oz	190	3	2
Latin Style Mango	6 oz	190	3	2
Latin Style Papaya	6 oz	190	3	2
Latin Style Passion Fruit	6 oz	190	3	2
Latin Style Strawberry Kiwi	6 oz	180	3	2
Light N'Lively				
Free Blueberry	4.4 oz	70	0	0
Free Peach	4.4 oz	70	0	0
Free Strawberry	4.4 oz	70	0	0
Free Strawberry Banana Cream	4.4 oz	70	0	0
Free Strawberry Fruit Cup	4.4 oz	70	0	0
Lowfat Blueberry	4.4 oz	130	1	1
Lowfat Peach	4.4 oz	130	1	1
Lowfat Pineapple	4.4 oz	130	1	1
Lowfat Red Raspberry	4.4 oz	120	1	1
Lowfat Strawberry	4.4 oz	130	1	1
Lowfat Strawberry Banana Cream	4.4 oz	130	1	1
Lowfat Strawberry Fruit Cup	4.4 oz	130	1	1

FOOD	PORTION	CALS	FAT	SAT FAT
Oberweis				
Peach	1 pkg (8 oz)	210	3	2
Pascual				
Nonfat Cherries & Berries	1 pkg (4.4 oz)	100	0	0
Nonfat Peach	1 pkg (4.4 oz)	100	0	0
Silk				
Organic Soy Strawberry	1 pkg (6 oz)	160	2	0
Soy Apricot Mango	1 pkg	160	2	0
Soy Banana Strawberry	1 pkg	160	2	0
Soy Black Cherry	1 pkg	160	2	0
Soy Blueberry	1 pkg	160	2	0
Soy Key Lime	1 pkg	170	2	0
Soy Lemon	1 pkg	160	2	0
Soy Lemon Kiwi	1 pkg	150	2	0
Soy Peach	1 pkg	170	2	0
Soy Plain	8 oz	120	3	0
Soy Raspberry	1 pkg	160	2	0
Soy Vanilla	1 pkg (8 oz)	120	2	0
Stonyfield Farm				
Creamy Maple	1 pkg	160	6	4
Mocho-Ccino	1 pkg	170	6	4
Nonfat Apricot Mango	1 pkg (8 oz)	160	0	0
Nonfat Black Cherry	1 pkg (8 oz)	160	0	0
Nonfat Cappuccino	1 pkg (8 oz)	160	0	0
Nonfat Cherry Vanilla	1 pkg (8 oz)	190	0	0
Nonfat Chocolate Underground	1 pkg (8 oz)	200	0	0
Nonfat French Vanilla	1 pkg (8 oz)	180	0	0
Nonfat Lotsa Lemon	1 pkg (8 oz)	160	0	0
Nonfat Peach	1 pkg (8 oz)	150	0	0
Nonfat Plain	1 pkg (8 oz)	100	0	0
Nonfat Raspberry	1 pkg (8 oz)	160	0	0
Nonfat Strawberry	1 pkg (8 oz)	180	0	0
Organic French Vanilla	1 pkg	170	6	4
Organic Wild Blueberry	1 pkg	160	6	4
Organic Lowfat Blueberry	1 pkg (6 oz)	130	2	1
Organic Lowfat Luscious Lemon	1 pkg (6 oz)	130	2	1
Organic Lowfat Maple Vanilla	1 pkg (6 oz)	120	2	1
Organic Lowfat Mocha Latte	1 pkg (6 oz)	120	2	1
Organic Lowfat Plain	1 cup (8 oz)	110	2	2
Organic Lowfat Raspberry	1 pkg (6 oz)	130	2	1

FOOD	PORTION	CALS	FAT	SAT FAT
Organic Lowfat Strawberry	1 pkg (6 oz)	130	2	1
Organic Lowfat Vanilla	1 pkg (6 oz)	120	2	1
Strawberries & Cream	1 pkg	160	5	4
Vanilla Truffle	1 pkg	220	5	3
YoSelf Organic Chocolate	1 (4 oz)	110	1	1
YoSelf Organic Creme Caramel	1 (4 oz)	110	1	1
Yosqueeze Strawberry	1 tube (2 oz)	60	1	1
Total				
Greek Yogurt	1 pkg (5 oz)	180	12	6
Greek Yogurt 0% Fat	1 pkg (5 oz)	80	0	0
Greek Yogurt 1% Fat	1 pkg (5 oz)	120	8	6
Yoplait				
99% Fat Free Blueberry	6 oz	180	2	1
99% Fat Free Boysenberry	6 oz	180	2	1
99% Fat Free Cherry	6 oz	180	2	1
99% Fat Free Harvest Peach	4 oz	120	1	1
99% Fat Free Harvest Peach	6 oz	180	2	1
99% Fat Free Key Lime Pie	6 oz	180	2	1
99% Fat Free Lemon	6 oz	180	2	1
99% Fat Free Mixed Berry	6 oz	180	2	1
99% Fat Free Mixed Berry	6 oz	120	1	1
99% Fat Free Orange	6 oz	180	2	1
99% Fat Free Pina Colada	6 oz	180	2	1
99% Fat Free Pineapple	6 oz	180	2	1
99% Fat Free Raspberry	6 oz	180	2	1
99% Fat Free Strawberry	4 oz	120	1	1
99% Fat Free Strawberry	6 oz	180	2	1
99% Fat Free Strawberry Banana	4 oz	120	1	1
99% Fat Free Strawberry Banana	6 oz	180	2	1
99% Fat Free Strawberry Cheesecake	6 oz	180	2	1
Custard Style Banana	6 oz	190	4	2
Custard Style Blueberry	6 oz	190	4	2
Custard Style Cherry Vanilla	6 oz	190	4	2
Custard Style Key Lime Pie	6 oz	190	4	2
Custard Style Lemon	6 oz	190	4	2
Custard Style Peaches'n Cream	6 oz	190	4	2
Custard Style Raspberry	6 oz	190	4	2
Custard Style Raspberry Cheesecake	6 oz	190	4	2
Custard Style Strawberry	6 oz	190	4	2
Custard Style Strawberry Banana	6 oz	190	4	2

FOOD	PORTION	CALS	FAT	SAT FAT
Custard Style Strawberry Vanilla	4 oz	120	2	2
Custard Style Vanilla	6 oz	190	4	2
Go-Gurt Strawberry Banana Burst	1 pkg (2.25 oz)	80	2	1
Go-Gurt Watermelon Meltdown	1 pkg (2.25 oz)	80	2	1
Light Amaretto Cheesecake	6 oz	90	0	0
Light Apricot Mango	6 oz	90	0	0
Light Banana Cream	6 oz	90	0	0
Light Blueberry	6 oz	90	0	0
Light Boston Cream Pie	6 oz	90	0	0
Light Caramel Apple	6 oz	90	0	0
Light Cherry	6 oz	90	0	0
Light Key Lime Pie	6 oz	90	0	0
Light Lemon Cream Pie	6 oz	90	0	0
Light Peach	6 oz	90	0	0
Light Peach Melba	6 oz	90	0	0
Light Raspberry	6 oz	90	0	0
Light Strawberry	6 oz	90	0	0
Light Strawberry Banana	6 oz	90	0	0
Light White Chocolate Strawberry	6 oz	90	0	0
Original Cafe Au Lait	6 oz	170	2	1
Original Coconut Cream Pie	6 oz	200	4	3
Original French Vanilla	6 oz	180	2	1
Trix Rainbow Punch	6 oz	190	2	1
Trix Raspberry Rainbow	6 oz	190	2	1
Trix Strawberry Banana Bash	6 oz	190	2	1
Trix Strawberry Punch	4 oz	130	2	1
Trix Triple Cherry	6 oz	190	2	1
Trix Watermelon Burst	4 oz	130	2	1
Trix Wild Berry Blue	4 oz	130	2	1
Whips! Orange Creme	1 pkg (4 oz)	140	3	2
Whips! Raspberry Mousse	1 pkg (4 oz)	140	3	2

YOGURT DRINKS
Dannon
Frusion Smoothie Peach Passion Fruit	1 bottle (10 oz)	270	4	2
Frusion Smoothie Tropical Fruit	1 bottle (10 oz)	270	4	2

Yo-Goat
Blueberry	8 oz	150	8	5

Yoplait
Nouriche All Flavors	1 bottle (11 oz)	290	0	0

FOOD	PORTION	CALS	FAT	SAT FAT
YOGURT FROZEN				
chocolate soft serve	½ cup (4 fl oz)	115	4	3
vanilla soft serve	½ cup (4 fl oz)	114	4	2
Breyers				
Chocolate	½ cup	150	5	3
Vanilla	½ cup	140	5	3
Vanilla No Sugar Added	½ cup	100	5	3
Dannon				
Light Cappuccino	½ cup (2.8 oz)	80	0	0
Light Cherry Vanilla Swirl	½ cup (2.8 oz)	90	0	0
Light Chocolate	½ cup (2.7 oz)	80	0	0
Light Mint Chocolate Fudge	½ cup (2.8 oz)	90	0	0
Light Peach Raspberry Melba	½ cup (2.8 oz)	90	0	0
Light Strawberry Cheesecake	½ cup (2.8 oz)	90	0	0
Light Vanilla	½ cup (2.8 oz)	80	0	0
Light Duets Strawberry Sundae	6 oz	90	0	0
Light Nonfat Cappuccino	8 oz	100	0	0
Light'N Crunchy Banana Cream Pie	½ cup (2.8 oz)	110	1	0
Light'N Crunchy Caramel Toffee Crunch	½ cup (2.8 oz)	110	1	1
Light'N Crunchy Mocha Chocolate Chunk	½ cup (2.8 oz)	110	1	1
Light'N Crunchy Peanut Chocolate Crunch	½ cup (2.8 oz)	110	1	1
Light'N Crunchy Rocky Road	½ cup (2.8 oz)	110	1	0
Light'N Crunchy Triple Chocolate	½ cup (2.8 oz)	110	1	1
Light'N Crunchy Vanilla Streusel	½ cup (2.8 oz)	110	1	1
Edy's				
Black Cherry Vanilla Swirl	½ cup	90	0	0
Caramel Fudge Cosmo	½ cup	140	4	3
Caramel Praline Crunch	½ cup	100	0	0
Chocolate Decadence	½ cup	120	4	2
Chocolate Fudge	½ cup	100	0	0
Coffee Fudge Sundae	½ cup	100	0	0
Cookies'N Cream	½ cup	120	4	2
Heath Toffee Crunch	½ cup	120	4	2
Raspberry	½ cup	90	3	2
Ultimate Tin Roof Sundae	½ cup	130	4	2
Vanilla	½ cup	90	0	0
Vanilla Chocolate Swirl	½ cup	90	0	0

FOOD	PORTION	CALS	FAT	SAT FAT
Friendly's				
Apple Bettie	½ cup (2.6 oz)	140	3	2
Fabulous Fudge Swirl	½ cup (2.6 oz)	140	3	3
Fudge Berry Swirl	½ cup (2.6 oz)	150	4	3
Lowfat Perfectly Peach	½ cup (2.6 oz)	110	2	1
Lowfat Purely Chocolate	½ cup (2.6 oz)	120	3	2
Lowfat Raspberry Delight	½ cup (2.6 oz)	120	3	2
Lowfat Simply Vanilla	½ cup (2.6 oz)	120	3	2
Lowfat Strawberry Patch	½ cup (2.6 oz)	110	2	1
Mint Chocolate Chip	½ cup (2.6 oz)	130	4	2
Strawberry Cheesecake Blast	½ cup (2.6 oz)	140	4	2
Toffee Almond Crunch	½ cup (2.6 oz)	160	5	2
Häagen-Dazs				
Lowfat Dulce De Leche	½ cup	190	3	2
Nonfat Chocolate	½ cup	140	0	0
Nonfat Coffee	½ cup	140	0	0
Nonfat Strawberry	½ cup	140	0	0
Nonfat Vanilla	½ cup	140	0	0
Nonfat Vanilla Raspberry Swirl	½ cup	130	0	0
Nonfat Vanilla Fudge	½ cup	160	0	0
Hood				
Bavarian Truffle & Twist	½ cup (2.6 oz)	150	4	3
Coffee Toffee Chunk Sundae	½ cup (2.6 oz)	150	4	3
Combo Bars	1 (2.2 oz)	90	2	1
Cookies & Cream	½ cup (2.6 oz)	140	4	2
Grandma's Raisin Oatmeal Cookie Dough	½ cup (2.6 oz)	140	3	2
Mixed Berry Swirl	½ cup (2.6 oz)	120	2	2
Natural Strawberry	½ cup (2.6 oz)	110	3	2
Natural Strawberry Banana	½ cup (2.6 oz)	110	3	2
Natural Vanilla	½ cup (2.6 oz)	120	3	2
Nonfat Caramel & Brownie Sundae	½ cup (2.6 oz)	120	0	0
Nonfat Chocolate Marshmallow	½ cup (2.6 oz)	110	0	0
Nonfat Double Raspberry	½ cup (2.6 oz)	120	0	0
Nonfat Mocha Fudge	½ cup (2.6 oz)	120	0	0
Nonfat Olde Fashioned Vanilla	½ cup (2.6 oz)	110	0	0
Nonfat Peach Cobbler A La Mode	½ cup (2.6 oz)	110	0	0
Nonfat Strawberry	½ cup (2.6 oz)	100	0	0
Nonfat Vanilla Fudge	½ cup (2.6 oz)	120	0	0
Raspberry Swirl	½ cup (2.6 oz)	130	2	2

FOOD	PORTION	CALS	FAT	SAT FAT
Sundae Cups Chocolate & Strawberry	1 (2.2 oz)	110	2	1
Vanilla Chocolate Strawberry	½ cup (2.6 oz)	120	3	2
Vanilla Swiss Almond Sundae	½ cup (2.6 oz)	150	4	2
Turkey Hill				
Black Raspberry	½ cup	110	3	—
Caramel Cashew Crunch	½ cup	160	9	—
Chocolate Chip Cookie Dough	½ cup	140	5	3
Chocolate Chip Cookie Dough	½ cup	190	10	—
Clark Bar	½ cup	140	5	—
Fat Free Chocolate Cherry Cordial	½ cup	100	0	0
Fat Free Chocolate Marshmallow	½ cup	130	0	0
Fat Free Mint Cookie 'N Cream	½ cup	110	0	0
Fat Free Neapolitan	½ cup	100	0	0
Fat Free Orange Swirl	½ cup	100	0	0
Fat Free Vanilla Fudge	½ cup	110	0	0
Peach Raspberry	½ cup	110	2	2
Tin Roof Sundae	½ cup	140	5	3
Vanilla & Chocolate	½ cup	110	3	2
Vanilla Bean	½ cup	110	3	2
ZUCCHINI				
baby raw	1 (0.5 oz)	3	tr	tr
canned italian style	½ cup	33	tr	tr
frzn cooked	½ cup	19	tr	tr
raw sliced	½ cup	9	tr	tr
sliced cooked	½ cup	14	tr	tr
Progresso				
Italian Style	½ cup (4.2 oz)	50	2	0
TAKE-OUT				
indian paalkora	1 serv	46	2	tr

PART TWO

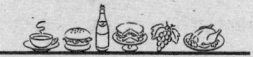

Restaurant Chains

FOOD	PORTION	CALS	FAT	SAT FAT
APPLEBEE'S				
DESSERTS				
Apple Betty Cobbler Ala Mode	1 serv	598	22	–
Fudge Brownie Sundae	1 serv	739	40	–
Low Fat Bikini Banana Strawberry Shortcake	1 serv	248	2	tr
Low Fat Brownie Sundae	1 serv	415	2	tr
Low Fat Marble Cheesecake	1 serv	261	2	1
MAIN MENU SELECTIONS				
Applebee's Burger w/ Fries	1 serv	1274	79	–
Basic Hamburger w/ Fries	1 serv	980	58	–
Beef Fajita Quesadilla	1 serv	1205	86	–
Bourbon Street Steak w/ Fried New Potatoes	1 serv	1115	94	–
Low Fat Asian Chicken Salad	1 serv (5 oz)	623	9	2
Low Fat Asian Chicken Salad	1 med serv (2.5 oz)	370	6	1
Low Fat Blackened Chicken Salad	1 med serv (2.5 oz)	287	3	1
Low Fat Blackened Chicken Salad	1 serv (5 oz)	411	5	1
Low Fat Garlic Chicken Pasta	1 serv	587	8	2
Low Fat Lemon Chicken Pasta	1 serv	528	11	4
Low Fat Quesadilla Chicken Fajita	1 serv	518	11	tr
Low Fat Quesadilla Veggie	1 serv	344	8	tr
Mozzarella Stix	8 pieces	963	57	–
Quesadillas	1 serv	684	46	–
Riblet Basket w/ Fries	1 serv	1317	92	–
Salad Dinner w/o Dressing	1 serv	303	18	–
Salad Santa Fe Chicken	1 med	724	42	–
Sandwich Bacon Cheese Chicken Grill w/o Fries	1	746	46	–
Sandwich Gyro	1	880	69	–
Stir Fry Chicken	1 serv	566	7	–
ARBY'S				
BEVERAGES				
Chocolate Shake	1 (14 oz)	480	16	8
Hot Chocolate	1 serv (8.6 oz)	110	1	1
Jamocha Shake	1 (14 oz)	470	15	7
Milk	1 serv (8 oz)	120	5	3

FOOD	PORTION	CALS	FAT	SAT FAT
Orange Juice	1 serv (10 oz)	140	0	0
Strawberry Shake	1 (14 oz)	500	13	8
Vanilla Shake	1 (14 oz)	470	15	7
BREAKFAST SELECTIONS				
Add Egg	1 serv (2 oz)	110	9	2
Add Swiss Cheese Slice	1 slice (0.5 oz)	45	3	2
Biscuit w/ Bacon	1 (3.2 oz)	320	21	5
Biscuit w/ Butter	1 (2.9 oz)	280	17	4
Biscuit w/ Ham	1 (4.3 oz)	330	20	5
Biscuit w/ Sausage	1 (4.2)	460	33	9
Croissant w/ Bacon	1 (2.5 oz)	300	20	11
Croissant w/ Ham	1 (3.7 oz)	310	19	11
Croissant w/ Sausage	1 (3.6 oz)	420	32	15
French Toast Syrup	1 serv (0.5 oz)	130	0	0
Sourdough w/ Bacon	1 (5 oz)	380	7	2
Sourdough w/ Ham	1 (4 oz)	220	7	2
Sourdough w/ Sausage	1 (4 oz)	330	19	6
Toastix w/o Syrup	1 serv (4.4 oz)	370	17	4
DESSERTS				
Apple Turnover Iced	1 (4.5 oz)	420	16	5
Cherry Turnover Iced	1 (4.5 oz)	410	16	5
MAIN MENU SELECTIONS				
Arby's Sauce	1 serv (0.5 oz)	15	0	0
Au Jus Sauce	1 serv (3 oz)	5	1	tr
BBQ Dipping Sauce	1 serv (1 oz)	40	0	0
Baked Potato Broccoli'N Cheddar	1 (14 oz)	540	24	12
Baked Potato Deluxe	1 (13 oz)	650	34	20
Baked Potato w/ Butter & Sour Cream	1 (11.2 oz)	500	24	15
Bronco Berry Sauce	1 serv (1.5 oz)	90	0	0
Chicken Finger 4-Pak	1 serv (6.77 oz)	640	38	8
Chicken Finger Snack w/ Curly Fries	1 serv (6.4 oz)	580	32	7
Curly Fries	1 lg (7 oz)	620	30	7
Curly Fries	1 med (4.5 oz)	400	20	5
Curly Fries	1 sm (3.8 oz)	310	15	4
Curly Fries Cheddar	1 serv (6 oz)	460	24	6
German Mustard	1 pkg (0.25 oz)	5	0	0
Homestyle Fries	1 med (5 oz)	370	16	4
Homestyle Fries	1 sm (4 oz)	300	13	4
Homestyle Fries	1 lg (7.5 oz)	560	24	6
Homestyle Fries Child-Size	1 serv (3 oz)	220	10	3

FOOD	PORTION	CALS	FAT	SAT FAT
Honey Mustard	1 serv (1 oz)	130	12	2
Horsey Sauce	1 pkg (0.5 oz)	60	5	1
Jalapeno Bites	1 serv (4 oz)	330	21	9
Ketchup	1 pkg (0.3 oz)	10	0	0
Marinara Sauce	1 serv (1.5 oz)	35	1	0
Mayonnaise	1 pkg (0.4 oz)	90	10	2
Mayonnaise Light Cholesterol Free	1 pkg (0.4 oz)	20	2	0
Mozzarella Sticks	4 (4.8 oz)	470	29	14
Onion Petals	1 serv (4 oz)	410	24	4
Potato Cakes	2 (3.5 oz)	250	16	4
Sandwich Chicken Bacon'N Swiss	1 (7.4 oz)	610	33	8
Sandwich Chicken Breast Fillet	1 (7.2 oz)	540	30	5
Sandwich Chicken Cordon Bleu	1 (8.4 oz)	630	35	8
Sandwich Grilled Chicken Deluxe	1 (8.7 oz)	450	22	4
Sandwich Hot Ham 'N Swiss	1 (5.9 oz)	340	13	5
Sandwich Market Fresh Roast Beef & Swiss	1 (12.5 oz)	810	42	13
Sandwich Market Fresh Roast Beef Ranch & Bacon	1 (13.5 oz)	880	44	10
Sandwich Market Fresh Roast Chicken Caesar	1 (12.7 oz)	820	38	9
Sandwich Market Fresh Roast Ham & Swiss	1 (12.5 oz)	730	34	8
Sandwich Market Fresh Roast Turkey & Swiss	1 (12.5 oz)	760	33	6
Sandwich Market Fresh Ultimate BLT	1 (10.5 oz)	820	49	11
Sandwich Roast Beef Arby-Q	1 (6.4 oz)	360	14	4
Sandwich Roast Beef Beef'N Cheddar	1 (6.9 oz)	480	24	8
Sandwich Roast Beef Big Montana	1 (11 oz)	630	32	15
Sandwich Roast Beef Giant	1 (7.9 oz)	480	23	10
Sandwich Roast Beef Junior	1 (4.4 oz)	310	13	5
Sandwich Roast Beef Melt w/ Cheddar	1 (5.2 oz)	340	15	5
Sandwich Roast Beef Regular	1 (5.4 oz)	350	16	6
Sandwich Roast Beef Super	1 (8.5 oz)	470	23	7
Sandwich Roast Chicken Club	1 (8.4 oz)	520	28	7
Sub Sandwich French Dip	1 (10 oz)	440	18	8
Sub Sandwich Hot Ham'N Swiss	1 (9.7 oz)	530	27	8
Sub Sandwich Italian	1 (11 oz)	780	53	15
Sub Sandwich Philly Beef'N Swiss	1 (10.8 oz)	700	42	15
Sub Sandwich Roast Beef	1 (11.6 oz)	760	48	16

FOOD	PORTION	CALS	FAT	SAT FAT
Sub Sandwich Roast Beef	1 (11.6 oz)	760	48	16
Sub Sandwich Turkey	1 (10.6 oz)	630	37	9
Tangy Southwest Sauce	1 serv (1.5 oz)	250	26	5
SALAD DRESSINGS				
Bleu Cheese	1 serv (2 oz)	300	31	6
Buttermilk Ranch	1 serv (2 oz)	290	30	5
Buttermilk Ranch Light	1 serv (2 oz)	100	6	1
Caesar	1 serv (2 oz)	310	34	5
Honey French	1 serv (2 oz)	290	24	4
Italian Reduced Calorie	1 serv (2 oz)	25	1	1
Italian Parmesan	1 serv (2 oz)	240	24	4
Thousand Island	1 serv (2 oz)	290	28	5
SALADS AND SALAD BARS				
Caesar Side Salad	1 (5 oz)	45	2	1
Caesar Salad w/o Dressing	1 serv (8 oz)	90	4	3
Chicken Finger w/o Dressing	1 serv (13 oz)	570	34	9
Croutons Seasoned	1 serv (0.25 oz)	30	1	0
Croutons Cheese & Garlic	1 serv (0.63 oz)	100	6	—
Garden Salad	1 (12.3 oz)	70	1	0
Grilled Chicken	1 serv (16.3 oz)	210	5	2
Grilled Chicken Caesar w/o Dressing	1 serv (12 oz)	230	8	4
Roast Chicken	1 serv (14.8 oz)	160	3	0
Side Salad	1 (5.7 oz)	25	0	0
Turkey Club Salad w/o Dressing	1 serv (12 oz)	350	21	10
AU BON PAIN				
BAKED SELECTIONS				
Bagel Cinnamon Crisp	1 (6 oz)	540	7	1
Baguette	1 loaf (10.6 oz)	680	3	0
Bread Stick	1 (2.3 oz)	200	3	0
Cinnamon Roll	1 (4 oz)	300	5	2
Cookie Chocolate Chip	1 (2 oz)	230	7	4
Cookie Chocolate Chunk Macadamia	1 (2 oz)	250	13	4
Cookie Gingerbread Man w/ Raisins & Icing	1 (2.7 oz)	280	7	2
Cookie Oatmeal Raisin	1 (2 oz)	210	6	2
Cookie Peanut Butter	1 (2 oz)	240	12	3
Cookie Shortbread	1 (2.3 oz)	240	7	4
Cookie Walnut Raisin	1 (2 oz)	250	13	4
Cookie English Toffee	1 (2 oz)	230	7	4

FOOD	PORTION	CALS	FAT	SAT FAT
Creme De Fleur	1 serv (5.55 oz)	470	19	11
Croissant Almond	1 (4.7 oz)	480	25	9
Croissant Apple	1 (3.5 oz)	200	3	2
Croissant Chocolate	1 (3.1 oz)	330	10	6
Croissant Cinnamon Raisin	1 (3.8 oz)	300	5	3
Croissant Raspberry Cheese	1 (3.6 oz)	290	9	5
Croissant Sweet Cheese	1 (3.6 oz)	320	12	7
Danish Cranberry	1 (4.5 oz)	350	9	4
Danish Lemon	1 (4.3 oz)	340	9	4
Danish Sweet Cheese	1 (4.2 oz)	390	16	7
Focaccia	1 piece (5.4 oz)	430	16	2
Four Grain Bread	1 serv (4.7 oz)	400	4	1
French Roll	1 (4.2 oz)	260	1	0
French Roll Roast Beef	1 (11 oz)	540	19	4
Hearth Roll	1 (3 oz)	210	2	1
Holiday Cookie w/ Icing & Sprinkles	1 (1.6 oz)	150	3	1
Loaf Multigrain	1 slice (1.8 oz)	130	1	0
Muffin Banana Walnut	1 (5.4 oz)	430	21	4
Muffin Blueberry	1 (5.6 oz)	470	15	3
Muffin Bran Raisin	1 (5.5 oz)	400	12	5
Muffin Carrot	1 (5.8 oz)	520	25	5
Muffin Corn	1 (5.7 oz)	390	16	3
Muffin Cranberry Walnut	1 (5.4 oz)	500	27	5
Muffin Milk Chocolate Chunk	1 (5.3 oz)	530	23	8
Muffin Pumpkin	1 (6 oz)	510	18	3
Muffin Low Fat 3 Berry	1 (4.4 oz)	270	3	0
Muffin Low Fat Chocolate Cake	1 (4.2 oz)	470	0	0
Parisienne Loaf	1 loaf (19 oz)	1210	5	1
Petit Pain	1 (2.9 oz)	180	1	0
Roll Braided w/ Topping	1 (10 oz)	430	14	3
Roll Pecan	1 (6 oz)	620	24	6
Sandwich Loaf Country White	1 serv (1.75 oz)	110	1	0
Sandwich Loaf Tomato Herb	1 serv (1.75 oz)	120	1	0
Scone Chocolate Walnut	1 (4 oz)	420	19	8
Scone Cranberry Orange Almond	1 (4 oz)	400	15	7
Scone Maple Oat Pecan Date	1 (4 oz)	410	17	8
Scone Orange	1 (4.2 oz)	370	13	7
Shortbread Heart ½ Chocolate	1 (2.7 oz)	290	10	6
Shortbread Heart w/ Red Sugar	1 (2.5 oz)	270	7	4
Sourdough Bagel Asiago Cheese	1 (4.8 oz)	340	5	3

FOOD	PORTION	CALS	FAT	SAT FAT
Sourdough Bagel Cheddar Scallion	1 (4.1 oz)	310	5	3
Sourdough Bagel Cinnamon Crisp	1 (4.6 oz)	360	5	1
Sourdough Bagel Cinnamon Raisin	1 (4.5 oz)	300	1	0
Sourdough Bagel Cranberry Nut	1 (4.7 oz)	400	7	1
Sourdough Bagel Cranberry Nut	1 (4.7 oz)	400	7	1
Sourdough Bagel Double Cheddar Jalapeno	1 serv (4.1 oz)	320	6	4
Sourdough Bagel Dutch Apple	1 (4.7 oz)	380	3	1
Sourdough Bagel Everything	1 (4.4 oz)	330	3	0
Sourdough Bagel Focaccia	1 (4.1 oz)	320	5	1
Sourdough Bagel Honey 9 Grain	1 (4.8 oz)	310	2	0
Sourdough Bagel Plain	1 (4 oz)	300	1	0
Sourdough Bagel Poppy Seed	1 (4.4 oz)	330	3	0
Sourdough Bagel Sesame	1 (4.4 oz)	340	4	1
Sourdough Bagel Wild Blueberry	1 (4.1 oz)	280	1	0
Sourdough bagel Onion	1 (4.4 oz)	320	1	0
Streudel Cherry	1 serv (4 oz)	380	23	2
Streudel Apple	1 serv (4.35 oz)	400	23	0
SALADS AND SALAD BARS				
Caesar w/o Dressing	1 serv (7.8 oz)	240	12	6
Chef's	1 serv (10.3 oz)	290	15	7
Chicken Caesar	1 serv (10.2 oz)	380	18	8
Chicken Oriental	1 serv (8.6 oz)	220	6	2
Chicken Pesto Salad	1 serv (8 oz)	400	23	6
Garden	1 serv (9.3 oz)	160	5	1
Garden Side	1 serv (5.1 oz)	90	2	1
Gorgonzola & Walnut	1 serv (5 oz)	330	28	7
Mozzarella & Red Pepper Salad	1 serv (10.5 oz)	360	25	16
Tuna	1 serv (13.2 oz)	440	24	4
SANDWICHES AND FILLINGS				
Chicken Tarragon	1 serv (4 oz)	240	17	3
Club Hot Roasted Turkey	1 (11.7 oz)	630	28	9
Country Ham	1 serv (3.7 oz)	150	7	3
Cracked Pepper Chicken	1 serv (3.9 oz)	140	2	0
Cream Cheese Plain	1 serv (2 oz)	190	10	11
Cream Cheese Reduced Fat Honey Walnut	1 serv (2 oz)	150	10	7
Cream Cheese Reduced Fat Sundried Tomato	1 serv (2 oz)	140	12	7
Cream Cheese Reduced Fat Veggie	1 serv (2 oz)	140	12	7

FOOD	PORTION	CALS	FAT	SAT FAT
Croissant Spinach & Cheese	1 (3.6 oz)	220	9	5
Croque Madame	1 (11 oz)	570	22	15
Croque Monsieur	1 (11 oz)	590	25	16
Egg On A Bagel	1 serv (7.1 oz)	500	5	1
Egg On A Bagel w/ Bacon	1 serv (7.6 oz)	580	12	4
Egg On A Bagel w/ Cheese	1 serv (7.85 oz)	590	12	5
Egg On A Bagel w/ Cheese & Bacon	1 serv (8.35 oz)	670	19	7
Fo-Ca-Cha-Cha Chicken	1 serv (11.15 oz)	730	17	3
Focaccia Chicken & Mozzarella	1 serv (13.75 oz)	800	14	2
Focaccia Chicken Tarragon w/ Field Greens	1 (12.5 oz)	870	47	8
Focaccia Garden Vegetable Goat Cheese w/ Artichoke Spread	1 (14.25 oz)	570	21	6
Focaccia Hickory Smoked Ham & Brie	1 (13.3 oz)	620	27	9
Focaccia Smoked Turkey & Swiss w/ Cilantro	1 (13.25 oz)	810	40	14
French Roll Ham	1 (11 oz)	390	16	3
French Roll Hot Grilled Chicken	1 (11 oz)	620	23	5
French Roll Hot Roast Turkey	1 (11 oz)	500	15	2
French Roll Tuna	1 (10.6 oz)	550	21	3
Grilled Chicken	1 serv (3.9 oz)	140	2	0
Hot Croissant Spinach & Cheese	1 (4 oz)	290	9	5
Pane Bagniate	1 (12 oz)	670	28	5
Roast Beef	1 serv (3.7 oz)	140	5	0
Sandwich Arizona Chicken	1 (12 oz)	600	15	6
Sandwich Cheese	1 (7.2 oz)	590	26	18
Sandwich Fresh Mozzarella Tomato & Pesto	1 (11 oz)	790	43	21
Sandwich Honey Dijon Chicken	1 (13.6 oz)	750	24	9
Sandwich Thai Chicken	1 (11.4 oz)	550	12	3
Tuna Salad	1 serv (4.5 oz)	360	29	5
Turkey Breast	1 serv (3.7 oz)	120	1	0
Wrap Chicken Caesar	1 (10.5 oz)	640	26	9
Wrap Fields & Feta	1 (13.5 oz)	620	19	5
Wrap Honey Smoked Turkey	1 (15 oz)	520	7	1
Wrap Roast Beef & Brie	1 (14 oz)	570	28	11
SOUPS				
Autumn Pumpkin	1 serv (8 oz)	170	9	5
Black Bean	1 serv (8 oz)	180	1	0
Chicken Florentine	1 serv (8 oz)	140	8	4

FOOD	PORTION	CALS	FAT	SAT FAT
Chicken Noodle	1 serv (8 oz)	100	2	1
Clam Chowder	1 serv (8 oz)	220	15	6
Corn & Green Chili Bisque	1 serv (8 oz)	200	10	6
Corn Chowder	1 serv (8 oz)	270	15	9
Curried Rice & Lentil	1 serv (8 oz)	140	2	0
French Moroccan Tomato Lentil	1 serv (8 oz)	130	2	1
Garden Vegetable	1 serv (8 oz)	50	1	0
Low Sodium Mediterranean Pepper	1 serv (12 oz)	280	6	0
Low Sodium Southwest Vegetable	1 serv (12 oz)	220	5	0
Old Fashioned Tomato	1 serv (8 oz)	140	6	2
Pasta E Fagioli	1 serv (8 oz)	240	7	2
Potato Cheese	1 serv (8 oz)	190	10	1
Potato Leek	1 serv (8 oz)	200	13	8
Red Beans & Rice	1 serv (8 oz)	200	5	1
Soup Bread Bowl	1 (9.25 oz)	600	3	0
Southern Black Eyed Pea	1 serv (8 oz)	320	2	0
Split Pea	1 serv (8 oz)	160	1	0
Tomato Florentine	1 serv (8 oz)	120	3	1
Tuscan Vegetable	1 serv (8 oz)	140	4	2
Vegetable Beef Barley	1 serv (8 oz)	110	3	1
Vegetarian Lentil	1 serv (8 oz)	120	1	0
Vegetarian Chili	1 serv (8 oz)	170	2	0
Vegetarian Chili	1 serv (8 oz)	170	2	0
Wild Mushroom Bisque	1 serv (8 oz)	140	7	2

AUNTIE ANNE'S
BEVERAGES

FOOD	PORTION	CALS	FAT	SAT FAT
Dutch Smoothie Pina Colada	1 (14 oz)	260	8	5
Dutch Ice Blue Raspberry	1 (14 oz)	165	0	0
Dutch Ice Grape	1 (14 oz)	180	0	0
Dutch Ice Kiwi Banana	1 (14 oz)	190	0	0
Dutch Ice Lemonade	1 (14 oz)	315	0	0
Dutch Ice Mocha	1 (14 oz)	400	10	9
Dutch Ice Orange Creme	1 (14 oz)	280	0	0
Dutch Ice Pina Colada	1 (14 oz)	220	0	0
Dutch Ice Strawberry	1 (14 oz)	220	0	0
Dutch Ice Wild Cherry	1 (14 oz)	210	0	0
Dutch Shake Chocolate	1 (14 oz)	580	27	18
Dutch Shake Coffee	1 (14 oz)	590	27	18
Dutch Shake Strawberry	1 (14 oz)	610	27	18

FOOD	PORTION	CALS	FAT	SAT FAT
Dutch Shake Vanilla	1 (14 oz)	510	27	17
Dutch Smoothie Blue Raspberry	1 (14 oz)	230	8	5
Dutch Smoothie Grape	1 (14 oz)	230	8	5
Dutch Smoothie Kiwi Banana	1 (14 oz)	240	8	5
Dutch Smoothie Lemonade	1 (14 oz)	300	8	5
Dutch Smoothie Mocha	1 (14 oz)	330	13	9
Dutch Smoothie Orange Creme	1 (14 oz)	280	8	5
Dutch Smoothie Strawberry	1 (14 oz)	250	8	5
Dutch Smoothie Wild Cherry	1 (14 oz)	250	8	5
Lemonade	1 (22 oz)	180	0	0
Lemonade Strawberry	1 (22 oz)	190	0	0
DIPPING SAUCES				
Caramel Dip	1 serv (1.5 oz)	135	3	2
Cheese Sauce	1 serv (1.25 oz)	100	8	4
Chocolate Dip	1 serv (1.25 oz)	130	4	2
Cream Cheese Light	1 serv (1.25 oz)	70	6	4
Cream Cheese Strawberry	1 serv (1.25 oz)	110	10	6
Hot Salsa Cheese	1 serv (1.25 oz)	100	8	4
Marinara Sauce	1 serv (1.25 oz)	10	0	0
Sweet Mustard	1 serv (1.25 oz)	60	2	1
PRETZELS				
Almond	1	400	8	5
Almond w/o Butter	1	350	2	1
Cinnamon Raisin w/o Butter	1	350	2	0
Cinnamon Sugar	1	450	9	5
Garlic	1	350	5	3
Garlic w/o Butter	1	320	1	0
Glazin' Raisin	1	510	4	2
Glazin' Raisin w/o Butter	1	470	1	0
Jalapeno	1	310	5	3
Jalapeno w/o Butter	1	270	1	0
Maple Crumb	1	550	6	2
Maple Crumb w/o Butter	1	520	3	0
Original	1	370	4	2
Original w/o Butter	1	340	1	0
Parmesan Herb	1	440	13	7
Parmesan Herb w/o Butter	1	390	5	3
Sesame	1	410	12	4
Sesame w/o Butter	1	350	6	1
Sour Cream & Onion w/o Butter	1	310	1	0

FOOD	PORTION	CALS	FAT	SAT FAT
Sour Cream & Onion	1	340	5	3
Stixs	4	247	3	1
Stixs w/o Butter	4	227	1	0
Whole Wheat	1	370	5	2
Whole Wheat w/o Butter	1	350	2	0

BAJA FRESH
MAIN MENU SELECTIONS

FOOD	PORTION	CALS	FAT	SAT FAT
Baja Burrito Chicken	1 serv	820	35	14
Baja Burrito Steak	1 serv	920	42	17
Black Beans	1 serv	360	3	1
Burrito Bean & Cheese Chicken	1 serv	1000	33	15
Burrito Bean & Cheese Steak	1 serv	1100	41	19
Burrito Bean & Cheese Vegetarian	1 serv	870	31	15
Burrito Dos Manos Chicken	1 full serv	1480	40	16
Burrito Dos Manos Steak	1 full serv	1580	48	18
Burrito Mexicano Chicken	1 serv	830	13	3
Burrito Mexicano Steak	1 serv	920	20	6
Burrito Ultimo Chicken	1 serv	860	30	13
Burrito Ultimo Steak	1 serv	950	37	16
Cebollitas	1 serv	40	2	0
Chips & Salsa Baja	1 serv	1100	50	5
Enchiladas Cheese	1 serv	850	37	17
Enchiladas Chicken	1 serv	780	25	10
Enchiladas Steak	1 serv	890	33	15
Enchiladas Verde Cheese	1 serv	840	35	17
Enchiladas Verde Chicken	1 serv	770	23	10
Enchiladas Verde Vegetarian	1 serv	720	22	10
Fajitas Chicken Corn Tortillas	1 serv	1200	29	9
Fajitas Chicken Flour Tortillas	1 serv	1360	37	12
Fajitas Steak Corn Tortillas	1 serv	1360	42	15
Fajitas Steak Flour Tortillas	1 serv	1530	50	18
Grilled Vegetarian	1 serv	770	27	12
Mini Quesa-Dita Cheese	1 serv	620	20	9
Mini Quesa-Dita Chicken	1 serv	670	21	9
Mini Quesa-Dita Steak	1 serv	700	23	11
Mini Tosta-Dita Chicken	1 serv	570	17	4
Mini Tosta-Dita Steak	1 serv	630	22	6
Nachos Cheese	1 serv	1880	103	37
Nachos Chicken	1 serv	2010	105	38

FOOD	PORTION	CALS	FAT	SAT FAT
Nachos Steak	1 serv	2100	113	41
Pinto Beans	1 serv	320	1	0
Quesadilla	1 serv	1180	70	35
Quesadilla Cheese	1 serv	1130	69	35
Quesadilla Chicken	1 serv	1260	71	35
Quesadilla Steak	1 serv	1350	79	39
Taco Baja Style Chicken	1 serv	190	5	1
Taco Baja Style Steak	1 serv	220	7	2
Taco Baja Style Wild Gulf Shrimp	1 serv	190	5	1
Taco Chilito Chicken	1 serv	320	10	4
Taco Chilito Steak	1 serv	340	12	5
Taco Fish	1 serv	270	13	2
Taco Mahi Mahi	1 serv	260	10	2
Taquitos Chicken w/ Beans	1 serv	750	36	12
Taquitos Chicken w/ Rice	1 serv	710	36	11
Taquitos Steak w/ Beans	1 serv	820	42	16
Taquitos Steak w/ Rice	1 serv	790	42	15
Tostada Chicken	1 serv	1140	52	14
Tostada Steak	1 serv	1230	60	17
Tostada Vegetarian	1 serv	1010	50	14
SALAD DRESSINGS				
Fat Free Salsa Verde	1 serv (2.6 oz)	15	0	0
Guacamole	2 oz	70	6	1
Olive Oil Vinaigrette	1 serv (2.6 oz)	230	25	4
Pico De Gallo	1 serv	50	1	0
Pronto Guacamole	1 serv	550	30	4
Ranch	1 serv (2.6 oz)	220	19	4
Salsa Baja	1 serv	70	3	0
Salsa Roja	1 serv	70	1	0
Salsa Verde	1 serv	50	0	0
Sour Cream	1 oz	60	5	4
SALADS AND SALAD BARS				
Baja Ensalada Chicken	1 serv	310	18	2
Baja Ensalada Fish	1 serv	360	15	4
Baja Ensalada Steak	1 serv	460	18	7
Side Salad	1 serv	70	3	1

BASKIN-ROBBINS
FROZEN YOGURT

Cafe Mocha Truly Free Soft Serve	1 reg	140	1	1

FOOD	PORTION	CALS	FAT	SAT FAT
Chocolate Nonfat Soft Serve	1 reg	190	1	0
Lowfat Maui Brownie Madness	1 reg	250	9	4
ICE CREAM				
Cappuccino Blast w/ Whipped Cream	1 reg	340	16	10
Chocolate	1 reg	270	16	10
Chocolate Chip	1 reg	270	17	11
Espresso'n Cream Lowfat	1 reg	180	3	2
Jamoca Almond Fudge	1 reg	280	16	8
Peach Crumb Pie No Sugar Added	1 reg	180	5	3
Pralines'n Cream	1 reg	280	15	8
Shake Chocolate	16 oz	750	43	21
Shake Vanilla	16 oz	630	35	22
Smoothie Very Strawberry w/ Soft Serve Ice Cream	1 reg	320	1	1
Thin Mint No Sugar Added	1 reg	160	4	3
Vanilla	1 reg	270	16	10
ICES				
Daiquiri Ice	1 reg	130	0	0
Sherbet Rainbow	1 reg	160	2	2
Sorbet Peachy Keen	1 reg	110	0	0
BEN & JERRY'S				
Sugar Cone	1	48	tr	tr
FROZEN YOGURT				
Black Raspberry Low Fat	½ cup	140	2	1
Cherry Garcia	½ cup	170	3	2
Chocolate Fudge Brownie	½ cup	190	3	2
Half Baked	½ cup	210	4	2
Phish Food	½ cup	230	5	4
ICE CREAM				
Brownie Batter	½ cup	310	18	10
Butter Pecan	½ cup	290	21	10
Cherry Garcia	½ cup	250	15	11
Chocolate Chip Cookie Dough	½ cup	280	16	9
Chocolate Chocolate Cookie	½ cup	280	14	9
Chocolate For A Change	½ cup	270	17	11
Chocolate Fudge Brownie	½ cup	280	14	9
Chubby Hubby	½ cup	330	21	12
Chunky Monkey	½ cup	300	19	11
Coffee For A Change	½ cup	240	15	10

FOOD	PORTION	CALS	FAT	SAT FAT
Coffee Heath Bar Crunch	½ cup	310	18	12
Everything But The	½ cup	320	19	12
Fudge Central	½ cup	300	18	12
Half Baked	½ cup	280	14	9
Karamel Sutra	½ cup	290	15	10
Makin' Whoopie Pie	½ cup	270	14	9
Mint Chocolate Cookie	½ cup	270	16	10
New York Super Fudge Chunk	½ cup	270	20	11
Oatmeal Cookie Chunk	½ cup	280	16	10
One Sweet Whirled	½ cup	280	15	11
Organic Chocolate Fudge Brownie	½ cup	260	13	9
Organic Strawberry	½ cup	200	12	8
Organic Sweet Cream & Cookies	½ cup	240	15	9
Organic Vanilla	½ cup	220	14	10
Peanut Butter Cup	½ cup	380	26	13
Peanut Butter Me Up	½ cup	330	21	11
Phish Food	½ cup	280	13	10
Pistachio Pistachio	½ cup	280	19	12
Uncanny Cashew	½ cup	290	19	13
Vanilla Heath Bar Crunch	½ cup	300	19	11
Vanilla For A Change	½ cup	240	16	11
SORBETS				
Berry Berry Extraordinary	½ cup	100	0	0
Mango Lime	½ cup	100	0	0
Strawberry Kiwi	½ cup	100	0	0

BIG BOY
DESSERTS

FOOD	PORTION	CALS	FAT	SAT FAT
Frozen Yogurt Fat Free	1 serv	118	0	—
Frozen Yogurt Shake	1	156	1	—
MAIN MENU SELECTIONS				
Baked Cod w/ Salad Baked Potato Roll & Margarine	1 meal	744	21	—
Baked Potato	1	163	2	—
Breast of Chicken Pita w/ Mozzarella & Ranch Dressing	1	361	11	—
Breast of Chicken w/ Mozzarella Salad Baked Potato Roll & Margarine	1 meal	697	20	—
Cabbage Soup	1 cup	34	4	—
Cabbage Soup	1 bowl	40	5	—

FOOD	PORTION	CALS	FAT	SAT FAT
Cajun Cod w/ Salad Baked Potato Roll & Margarine	1 meal	736	21	—
Chicken & Pasta Primavera w/ Salad Roll & Margarine	1 meal	676	14	—
Chicken 'n Vegetable Stir Fry w/ Salad Baked Potato Roll & Margarine	1 meal	795	18	—
Dinner Roll	1	210	5	—
Plain Egg Beaters Omelette w/ Whole Wheat Bread & Margarine	1 meal	305	10	—
Promise Margarine	1 pat	25	3	—
Rice Pilaf	1 serv	153	4	—
Scrambled Egg Beaters w/ Whole Wheat Bread & Margarine	1 meal	305	10	—
Southwest Chicken w/ Salad Baked Potato Roll & Margarine	1 meal	702	18	—
Spaghetti Marinara w/ Salad Roll & Margarine	1 meal	754	11	—
Turkey Pita w/ Ranch Dressing	1	245	6	—
Vegetable Stir Fry w/ Salad Baked Potato Roll & Margarine	1 meal	616	14	—
Vegetarian Egg Beaters Omelette w/ Whole Wheat Bread & Margarine	1 meal	330	10	—
SALAD DRESSINGS				
Italian Fat Free	1 oz	11	0	—
Lo Cal Oriental	1 oz	20	2	—
Lo Cal Ranch	1 oz	41	3	—
SALADS AND SALAD BARS				
Chicken Breast Salad w/ Roll & Margarine	1 serv	523	16	—
Oriental Chicken Breast Salad w/ Dinner Roll & Margarine	1 serv	660	20	—
Tossed Salad	1	35	2	—

BLIMPIE
COOKIES

FOOD	PORTION	CALS	FAT	SAT FAT
Chocolate Chunk	1	200	10	6
Macadamia White Chunk	1	210	10	5
Oatmeal Raisin	1	190	8	2
Peanut Butter	1	220	12	5
Sugar	1	330	17	5

FOOD	PORTION	CALS	FAT	SAT FAT
SALAD DRESSINGS AND TOPPINGS				
Caesar Dressing	1 serv (1.5 oz)	208	22	4
Cracked Peppercorn Dressing	1 serv (1.5 oz)	237	25	1
Frank's Red Hot Buffalo Sauce	1 serv (1 oz)	13	tr	tr
French's Honey Mustard	1 tbsp	5	0	0
GourMayo Chipotle Chili	1 tbsp	50	5	1
GourMayo Sun Dried Tomato	1 tbsp	50	5	1
GourMayo Wasabi Horseradish	1 tbsp	50	5	1
Guacamole	1 serv (1.5 oz)	194	18	3
Oil & Vinegar	1 serv	36	4	1
Pesto Dressing	1 serv (1 oz)	132	13	2
SALADS AND SALAD BARS				
Antipasto	1 reg serv	244	13	6
Chef	1 reg serv	212	9	5
Chili Ole	1 reg serv	480	27	11
Grilled Chicken w/ Caesar Dressing	1 reg serv	347	27	5
Grilled Chicken w/o Dressing	1 serv	139	5	2
Roast Beef 'N Blue	1 reg serv	390	16	10
Seafood	1 reg serv	122	4	1
Tuna	1 reg serv	261	20	3
Zesto Pesto Turkey	1 reg serv	370	19	8
SANDWICHES				
6 Inch Hot Sub BLT	1	588	32	10
6 Inch Hot Sub Buffalo Chicken	1	400	13	7
6 Inch Hot Sub Buffalo Chicken w/o Cheese	1	320	7	3
6 Inch Hot Sub ChiliMax	1	511	13	2
6 Inch Hot Sub Grilled Chicken	1	373	9	3
6 Inch Hot Sub Meatball	1	572	27	10
6 Inch Hot Sub MexiMelt	1	425	9	2
6 Inch Hot Sub Pastrami	1	507	17	7
6 Inch Hot Sub Steak & Onion Melt	1	440	16	6
6 Inch Hot Sub VegiMax	1	395	7	2
6 Inch Sub Blimpie Best	1	476	16	7
6 Inch Sub Club	1	440	12	6
6 Inch Sub Ham & Cheese	1	436	13	6
6 Inch Sub Roast Beef	1	468	14	6
6 Inch Sub Roast Beef w/o Cheese	1	388	8	2
6 Inch Sub Seafood	1	355	8	2
6 Inch Sub Tuna	1	493	23	4

FOOD	PORTION	CALS	FAT	SAT FAT
6 Inch Sub Turkey w/o Cheese	1	344	5	1
6 inch Sub Turkey	1	424	11	5
Cheddar	1 slice	52	5	3
Grilled Subs Beef Turkey & Cheddar	1	600	31	10
Grilled Subs Cuban	1	462	12	6
Grilled Subs Pastrami	1	462	14	6
Grilled Subs Reuben	1	630	33	5
Provolone	1 slice	80	6	4
Swiss	1 slice	80	6	4
Wraps Southwestern	1	674	35	8
Wraps Beef & Cheddar	1	714	37	11
Wraps Chicken Caesar	1	646	35	7
Wraps Steak & Onions	1	716	37	10
Wraps Ultimate BLT	1	831	50	15
Wraps Zesty Italian	1	638	33	10
SIDE ORDERS				
Cole Slaw	1 serv (5 oz)	180	13	2
Macaroni Salad	1 serv (5 oz)	360	25	4
Mustard Potato Salad	1 serv (5 oz)	160	5	1
Potato Chips Cheddar & Sour Cream	1 bag	210	11	2
Potato Chips Jalapeno	1 bag	210	11	2
Potato Chips Lea & Perrins Barbecue	1 bag	210	10	2
Potato Chips Regular	1 bag	210	11	2
Potato Chips Romano & Garlic	1 bag	210	11	2
Potato Chips Sour Cream & Onion	1 bag	210	11	2
Potato Salad	1 serv (5 oz)	270	19	3
SOUPS				
Chicken w/ White & Wild Rice	1 serv (8 oz)	230	12	2
Cream Of Broccoli & Cheese	1 serv (8 oz)	190	12	5
Cream Of Potato	1 serv (8 oz)	190	9	3
Garden Vegetable	1 serv (8 oz)	80	1	0
Grande Chili w/ Beans & Beef	1 serv (8 oz)	250	7	4
Homestyle Chicken Noodle	1 serv (8 oz)	120	3	1
Tomato Basil w/ Raviolini	1 serv (8 oz)	110	1	0
Vegetable Beef	1 serv (8 oz)	80	2	1
BOJANGLES				
Biscuit	1	243	12	3
Biscuit + Bacon	1	290	17	5
Biscuit + Bacon Egg Cheese	1	550	42	14

FOOD	PORTION	CALS	FAT	SAT FAT
Biscuit + Cajun Filet	1	454	21	6
Biscuit + Country Ham	1	270	15	4
Biscuit + Egg	1	400	30	6
Biscuit + Sausage	1	350	23	7
Biscuit + Smoked Sausage	1	380	26	9
Biscuit + Steak	1	649	49	13
Botato Rounds	1 serv	235	11	4
Buffalo Bites	1 serv	180	5	2
Cajun Pintos	1 serv	110	0	0
Cajun Spiced Breast	1 serv	278	17	—
Cajun Spiced Leg	1 serv	284	19	—
Cajun Spiced Thigh	1 serv	310	23	—
Cajun Spiced Wing	1 serv	355	25	—
Chicken Supremes	1 serv	337	16	6
Corn On The Cob	1 serv	140	2	0
Dirty Rice	1 serv	166	6	2
Green Beans	1 serv	25	0	0
Macaroni & Cheese	1 serv	198	14	5
Marinated Cole Slaw	1 serv	136	3	0
Potatoes w/o Gravy	1 serv	80	1	0
Sandwich Cajun Filet w/o Mayo	1	337	11	5
Sandwich Cajun Filet w/ Mayo	1	437	22	7
Sandwich Grilled Filet w/ Mayo	1	335	16	5
Sandwich Grilled Filet w/o Mayo	1 serv	235	5	3
Seasoned Fries	1 serv	344	19	5
Southern Style Breast	1 serv	261	16	—
Southern Style Leg	1 serv	254	15	—
Southern Style Thigh	1 serv	308	21	—
Southern Style Wing	1 serv	337	21	—
Sweet Biscuit Bo Berry	1	220	10	3
Sweet Biscuit Cinnamon	1	320	18	4

BOSTON MARKET

BAKED SELECTIONS

FOOD	PORTION	CALS	FAT	SAT FAT
Brownie	1 (3.3 oz)	450	27	7
Cinnamon Apple Pie	⅓ pie (4.8 oz)	390	23	4
Cookie Chocolate Chip	1 (2.8 oz)	340	17	6

MAIN MENU SELECTIONS

FOOD	PORTION	CALS	FAT	SAT FAT
½ Chicken w/ Skin	1 serv (9.7 oz)	590	33	10
¼ Dark Meat Chicken No Skin	1 serv (3.3 oz)	190	10	3

FOOD	PORTION	CALS	FAT	SAT FAT
¼ Dark Meat Chicken w/ Skin	1 serv (4.4 oz)	320	21	6
¼ White Meat Chicken No Skin Or Wing	1 serv (4.9 oz)	170	4	1
¼ White Meat Chicken w/ Skin And Wing	1 serv (5.3 oz)	280	12	4
BBQ Baked Beans	¾ cup (7.1 oz)	270	5	2
BBQ Chicken Sandwich	1 (9.9 oz)	540	9	3
Baked Sweet Potato Low Fat	1 (12.5 oz)	460	7	1
Black Beans And Rice	1 cup (8 oz)	300	10	2
Boston Hearth Ham Lean	1 serv (5 oz)	210	9	4
Broccoli Cauliflower Au Gratin	¾ cup (6.1 oz)	200	11	7
Broccoli Rice Casserole	¾ cup (6 oz)	240	12	8
Broccoli With Red Peppers	¾ cup (3.4 oz)	60	4	1
Butternut Squash Low Fat	¾ cup (6.8 oz)	160	6	4
Chicken Gravy	1 serv (1 oz)	15	1	0
Chicken Salad Sandwich	1 (11.5 oz)	680	30	5
Chicken Sandwich w/ Cheese & Sauce	1 (12.4 oz)	750	33	12
Chicken Sandwich w/o Cheese & Sauce Low Fat	1 (10 oz)	430	5	1
Chunky Chicken Salad	¾ cup (5.5 oz)	370	27	5
Chunky Cinnamon Apple Sauce No Fat	¾ cup (6.4 oz)	250	0	0
Cole Slaw	¾ cup (6.5 oz)	300	19	3
Corn Bread	1 (2.4 oz)	200	6	2
Coyote Bean Salad	¾ cup (5.3 oz)	190	9	1
Cranberry Relish Low Fat	¾ cup (7.9 oz)	370	5	1
Creamed Spinach	¾ cup (6.4 oz)	260	20	13
Fruit Salad Low Fat	¾ cup (5.5 oz)	70	1	0
Green Bean Casserole	¾ cup (6 oz)	130	9	5
Green Beans	¾ cup (3 oz)	80	6	1
Ham Sandwich w/ Cheese & Sauce	1 (11.8 oz)	760	34	12
Ham Sandwich w/o Cheese & Sauce	1 (9.3 oz)	440	8	3
Homestyle Mashed Potatoes & Gravy	¾ cup (6.6 oz)	210	10	6
Honey Glazed Carrots	¾ cup (5.4 oz)	280	15	3
Hot Cinnamon Apples	¾ cup (6.4 oz)	250	5	1
Macaroni & Cheese	¾ cup (6.7 oz)	280	11	6
Mashed Potatoes	⅔ cup (5.6 oz)	190	9	6
Meat Loaf & Brown Gravy	1 serv (7 oz)	390	22	8
Meat Loaf & Chunky Tomato Sauce	1 serv (8 oz)	370	18	8
Meat Loaf Sandwich w/ Cheese	1 (13.8 oz)	860	33	16

FOOD	PORTION	CALS	FAT	SAT FAT
Meat Loaf Sandwich w/o Cheese	1 (12.3 oz)	690	21	7
New Potatoes Low Fat	¾ cup (4.6 oz)	130	3	0
Old Fashioned Potato Salad	¾ cup (6.2 oz)	340	24	4
Open Face Turkey Sandwich	1 (13.4 oz)	500	12	2
Original Chicken Pot Pie	1 pie (14.9 oz)	780	46	13
Oven Roasted Potato Planks Low Fat	5 pieces (5.8 oz)	180	5	1
Pastry Sandwich BBQ Chicken	1 (7.2 oz)	640	39	12
Pastry Sandwich Broccoli Chicken Cheddar	1 (7.2 oz)	690	47	13
Pastry Sandwich Ham & Cheddar	1 (6.6 oz)	640	41	13
Pastry Sandwich Italian Chicken	1 (7.2 oz)	630	41	12
Red Beans And Rice Low Fat	1 cup (8 oz)	260	5	0
Rice Pilaf	⅔ cup (5.1 oz)	180	5	1
Rotisserie Turkey Breast Skinless Low Fat	1 serv (5 oz)	170	1	1
Savory Stuffing	¾ cup (6.1 oz)	310	12	2
Southwest Savory Chicken	1 serv (9.6 oz)	400	15	5
Squash Casserole	¾ cup (6.6 oz)	330	24	13
Steamed Vegetables Low Fat	⅔ cup (3.7 oz)	35	1	0
Sweet Potato Casserole	¾ cup (6.4 oz)	280	18	5
Tabasco BBQ Drumstick	1 (2.4 oz)	130	6	2
Tabasco BBQ Wing	1 (1.8 oz)	110	7	2
Teriyaki Chicken ¼ White w/ Skin	1 serv (6.8 oz)	340	12	4
Teriyaki Chicken ¼ w/ Skin	1 serv (5.9 oz)	380	21	6
Triple Topped Chicken	1 serv (9.2 oz)	470	22	12
Turkey Club Sandwich	1 (11.1 oz)	650	26	8
Turkey Sandwich w/ Cheese & Sauce	1 (11.8 oz)	710	28	10
Turkey Sandwich w/o Cheese & Sauce	1 (9.3 oz)	400	4	1
Whole Kernel Corn	¾ cup (5.8 oz)	180	4	1
Zucchini Marinara Low Fat	¾ cup (6.6 oz)	60	3	0
SALADS AND SALAD BARS				
Caesar Salad Entree	1 serv (10 oz)	510	42	11
Caesar Salad w/o Dressing	1 serv (8 oz)	230	12	6
Caesar Side Salad	1 (4 oz)	200	17	5
Chicken Caesar Salad	1 serv (13 oz)	650	45	12
Tossed Salad w/ Caesar Dressing	1 serv (8 oz)	380	31	5
Tossed Salad w/ Fat Free Ranch	1 serv (8 oz)	160	3	0
Tossed Salad w/ Old Venice Dressing	1 serv (8 oz)	340	27	4
SOUPS				
Chicken Chili	1 cup (8.7 oz)	220	7	2

FOOD	PORTION	CALS	FAT	SAT FAT
Chicken Noodle	1 cup (8.4 oz)	130	5	1
Chicken Tortilla	1 cup (8.4 oz)	220	11	4
Potato	1 cup (8 oz)	270	16	8
Tomato Bisque	1 cup (8 oz)	280	23	10

BOSTON PIZZA
CHILDREN'S MENU SELECTIONS

FOOD	PORTION	CALS	FAT	SAT FAT
Corkscrews n' Cheese	1 serv	870	33	—
Dino Fingers & Fries w/ Ketchup	1 serv	680	35	—
Grill Cheese Sandwich w/ Fries & Ketchup	1 serv	770	32	—
Mini Lasagna	1 serv	400	14	—
Pint Sized Ham Pizza	1 serv	430	8	—
Potato Smiles	1 serv	580	30	—
Stuffed Pizza w/ Fries & Ketchup	1 serv	850	31	—
Super Spaghetti	1 serv	340	6	—

MAIN MENU SELECTIONS

FOOD	PORTION	CALS	FAT	SAT FAT
BBQ Ribs w/ Fries	1 serv	2220	148	—
BBQ Ribs w/ Garlic Mashed Potatoes	1 serv	1760	122	—
BBQ Ribs w/ Spaghetti	1 serv	1870	121	—
Baked Onion Soup	1 serv	210	7	—
Bayou Chicken Strips w/ Dipping Sauce	1 serv	370	16	—
Boston's Extreme Double Order	1 serv	1660	107	—
Boston's Extreme Starter Order	1 serv	940	61	—
Bruschetta	1 serv	640	39	—
Buffalo Chicken Fingers w/ Caesar Salad	1 serv	650	38	—
Buffalo Chicken Fingers w/ Fries	1 serv	1430	82	—
Buffalo Chicken Fingers w/ Light Ranch	1 serv	600	34	—
Cactus Cuts & Dip	1 serv	1380	83	—
Carne Amore	1 full order	1250	50	—
Cheese Toast	1 basket	800	41	—
Cheese Toast	1 serv	400	21	—
Chicken & Rib Combo	1 serv	1470	90	—
Chicken & Rib Combo w/ Fries	1 serv	1920	116	—
Chicken & Rib Combo w/ Spaghetti	1 serv	1590	90	—
Chicken Fingers w/ Caesar Salad	1 serv	640	38	—
Chicken Fingers w/ Fries	1 serv	1420	82	—

FOOD	PORTION	CALS	FAT	SAT FAT
Chicken Fingers w/ Light Ranch	1 serv	590	34	–
Chips & Salsa	1 serv	830	41	–
Deluxe Cheese Bread	1 basket	890	42	–
Deluxe Cheese Toast	1 serv	420	21	–
Fettuccini Cajun Shrimp	1 full order	1200	43	–
Fettuccini Four Cheese	1 full order	1370	64	–
Fettuccini Jambalaya	1 full order	1360	50	–
Fettuccini Spicy Chicken & Spinach	1 full order	1330	53	–
Fries	1 serv	700	33	–
Garlic Toast w/ Garlic Margarine	1 slice	170	6	–
Garlic Twist Bread	1 serv	540	15	–
Garlic Twist Bread	1 basket	1080	30	–
Homestyle Macaroni	1 full order	1490	83	–
Italian Pizza Bread w/ Dip	1 serv	1000	53	–
Ketchup	1 serv (2 oz)	20	1	–
Lasagna Boston's	1 full order	820	30	–
Lasagna Mediterranean	1 full order	870	35	–
Lasagna Seafood	1 full order	970	45	–
Linguini Chicken & Mushroom	1 full order	1320	53	–
Mashed Potatoes	1 serv	240	8	–
Mexican Beef w/ Sour Cream	1 serv	970	57	–
Mini Tortellini	1 serv	490	15	–
NY Steak Sandwich w/ Fries	1 serv	1580	96	–
Nachos	1 full order	1540	95	–
Nachos Beef	1 full order	1760	106	–
Nachos Chicken	1 full order	1630	96	–
Penne Baked 3 Cheese	1 full order	990	37	–
Penne Italiano	1 full order	1160	46	–
Penne Pisa Pesto	1 full order	1270	63	–
Penne Roast Veggie	1 full order	900	31	–
Pizza Bread w/o Meat Sauce	1 serv	520	14	–
Plain Pasta w/ Alfredo Sauce	1 full order	1200	52	–
Plain Pasta w/ Creamy Tomato Sauce	1 full order	1070	38	–
Plain Pasta w/ Marinara Sauce	1 full order	870	20	–
Plain Pasta w/ Meatsauce	1 full order	910	22	–
Plain Pasta w/ Seafood Sauce	1 full order	1050	36	–
Plain Pasta w/ Spicy Tomato Sauce	1 full order	880	20	–
Plain Pasta w/ Tex Mex Sauce	1 full order	940	23	–
Potato Skins	1 full order	860	53	–
Quesadilla Chicken w/ Sour Cream	1 serv	770	40	–

FOOD	PORTION	CALS	FAT	SAT FAT
Quesadilla Garden Veggie w/ Sour Cream	1 serv	750	40	—
Quesadilla Sundried Tomato w/ Sour Cream	1 serv	890	50	—
Shrimp Dinner w/ Fries	1 serv	1510	82	—
Shrimp Dinner w/ Garlic Mashed Potatoes	1 serv	1050	57	—
Shrimp Dinner w/ Spaghetti	1 serv	1180	56	—
Side Tossed Salad w/ House Dressing	1 serv	170	14	—
Sirloin Steak Dinner w/ Fries	1 serv	1910	113	—
Sirloin Steak Dinner w/ Garlic Mashed Potatoes	1 serv	1450	88	—
Sirloin Steak Dinner w/ Spaghetti	1 serv	1580	87	—
Smokey Mountain Spaghetti	1 full order	1860	71	—
Spaghetti w/ Meatsauce	1 serv	370	8	—
Spinach & Artichoke Dip w/ Tortilla Chips	1 serv	890	57	—
Steak & Shrimp Dinner w/ Fries	1 serv	1760	108	—
Steak & Shrimp Dinner w/ Garlic Mashed Potatoes	1 serv	1310	83	—
Steak & Shrimp Dinner w/ Spaghetti	1 serv	1430	82	—
The Ribber w/ Fries	1 serv	1470	85	—
The Ribber w/ Garlic Mashed Potatoes	1 serv	1010	60	—
The Ribber w/ Spaghetti	1 serv	1140	60	—
Tortellini w/ Alfredo Sauce	1 full order	1220	40	—
Tortellini w/ Creamy Tomato Sauce	1 full order	1370	57	—
Tortellini w/ Marinara Sauce	1 full order	1180	39	—
Tortellini w/ Meatsauce	1 full order	1500	71	—
Tortellini w/ Seafood Sauce	1 full order	1360	55	—
Tortellini w/ Spicy Tomato Sauce	1 full order	1180	39	—
Tortellini w/ Tex Mex Sauce	1 full order	1240	42	—
Veal Parmigan w/ Fries	1 serv	1550	88	—
Veal Parmigan w/ Garlic Mashed Potatoes	1 serv	1090	63	—
Veal Parmigan w/ Spaghetti	1 serv	1220	62	—
Wings BBQ Double Order	1 serv	1700	107	—
Wings BBQ Starter Size	1 serv	960	61	—
Wings Cajun Double Order	1 serv	1610	107	—
Wings Cajun Starter Size	1 serv	910	60	—

FOOD	PORTION	CALS	FAT	SAT FAT
Wings Honey Garlic Double Order	1 serv	1720	107	—
Wings Honey Garlic Starter Size	1 serv	970	60	—
Wings Screamin' Hot Double Order	1 serv	1630	107	—
Wings Screamin' Hot Starter Size	1 serv	920	60	—
Wings Teriyaki Double Order	1 serv	1690	107	—
Wings Teriyaki Starter Size	1 serv	950	60	—
Wings Thai Double Order	1 serv	1870	123	—
Wings Thai Starter Size	1 serv	1040	69	—
PIZZA				
Bacon Double Cheeseburger Individual	1 pie	1210	56	—
Bacon Double Cheeseburger Large	1 slice	350	15	—
Bacon Double Cheeseburger Medium	1 slice	300	13	—
Boston Royal Individual	1 pie	770	23	—
Boston Royal Large	1 slice	230	6	—
Boston Royal Medium	1 slice	200	6	—
Cajun Chicken Individual	1 pie	780	25	—
Cajun Chicken Large	1 slice	250	8	—
Cajun Chicken Medium	1 slice	200	7	—
Californian Individual	1 pie	580	8	—
Californian Large	1 slice	190	3	—
Californian Medium	1 slice	160	2	—
Four Cheese Individual	1 pie	800	29	—
Four Cheese Large	1 slice	260	10	—
Four Cheese Medium	1 slice	240	10	—
Great White Individual	1 pie	880	34	—
Great White Large	1 slice	260	9	—
Great White Medium	1 slice	220	8	—
Hawaiian Individual	1 pie	690	16	—
Hawaiian Large	1 slice	220	5	—
Hawaiian Medium	1 slice	180	4	—
Meat Lovers Individual	1 pie	1120	55	—
Meat Lovers Large	1 slice	330	15	—
Meat Lovers Medium	1 slice	280	14	—
Pepperoni Individual	1 pie	760	27	—
Pepperoni Large	1 slice	240	9	—
Pepperoni Medium	1 slice	200	7	—
Pepperoni & Mushroom Individual	1 pie	760	27	—
Pepperoni & Mushroom Large	1 slice	250	9	—

FOOD	PORTION	CALS	FAT	SAT FAT
Pepperoni & Mushroom Medium	1 slice	200	7	—
Perogy Individual	1 pie	1010	45	—
Perogy Large	1 slice	330	15	—
Perogy Medium	1 slice	280	13	—
Popeye Individual	1 pie	730	21	—
Popeye Large	1 slice	240	7	—
Popeye Medium	1 slice	200	6	—
Rustic Italian Individual	1 pie	940	37	—
Rustic Italian Large	1 slice	310	12	—
Rustic Italian Medium	1 slice	250	10	—
Sante Fe Chicken Individual	1 pie	800	27	—
Sante Fe Chicken Large	1 slice	260	9	—
Sante Fe Chicken Medium	1 slice	220	7	—
Super Veggie Individual	1 pie	850	29	—
Super Veggie Large	1 slice	280	10	—
Super Veggie Medium	1 slice	230	7	—
Thai Chicken Individual	1 pie	870	29	—
Thai Chicken Large	1 slice	280	10	—
Thai Chicken Medium	1 slice	240	8	—
The Basic Individual	1 pie	620	15	—
The Basic Large	1 slice	200	5	—
The Basic Medium	1 slice	160	4	—
The Deluxe Individual	1 pie	780	26	—
The Deluxe Large	1 slice	240	7	—
The Deluxe Medium	1 slice	190	6	—
Tropical Chicken Individual	1 pie	1060	50	—
Tropical Chicken Large	1 slice	340	16	—
Tropical Chicken Medium	1 slice	280	13	—
Tuscan Individual	1 pie	900	32	—
Tuscan Large	1 slice	290	11	—
Tuscan Medium	1 slice	240	8	—
Vegetarian Individual	1 pie	670	15	—
Vegetarian Large	1 slice	220	5	—
Vegetarian Medium	1 slice	170	4	—
Zorba The Greek Individual	1 pie	810	27	—
Zorba The Greek Large	1 slice	270	9	—
Zorba The Greek Medium	1 slice	220	7	—
SALADS AND SALAD BARS				
Boston's Cobb Salad	1 serv	1100	80	—
Caesar Salad	1 reg	260	21	—

FOOD	PORTION	CALS	FAT	SAT FAT
Caesar Salad Meal Sized	1 serv	690	48	–
Greek Salad	1 serv	500	44	–
Greek Salad Meal Sized	1 serv	1110	90	–
House Dressing	1 serv (2 oz)	136	13	–
Spinach Salad	1 serv	190	14	–
Spinach Salad Meal Sized	1 serv	500	31	–
Taco Salad Beef w/ Sour Cream & Salsa	1 serv	640	41	–
Taco Salad Chicken w/ Sour Cream & Salsa	1 serv	520	28	–
Thai Chicken Salad	1 serv	730	21	–
Tossed Garden Greens w/ House Dressing	1 serv	170	14	–
Veggie Plate w/ Low Fat Ranch Dressing	1 serv	180	7	–
SANDWICHES				
BBQ Beef w/ Fries	1 serv	1580	62	–
Beef Dip w/ Fries & Au Jus	1 serv	1560	72	–
Boston Cheesesteak w/ Fries & Au Jus	1 serv	1790	87	–
Boston Brute w/ Fries	1 serv	1420	60	–
Buffalo Chicken w/ Fries	1 serv	1720	80	–
Chicken Foccacia w/ Fries	1 serv	1350	65	–
Spicy Italian Sausage w/ Caesar Salad	1 serv	1070	51	–
Stromboli Chicken w/ Caesar Salad	1 serv	1020	44	–
Stromboli Perogy w/ Caesar Salad	1 serv	1120	58	–
Stromboli Sante Fe w/ Caesar Salad	1 serv	1000	45	–
Super Ham & Cheese w/ Fries	1 serv	1370	71	–
Tango Chicken Wrap w/ Caesar Salad	1 serv	740	42	–
BROWN'S CHICKEN				
Breadsticks w/ Garlic Butter	1	199	4	–
Breast	3.5 oz	284	15	–
Coleslaw	3.5 oz	131	10	–
Corn Fritters	3.5 oz	415	25	–
Corn On Cob	1 ear (3 inch)	126	3	–
Fettucini Alfredo	1 serv (12 oz)	1507	64	–
French Fries	3.5 oz	503	22	–
Gizzard	3.5 oz	387	20	–
Leg	3.5 oz	287	16	–

FOOD	PORTION	CALS	FAT	SAT FAT
Liver	3.5 oz	341	19	—
Mostaccioli w/ Meat	1 serv (12 oz)	835	14	—
Mostaccioli w/o Meat	1 serv (12 oz)	792	10	—
Mushrooms	3.5 oz	289	16	—
Potato Salad	3.5 oz	94	4	—
Ravioli w/ Meat	1 serv (12 oz)	865	20	—
Ravioli w/o Meat	1 serv (12 oz)	822	16	—
Shrimp	3.5 oz	277	10	—
Thigh	3.5 oz	355	24	—
Wing	3.5 oz	385	25	—

BRUEGGER'S BAGELS
BAGELS

FOOD	PORTION	CALS	FAT	SAT FAT
Blueberry	1	330	2	0
Chocolate Chip	1	310	5	2
Cinnamon Raisin	1	320	2	0
Cinnamon Sugar	1	340	2	0
Everything	1	310	2	0
Garlic	1	310	2	0
Honey Grain	1	330	3	0
Jalapeno Bagel	1	310	2	0
Onion	1	310	2	0
Orange Cranberry	1	330	2	0
Plain	1	300	2	0
Poppy Seed	1	310	3	0
Pumpernickel	1	320	3	0
Rosemary Olive Oil	1	350	6	1
Salt	1	300	2	0
Sesame	1	320	2	0
Sun Dried Tomato	1	320	2	0

DESSERTS

FOOD	PORTION	CALS	FAT	SAT FAT
Blondies	1	370	23	6
Brownie Chocolate Chunk	1	330	19	7
Brownie Mint	1	300	17	7
Bruegger Bar	1	420	24	11
Cappuccino Bar	1	420	25	9
Luscious Lemon Bar	1	350	20	7
Oatmeal Cranberry Mountains	1	430	24	13
Raspberry Sammies	1	270	13	8

FOOD	PORTION	CALS	FAT	SAT FAT
SANDWICH FILLINGS				
Atlantic Smoked Salmon	2 oz	90	3	1
Cream Cheese Bacon Scallion	2 tbsp	100	8	5
Cream Cheese Chive	2 tbsp	100	9	5
Cream Cheese Garden Veggie	2 tbsp	90	8	5
Cream Cheese Garden Veggie Light	2 tbsp	60	4	3
Cream Cheese Herb Garlic Light	2 tbsp	70	5	3
Cream Cheese Honey Walnut	2 tbsp	110	8	5
Cream Cheese Jalapeno	2 tbsp	100	9	5
Cream Cheese Light Strawberry	2 tbsp	70	4	3
Cream Cheese Olive Pimento	2 tbsp	100	9	4
Cream Cheese Plain	2 tbsp	90	8	5
Cream Cheese Plain Light	2 tbsp	70	5	2
Cream Cheese Smoked Salmon	2 tbsp	100	9	5
Cream Cheese Wildberry	2 tbsp	100	9	5
Hummus	2 tbsp	60	4	1
Tuna Salad	1 serv (2.5 oz)	180	14	2
SANDWICHES				
Chicken Breast	1	440	6	2
Chicken Fajita	1	500	12	5
Chicken Salad w/ Mayo	1	460	12	2
Deli-Style Ham w/ Honey Mustard	1	440	5	1
Egg Cheese	1	480	15	6
Egg Cheese Sausage	1	680	33	12
Egg Cheese Bacon	1	560	22	9
Egg Cheese Ham	1	520	17	7
Garden Veggie	1	390	3	0
Herby Turkey	1	530	14	7
Leonardo Da Veggie	1	460	11	6
Santa Fe Turkey	1	480	10	4
Turkey w/ Mayo	1	480	14	2
BURGER KING				
BEVERAGES				
Cocoa Cola Classic	1 med (22 fl oz)	280	0	0
Coffee	1 serv (12 oz)	5	0	0
Diet Coke	1 med (22 fl oz)	1	0	0
Milk 2%	1 (8 oz)	130	5	3
Shake Chocolate	1 med (13.9 oz)	440	10	6
Shake Chocolate	1 sm (10.7 oz)	330	7	4

FOOD	PORTION	CALS	FAT	SAT FAT
Shake Chocolate Syrup Added	1 med (15.9 oz)	570	10	6
Shake Chocolate Syrup Added	1 sm (11.7 oz)	390	7	4
Shake Strawberry Syrup Added	1 med (15.9 oz)	550	9	5
Shake Strawberry Syrup Added	1 sm (11.7 oz)	390	7	4
Shake Vanilla	1 med (13.9 oz)	430	9	5
Shake Vanilla	1 sm (10.7 oz)	330	7	4
Sprite	1 med (22 fl oz)	260	0	0
Tropicana Orange Juice	1 serv (10 oz)	140	0	0
BREAKFAST SELECTIONS				
AM Express Dip	1 serv (1 oz)	80	0	0
AM Express Grape Jam	1 serv (0.4 oz)	30	0	0
AM Express Strawberry Jam	1 serv (0.4 oz)	30	0	0
Bacon	3 strips (0.3 oz)	40	3	1
Biscuit	1 (3.3 oz)	300	15	3
Biscuit w/ Bacon Egg & Cheese	1 (6.6 oz)	620	43	14
Biscuit w/ Egg	1 (4.6 oz)	380	21	5
Biscuit w/ Sausage	1 (4.6 oz)	490	33	10
Cini-minis w/o Icing	4 (3.8 oz)	440	23	6
Croissan'wich Sausage Egg & Cheese	1 (5.3 oz)	530	41	13
Croissan'wich w/ Sausage & Cheese	1 (3.7 oz)	450	35	12
French Toast Sticks	5 sticks (4 oz)	440	23	5
Ham	1 serv (1.2 oz)	35	1	0
Hash Browns	1 sm (2.6 oz)	240	15	6
Land O'Lakes Whipped Classic Blend	1 serv (0.4 oz)	65	7	1
Vanilla Icing Cini-Minis	1 serv (1 oz)	110	3	tr
MAIN MENU SELECTIONS				
American Cheese	2 slices (0.9 oz)	90	8	5
BK Big Fish Sandwich	1 (8.8 oz)	720	43	9
BK Broiler Chicken Breast Patty	1 (3.5 oz)	140	4	1
BK Broiler Chicken Sandwich	1 (8.7 oz)	530	16	5
BK Broiler Chicken Sandwich w/o Mayo	1 (8.7 oz)	370	9	5
Bacon Cheeseburger	1 (4.9 oz)	400	22	10
Bacon Double Cheeseburger	1 (7.2 oz)	630	38	18
Big King Sandwich	1 (7.6 oz)	640	42	18
Bull's Eye Barbecue Sauce	1 serv (0.5 oz)	20	0	0
Cheeseburger	1 (4.7 oz)	360	19	9
Chick'N Crisp Sandwich	1 (4.9 oz)	460	27	6
Chick'N Crisp Sandwich w/o Mayo	1 (4.9 oz)	360	16	6
Chicken Sandwich	1 (8 oz)	710	43	9

FOOD	PORTION	CALS	FAT	SAT FAT
Chicken Sandwich w/o Mayo	1 (8 oz)	500	20	9
Chicken Tenders	4 (2.2 oz)	180	11	3
Chicken Tenders	8 (4.3 oz)	350	22	7
Chicken Tenders	5 (2.7 oz)	230	14	4
Dipping Sauce Barbecue	1 serv (1 oz)	35	0	0
Dipping Sauce Honey	1 serv (1 oz)	90	0	0
Dipping Sauce Honey Mustard	1 serv (1 oz)	90	6	1
Dipping Sauce Ranch	1 serv (1 oz)	170	17	3
Dipping Sauce Sweet & Sour	1 serv (1 oz)	45	0	0
Double Cheeseburger	1 (6.9 oz)	580	36	17
Double Whopper	1 (12.2 oz)	920	59	21
Double Whopper w/ Cheese	1 (13.1 oz)	1010	67	26
Double Whopper w/ Mayo	1 (13.1 oz)	850	50	26
Double Whopper w/o Mayo	1 (12.2 oz)	760	42	21
Dutch Apple Pie	1 serv (4 oz)	300	15	3
French Fries No Salt	1 king size (6 oz)	590	30	12
French Fries No Salt	1 sm (2.6 oz)	250	13	5
French Fries No Salt	1 med (4.1 g)	400	21	8
French Fries Salted	1 sm (2.6 oz)	250	13	5
French Fries Salted	1 med (4.1 oz)	400	21	8
French Fries Salted	1 king size (6 oz)	590	30	12
Hamburger	1 (4.2 oz)	320	15	6
Hamburger Bun	1 (4.6 oz)	130	2	0
Hamburger Patty	1 (1.9 oz)	170	13	6
Hash Browns	1 lg (4.5 oz)	410	26	10
Ketchup	1 serv (0.5 oz)	15	0	0
King Sauce	1 serv (0.5 oz)	70	7	1
Lettuce	1 leaf (0.7 oz)	0	0	0
Mustard	1 serv (3 g)	0	0	0
Onion	1 serv (0.5 oz)	5	0	0
Onion Rings	1 med serv (3.3 oz)	380	19	4
Onion Rings	1 king serv (5.3 oz)	600	30	7
Pickles	4 slices (0.5 oz)	0	0	0
Tartar Sauce	1 serv (1.5 oz)	260	29	4
Tomato	2 slices (1 oz)	5	0	0
Whopper	1 (9.5 oz)	660	40	12
Whopper Bun	1 (2.7 oz)	220	4	1
Whopper Jr.	1 (5.5 oz)	400	24	8

FOOD	PORTION	CALS	FAT	SAT FAT
Whopper Jr. w/ Cheese	1 (6 oz)	450	28	10
Whopper Jr. w/ Cheese w/o Mayo	1 (6 oz)	370	19	10
Whopper Jr. w/o Mayo	1 (5.5 oz)	320	15	8
Whopper Patty	1 (2.8 oz)	250	19	9
Whopper w/ Cheese	1 (10.4 oz)	760	48	17
Whopper w/ Cheese w/o Mayo	1 (10.4 oz)	600	31	17
Whopper w/o Mayo	1 (9.5 oz)	510	23	12

CARL'S JR.
BAKED SELECTIONS

FOOD	PORTION	CALS	FAT	SAT FAT
Cheese Danish	1	400	23	6
Cheesecake Strawberry Swirl	1 serv	290	17	9
Chocolate Cake	1 serv	300	12	3
Chocolate Chip Cookie	1	350	18	7
Muffin Blueberry	1	340	14	2
Muffin Bran Raisin	1	370	13	2

BEVERAGES

FOOD	PORTION	CALS	FAT	SAT FAT
Coca-Cola Classic	1 reg (21 oz)	220	0	0
Coffee	1 reg (12 oz)	2	tr	0
Diet Coke	1 reg (21 oz)	tr	0	0
Dr. Pepper	1 reg (21 oz)	200	0	0
Hot Chocolate	1 serv (12 oz)	120	2	2
Iced Tea	1 reg (12 oz)	5	0	0
Lemonade Minute Maid Orange	1 reg (21 oz)	200	0	0
Milk 1%	1 (10 fl oz)	150	3	2
Minute Maid Orange Soda	1 reg (21 oz)	200	0	0
Nestea Raspberry	1 reg (21 oz)	160	0	0
Orange Juice	1 (10 oz)	150	0	0
Ramblin' Root Beer	1 reg (21 oz)	220	0	0
Shake Chocolate	1 reg (32 oz)	770	15	10
Shake Strawberry	1 reg (32 oz)	750	15	10
Shake Vanilla	1 reg (32 oz)	700	16	11
Sprite	1 reg (21 oz)	200	0	0

BREAKFAST SELECTIONS

FOOD	PORTION	CALS	FAT	SAT FAT
Bacon	2 strips	45	4	2
Breakfast Burrito	1	560	32	11
Breakfast Quesadilla	1	370	17	5
English Muffin w/ Margarine	1	210	9	2
French Toast Dips w/o Syrup	1 serv	370	20	3
Grape Jelly	1 serv (0.5 oz)	40	0	0

FOOD	PORTION	CALS	FAT	SAT FAT
Hash Brown Nuggets	1 serv	330	21	5
Sausage	1 patty	190	18	6
Scrambed Eggs	1 serv	180	14	3
Sourdough Breakfast	1 serv	410	20	10
Strawberry Jam	1 serv (0.5 oz)	40	0	0
Sunrise Sandwich w/o Meat	1	360	21	8
Table Syrup	1 serv (1 oz)	90	0	0
MAIN MENU SELECTIONS				
American Cheese	1 sm	50	4	3
BBQ Sauce	1 serv (1.1 oz)	50	0	0
Breadstick	1 (0.3 oz)	35	1	0
Carl's Famous Star	1	590	32	9
Chicken Stars	6 pieces	260	16	5
CrissCut Fries	1 serv	410	24	5
Croutons	1 serv (0.5 oz)	30	1	0
Double Sourdough Bacon Cheeseburger	1	880	59	24
Double Western Bacon Cheeseburger	1	920	50	21
Famous Bacon Cheeseburger	1	700	41	13
French Fries	1 med	460	22	5
French Fries	1 kid size	250	12	3
Hamburger	1	280	9	4
Honey Sauce	1 serv (1 oz)	90	0	0
Mustard Sauce	1 serv (1 oz)	50	0	0
Onion Rings	1 serv	430	22	5
Potato Bacon & Cheese	1	640	29	9
Potato Broccoli & Cheese	1 serv	530	21	5
Potato Plain w/o Margarine	1	290	0	0
Potato Sour Cream & Chives	1	430	14	4
Salsa	1 serv (0.9 oz)	10	0	0
Sandwich Bacon Swiss Crispy Chicken	1	760	38	11
Sandwich Carl's Catch Fish	1	530	28	7
Sandwich Charbroiled Sirloin Steak	1	550	24	5
Sandwich Chargrilled Chicken Club	1	470	23	7
Sandwich Chargrilled Santa Fe Chicken	1	540	31	8
Sandwich Chargrilled BBQ Chicken	1	290	4	1
Sandwich Ranch Crispy Chicken	1	660	31	7
Sandwich Southwest Spicy Chicken	1	620	41	10

FOOD	PORTION	CALS	FAT	SAT FAT
Sandwich Spicy Chicken	1	480	26	5
Sandwich Western Bacon Crispy Chicken	1	750	28	11
Sourdough Bacon Cheeseburger	1	640	41	15
Sourdough Ranch Bacon Cheeseburger	1	720	46	16
Super Star	1	790	47	15
Sweet N'Sour Sauce	1 serv (1 oz)	50	0	0
Swiss Cheese	1 serv	50	4	3
Western Bacon Cheeseburger	1	660	30	12
Zucchini	1 serv	320	19	5
SALAD DRESSINGS				
1000 Island	1 serv (2 oz)	230	23	4
Blue Cheese	1 serv (2 oz)	320	35	7
French Fat Free	1 serv (2 oz)	60	0	0
House	1 serv (2 oz)	220	22	4
Italian Fat Free	1 serv (2 oz)	15	0	0
SALADS AND SALAD BARS				
Salad-To-Go Charbroiled Chicken	1 serv	200	7	3
Salad-To-Go Garden	1	50	3	2

CARVEL
BEVERAGES

FOOD	PORTION	CALS	FAT	SAT FAT
Carvelanche w/ Topping	1 (16 oz)	600	30	18
Regular Fizzlers	1 (16 oz)	340	5	3
Thick Shake Chocolate	1 (16 oz)	720	31	18
Thick Shake Reduced Fat Chocolate	1 (16 oz)	520	8	5
Thick Shake Reduced Fat Vanilla	1 (16 oz)	460	7	4
Thick Shake Vanilla	1 (16 oz)	657	30	18
ICE CREAM				
Cake Butterscotch Dream	1 slice (4 oz)	260	10	6
Cake Celebration	1 slice (4 oz)	200	10	7
Cake Cookies & Cream	1 serv (4 oz)	240	12	7
Cake Fudge Drizzle	1 slice (4 oz)	240	11	7
Cake Fudgie The Whale	1/14 cake (3.6 oz)	290	16	7
Cake Game Ball	1 slice (4 oz)	330	17	10
Cake Holiday	1 slice (4 oz)	200	10	7
Cake Lil'Love	1 piece (4 oz)	200	10	7
Cake Lil'Love All Vanilla	1 piece (4.4 oz)	330	16	10
Cake Sinfully Chocolate	1 slice (4 oz)	240	10	6

FOOD	PORTION	CALS	FAT	SAT FAT
Cake Strawberries & Cream	1 slice (4 oz)	270	10	6
Chocolate	4 oz	190	10	6
Chocolate No Fat	4 oz	120	0	0
Flying Saucer 98% Fat Free Black Raspberry	1	170	2	0
Flying Saucer 98% Fat Free Chocolate	1	170	2	0
Flying Saucer 98% Fat Free Coffee	1	190	2	0
Flying Saucer 98% Fat Free Maple	1	190	2	0
Flying Saucer 98% Fat Free Mint	1	190	2	0
Flying Saucer 98% Fat Free Pistachio	1	190	2	0
Flying Saucer 98% Fat Free Strawberry	1	190	2	0
Flying Saucer 98% Fat Free Vanilla	1	190	2	0
Flying Saucer Chocolate	1	230	9	5
Flying Saucer Vanilla	1	240	10	5
Vanilla	4 oz	200	10	6
Vanilla No Fat	4 oz	120	0	0
Vanilla No Sugar Added	4 oz	130	3	2
ICES				
Italian Ice Blue Raspberry	4 oz	70	0	0
Italian Ice Bubble Gum	4 oz	70	0	0
Italian Ice Cherry	4 oz	100	0	0
Italian Ice Chocolate Ice Cream	4 oz	90	1	0
Italian Ice Cotton Candy	4 oz	70	0	0
Italian Ice Lemon	4 oz	70	0	0
Italian Ice Mango	4 oz	70	0	0
Italian Ice Orange	4 oz	70	0	0
Italian Ice Vanilla Ice Cream	4 oz	90	2	0
Italian Ice Watermelon	4 oz	70	0	0
Sherbet All Flavors	4 oz	140	1	1
CHICK-FIL-A				
BEVERAGES				
Coca-Cola Classic	1 sm	110	0	0
Diet Coke	1 sm	0	0	0
Diet Lemonade	1 sm	25	0	0
Ice Tea Sweetened	1 sm	80	0	0
Iced Tea Unsweetened	1 serv	0	0	0
Lemonade	1 sm	170	1	0

FOOD	PORTION	CALS	FAT	SAT FAT
DESSERTS				
Cheesecake w/ Blueberry Topping	1 slice	370	21	12
Cheesecake w/ Strawberry Topping	1 slice	360	21	12
Fudge Nut Brownie	1	330	15	4
IceDream Cup	1 sm	230	6	4
IceDream Cone	1 sm	160	4	2
Lemon Pie	1 slice	320	10	4
MAIN MENU SELECTIONS				
Barbecue Sauce	1 pkg	45	0	0
Carrot & Raisin Salad	1 sm	130	6	1
Chargrilled Chicken Caesar Salad	1 serv	240	10	6
Chargrilled Chicken Club Sandwich w/o Sauce	1	360	13	5
Chargrilled Chicken Deluxe Sandwich	1	280	7	2
Chargrilled Chicken Filet	1	100	2	0
Chargrilled Chicken Sandwich	1	280	7	2
Chargrilled Chicken Sandwich w/o Butter	1	240	4	1
Chick-N-Strips	4	250	11	3
Chicken Deluxe Sandwich	1	420	16	4
Chicken Sandwich	1	410	16	4
Chicken Sandwich w/o Butter	1	380	13	3
Chicken Filet	1	230	11	3
Chicken Salad Sandwich On Whole Wheat	1	350	15	3
Cole Slaw	1 sm	210	17	3
Cool Wrap Chargrilled Chicken	1	390	7	8
Cool Wrap Chicken Caesar	1	460	11	6
Cool Wrap Spicy Chicken	1	390	7	4
Dijon Honey Mustard Sauce	1 pkg	50	5	1
Hearty Breast of Chicken Soup	1 cup	100	2	0
Honey Mustard Sauce	1 pkg	45	0	0
Nuggets	8	260	12	3
Polynesian Sauce	1 pkg	110	6	1
Waffle Fries w/o Salt	1 sm	280	14	5
Waffle Potato Fries	1 sm	280	14	5
SALAD DRESSINGS				
Basil Vinaigrette	1 pkg	210	21	4
Blue Cheese	1 pkg	190	20	4
Buttermilk Ranch	1 pkg	190	20	3

FOOD	PORTION	CALS	FAT	SAT FAT
Caesar	1 pkg	200	21	4
Fat Free Dijon Honey Mustard	1 pkg	60	0	0
Light Italian	1 pkg	20	1	0
Spicy	1 pkg	210	22	4
Thousand Island	1 pkg	170	16	3
SALADS AND SALAD BARS				
Chargrilled Chicken Garden Salad	1 serv	180	6	3
Chick-N-Strips Salad	1 serv	340	16	5
Croutons Garlic & Butter	1 pkg	90	4	0
Roasted Sunflower Kernels Unsalted	1 pkg	80	7	1
Side Salad	1 serv	80	5	3

CHILI'S
DESSERTS

FOOD	PORTION	CALS	FAT	SAT FAT
Diet By Chocolate Cake	1 serv	370	2	1
Diet By Chocolate Cake w/ Yogurt	1 serv	465	2	1
Diet By Chocolate Cake w/ Yogurt & Fudge Topping	1 serv	534	3	1
MAIN MENU SELECTIONS				
Guiltless Grill Chicken Fajitas	1 serv	726	13	4
Guiltless Grill Chicken Platter	1 serv	563	7	3
Guiltless Grill Chicken Salad w/ Dressing	1 serv	254	3	1
Guiltless Grill Chicken Sandwich	1	527	7	2
Guiltless Grill Veggie Pasta	1 serv	590	11	3
Guiltless Grill Veggie Pasta w/ Chicken	1 serv	696	13	4

CHURCH'S CHICKEN
DESSERTS

FOOD	PORTION	CALS	FAT	SAT FAT
Apple Pie	1 pie	280	12	–
Edward's Double Lemon Pie	1 pie	300	14	–
Edward's Strawberry Cream Cheese Pie	1 pie	280	15	–
MAIN MENU SELECTIONS				
Breast	1 serv	200	12	–
Cajun Rice	1 reg	130	7	–
Chicken Fried Steak w/ White Gravy	1 serv	470	28	–
Cole Slaw	1 reg	92	6	–
Collard Greens	1 reg	25	0	0
Corn On The Cob	1 ear	139	3	–

FOOD	PORTION	CALS	FAT	SAT FAT
French Fries	1 reg	210	11	—
Honey Butter Biscuit	1	250	16	—
Jalapeno Cheese Bombers	4 pieces	240	10	—
Krispy Tender Strips	1 piece	137	5	—
Leg	1 serv	140	9	—
Macaroni & Cheese	1 reg	210	11	—
Mashed Potatoes & Gravy	1 reg	90	3	—
Okra	1 reg	210	16	—
Sweet Corn Nuggets	1 reg	250	12	—
Tender Crunchers	6-8 pieces	411	15	—
Thigh	1 serv	230	16	—
Whole Jalapeno Peppers	2	10	0	0
Wing	1 serv	250	16	—
SAUCES				
BBQ	1 pkg	29	0	0
Creamy Jalapeno	1 pkg	102	11	—
Honey Mustard	1 pkg	111	11	—
Purple Pepper	1 pkg	21	0	0
Sweet & Sour	1 pkg	31	0	0
CINNABON				
Caramel Pecanbon	1	890	41	13
Cinnabon	1 reg	670	34	14
COLOMBO FROZEN YOGURT				
Strawberry Lowfat	½ cup	110	2	1
Strawberry Nonfat	½ cup	100	0	0
D'ANGELO'S SANDWICH SHOP				
CHILDREN'S MENU SELECTIONS				
D'Lite Turkey	1 kidz	217	3	0
Sub Cheeseburger	1 kidz	294	13	6
Sub Ham & Cheese	1 kidz	214	4	2
Sub Meatball	1 kidz	330	15	5
Sub Tuna	1 kidz	450	30	4
SALAD DRESSINGS AND TOPPINGS				
Bacon	1 serv	64	5	2
Bleu Cheese	1 serv (1 oz)	152	15	3
Buffalo Sauce	1 serv (1 oz)	10	0	0
Caesar	1 serv (1 oz)	140	15	3
Caesar Fat Free	1 serv (1 oz)	20	0	0

FOOD	PORTION	CALS	FAT	SAT FAT
Creamy Italian	1 serv (1 oz)	122	13	2
Cucumbers	3 slices	2	0	0
Greek Dressing w/ Feta	1 serv (3 oz)	227	26	4
Honey Mustard Dressing	1 serv (1 oz)	150	142	2
Hot Peppers	1 serv	0	0	0
Mayonnaise	2 tbsp	236	26	3
Mayonnaise Fat Free	1 pkg	10	0	0
Mustard Honey Dijon	2 tbsp	60	0	0
Mustard Yellow	2 tbsp	20	1	0
Olive Oil Vinaigrette	1 serv (3 oz)	170	17	3
Olive Oil Blend	2 tbsp	239	27	4
Ranch Lite	1 serv (3 oz)	240	19	3
Sesame Ginger	1 serv (1 oz)	170	7	1
SALADS				
Antipasto Salad w/o Dressing	1 serv	275	16	6
Asian Chicken w/o Dressing	1 serv	224	4	1
Caesar w/ Dressing	1 serv	474	39	7
Chef w/o Dressing	1 serv	273	12	5
Chicken Caesar w/ Dressing	1 serv	532	38	8
Chicken Stir Fry w/o Dressing	1 serv	166	3	1
Cobb w/o Dressing	1 serv	289	17	8
Greek w/o Dressing	1 serv	298	23	9
Lobster w/o Dressing	1 serv	385	27	3
Roast Beef w/o Dressing	1 serv	146	3	1
Tossed Garden w/o Dressing	1 serv	47	1	tr
Turkey w/o Dressing	1 serv	157	2	tr
SANDWICHES				
D'Lite Chicken Stir Fry	1 sm	426	6	1
D'Lite Fresh Veggie	1	348	7	3
D'Lite Grilled Chicken Breast	1 sm	387	7	1
D'Lite Ham & Cheese	1 sm	351	6	2
D'Lite Roast Beef	1 sm	353	5	1
D'Lite Turkey	1 sm	364	4	0
D'Lite Turkey Cranberry	1 sm	460	4	0
Pokket Caesar Salad	1 sm	643	40	7
Pokket Capacola & Cheese	1 sm	426	14	6
Pokket Cheeseburger	1 sm	481	25	11
Pokket Chicken Caesar Salad	1 sm	701	39	1
Pokket Chicken Club	1 sm	559	28	5
Pokket Chicken Honey Dijon	1 sm	527	20	7

FOOD	PORTION	CALS	FAT	SAT FAT
Pokket Chicken Salad	1 sm	705	42	6
Pokket Chicken Stir Fry	1 sm	425	10	5
Pokket Classic Veggie No Cheese	1 sm	238	2	tr
Pokket Greek	1 sm	812	61	14
Pokket Grilled Chicken	1 sm	328	5	1
Pokket Ham & Cheese	1 sm	349	9	5
Pokket Ham & Salami	1 sm	412	17	8
Pokket Hamburger	1 sm	422	21	8
Pokket Italian	1 sm	574	33	13
Pokket Lobster	1 sm	568	32	4
Pokket Meatball	1 sm	600	31	10
Pokket Mortadella & Cheese	1 sm	505	28	11
Pokket Seafood Salad	1 sm	532	28	3
Pokket Steak	1 sm	335	13	5
Pokket Steak & Cheese	1 sm	407	18	9
Pokket Tuna	1 sm	791	58	7
Sub Cheeseburger	1 sm	542	27	11
Sub Chicken Club	1 sm	619	30	5
Sub Chicken Honey Dijon	1 sm	587	22	7
Sub Chicken Salad	1 sm	769	44	6
Sub Chicken Stir Fry	1 sm	487	11	5
Sub Classic Veggie	1 sm	465	15	8
Sub Grilled Chicken	1 sm	387	7	1
Sub Ham & Cheese	1 sm	412	11	5
Sub Ham & Salami	1 sm	474	19	8
Sub Hamburger	1 sm	482	22	8
Sub Italian	1 sm	637	34	13
Sub Lobster	1 sm	628	33	4
Sub Meatball	1 sm	663	33	10
Sub Mortadella & Cheese	1 sm	568	29	11
Sub Number 9	1 sm	475	19	9
Sub Pastrami	1 sm	526	27	9
Sub Pepperoni	1 sm	614	34	13
Sub Roast Beef	1 sm	350	5	1
Sub Salad	1 sm	298	3	tr
Sub Salami & Cheese	1 sm	597	32	13
Sub Seafood Salad	1	595	29	3
Sub Steak	1 sm	383	14	5
Sub Steak & Cheese	1 sm	455	19	9
Sub Steak Tip	1 sm	486	14	3

FOOD	PORTION	CALS	FAT	SAT FAT
Sub Stuffed Turkey	1 sm	1036	37	9
Sub Tuna	1 sm	853	59	7
Sub Turkey	1 sm	361	4	0
Sub Turkey Club	1 sm	360	8	2
Wrap Asian Chicken Salad	1	914	24	5
Wrap BLT & Cheese	1	500	18	8
Wrap Buffalo Chicken Salad	1	778	36	5
Wrap Caesar Salad	1	669	37	7
Wrap Capacola & Cheese	1	451	12	6
Wrap Cheese	1	631	27	18
Wrap Cheeseburger	1	569	26	11
Wrap Chef	1	832	40	9
Wrap Chicken Caesar Salad	1	788	39	8
Wrap Chicken Cobb	1	855	46	12
Wrap Chicken Filet & Bacon	1	643	28	5
Wrap Chicken Honey Dijon	1	619	20	7
Wrap Chicken Salad	1	780	41	6
Wrap Chicken Stir Fry	1	511	10	5
Wrap Classic Veggie	1	490	14	8
Wrap Greek	1	761	61	14
Wrap Grilled Chicken	1	420	5	1
Wrap Ham & Cheese	1	436	9	5
Wrap Ham & Salami	1	499	17	8
Wrap Hamburger	1	509	21	8
Wrap Italian	1	654	32	13
Wrap Lobster	1	766	44	5
Wrap Meatball	1	687	31	10
Wrap Mortadella & Cheese	1	592	28	11
Wrap Number 9	1	494	18	9
Wrap Pastrami	1	550	25	9
Wrap Pepperoni	1	638	33	13
Wrap Roast Beef	1	374	4	1
Wrap Salad	1	322	2	tr
Wrap Salami & Cheese	1	605	29	12
Wrap Steak	1	402	13	5
Wrap Steak & Cheese	1	474	18	9
Wrap Steak Tip	1	374	12	3
Wrap Tuna	1	881	58	7
Wrap Turkey	1	385	3	0
Wrap Turkey Club	1	435	8	2

FOOD	PORTION	CALS	FAT	SAT FAT
SOUPS				
#9 Steak & Cheese	1 sm	280	21	12
Chicken Noodle	1 sm	130	2	1
Hearty Vegetable	1 sm	40	0	0
Lobster Bisque	1 sm	360	29	18
New England Clam Chowder	1 sm	270	20	12
Santa Fe Chipotle Vegetable	1 sm	130	1	0
Shrimp & Roasted Corn	1 sm	250	16	8
Thanksgiving Everyday	1 sm	250	17	9
DAIRY QUEEN				
FOOD SELECTIONS				
Chicken Breast Fillet Sandwich	1 (6.7 oz)	430	20	4
Chicken Strip Basket	1 serv (14.5 oz)	1000	50	13
Chili 'n' Cheese Dog	1 (5 oz)	330	21	9
DQ Homestyle Bacon Double Cheeseburger	1 (8.9 oz)	610	36	18
DQ Homestyle Cheeseburger	1 (5.3 oz)	340	17	8
DQ Homestyle Double Cheeseburger	1 (7.7 oz)	540	31	16
DQ Homestyle Hamburger	1 (4.8 oz)	290	12	5
DQ Ultimate Burger	1 (9.4 oz)	670	43	19
French Fries	1 sm (4 oz)	350	18	4
French Fries	1 med (3.9 oz)	440	23	5
Grilled Chicken Sandwich	1 (6.5 oz)	310	10	3
Hot Dog	1 (3.5 oz)	240	14	5
Onion Rings	1 serv (4 oz)	320	16	4
The Great Steakmelt Basket	1 serv (13.2 oz)	770	38	13
ICE CREAM				
Banana Split	1 (12.9 oz)	510	12	8
Blizzard Chocolate Sandwich Cookie	1 med (11.4 oz)	640	23	11
Blizzard Chocolate Sandwich Cookie	1 sm (12 oz)	520	18	9
Blizzard Chocolate Chip Cookie Dough	1 med (15.4 oz)	950	36	19
Blizzard Chocolate Chip Cookie Dough	1 sm (12 oz)	660	24	13
Breeze Heath	1 sm (10.2 oz)	470	10	6
Breeze Heath	1 med (14.2 oz)	710	18	11
Breeze Strawberry	1 sm (12 oz)	320	1	1
Breeze Strawberry	1 med (13.4 oz)	460	1	1
Buster Bar	1 (5.2 oz)	450	28	12

FOOD	PORTION	CALS	FAT	SAT FAT
Chocolate Malt	1 sm (14.7 oz)	650	16	10
Chocolate Malt	1 med (19.9 oz)	880	22	14
Cone Chocolate	1 sm (5 oz)	240	8	5
Cone Chocolate	1 med (6.9 oz)	340	11	7
Cone Vanilla	1 lg (8.9 oz)	410	12	8
Cone Vanilla	1 med (6.9 oz)	330	9	6
Cone Vanilla	1 sm (5 oz)	230	7	5
Cone Yogurt	1 med (6.9 oz)	260	1	1
Cone Dipped	1 med (7.7 oz)	490	24	13
Cone Dipped	1 sm (5.5 oz)	340	17	9
Cup Of Yogurt	1 med (6.7 oz)	230	1	0
DQ 8 Inch Round Cake Undecorated	⅛ of cake (6.2 oz)	340	13	8
DQ Fudge Bar No Sugar Added	1 (2.3 oz)	50	0	0
DQ Lemon Freez'r	½ cup (3.2 oz)	80	0	0
DQ Nonfat Frozen Yogurt	½ cup (3 oz)	100	0	0
DQ Sandwich	1 (2.1 oz)	200	6	3
DQ Soft Serve Chocolate	½ cup (3.3 oz)	150	5	4
DQ Soft Serve Vanilla	½ cup (3.3 oz)	140	5	3
DQ Treatzza Pizza Heath	⅛ of pie (2.3 oz)	180	7	4
DQ Treatzza Pizza M&M	⅛ of pie (2.4 oz)	190	7	4
DQ Vanilla Orange Bar No Sugar Added	1 (2.3 oz)	60	0	0
Dilly Bar Chocolate	1 (3 oz)	210	13	7
Frozen Hot Chocolate	1 (20.9 oz)	860	35	16
Misty Slush	1 sm (15.9 oz)	220	0	0
Misty Slush	1 med (20.9 oz)	290	0	0
Peanut Buster Parfait	1 (10.7 oz)	730	31	17
Pecan Mudslide Treat	1 (4.6 oz)	650	30	12
S'more Galore Parfait	1 (10.7 oz)	730	30	10
Shake Chocolate	1 med (18.9 oz)	770	20	13
Shake Chocolate	1 sm (13.9 oz)	560	15	10
Starkiss	1 (3 oz)	80	0	0
Strawberry Shortcake	1 (8.5 oz)	430	14	9
Sundae Chocolate	1 med (8.2 oz)	400	10	6
Sundae Chocolate	1 sm (5.7 oz)	280	7	5
Yogurt Sundae Strawberry	1 med (8.2 oz)	280	1	0

DELTACO
BEVERAGES

FOOD	PORTION	CALS	FAT	SAT FAT
Coffee	1 serv (8 oz)	0	0	0

FOOD	PORTION	CALS	FAT	SAT FAT
Coke Classic	1 med (12 oz)	150	0	0
Coke Classic	1 sm (10 oz)	120	0	0
Coke Classic	1 lg (20 oz)	230	0	0
Coke Classic Best Value	1 serv (27 oz)	320	0	0
Diet Coke	1 med (12 oz)	0	0	0
Diet Coke	1 lg (20 oz)	5	0	0
Diet Coke	1 sm (10 oz)	0	0	0
Diet Coke Best Value	1 serv (27 oz)	10	0	0
Iced Tea	1 med (12 oz)	0	0	0
Iced Tea	1 sm (10 oz)	0	0	0
Iced Tea	1 lg (20 oz)	5	0	0
Iced Tea Best Value	1 serv (27 oz)	10	0	0
Milk 1% Lowfat	1 serv (11 oz)	130	3	2
Mr Pibb	1 lg (20 oz)	230	0	0
Mr Pibb	1 sm (10 oz)	120	0	0
Mr Pibb	1 med (12 oz)	150	0	0
Mr Pibb Best Value	1 serv (27 oz)	320	0	0
Orange Juice	1 serv (11 oz)	140	0	0
Shake Chocolate	1 lg (15 oz)	680	16	12
Shake Chocolate	1 sm (11.4 oz)	520	12	9
Shake Strawberry	1 lg (15 oz)	540	8	6
Shake Strawberry	1 sm (11.4 oz)	410	6	4
Shake Vanilla	1 lg (15 oz)	550	10	6
Shake Vanilla	1 sm (11.4 oz)	420	7	5
Sprite	1 sm (10 oz)	110	0	0
Sprite	1 med (12 oz)	140	0	0
Sprite	1 lg (20 oz)	230	0	0
Sprite Best Value	1 serv (27 oz)	310	0	0
BREAKFAST SELECTIONS				
Burrito Breakfast	1 (3.8 oz)	250	11	6
Burrito Egg & Cheese	1 (7.5 oz)	450	24	13
Burrito Macho Bacon & Egg	1 (15.9 oz)	1030	60	20
Burrito Steak & Egg	1 (9 oz)	580	34	16
Quesadilla Bacon & Egg	1 (6.1 oz)	450	23	12
Side of Bacon	2 strips (0.3 oz)	50	4	2
MAIN MENU SELECTIONS				
Beans 'n Cheese Cup	1 serv (7.7 oz)	260	3	2
Burrito Combo	1 (8.2 oz)	490	21	13
Burrito Del Beef	1 (8 oz)	550	30	17
Burrito Del Classic Chicken	1 (8.5 oz)	580	38	13

FOOD	PORTION	CALS	FAT	SAT FAT
Burrito Deluxe Combo	1 (10.7 oz)	530	25	15
Burrito Deluxe Del Beef	1 (10.5 oz)	590	33	19
Burrito Green	1 (5 oz)	280	8	5
Burrito Macho Beef	1 (18.9 oz)	1170	62	29
Burrito Macho Combo	1 (19.4 oz)	1050	44	21
Burrito Red	1 (5 oz)	270	8	5
Burrito Red Regular	1 (7.5 oz)	390	12	9
Burrito Regular Green	1 (7.5 oz)	400	12	9
Burrito Spicy Chicken	1 (8.7 oz)	480	16	10
Burrito The Works	1 (10.2 oz)	480	18	11
Cheeseburger	1 (4.6 oz)	330	13	6
Del Cheeseburger	1 (5.6 oz)	430	25	7
Double Del Cheeseburger	1 (7.1 oz)	560	35	12
Fries	1 sm (3 oz)	210	14	2
Fries	1 reg (5 oz)	350	23	4
Fries Best Value	1 serv (7 oz)	490	32	5
Fries Chili Cheese	1 serv (10.5 oz)	670	46	15
Fries Deluxe Chili Cheese	1 serv (11.9 oz)	710	49	16
Get A Lot Meals #1 Combo Burrito Fries Drink	1 meal	980	44	16
Get A Lot Meals #2 Del Classic Chicken Burrito Fries Drink	1 meal	1080	61	17
Get A Lot Meals #3 Regular Red Burrito Fries Drink	1 meal	890	35	12
Get A Lot Meals #4 Two Chicken Soft Tacos Fries Drink	1 meal	910	46	11
Get A Lot Meals #5 Taco Combo Burrito Drink	1 meal	790	31	17
Get A Lot Meals #6 Two Tacos Quesadilla Drink	1 meal	960	47	29
Get A Lot Meals #7 Macho Combo Burrito Fries Drink	1 meal	1530	67	25
Get A Lot Meals #8 Two Big Fat Tacos Fries Drink	1 meal	802	45	14
Get A Lot Meals #9 Double Del Cheeseburger Fries Drink	1 meal	1050	58	16
Nachos	1 serv (4 oz)	380	24	8
Nachos Macho	1 serv (17 oz)	1200	66	26
Quesadilla Chicken	1 (6.8 oz)	580	31	21
Quesadilla Regular	1 (5.3 oz)	500	27	20

FOOD	PORTION	CALS	FAT	SAT FAT
Quesadilla Spicy Jack Chicken	1 (6.8 oz)	570	30	16
Quesadilla Spicy Jack Regular	1 (5.3 oz)	490	26	17
Rice Cup	1 serv (4 oz)	150	2	1
Soft Taco	1 (2.8 oz)	160	8	4
Soft Taco Chicken	1 (3.3 oz)	210	12	4
Taco	1 (2.2 oz)	160	10	4
Taco Big Fat	1 (5.4 oz)	320	11	5
Taco Big Fat Chicken	1 (5.4 oz)	340	13	4
Taco Big Fat Steak	1 (5.4 oz)	390	19	6
Taco Salad Deluxe	1 (18.8 oz)	760	37	17
Tostada Salad	1 (4.5 oz)	210	9	5

DOMINO'S PIZZA
12 INCH MEDIUM PIZZAS

FOOD	PORTION	CALS	FAT	SAT FAT
Add A Topping Anchovies	1 topping serv	23	1	tr
Add A Topping Bacon	1 topping serv	81	7	2
Add A Topping Banana Peppers	1 topping serv	3	tr	–
Add A Topping Canned Mushrooms	1 topping serv	4	tr	tr
Add A Topping Cheddar Cheese	1 topping serv	57	5	3
Add A Topping Cooked Beef	1 topping serv	56	5	2
Add A Topping Extra Cheese	1 topping serv	48	4	2
Add A Topping Fresh Mushrooms	1 topping serv	4	tr	tr
Add A Topping Green Olives	1 topping serv	12	1	tr
Add A Topping Green Peppers	1 topping serv	3	tr	–
Add A Topping Ham	1 topping serv	18	1	tr
Add A Topping Italian Sausage	1 topping serv	55	4	2
Add A Topping Onion	1 topping serv	4	tr	–
Add A Topping Pepperoni	1 topping serv	62	6	2
Add A Topping Pineapple Tidbits	1 topping serv	10	0	0
Add A Topping Ripe Olives	1 topping serv	14	1	tr
Deep Dish Cheese	2 slices (6.3 oz)	477	22	8
Hand Tossed Cheese	2 slices (5.2 oz)	347	11	5
Thin Crust Cheese	¼ pie (3.7 oz)	271	12	5

14 INCH LARGE PIZZAS

FOOD	PORTION	CALS	FAT	SAT FAT
Add A Topping Anchovies	1 topping serv	23	1	tr
Add A Topping Bacon	1 topping serv	75	6	2
Add A Topping Banana Peppers	1 topping serv	3	tr	–
Add A Topping Canned Mushrooms	1 topping serv	3	tr	tr
Add A Topping Cheddar Cheese	1 topping serv	48	4	2
Add A Topping Cheddar Cheese	1 topping serv	48	4	2

FOOD	PORTION	CALS	FAT	SAT FAT
Add A Topping Cooked Beef	1 topping serv	44	4	2
Add A Topping Extra Cheese	1 topping serv	45	4	2
Add A Topping Fresh Mushrooms	1 topping serv	3	tr	tr
Add A Topping Green Olives	1 topping serv	11	1	tr
Add A Topping Green Peppers	1 topping serv	2	tr	—
Add A Topping Ham	1 topping serv	17	1	tr
Add A Topping Italian Sausage	1 topping serv	44	3	1
Add A Topping Onion	1 topping serv	3	tr	—
Add A Topping Pepperoni	1 topping serv	55	5	2
Add A Topping Pineapple Tidbits	1 topping serv	8	0	0
Add A Topping Ripe Olives	1 topping serv	12	1	tr
Deep Dish Cheese	2 slices (6.1 oz)	455	20	8
Hand-Tossed Cheese	2 slices (4.8 oz)	317	10	5
Thin Crust Cheese	⅙ pie (3.5 oz)	253	11	5
6 INCH DEEP DISH PIZZAS				
Add A Topping Anchovies	1 topping serv	45	2	tr
Add A Topping Bacon	1 topping serv	82	7	2
Add A Topping Banana Peppers	1 topping serv	3	tr	—
Add A Topping Canned Mushrooms	1 topping serv	2	tr	0
Add A Topping Cheddar Cheese	1 topping serv	86	7	4
Add A Topping Cooked Beef	1 topping serv	44	4	2
Add A Topping Extra Cheese	1 topping serv	57	5	3
Add A Topping Fresh Mushrooms	1 topping serv	2	tr	0
Add A Topping Green Olives	1 topping serv	10	1	tr
Add A Topping Green Peppers	1 topping serv	2	tr	—
Add A Topping Ham	1 topping serv	17	1	tr
Add A Topping Italian Sausage	1 topping serv	44	3	1
Add A Topping Onion	1 topping serv	3	tr	—
Add A Topping Pepperoni	1 topping serv	50	5	2
Add A Topping Pineapple Tidbits	1 topping serv	5	0	0
Add A Topping Ripe Olives	1 topping serv	11	1	tr
Cheese	1 pie (7.6 oz)	595	27	11
MAIN MENU SELECTIONS				
Breadstick	1 (0.8 oz)	78	3	1
Buffalo Wings Barbeque	1 piece (0.9 oz)	50	2	1
Buffalo Wings Hot	1 piece (0.9 oz)	45	2	1
Cheesy Bread	1 piece (1 oz)	103	5	2
Garden Salad	1 lg (7.7 oz)	39	tr	tr
Garden Salad	1 sm (4.3 oz)	22	tr	tr

FOOD	PORTION	CALS	FAT	SAT FAT
SALAD DRESSINGS				
Marzetti Blue Cheese	1 serv (1.5 oz)	220	24	4
Marzetti Creamy Caesar	1 serv (1.5 oz)	200	22	3
Marzetti Fat Free Ranch	1 serv (1.5 oz)	40	0	0
Marzetti Honey French	1 serv (1.5 oz)	210	18	3
Marzetti House Italian	1 serv (1.5 oz)	220	24	3
Marzetti Light Italian	1 serv (1.5 oz)	20	1	0
Marzetti Ranch	1 serv (1.5 oz)	260	29	4
Marzetti Thousand Island	1 serv (1.5 oz)	200	20	3
DONATOS PIZZA				
PIZZA				
Dessert Apple	¼ pie	722	20	4
Dessert Cherry	¼ pie	818	20	4
Original	¼ pie	660	33	14
Original Chicken Vegy Medley	¼ pie	500	19	8
Original Chicken Vegy Medley No Cheese	¼ pie	392	10	3
Original Founders	¼ pie	737	42	17
Original Hawaiian	¼ pie	620	30	10
Original Hawaiian No Cheese	¼ pie	411	13	2
Original Mariachi Beef	¼ pie	613	30	14
Original Mariachi Chicken	¼ pie	580	25	12
Original Serious Cheese	¼ pie	640	28	20
Original Serious Meat	¼ pie	817	47	20
Original Vegy	¼ pie	564	24	10
Original Vegy No Cheese	¼ pie	370	9	2
Original Works	¼ pie	729	41	17
Traditional Chicken Vegy Medley	¼ pie	647	17	8
Traditional Founders	¼ pie	900	40	17
Traditional Hawaiian	¼ pie	794	30	12
Traditional Mariachi Beef	¼ pie	797	31	15
Traditional Mariachi Chicken	¼ pie	770	26	13
Traditional Serious Meat	¼ pie	977	46	20
Traditional Vegy	¼ pie	752	26	12
Traditional Works	¼ pie	892	39	17
Traditional Original	¼ pie	928	39	28
Traditional Serious Cheese	¼ pie	830	36	30

FOOD	PORTION	CALS	FAT	SAT FAT
SALAD DRESSINGS				
Italian	1 serv (1.5 oz)	230	24	4
Italian Lite	1 serv (1.5 oz)	20	1	0
SALADS				
Grilled Chicken w/o Dressing	1 serv	314	18	7
Italian Chef w/o Dressing	1 serv	338	23	9
Side w/o Dressing	1 serv	106	7	3
SIDE ORDERS				
Breadsticks	2	220	5	1
Chicken Wings Hot	5	449	29	—
Chicken Wings Mild	5	451	29	—
Three Cheese Garlic Bread	1 bun	605	28	8
SUBS				
Big Don Italian	1 serv	705	33	10
Big Don Lite Italian	1 serv	631	25	9
Grilled Chicken	1 serv	786	43	12
Ham & Cheese Italian	1 serv	609	22	5
Ham & Cheese Lite Italian	1 serv	534	14	4
Southwest Turkey	1 serv	710	33	7
Steak & Cheese	1 serv	929	52	18
Vegy Italian	1 serv	730	36	9
Vegy Lite Italian	1 serv	661	28	8
DUNKIN' DONUTS				
BAGELS AND CREAM CHEESE				
Bagel Blueberry	1	340	1	0
Bagel Cinnamon Raisin	1	340	1	0
Bagel Egg	1	350	2	0
Bagel Everything	1	360	2	0
Bagel Garlic	1	360	1	0
Bagel Onion	1	330	1	0
Bagel Plain	1	340	1	0
Bagel Poppyseed	1	360	3	0
Bagel Pumpernickel	1	350	2	0
Bagel Salt	1	340	1	0
Bagel Sesame	1	380	5	1
Bagel Wheat	1	330	2	0
Cream Cheese Chive	1 pkg	190	19	13
Cream Cheese Garden Vegetable	1 pkg	180	17	11
Cream Cheese Lite	1 pkg	130	11	7

FOOD	PORTION	CALS	FAT	SAT FAT
Cream Cheese Plain	1 pkg	200	19	13
Cream Cheese Salmon	1 pkg	180	17	11
BAKED SELECTIONS				
Bow Tie Donut	1	300	17	4
Cake Donut Blueberry	1	290	16	4
Cake Donut Butternut	1	300	16	5
Cake Donut Chocolate Coconut	1	300	19	6
Cake Donut Chocolate Frosted	1	300	16	3
Cake Donut Chocolate Glazed	1	290	16	4
Cake Donut Cinnamon	1	270	15	3
Cake Donut Coconut	1	290	17	5
Cake Donut Double Chocolate	1	310	17	4
Cake Donut Glazed	1	270	15	3
Cake Donut Old Fashioned	1	250	15	3
Cake Donut Powdered	1	270	15	3
Cake Donut Toasted Coconut	1	300	17	5
Cake Donut Whole Wheat Glazed	1	310	19	4
Chocolate Frosted Donut	1	200	9	2
Chocolate Kreme Filled Donut	1	270	13	3
Cinnamon Bun	1	510	15	4
Coffee Roll	1	270	14	3
Coffee Roll Chocolate Frosted	1	290	15	3
Coffee Roll Maple Frosted	1	290	14	3
Coffee Roll Vanilla Frosted	1	290	14	3
Cookie Chocolate Chocolate Chunk	1	210	11	7
Cookie Chocolate Chunk	1	220	11	7
Cookie Chocolate Chunk w/ Nut	1	230	12	6
Cookie Chocolate White Chocolate Chunk	1	230	12	7
Cookie Oatmeal Raisin Pecan	1	220	10	5
Cookie Peanut Butter Chocolate Chunk w/ Nuts	1	240	14	6
Cookie Peanut Butter w/ Nuts	1	240	14	6
Croissant Almond	1	350	22	5
Croissant Chocolate	1	400	25	9
Croissant Plain	1	290	18	6
Cruller Glazed	1	290	15	2
Cruller Glazed Chocolate	1	280	15	3
Cruller Plain	1	240	15	3
Cruller Powdered	1	270	15	3

FOOD	PORTION	CALS	FAT	SAT FAT
Cruller Sugar	1	250	15	3
Donut Apple Crumb	1	230	10	3
Donut Apple N' Spice	1	200	8	2
Donut Bavarian Kreme	1	210	9	2
Donut Black Raspberry	1	210	8	2
Donut Blueberry Crumb	1	240	10	3
Donut Boston Kreme	1	240	9	2
Donut Chocolate Iced Bismark	1	340	15	4
Dunkin' Donut	1	240	15	3
Eclair Donut	1	270	11	3
Fritter Glazed	1	260	14	3
Glazed Donut	1	180	8	2
Jelly Filled Donut	1	210	8	2
Jelly Stick	1	290	12	3
Lemon Donut	1	200	9	2
Maple Frosted Donut	1	210	9	2
Marble Frosted Donut	1	200	9	2
Muffin Apple Cinnamon Pecan	1	510	21	6
Muffin Apple N'Spice	1	350	12	3
Muffin Banana Nut	1	360	15	3
Muffin Blueberry	1 (4 oz)	320	12	3
Muffin Blueberry	1 (6 oz)	490	17	6
Muffin Bran	1	390	12	2
Muffin Cherry	1	340	12	3
Muffin Chocolate Hazelnut	1	610	26	8
Muffin Chocolate Chip	1 (6 oz)	590	24	10
Muffin Chocolate Chip	1 (4 oz)	400	17	6
Muffin Corn	1 (4 oz)	390	15	3
Muffin Corn	1 (6 oz)	500	16	5
Muffin Cranberry Orange	1	470	15	5
Muffin Cranberry Orange Nut	1	350	15	3
Muffin Lemon Poppyseed	1	360	13	3
Muffin Oat Bran	1	370	13	2
Muffin Lowfat Apple & Spice	1	240	2	0
Muffin Lowfat Banana	1	250	2	0
Muffin Lowfat Blueberry	1	250	2	0
Muffin Lowfat Bran	1	240	1	0
Muffin Lowfat Cherry	1	250	2	0
Muffin Lowfat Chocolate	1	250	3	1
Muffin Lowfat Corn	1	240	3	1

FOOD	PORTION	CALS	FAT	SAT FAT
Muffin Lowfat Cranberry Orange	1	240	2	0
Muffin Reduced Fat Blueberry	1	450	12	9
Muffin Reduced Fat Corn	1	460	11	7
Munchkins Chocolate Cake Glazed	3	200	10	2
Munchkins Cake Butternut	3	200	11	3
Munchkins Cake Cinnamon	4	250	14	3
Munchkins Cake Coconut	3	200	12	4
Munchkins Cake Glazed	3	200	10	2
Munchkins Cake Plain	4	220	14	3
Munchkins Cake Powdered	4	250	14	3
Munchkins Cake Sugared	4	240	14	3
Munchkins Cake Toasted Coconut	3	200	11	—
Munchkins Yeast Glazed	5	200	9	2
Munchkins Yeast Jelly Filled	5	210	9	2
Munchkins Yeast Lemon Filled	4	170	8	2
Munchkins Yeast Sugar Raised	7	220	12	3
Strawberry Frosted Donut	1	210	9	2
Strawberry Donut	1	210	8	2
Sugar Raised Donut	1	170	8	2
Sugared Cake Donut	1	250	15	3
Vanilla Frosted Donut	1	210	9	2
Vanilla Kreme Filled Donut	1	270	13	3
BEVERAGES				
Coffee Coolatta w/ 2% Milk	1 (16 oz)	240	2	2
Coffee Coolatta w/ Cream	1 (16 oz)	410	22	14
Coffee Coolatta w/ Milk	1 (16 oz)	260	4	3
Coffee Coolatta w/ Skim Milk	1 (16 oz)	230	0	0
Coolatta Orange Mango Fruit	1 (16 oz)	290	0	0
Coolatta Pink Lemonade Fruit	1 (16 oz)	350	0	0
Coolatta Raspberry Lemonade	1 (16 oz)	280	0	0
Coolatta Strawberry Fruit	1 (16 oz)	280	0	0
Coolatta Vanilla	1 (16 oz)	450	7	4
Cream	1 serv (1 oz)	60	5	3
Dark Roast Coffee	1 serv (10 oz)	5	0	0
Decaf Coffee	1 serv (10 oz)	0	0	0
Dunkaccino	1 (20 oz)	510	23	7
Dunkaccino	1 (18.75 oz)	480	22	7
Dunkaccino	1 (10 oz)	250	11	4
Dunkaccino	1 (14 oz)	360	17	5
French Vanilla Coffee	1 serv (10 oz)	5	0	0

FOOD	PORTION	CALS	FAT	SAT FAT
Hazelnut Coffee	1 serv (10 oz)	5	0	0
Hot Cocoa	1 (10 oz)	230	8	2
Hot Cocoa	1 (14 oz)	330	11	3
Hot Cocoa	1 (18.75 oz)	440	15	4
Hot Cocoa	1 (20 oz)	470	16	4
Regular Coffee	1 serv (10 oz)	5	0	0
SANDWICHES				
Breakfast Sandwich Ham Egg Cheese	1	320	12	6
Omwich Bagel Bacon Cheddar	1	600	21	8
Omwich Bagel Spanish Cheese	1	570	18	6
Omwich Bagel Three Cheese	1	610	22	9
Omwich Croissant Spanish Cheese	1	530	36	11
Omwich Croissant Bacon Cheddar	1	560	38	13
Omwich Croissant Three Cheese	1	560	39	15
Omwich English Muffin Bacon Cheddar	1	400	21	8
Omwich English Muffin Spanish Cheese	1	370	18	6
Omwich English Muffin Three Cheese	1	400	22	9

EINSTEIN BROS BAGELS
BAGELS AND BREADS

FOOD	PORTION	CALS	FAT	SAT FAT
Bagel Asiago Cheese	1	360	3	2
Bagel Cranberry Special	1	350	1	0
Bagel Egg	1	340	3	1
Bagel Honey Whole Wheat	1	320	1	0
Bagel Jalapeno	1	330	1	0
Bagel Lucky Gree	1	320	1	0
Bagel Mango	1	360	1	0
Bagel Potato	1	350	5	1
Bagel Power	1	410	5	1
Bagel Power w/ Peanut Butter	1	750	34	6
Bagel Pumpkin	1	330	2	0
Bagel Roasted Red Pepper & Pesto	1	410	7	4
Bagel Six Cheese	1	390	6	3
Bagel Spicy Nacho	1	450	9	5
Bagel Spinach Florentine	1	410	7	4
Bagel Croutons	¼ cup	25	1	0
Bagel Twist	1	220	4	2

FOOD	PORTION	CALS	FAT	SAT FAT
Bread Ciabatta	1 serv	320	3	1
Chocolate Chip	1	370	3	2
Chopped Garlic	1	380	3	1
Chopped Onion	1	330	1	0
Cinnamon Raisin Swirl	1	350	1	0
Cinnamon Sugar	1	330	1	0
Dark Pumpernickel	1	320	1	0
Everything	1	340	2	0
Focaccia Cheese Pizza	1 serv	500	11	7
Focaccia Margherita	1 serv	400	17	2
Focaccia Pepperoni Pizza	1 serv	590	19	10
Nutty Banana	1	360	3	1
Plain	1	320	1	0
Poppy Dip'd	1	350	2	0
Roll Challah	1	300	5	1
Salt	1	330	1	0
Sesame Dip'd	1	380	5	1
Sun Dried Tomato	1	320	1	0
Wild Blueberry	1	350	1	0
BEVERAGES				
Americano	1 reg	1	0	0
Cafe Latte	1 reg	140	5	4
Cafe Latte Nonfat	1 reg	100	0	0
Cappuccino	1 reg	90	4	2
Cappuccino Nonfat	1 reg	60	0	0
Chai 2% Milk	1 reg	210	2	2
Chai Skim Milk	1 reg	190	0	0
Coffee	1 reg	0	0	0
Espresso	1 reg	1	0	0
Half & Half	2 tbsp	40	3	2
Hot Chocolate	1 reg	290	11	8
Hot Chocolate Lower Fat	1 reg	260	7	6
Hot Tea All Flavors	1 cup	0	0	0
Iced Americano	1 serv	1	0	0
Iced Coffee	1 serv	0	0	0
Iced Latte	1 serv	120	5	3
Iced Latte Nonfat	1 serv	90	0	0
Iced Mocha	1 serv	210	6	4
Iced Mocha Low Fat	1 serv	180	3	2
Mocha	1 reg	230	6	5

FOOD	PORTION	CALS	FAT	SAT FAT
Mocha Low Fat	1 reg	190	3	2
DESSERTS				
Brownie Iced	1	550	24	6
Brownie Iced w/ Walnuts	1	600	29	6
Cherry Figure 8	1	400	18	6
Cinnamon Roll	1	810	32	9
Cookie Chocolate Chunk	1	640	31	10
Cookie Oatmeal Raisin	1	600	27	6
Cookie Peanut Butter	1	640	34	7
Muffin Banana Nut	1	640	32	4
Muffin Blueberry	1	540	22	4
Muffin Chocolate Chip	1	620	27	8
Pound Cake Lemon Iced	1 slice	540	25	13
Pound Cake Marble	1 slice	460	24	12
Rice Krispy Bar	1	420	8	2
Scone Blueberry w/ Icing	1	450	18	8
Scone Lemon Currant	1	430	15	5
Strudel Cinnamon Walnut	1 piece	550	31	11
Sweetie Pie	1	620	20	2
SALAD DRESSINGS				
Asian Sesame	2 tbsp	80	2	0
Caesar	2 tbsp	150	16	3
Chipotle Vinaigrette	2 tbsp	110	10	2
Horseradish Sauce	2 tbsp	170	18	3
Raspberry Vinaigrette	2 tbsp	160	14	2
Thousand Island	2 tbsp	110	9	20
SALADS				
Asian Chicken Salad	1 serv (14.5 oz)	550	9	2
Bros Bistro	1 serv (9.5 oz)	520	43	10
Chicken Caesar	1 serv (12.5 oz)	750	53	11
Chicken Chipotle Salad	1 serv	710	43	9
Chicken Salad On Greens	1 serv (10.5 oz)	210	9	2
Egg Salad	1 serv (4 oz)	200	17	4
Fresh Fruit Cup	1 serv (8 oz)	110	1	0
Mixed Greens	1 serv (3.5 oz)	228	18	3
Potato	½ cup	290	21	3
Tuna Salad On Greens	1 serv (10.5 oz)	170	5	1
SANDWICHES				
12 Grain Bread Deli Chicken Salad	1	440	13	2
12 Grain Bread Deli Egg Salad	1	490	21	4

FOOD	PORTION	CALS	FAT	SAT FAT
12 Grain Bread Deli Ham	1	560	25	7
12 Grain Bread Deli Roast Beef	1	560	24	7
12 Grain Bread Deli Smoked Turkey	1	530	21	6
12 Grain Bread Deli Tuna Salad	1	440	13	2
12 Grain Bread Deli Turkey Pastrami	1	540	21	6
12 Grain Bread Ultimate Toasted Cheese w/ Tomato	1	870	50	25
Bagel Chicken Salad	1	500	10	2
Bagel Egg Bacon	1	580	19	7
Bagel Egg Ham	1	530	13	5
Bagel Egg Salad	1	560	18	5
Bagel Egg Sausage	1	550	14	5
Bagel Ham	1	450	6	2
Bagel Holey Cow	1	900	50	13
Bagel Hummus & Feta	1	540	13	4
Bagel New York Lox	1	660	27	19
Bagel Original	1	480	10	4
Bagel Roast Beef	1	460	4	2
Bagel Rueben Deli	1	660	19	6
Bagel Salmon & Shmear	1	650	22	12
Bagel Sante Fe	1	650	24	8
Bagel Smoked Turkey	1	420	2	0
Bagel Tasty Turkey	1	570	15	9
Bagel The Veg Out	1	490	13	7
Bagel Tuna Salad	1	470	6	2
Bagel Turkey Pastrami	1	440	2	0
Challah Club Mex	1	750	45	14
Challah Cobbie	1	630	33	12
Challah Deli Chicken Salad	1	480	14	3
Challah Deli Egg Salad	1	430	20	5
Challah Deli Pastrami	1	480	21	7
Challah Deli Roast Beef	1	500	23	8
Challah Deli Smoked Turkey	1	470	21	7
Challah Deli Tuna Salad	1	370	10	3
Challah Deli Turkey Ham	1	500	25	8
Challah BBQ Chicken	1	380	8	2
Challah Roasted Chicken & Smoked Gouda	1	440	13	6
Chicago Bagel Dog Asiago	1	740	34	15
Chicago Bagel Dog Chili Cheese	1	810	38	17

FOOD	PORTION	CALS	FAT	SAT FAT
Chicago Bagel Dog Everything	1	730	34	12
Chicago Bagel Dog Onion w/o Cheese	1	680	30	12
Country White Deli Chicken Salad	1	540	15	4
Country White Deli Egg Salad	1	590	23	6
Country White Deli Ham	1	660	27	9
Country White Deli Roast Beef	1	660	26	9
Country White Deli Smoked Turkey	1	630	23	8
Country White Deli Tuna Salad	1	510	11	3
Country White Deli Turkey Pastrami	1	640	23	8
Country White Ultimate Toasted Cheese w/ Tomato	1	870	51	26
Panini Cali Club	1	730	24	9
Panini Cuban Ham	1	700	31	11
Panini Denver Omelet Breakfast	1	740	33	13
Panini Italian Chicken	1	770	36	13
Panini Taos Turkey	1	740	25	9
Panini Ultimate Toasted Cheese	1	900	44	24
Roll Ups Albuquerque Turkey	1	790	39	15
Roll Ups Thai Vegetable w/ Chicken	1	670	18	1
Roll Ups Thai Vegetables	1	630	21	2
SOUPS				
Broccoli Sharp Cheddar	1 cup	230	15	8
Chicken & Wild Rice	1 cup	190	4	1
Chicken Noodle	1 cup	220	9	3
Clam Chowda	1 cup	160	11	6
Minestrone Low Fat	1 cup	180	3	1
Tomato Bisque	1 cup	190	10	3
Tortilla	1 cup	90	3	0
Turkey Chili	1 cup	140	5	1
SPREADS				
Butter	1 tbsp	100	11	8
Butter & Margarine Blend	1 tbsp	60	7	2
Cream Cheese Blueberry	1 tbsp	70	5	4
Cream Cheese Cappuccino	2 tbsp	70	5	4
Cream Cheese Garden Vegetable	2 tbsp	60	5	4
Cream Cheese Honey Almond Reduced Fat	2 tbsp	70	5	3
Cream Cheese Jalapeno Salsa	1 tbsp	60	5	3
Cream Cheese Maple Walnut Raisin	2 tbsp	60	5	4

FOOD	PORTION	CALS	FAT	SAT FAT
Cream Cheese Onion & Chive	2 tbsp	70	6	4
Cream Cheese Plain	2 tbsp	60	7	5
Cream Cheese Plain Reduced Fat	2 tbsp	60	5	4
Cream Cheese Pumpkin	2 tbsp	100	8	6
Cream Cheese Smoked Salmon	2 tbsp	60	5	4
Cream Cheese Strawberry	2 tbsp	70	5	4
Cream Cheese Sun Dried Tomato & Basil	2 tbsp	60	5	4
Fruit Spread Apricot	1 serv	75	0	0
Fruit Spread Grape	1 serv (1 oz)	75	0	0
Fruit Spread Strawberry	1 serv (1 oz)	75	0	0
Honey Butter	1 tbsp	90	8	4
Hummus	1 serv	110	7	1
Mayo Ancho Lime	1 tbsp	50	5	1
Mustard French Dijon	1 tsp	10	0	0
Mustard Grain Dijon	1 tsp	5	0	0
Mustard Honey	1 tsp	15	0	0
Mustard Raspberry	2 tbsp	50	2	0
Mustard Yellow	1 tbsp	5	0	0
Peanut Butter	2 tbsp	190	15	2
Salsa Ancho Lime	¼ cup	20	1	0

EL POLLO LOCO
DESSERTS

FOOD	PORTION	CALS	FAT	SAT FAT
Churro	1	179	11	3
Fosters Freeze Soft Serve	1 cup	180	5	3

MAIN MENU SELECTIONS

FOOD	PORTION	CALS	FAT	SAT FAT
Bowl Chicken Caesar	1 serv	535	28	5
Bowl Pollo	1 serv	545	10	1
Bowl Veggie	1 serv	570	16	4
Bowl Veggie w/o Cheese	1 serv	529	12	2
Burrito BRC	1 (9.3 oz)	482	15	5
Burrito Classic Chicken	1	580	22	7
Burrito Twice Grilled	1 serv	835	39	16
Burrito BRC	1 serv	530	15	5
Burrito Caesar	1 serv	895	45	7
Burrito Chicken Lover's	1 serv	525	18	6
Burrito Spicy	1 serv	555	19	6
Burrito Ultimate Chicken	1 serv	685	23	7
Chicken Breast	1 piece	153	4	1

FOOD	PORTION	CALS	FAT	SAT FAT
Chicken Leg	1 piece	86	3	0
Chicken Thigh	1 piece	120	7	2
Chicken Wing	1	83	3	1
Cole Slaw	1 serv	206	16	3
Corn Cobbette	1 serv	80	1	0
French Fries	1 serv	444	19	5
Fresh Vegetables	1 serv	70	4	1
Gravy	1 serv (1 oz)	107	4	1
Mashed Potatoes	1 serv	97	1	0
Nachos Chicken	1 serv	1420	91	26
Pinto Beans	1 serv	165	4	tr
Popcorn Chicken	1 serv	226	12	2
Potato Salad	1 serv	256	14	2
Quesadilla Cheese	1 serv	495	25	11
Quesadilla Chicken	1 serv	593	29	12
Smokey Black Beans	1 serv	306	16	6
Spanish Rice	1 serv	165	1	tr
Taco Al Carbon Chicken	1 serv	135	3	tr
Taco Soft Chicken	1	237	12	4
Taquitos Chicken	2	370	17	4
Tortilla Chips	1 serv	426	24	6
Tortilla Corn	1 (6 inches)	70	1	0
Tortilla Corn	1 (4.5 inch)	40	1	0
Tortilla Flour	1 (6.5 inch)	110	4	0
Tortilla Flour	1 (12 inches)	325	8	2
Tortilla Spicy Tomato	1 (12 inches)	270	7	1
Tostada Salad	1 serv	700	32	9
SALAD DRESSINGS AND TOPPINGS				
Bleu Cheese	1 serv (1.5 oz)	230	24	5
Buttermilk Ranch	1 serv (1.5 oz)	220	24	4
Creamy Chipotle	1 (0.5 oz)	75	8	1
Creamy Cilantro	1 serv (0.5 oz)	80	8	1
Guacamole	1 serv (1 oz)	30	2	0
Hot Sauce Jalapeno	1 pkg (0.5 oz)	5	0	0
Light Italian	1 serv (1.5 oz)	20	1	0
Salsa Avocado	1 serv (1 oz)	20	1	0
Salsa House	1 serv (1 oz)	6	tr	0
Salsa Pico De Gallo	1 serv (1 oz)	10	tr	0
Salsa Spicy Chipotle	1 serv (1 oz)	7	0	0
Sour Cream	1 serv (1 oz)	60	5	4

FOOD	PORTION	CALS	FAT	SAT FAT
Thousand Island	1 serv (1.5 oz)	220	21	3
SALADS				
Caesar	1 serv	565	45	8
Caesar w/o Dressing	1 serv	250	11	3
Fiesta Salad	1 serv	755	58	16
Fiesta Salad w/o Dressing	1 serv	450	26	11
Garden Salad	1 serv	110	7	3
Macaroni & Cheese	1 serv	381	26	16
Tostada Salad w/o Shell	1 serv	360	14	6

FAZOLI'S
DESSERTS

FOOD	PORTION	CALS	FAT	SAT FAT
Cheesecake	1 slice	290	22	14
Cheesecake Turtle	1 slice	420	34	17
Cookie Milk Chocolate Chunk	1	360	15	12
Lemon Ice	1 serv	190	0	0
Specialty Cheesecake	1 serv	300	22	14
Strawberry Topping	1 serv	35	0	0
MAIN MENU SELECTIONS				
Baked Chicken Parmesan	1 serv	740	20	4
Baked Spaghetti Parmesan	1 serv	700	25	13
Baked Ziti	1 sm	490	17	7
Baked Ziti	1 reg	750	26	11
Breadstick	1	140	6	1
Breadstick Dry	1	90	1	0
Broccoli Fettuccine Alfredo	1 sm	560	15	4
Broccoli Fettuccine Alfredo	1 reg	830	23	6
Cheese Ravioli w/ Marinara Sauce	1 serv	480	15	7
Cheese Ravioli w/ Meat Sauce	1 serv	510	17	8
Classic Sampler	1 serv	710	21	6
Fettuccine Alfredo	1 sm	530	15	4
Fettuccine Alfredo	1 reg	800	22	6
Fettuccine w/ Shrimp & Scallop	1 serv	590	16	5
Homestyle Lasagna	1 serv	440	19	6
Homestyle Lasagna w/ Broccoli	1 serv	420	18	5
Minestrone Soup	1 serv	120	1	0
Peppery Chicken Alfredo	1 serv	610	16	4
Pizza Cheese	1 serv	460	15	8
Pizza Combination Double Slice	1 serv	570	25	12
Pizza Pepperoni	1 serv	530	22	11

FOOD	PORTION	CALS	FAT	SAT FAT
Pizza Baked Spaghetti	1 serv	750	31	15
Spaghetti w/ Marinara Sauce	1 sm	420	6	1
Spaghetti w/ Marinara Sauce	1 reg	620	8	1
Spaghetti w/ Meat Sauce	1 reg	670	11	3
Spaghetti w/ Meat Sauce	1 sm	450	8	2
Spaghetti w/ Meatballs	1 reg	1020	42	14
Spaghetti w/ Meatballs	1 sm	730	31	11
SALAD DRESSINGS				
Honey French	1 serv	150	12	2
House Italian	1 serv	110	9	2
Ranch	1 serv	150	17	3
Reduced Calorie Italian	1 serv	50	5	1
Thousand Island	1 serv	130	13	2
SALADS AND SALAD BARS				
Caesar Side Salad	1	220	17	4
Chicken & Pasta Caesar Salad	1	500	27	7
Chicken Caesar Salad	1	420	29	6
Chicken Finger Salad	1	190	9	3
Chicken Finger Salad w/ Bacon & Honey Mustard	1	400	28	7
Garden Salad	1	25	0	0
Garden Salad w/ Balsamic Vinaigrette	1	120	9	2
Italian Chef Salad	1	260	21	9
Pasta Salad	1 serv	590	25	6
SANDWICHES				
Panini Chicken Caesar Club	1	660	35	11
Panini Chicken Pesto	1	510	20	6
Panini Four Cheese & Tomato	1	720	43	16
Panini Ham & Swiss	1	600	30	9
Panini Italian Club	1	670	37	11
Panini Italian Deli	1	660	35	13
Panini Smoked Turkey	1	710	38	12
Submarinos Club	half	1100	44	14
Submarinos Ham & Swiss	1	1000	37	11
Submarinos Meatball	half	1260	59	23
Submarinos Original	half	1160	55	17
Submarinos Pepperoni Pizza	half	1060	40	19
Submarinos Turkey	half	990	34	10

FOOD	PORTION	CALS	FAT	SAT FAT
FOSTERS FREEZE				
Soft Serve Vanilla	1 serv (4 oz)	152	4	–
GODFATHER'S PIZZA				
Golden Crust Cheese	⅒ lg (3.5 oz)	242	9	–
Golden Crust Cheese	⅛ med (3.1 oz)	212	8	–
Golden Crust Combo	⅛ med (4.4 oz)	271	12	–
Golden Crust Combo	⅒ lg (4.9 oz)	305	14	–
Original Crust Cheese	⅒ jumbo (5.8 oz)	382	9	–
Original Crust Cheese	¼ mini (1.9 oz)	131	3	–
Original Crust Cheese	⅛ med (3.5 oz)	231	5	–
Original Crust Cheese	⅒ lg (4 oz)	258	6	–
Original Crust Combo	¼ mini (2.9 oz)	176	7	–
Original Crust Combo	⅒ jumbo (8.3 oz)	503	18	–
Original Crust Combo	⅛ med (5.1 oz)	306	11	–
Original Crust Combo	⅒ lg (5.6 oz)	338	12	–
GREAT STEAK & POTATO COMPANY				
Baked Potato w/ Broccoli & Cheese	1 serv (12 oz)	340	5	2
Chicken Philadelphia	1 serv (10 oz)	640	27	7
Chicken Teriyaki	1 serv (11 oz)	580	17	5
Fresh Cut Fries	1 serv	920	48	12
Fresh Cut Fries	1 reg	540	29	7
Fresh Cut Fries	1 sm	460	24	6
Great Potato w/ Steak	1 serv (14 oz)	600	32	7
Great Potato w/ Turkey	1 serv (14 oz)	610	28	6
Great Salad Experience w/ Chicken w/o Dressing	1 serv (15 oz)	260	9	5
Great Steak	1 lg (18 oz)	1070	55	16
Great Steak	1 serv (11 oz)	660	34	10
Ham Delight	1 serv (11 oz)	710	33	9
Turkey Philadelphia	1 serv (10 oz)	690	28	7
Veggi Delight	1 serv (7 oz)	570	29	7
HÄAGEN-DAZS				
FROZEN YOGURT				
Pineapple Coconut	½ cup	230	13	8
Soft Serve Nonfat Chocolate	½ cup	110	0	0
Soft Serve Nonfat Chocolate Mousse	½ cup	80	0	0
Soft Serve Nonfat Coffee	½ cup	110	0	0
Soft Serve Nonfat Strawberry	½ cup	110	0	0

FOOD	PORTION	CALS	FAT	SAT FAT
Soft Serve Nonfat Vanilla	½ cup	110	0	0
Soft Serve Nonfat Vanilla Mousse	½ cup	70	0	0
Soft Serve Nonfat White Chocolate	½ cup	110	0	0
Vanilla Fudge	½ cup	160	0	0
Vanilla Raspberry Swirl	½ cup	130	0	0
ICE CREAM				
Bailey's Irish Cream	½ cup	270	17	10
Bar Chocolate	1 (2.7 oz)	200	12	8
Bar Chocolate & Dark Chocolate	1 (3.6 oz)	350	24	15
Bar Coffee	1 (2.7 oz)	190	13	8
Bar Coffee & Almond Crunch	1 (3.7 oz)	370	27	15
Bar Vanilla	1 (2.7 oz)	190	13	8
Bar Vanilla & Almonds	1 (3.7 oz)	380	28	14
Bar Vanilla & Milk Chocolate	1 (3.5 oz)	340	24	14
Belgian Chocolate Chocolate	½ cup	330	21	12
Brownies A La Mode	½ cup	280	16	10
Butter Pecan	½ cup	300	22	10
Cappuccino Commotion	½ cup	310	21	12
Chocolate	½ cup	269	17	10
Chocolate Chocolate Chip	½ cup	300	19	11
Chocolate Chocolate Mint	½ cup	300	20	11
Chocolate Swiss Almond	½ cup	300	20	11
Coffee	½ cup	250	17	10
Coffee Mocha Chip	½ cup	270	19	12
Cookie Dough Dynamo	½ cup	310	20	12
Cookies & Cream	½ cup	270	17	10
Cookies & Fudge	½ cup	180	3	2
Deep Chocolate Peanut Butter	½ cup	350	24	11
Dulce De Leche Caramel	½ cup	270	16	10
Lowfat Coffee Fudge	½ cup	170	3	2
Macadamia Brittle	½ cup	280	19	11
Macadamia Nut	½ cup	320	24	12
Mint Chip	½ cup	280	18	12
Pistachio	½ cup	280	19	10
Pralines & Cream	½ cup	280	17	9
Rum Raisin	½ cup	260	17	10
Strawberry	½ cup	250	16	9
Vanilla	½ cup	250	17	10
Vanilla Chocolate Chip	½ cup	290	19	12
Vanilla Swiss Almond	½ cup	290	20	11

FOOD	PORTION	CALS	FAT	SAT FAT
SORBET				
Bar Raspberry & Vanilla	1 (2.5 oz)	90	0	0
Mango	½ cup	120	0	0
Orange	½ cup	120	0	0
Raspberry	½ cup	120	0	0
Soft Serve Raspberry	½ cup	110	0	0
Strawberry	½ cup	120	0	0
Zesty Lemon	½ cup	120	0	0
HARDEE'S				
BEVERAGES				
Orange Juice	1 serv (11 oz)	140	tr	tr
Shake Chocolate	1 (12.2 oz)	370	5	3
Shake Peach	1 (12.1 oz)	390	4	3
Shake Strawberry	1 (12.7 oz)	420	4	3
Shake Vanilla	1 (12.2 oz)	350	5	3
BREAKFAST SELECTIONS				
Apple Cinnamon 'N' Raisin Biscuit	1 (2.18 oz)	200	8	2
Bacon & Egg Biscuit	1 (5.5 oz)	570	33	11
Bacon Egg & Cheese Biscuit	1 (5.9 oz)	610	37	13
Big Country Breakfast Bacon	1 serv (9.4 oz)	820	49	15
Big Country Breakfast Sausage	1 serv (11.4 oz)	1000	66	38
Biscuit 'N' Gravy	1 (7.8 oz)	510	28	9
Country Ham Biscuit	1 (3.8 oz)	430	22	5
Frisco Breakfast Sandwich Ham	1 (7.4 oz)	500	25	9
Ham Biscuit	1 (4 oz)	400	20	6
Ham Egg & Cheese Biscuit	1 (6.5 oz)	540	30	11
Hash Rounds	1 serv (2.8 oz)	230	14	3
Jelly Biscuit	1 (3.5 oz)	440	21	6
Rise 'N' Shine Biscuit	1 (2.9 oz)	390	21	6
Sausage Biscuit	1 (4.1 oz)	510	31	10
Sausage & Egg Biscuit	1 (6.3 oz)	630	40	22
Three Pancakes	1 serv (4.8 oz)	280	2	1
Ultimate Omelet Biscuit	1 (5.8 oz)	570	33	12
DESSERTS				
Big Cookie	1 (2.0 oz)	280	12	4
Cone Chocolate	1 (4.1 oz)	180	2	1
Cone Vanilla	1 (4.1 oz)	170	2	1
Cool Twist Cone Vanilla/ Chocolate	1 (4.1 oz)	180	2	1
Peach Cobbler	1 serv (6 oz)	310	7	1

FOOD	PORTION	CALS	FAT	SAT FAT
Sundae Hot Fudge	1 (5.5 oz)	290	6	3
Sundae Strawberry	1 (5.8 oz)	210	2	1
MAIN MENU SELECTIONS				
Baked Beans	1 serv (5 oz)	170	1	0
Big Roast Beef Sandwich	1 (6.5 oz)	460	24	9
Cheeseburger	1 (4.3 oz)	310	14	6
Chicken Fillet Sandwich	1 (7.5 oz)	480	18	3
Cole Slaw	1 serv (4 oz)	240	20	3
Cravin' Bacon Cheeseburger	1 (8.1 oz)	690	46	15
Fisherman's Fillet	1 (8.3 oz)	560	27	7
French Fries	1 lg (6 oz)	430	18	5
French Fries	1 sm (3.4 oz)	240	10	3
French Fries	1 med (5 oz)	350	15	4
Fried Chicken Breast	1 piece (5.2 oz)	370	15	4
Fried Chicken Leg	1 piece (2.4 oz)	170	7	2
Fried Chicken Thigh	1 piece (4.2 oz)	330	15	4
Fried Chicken Wing	1 piece (2.3 oz)	200	8	2
Frisco Burger	1 (8.1 oz)	720	46	16
Gravy	1 serv (1.5 oz)	20	tr	tr
Grilled Chicken Sandwich	1 (7.1 oz)	350	11	2
Hamburger	1 (3.9 oz)	270	11	3
Hot Ham 'N' Cheese	1 (5.1 oz)	310	12	6
Mashed Potatoes	1 serv (4 oz)	70	tr	tr
Mesquite Bacon Cheeseburger	1 (4.5 oz)	370	18	7
Mushroom 'N' Swiss Burger	1 (6.8 oz)	490	25	12
Quarter Pound Double Cheeseburger	1 (6 oz)	470	27	11
Regular Roast Beef	1 (4.3 oz)	320	16	6
The Boss	1 (7 oz)	570	33	12
The Works Burger	1 (8.1 oz)	530	30	12
SALAD DRESSINGS				
French Fat Free	1 serv (2 oz)	70	0	0
Ranch	1 serv (2 oz)	290	29	4
Thousand Island	1 serv (2 oz)	250	23	3
SALADS AND SALAD BARS				
Garden Salad	1 (10.2 oz)	220	13	9
Grilled Chicken Salad	1 (11.5 oz)	150	3	1
Side Salad	1 (4.6 oz)	25	tr	tr
HOT SAM'S PRETZELS				
Bavarian	1 reg (2.5 oz)	200	0	0

FOOD	PORTION	CALS	FAT	SAT FAT
Bavarian	1 lg (5.1 oz)	390	0	0
Bavarian Stix	10 (5 oz)	390	0	0
Sweet Dough	1 (4.5 oz)	360	3	1
Sweet Dough Blueberry	1 (4.5 oz)	400	4	2

HUNGRY HOWIE'S
MAIN MENU SELECTIONS

FOOD	PORTION	CALS	FAT	SAT FAT
Howie Wings	6 (3 oz)	180	14	4
Three Cheeser Bread	1 serv	370	14	5

PIZZA

FOOD	PORTION	CALS	FAT	SAT FAT
Large Cheese	1 slice	175	4	3
Large Cheese + Bacon	1 slice	208	5	3
Large Cheese + Beef	1 slice	197	6	3
Large Cheese + Black Olives	1 slice	181	5	3
Large Cheese + Green Olives	1 slice	181	5	3
Large Cheese + Green Peppers	1 slice	175	4	3
Large Cheese + Ham	1 slice	179	6	3
Large Cheese + Mushrooms	1 slice	175	4	3
Large Cheese + Onions	1 slice	175	5	3
Large Cheese + Pepperoni	1 slice	191	4	3
Large Cheese + Pineapple	1 slice	388	5	3
Large Cheese + Sausage	1 slice	195	6	3
Medium Cheese	1 slice	153	5	2
Medium Cheese + Bacon	1 slice	179	5	3
Medium Cheese + Beef	1 slice	177	6	3
Medium Cheese + Black Olives	1 slice	159	5	3
Medium Cheese + Green Olives	1 slice	159	4	3
Medium Cheese + Green Peppers	1 slice	155	5	3
Medium Cheese + Ham	1 slice	159	6	2
Medium Cheese + Mushrooms	1 slice	155	5	2
Medium Cheese + Onions	1 slice	155	5	3
Medium Cheese + Pepperoni	1 slice	171	6	3
Medium Cheese + Pineapple	1 slice	158	5	3
Medium Cheese + Sausage	1 slice	175	6	2
Small Cheese	1 slice	121	3	2
Small Cheese + Bacon	1 slice	138	3	2
Small Cheese + Beef	1 slice	137	4	2
Small Cheese + Black Olives	1 slice	125	3	2
Small Cheese + Green Olives	1 slice	125	3	2
Small Cheese + Green Peppers	1 slice	122	3	2

FOOD	PORTION	CALS	FAT	SAT FAT
Small Cheese + Ham	1 slice	126	3	2
Small Cheese + Mushrooms	1 slice	123	3	2
Small Cheese + Onions	1 slice	122	3	2
Small Cheese + Pepperoni	1 slice	136	4	3
Small Cheese + Pineapple	1 slice	124	3	2
Small Cheese + Sausage	1 slice	136	3	2
SALADS AND SALAD BARS				
Antipasto Salad w/o Dressing	1 lg	101	7	3
Chef Salad w/o Dressing	1 lg	99	6	3
Garden Salad w/o Dressing	1 lg	17	tr	0
Greek Salad w/o Dressing	1 lg	109	7	4
SANDWICHES				
Sub Deluxe Italian	½ sub	506	18	8
Sub Ham & Cheese	½ sub	475	15	7
Sub Pizza	½ sub	689	34	14
Sub Pizza Special	½ sub	606	24	11
Sub Steak Cheese Mushroom	½ sub	491	15	7
Sub Turkey	½ sub	466	13	6
Sub Turkey Club	½ sub	556	18	8
Sub Vegetarian	½ sub	530	21	11
IHOP				
Pancake Buckwheat	1 (2.5 oz)	134	5	1
Pancake Buttermilk	1 (2 oz)	108	3	1
Pancake Country Griddle	1 (2.25 oz)	134	4	1
Pancake Egg	1 (2 oz)	102	5	1
Pancake Harvest Grain 'N Nut	1 (2.25 oz)	160	8	1
Waffle	1 (4 oz)	305	15	3
Waffle Belgian	1 (6 oz)	408	20	11
Waffle Belgian Harvest Grain 'N Nut	1 (6 oz)	445	28	12
JACK IN THE BOX				
BEVERAGES				
Barq's Root Beer	1 serv (20 oz)	180	0	0
Coca-Cola Classic	1 serv (20 oz)	170	0	0
Coffee	1 serv (12 oz)	5	0	0
Diet Coke	1 serv (20 oz)	0	0	0
Dr Pepper	1 serv (20 oz)	190	0	0
Ice Cream Shake Caramel	1 serv (16 oz)	660	30	19
Ice Cream Shake Chocolate	1 (16 oz)	660	29	18
Ice Cream Shake Oreo	1 serv (16 oz)	670	33	19

FOOD	PORTION	CALS	FAT	SAT FAT
Ice Cream Shake Strawberry	1 serv (16 oz)	640	28	18
Ice Cream Shake Strawberry Banana	1 serv (16 oz)	700	28	18
Ice Cream Shake Vanilla	1 (16 oz)	570	29	18
Iced Tea	1 serv (20 oz)	0	0	0
Lowfat Milk 2%	1 serv (8 oz)	140	5	3
Orange Juice	1 serv (10 oz)	140	0	0
Sprite	1 serv (20 oz)	160	0	0
BREAKFAST SELECTIONS				
Breakfast Sandwich Sourdough	1	440	26	8
Breakfast Sandwich Ultimate	1	730	40	11
Breakfast Jack	1	310	14	5
Croissant Sausage	1	680	50	15
Croissant Supreme	1	570	37	9
French Toast Sticks	4 pieces	430	18	4
Hash Brown	1 serv	150	10	3
Pancakes w/ Bacon	1 serv (5.6 oz)	400	12	3
Sandwich Extreme Sausage	1	720	53	18
DESSERTS				
Cheesecake	1 serv	310	16	9
Double Fudge Cake	1 serv	310	11	3
MAIN MENU SELECTIONS				
American Cheese	1 slice	45	4	2
Bacon Cheddar Potato Wedges	1 serv	770	53	16
Cheeseburger	1 (4 oz)	330	15	6
Cheeseburger Bacon Bacon	1	910	59	19
Cheeseburger Bacon Ultimate	1	1120	75	28
Cheeseburger Junior Bacon	1	540	36	10
Cheeseburger Ultimate	1	990	66	28
Chicken Breast Pieces	4	360	17	3
Chicken Breast Strips	1 serv	500	25	6
Chicken Fajita Pita	1	330	11	5
Chicken Sandwich	1	410	21	5
Dipping Sauce Barbeque	1 serv (1.6 oz)	45	0	0
Double Cheeseburger	1 (5.3 oz)	450	24	12
Egg Rolls	5 pieces (10 oz)	730	41	10
Egg Rolls	1	130	6	2
Fish & Chips	1 serv	610	31	7
French Fries	1 med	410	20	5
French Fries	1 lg	580	28	6
French Fries	1 sm	330	16	4

FOOD	PORTION	CALS	FAT	SAT FAT
Hamburger	1	310	14	6
Hamburger w/ Cheese	1	360	18	8
Jumbo Jack	1	600	31	11
Jumbo Jack w/ Cheese	1	690	38	16
Onion Rings	1 serv	500	30	5
Philly Cheesesteak	1	580	22	11
Salsa	1 serv (1 oz)	10	0	0
Sandwich Roasted Turkey	1	580	25	8
Sandwich Ultimate Club	1	640	30	9
Seasoned Curly Fries	1 serv	400	23	5
Sour Cream	1 serv (1 oz)	60	5	3
Sourdough Grilled Chicken Club	1	520	28	6
Sourdough Jack	1	700	49	16
Spicy Crispy Chicken	1	730	37	10
Stuffed Jalapeno	3 pieces	230	13	6
Swiss Style Cheese	1 slice	40	3	2
Taco	1	170	9	3
Taco Monster	1	260	15	5
Turkey Jack	1	700	32	11
SALAD DRESSINGS AND TOPPINGS				
Almonds Roasted Slivered	1 serv (0.7 oz)	130	11	1
Asian Sesame	1 serv (2.5 oz)	230	17	3
Bacon Ranch	1 serv (2.5 oz)	320	33	5
Balsamic Vinaigrette Low Fat	1 serv (2.5 oz)	40	2	0
Country Crock Spread	1 pkg	25	3	1
Creamy Southwest Dressing	1 serv (2.5 oz)	270	26	4
Croutons	1 serv (0.5 oz)	60	2	0
Dipping Sauce Buttermilk House	1 serv (0.9 oz)	130	13	2
Dipping Sauce Frank's Red Hot Buffalo	1 serv (1 oz)	10	0	0
Dipping Sauce Sweet & Sour	1 serv (1 oz)	45	0	0
Grape Jelly	1 serv (0.5 oz)	35	0	0
Herb Mayo Sauce Low Fat	1 serv (1.5 oz)	45	4	1
Ketchup	1 pkg (0.3 oz)	10	0	0
Marinara Sauce	1 serv (0.9 oz)	15	0	0
Mustard	1 pkg	0	0	0
Ranch	1 serv (2.5 oz)	390	41	6
Ranch Lite	1 serv (2.5 oz)	190	18	3
Soy Sauce	1 serv (0.3 oz)	5	0	0
Syrup	1 serv (1.5 oz)	130	0	0

FOOD	PORTION	CALS	FAT	SAT FAT
Taco Sauce	1 serv (0.3 oz)	0	0	0
Tartar Sauce	1 serv (1.5 oz)	210	22	4
Thousand Island	1 serv (2 oz)	160	12	2
Vinegar	1 serv	0	0	0
Wonton Strips	1 serv (0.7 oz)	110	6	2
SALADS				
Asian Salad	1 serv	140	2	0
Chicken Club Salad	1 serv	290	16	6
Side Salad	1 serv	50	3	2
Southwest Chicken	1 serv	320	13	6

JAMBA JUICE

FOOD	PORTION	CALS	FAT	SAT FAT
Jambolas Honey Nut Energy	1 serv	192	1	—
Jambolas Mighty Multi Grain	1 serv	208	3	—
Jambolas Mind Over Blueberry	1 serv	170	1	—
Jambolas Pizza Protein	1 serv	199	3	—
Mango-A-Go-Go	1 reg (24 oz)	460	2	—
Orchard Oasis	1 reg (24 oz)	440	2	—
Protein Berry Pizazz	1 reg (24 oz)	470	1	—
Razzmatazz	1 reg (24 oz)	440	2	—

JERSEY MIKE'S

FOOD	PORTION	CALS	FAT	SAT FAT
Ham On Wheat	1	240	4	2
Ham On White	1	240	5	2
Ham/Turkey Wheat	1	230	3	1
Ham/Turkey White	1	240	4	1
Roast Beef Wheat	1	290	5	2
Roast Beef White	1	280	5	2
Turkey On Wheat	1	230	2	1
Turkey On White	1	230	3	1
Veggie On Wheat	1	170	2	0
Veggie On White	1	170	2	1

KFC

FOOD	PORTION	CALS	FAT	SAT FAT
BBQ Baked Beans	1 serv (5.5 oz)	190	3	1
Biscuit	1 (2 oz)	180	10	3
Chicken Pot Pie	1 (13 oz)	770	42	13
Chicken Twister	1 (8.7 oz)	550	32	7
Cole Slaw	1 serv (5 oz)	180	9	2
Corn On The Cob	1 ear (5.7 oz)	150	2	0
Cornbread	1 (2 oz)	228	13	2

FOOD	PORTION	CALS	FAT	SAT FAT
Crispy Strips Colonel's	3 (3.25 oz)	261	16	4
Crispy Strips Spicy Buffalo	3 (4.2 oz)	350	19	4
Extra Tasty Crispy Breast	1 (5.9 oz)	470	28	7
Extra Tasty Crispy Drumstick	1 (2.4 oz)	190	11	3
Extra Tasty Crispy Thigh	1 (4.2 oz)	370	25	6
Extra Tasty Crispy Whole Wing	1 (1.9 oz)	200	13	4
Green Beans	1 serv (4.7 oz)	45	2	1
Hot & Spicy Breast	1 (6.5 oz)	530	35	8
Hot & Spicy Drumstick	1 (2.3 oz)	190	11	3
Hot & Spicy Thigh	1 (3.8 oz)	370	27	7
Hot & Spicy Whole Wing	1 (1.9 oz)	210	15	4
Hot Wings	6 (4.8 oz)	471	33	8
Macaroni & Cheese	1 serv (5.4 oz)	180	8	3
Mashed Potatoes With Gravy	1 serv (4.8 oz)	120	6	1
Mean Greens	1 serv (5.4 oz)	70	3	1
Original Recipe Breast	1 (5.4 oz)	400	24	6
Original Recipe Chicken Sandwich	1 (7.3 oz)	497	22	5
Original Recipe Drumstick	1 (2.2 oz)	140	9	2
Original Recipe Thigh	1 (3.2 oz)	250	18	5
Original Recipe Whole Wing	1 (1.6 oz)	140	10	3
Potato Salad	1 serv (5.6 oz)	230	14	2
Potato Wedges	1 serv (4.8 oz)	280	13	4
Tender Roast Breast w/ Skin	1 (4.9 oz)	251	11	3
Tender Roast Breast w/o Skin	1 (4.2 oz)	169	4	1
Tender Roast Drumstick w/ Skin	1 (1.9 oz)	97	4	1
Tender Roast Drumstick w/o Skin	1 (1.2 oz)	67	2	1
Tender Roast Thigh w/ Skin	1 (3.2 oz)	207	12	4
Tender Roast Thigh w/o Skin	1 (2.1 oz)	106	6	2
Tender Roast Wing w/ Skin	1 (1.8 oz)	121	8	2
Value BBQ Chicken Sandwich	1 (5.3 oz)	256	8	1

KOO-KOO-ROO

FOOD	PORTION	CALS	FAT	SAT FAT
Original Breast	1 piece	187	6	1
Original Chicken Dark	3 pieces	320	16	5
Rotisserie Chicken Breast & Wing	1 serv	355	16	4
Rotisserie Chicken Leg & Thigh	1 serv	300	18	5
Rotisserie Half Chicken	1 serv	655	34	9
Sandwich BBQ Chicken	1	562	12	4
Sandwich Chicken Caesar	1	781	36	11
Sandwich Original Chicken	1	661	29	5

FOOD	PORTION	CALS	FAT	SAT FAT
Traditional Turkey Dinner	1 serv	692	29	10
Turkey Pot Pie	1 serv	883	44	12
Turkey Sandwich Hand Carved	1	599	32	8
Wrap Caesar Chicken	1	757	39	8
Wrap Chipotle Chicken	1	924	43	15

KRISPY KREME

FOOD	PORTION	CALS	FAT	SAT FAT
Chocolate Iced	1 (2 oz)	260	14	5
Chocolate Iced Cake	1 (2 oz)	230	12	3
Chocolate Iced Creme Filled	1 (2.3 oz)	270	14	3
Chocolate Iced Cruller	1 (1.7 oz)	240	14	4
Chocolate Iced Custard Filled	1 (2.7 oz)	250	9	3
Chocolated Iced w/ Sprinkles	1 (2 oz)	220	10	3
Cinnamon Apple Filled	1 (2.3 oz)	210	9	3
Cinnamon Bun	1 (2.1 oz)	220	11	3
Glazed Blueberry	1 (2.4 oz)	300	15	3
Glazed Creme Filled	1 (2.3 oz)	270	14	3
Glazed Cruller	1 (1.5 oz)	220	14	3
Glazed Devil's Food	1 (1.9 oz)	240	13	3
Lemon Filled	1 (2.2 oz)	210	10	3
Maple Iced	1 (1.8 oz)	200	9	3
Original Glazed	1 (1.3 oz)	180	10	3
Powdered Blueberry Filled	1 (2.1 oz)	200	9	3
Powdered Cake	1 (1.8 oz)	220	11	3
Raspberry Filled	1 (2 oz)	210	10	3
Traditional Cake	1 (1.7 oz)	200	11	3

KRYSTAL
BEVERAGES

FOOD	PORTION	CALS	FAT	SAT FAT
Chocolate Shake	1 (16 fl oz)	275	10	5

BREAKFAST SELECTIONS

FOOD	PORTION	CALS	FAT	SAT FAT
Biscuit	1 (2.5 oz)	244	12	2
Biscuit Bacon	1 (2.9 oz)	306	17	5
Biscuit Bacon, Egg & Cheese	1 (4.7 oz)	421	26	8
Biscuit Country Ham	1 (3.7 oz)	334	17	4
Biscuit Egg	1 (4 oz)	327	19	4
Biscuit Gravy	1 (7.5 oz)	419	26	7
Biscuit Sausage	1 (4.1 oz)	437	30	8
Sunriser	1 (3.8 oz)	259	17	5

DESSERTS

FOOD	PORTION	CALS	FAT	SAT FAT
Apple Pie	1 serv (4.5 oz)	300	10	4

FOOD	PORTION	CALS	FAT	SAT FAT
Donut Plain	1 (1.3 oz)	150	9	2
Donut w/ Chocolate Icing	1 (1.8 oz)	212	11	3
Donut w/ Vanilla Icing	1 (1.8 oz)	198	9	2
Lemon Meringue Pie	1 serv (4 oz)	340	9	3
Pecan Pie	1 serv (4 oz)	450	23	6
MAIN MENU SELECTIONS				
Big K	1 (8 oz)	540	35	14
Burger Plus	1 (6.5 oz)	415	26	10
Burger Plus w/ Cheese	1 (7.1 oz)	473	31	13
Cheese Krystal	1 (2.5 oz)	187	10	4
Chili	1 lg (12 oz)	327	12	5
Chili	1 reg (8 oz)	218	8	3
Chili Cheese Pup	1 (2.7 oz)	211	13	7
Chili Pup	1 (2.5 oz)	182	10	6
Corn Pup	1 (2.3 oz)	214	14	6
Crispy Crunchy Chicken Sandwich	1 (5.75 oz)	467	24	7
Double Cheese Krystal	1 (4.5 oz)	337	19	8
Double Krystal	1 (4 oz)	277	14	4
Fries	1 lg (5.3 oz)	463	23	8
Fries	1 reg (4.1 oz)	358	18	6
Fries	1 sm (3 oz)	262	13	5
Krys Kross Fries	1 serv (4.3 oz)	486	29	11
Krys Kross Fries Chili Cheese	1 serv (6.8 oz)	625	39	16
Krys Kross Fries w/ Cheese	1 serv (5.3 oz)	515	31	12
Krystal	1 (2.2 oz)	158	7	2
Plain Pup	1 (1.9 oz)	160	9	5
LITTLE CAESAR'S				
MAIN MENU SELECTIONS				
Crazy Bread	1 piece (1.4 oz)	106	3	1
Crazy Sauce	1 serv (6 oz)	170	tr	0
Deli-Style Sandwich Ham & Cheese	1 (11.6 oz)	728	35	13
Deli-Style Sandwich Italian	1 (11.9 oz)	740	37	12
Deli-Style Sandwich Veggie	1 (11.9 oz)	647	29	9
Hot Oven-Baked Sandwich Cheeser	1 (12.1 oz)	822	39	20
Hot Oven-Baked Sandwich Meatsa	1 (15 oz)	1036	56	24
Hot Oven-Baked Sandwich Pepperoni	1 (11.2 oz)	899	47	23
Hot Oven-Baked Sandwich Supreme	1 (13.1 oz)	894	46	21
Hot Oven-Baked Sandwich Veggie	1 (13.7 oz)	669	23	14

FOOD	PORTION	CALS	FAT	SAT FAT
PIZZA				
Baby Pan!Pan!	1 serv (8.4 oz)	616	24	12
Pan!Pan! Cheese	1 med slice (2.9 oz)	181	6	3
Pan!Pan! Pepperoni	1 med slice (3 oz)	199	8	4
Pizza!Pizza! Cheese	1 med slice (3.2 oz)	201	7	4
Pizza!Pizza! Pepperoni	1 med slice (3.3 oz)	220	9	4
SALAD DRESSINGS				
1000 Island	1 serv (1.5 oz)	183	17	3
Blue Cheese	1 serv (1.5 oz)	160	14	2
Caesar	1 serv (1.5 oz)	255	27	4
French	1 serv (1.5 oz)	166	16	2
Greek	1 serv (1.5 oz)	268	30	8
Italian	1 serv (1.5 oz)	200	21	3
Italian Fat Free	1 serv (1.5 oz)	15	0	0
Ranch	1 serv (1.5 oz)	221	22	3
SALADS AND SALAD BARS				
Antipasto Salad	1 serv (8.4 oz)	176	12	2
Caesar Salad	1 serv (5 oz)	140	5	3
Greek Salad	1 serv (10.3 oz)	168	10	tr
Tossed Salad	1 serv (8.5 oz)	116	3	tr
LONG JOHN SILVER'S				
MAIN MENU SELECTIONS				
Batter-Dipped Fish	1 piece (3 oz)	170	11	3
Breaded Chicken Strips	1 piece (1.15 oz)	100	5	1
Breaded Clams	1 serv (3 oz)	300	17	4
Breaded Fish	1 piece (1.6 oz)	110	5	1
Cheese Sticks	1 serv (1.6 oz)	160	9	4
Chicken Salsa	1 reg (11 oz)	690	32	7
Corn Cobbette w/ Butter	1 piece (3.3 oz)	140	8	2
Corn Cobbette w/o Butter	1 (3.1 oz)	80	1	0
Fish Cajun	1 lg (23 oz)	1450	70	15
Flavorbaked Chicken	1 piece (2.6 oz)	110	3	1
Flavorbaked Fish	1 piece (2.3 oz)	90	3	1
Fries	1 reg (3 oz)	250	15	3
Fries	1 lg (5 oz)	420	24	4

FOOD	PORTION	CALS	FAT	SAT FAT
Honey Mustard Sauce	1 serv (0.4 oz)	20	0	0
Hushpuppy	1 (0.8 oz)	60	3	0
Ketchup	1 serv (.32 oz)	10	0	0
Popcorn Chicken Munchers	1 serv (4 oz)	380	23	4
Popcorn Fish Munchers	1 serv (4 oz)	300	14	3
Popcorn Shrimp Munchers	1 serv (4 oz)	320	15	3
Rice	1 serv (3 oz)	140	3	1
Sandwich Batter Dipped Fish No Sauce	1 (5.4 oz)	320	13	4
Sandwich Flavorbaked Chicken	1 (5.8 oz)	290	10	2
Sandwich Flavorbaked Fish	1 (6 oz)	320	14	7
Sandwich Ultimate Fish	1 (6.4 oz)	430	21	7
Shrimp Sauce	1 serv (0.4 oz)	15	0	0
Side Salad	1 (4.3 oz)	25	0	0
Slaw	1 serv (3.4 oz)	140	6	—
Sweet'N'Sour Sauce	1 serv (0.4 oz)	20	0	0
Tartar Sauce	1 serv (0.4 oz)	35	2	—
Wraps Chicken Cajun	1 lg (22 oz)	1440	71	14
Wraps Chicken Cajun	1 reg (11 oz)	720	35	7
Wraps Chicken Ranch	1 lg (22 oz)	1450	72	14
Wraps Chicken Ranch	1 reg (11 oz)	730	36	7
Wraps Chicken Salsa	1 lg (22 oz)	1370	64	13
Wraps Chicken Tartar	1 reg (11 oz)	730	36	7
Wraps Chicken Tartar	1 lg (22 oz)	1450	72	14
Wraps Fish Cajun	1 reg (11.5 oz)	730	35	8
Wraps Fish Ranch	1 lg (23 oz)	1460	72	15
Wraps Fish Ranch	1 reg (11.5 oz)	730	36	8
Wraps Fish Salsa	1 reg (11.5 oz)	690	32	7
Wraps Fish Salsa	1 lg (23 oz)	1380	64	14
Wraps Fish Tartar	1 reg (11.5 oz)	730	36	8
Wraps Fish Tartar	1 lg (23 oz)	1470	72	15
Wraps Popcorn Shrimp Cajun	1 lg (22 oz)	1450	71	18
Wraps Popcorn Shrimp Cajun	1 reg (11 oz)	720	35	9
Wraps Popcorn Shrimp Ranch	1 reg (11 oz)	720	35	9
Wraps Popcorn Shrimp Ranch	1 lg (22 oz)	1460	72	18
Wraps Popcorn Shrimp Salsa	1 lg (22 oz)	1380	64	17
Wraps Popcorn Shrimp Salsa	1 reg (11 oz)	690	32	9
Wraps Popcorn Shrimp Tartar	1 reg (11 oz)	730	36	9
Wraps Popcorn Shrimp Tartar	1 lg (22 oz)	1460	72	18

FOOD	PORTION	CALS	FAT	SAT FAT
SALAD DRESSINGS				
Fat-Free French	1 serv (1.5 oz)	50	0	0
Fat-Free Ranch	1 serv (1.5 oz)	50	0	0
Italian	1 serv (1 oz)	130	14	2
Malt Vinegar	1 serv (0.3 oz)	0	0	0
Ranch Dressing	1 serv (1 oz)	170	18	3
Thousand Island	1 serv (1 oz)	110	10	2
MACHEEZMO MOUSE				
CHILDREN'S MENU SELECTIONS				
Quesadilla Kid Cheese	1 serv (5 oz)	360	13	—
Quesadilla Kid Chicken	1 serv (7 oz)	430	15	—
MAIN MENU SELECTIONS				
Broccoli	1 oz	4	0	—
Burrito Vegetarian	1 (14 oz)	655	8	—
Dinner Rice, Beans, Broccoli	1 serv (10 oz)	328	tr	—
Dinner Rice, Beans, Salad	1 serv (12 oz)	344	tr	—
Green Sauce	1 oz	5	0	—
Snack Famouse #5	1 serv (14 oz)	585	5	—
Snack Tacos Chicken	1 serv (6 oz)	290	8	—
Snack Tacos Veggie	1 serv (6 oz)	290	6	—
MANHATTAN BAGEL				
Blueberry	1	260	tr	0
Cheddar Cheese	1	270	4	2
Chocolate Chip	1	290	3	2
Cinnamon Raisin	1	280	tr	0
Egg	1	270	2	0
Everything	1	290	3	0
Jalapeno Cheddar	1	260	2	0
Marble	1	260	tr	0
Oat Bran	1	260	1	0
Oat Bran Raisin Walnut	1	270	3	0
Onion	1	270	tr	0
Plain	1	260	tr	0
Poppy	1	300	4	1
Pumpernickel	1	250	1	0
Rye	1	260	1	0
Salt	1	260	tr	0
Sesame	1	310	5	1
Spinach	1	270	tr	0

FOOD	PORTION	CALS	FAT	SAT FAT
Sun-Dried Tomato	1	260	1	0
Whole Wheat	1	260	tr	0

MAUI WOWI

Smoothie Rip Sticks All Flavors	1	88	0	0

MAX & ERMA'S

Black Bean Roll Up	1 serv	401	8	3
Black Bean Salsa	½ cup	215	15	2
Fruit Smoothie	1 serv	124	tr	tr
Garden Grill Sandwich w/ Tex Mex Dressing	1	569	7	tr
Garlic Breadstick	1	156	6	0
Hula Bowl w/ Fat Free Honey Mustard Dressing w/o Breadsticks	1 serv	583	10	1
Salad Dressing Fat Free French	2 tbsp	126	tr	0
Salad Dressing Fat Free Honey Mustard	2 tbsp	60	0	0
Salad Dressing Tex Mex	2 tbsp	33	tr	0
Sugar Snap Peas w/ Lemon Pepper Butter	1 serv (4 oz)	106	6	4

MCDONALD'S
BAKED SELECTIONS

Apple Pie Baked	1 (2.7 oz)	260	13	4
Cinnamon Roll	1 (3.5 oz)	340	15	5
Cookie Chocolate Chip	1 (1.4 oz)	170	9	3
McDonaldland Cookies	1 pkg (2 oz)	230	8	2

BEVERAGES

Coca-Cola Classic	1 sm (16 oz)	150	0	0
Coca-Cola Classic	1 lg (32 oz)	310	0	0
Coffee	1 sm (8 oz)	0	0	0
Coffee	1 lg (16 oz)	10	0	0
Diet Coke	1 sm (16 oz)	0	0	0
Diet Coke	1 lg (32 oz)	0	0	0
Half & Half Creamer	1 pkg	15	2	1
Hi-C Orange	1 sm (16 oz)	160	0	0
Hi-C Orange	1 lg (32 oz)	350	0	0
Iced Tea	1 lg (32 oz)	0	0	0
Iced Tea	1 sm (16 oz)	0	0	0
Milk Lowfat 1%	1 serv (8 oz)	100	3	2

FOOD	PORTION	CALS	FAT	SAT FAT
Orange Juice	1 (12 oz)	140	0	0
Shake Strawberry	1 (12 oz)	420	12	8
Sprite	1 sm (16 oz)	150	0	0
Sprite	1 lg (32 oz)	310	0	0
Triple Shake Chocolate	1 (12 oz)	430	12	8
Triple Shake Vanilla	1 (12 oz)	430	12	8
BREAKFAST SELECTIONS				
Bagel Ham Egg Cheese	1 (7.7 oz)	550	23	8
Bagel Spanish Omelet	1 (9.1 oz)	710	40	15
Bagel Steak Egg Cheese	1 (8.5 oz)	640	31	12
Big Breakfast	1 serv (9.4 oz)	710	48	13
Biscuit	1 (2.4 oz)	240	11	3
Biscuit Bacon Egg Cheese	1 (5.4 oz)	480	31	10
Biscuit Sausage	1 (4 oz)	410	28	8
Biscuit Sausage w/ Egg	1 (5.7 oz)	490	33	10
Breakfast Burrito Sausage	1 (4 oz)	290	16	6
English Muffin	1 (2 oz)	150	2	1
Hash Browns	1 serv (1.9 oz)	130	8	2
Hotcakes Margarine & Syrup	1 serv (8 oz)	600	17	3
McGriddles Bacon Egg & Cheese	1 (5.9 oz)	450	23	8
McGriddles Sausage Egg Cheese	1 (7 oz)	550	33	11
McMuffin Sausage	1 (4 oz)	370	23	9
McMuffin Sausage w/ Egg	1 (5.8 oz)	450	28	10
McMuffin Egg	1 (4.9 oz)	300	12	5
Sausage	1 (1.5 oz)	170	16	5
Scrambled Eggs	2 (3.6 oz)	160	11	4
DESSERTS				
Fruit 'n Yogurt Parfait	1 snack size (5.3 oz)	160	2	1
Fruit 'n Yogurt Parfait	1 serv (11.9 oz)	380	5	2
Fruit 'n Yogurt Parfait w/o Granola	1 serv (5 oz)	130	2	1
Fruit 'n Yogurt Parfait w/o Granola	1 serv (10.9 oz)	280	4	2
Kiddo Cone	1 (1 oz)	45	2	1
McDonaldland Chocolate Chip Cookies	1 pkg (2 oz)	280	14	8
McFlurry Butterfinger	1 (12 oz)	620	22	14
McFlurry M&M	1 (12 oz)	630	23	15
McFlurry Nestle Crunch	1 (12 oz)	630	24	16
McFlurry Oreo	1 (12 oz)	570	20	12
Nuts For Sundaes	1 serv (7 g)	40	4	0

FOOD	PORTION	CALS	FAT	SAT FAT
Reduced Fat Ice Cream Cone Vanilla	1 (3.2 oz)	150	5	3
Sundae Hot Caramel	1 (6.4 oz)	360	10	6
Sundae Hot Fudge	1 (6.3 oz)	340	12	9
Sundae Strawberry	1 (6.3 oz)	290	7	5
Triple Shake Chocolate	1 (32 oz)	1150	33	32
Triple Shake Raspberry	1 (12 oz)	420	12	8
Triple Shake Raspberry	1 (32 oz)	1120	32	22
Triple Shake Strawberry	1 (32 oz)	1120	32	22
Triple Shake Vanilla	1 (32 oz)	1140	32	22
MAIN MENU SELECTIONS				
Barbeque Sauce	1 pkg (1 oz)	45	0	0
Big Mac	1 (7.6 oz)	560	33	11
Big N' Tasty	1 (8.2 oz)	530	32	10
Big N' Tasty w/ Cheese	1 (8.7 oz)	580	37	12
Cheeseburger	1 (4.2 oz)	330	14	6
Cheeseburger Double	1 (6.1 oz)	480	27	12
Chicken McNuggets	4 pieces (2.5 oz)	210	13	3
Chicken McNuggets	6 pieces (3.8 oz)	310	20	4
Chicken McNuggets	20 pieces (12.7 oz)	1030	65	13
Chicken McNuggets	10 pieces (6.3 oz)	510	33	6
Chicken McGrill	1 (7.5 oz)	400	17	3
Crispy Chicken	1 serv (7.7 oz)	500	26	5
Filet-O-Fish	1 (5.5 oz)	470	26	5
French Fries	1 sm (2.4 oz)	210	10	2
French Fries	1 lg (6.2 oz)	540	26	5
French Fries	1 med (5.2 oz)	450	22	4
French Fries	1 McValue (3.7 oz)	320	16	3
Hamburger	1 (3.7 oz)	280	10	4
Honey	1 pkg (0.5 oz)	45	0	0
Honey Mustard	1 pkg (0.5 oz)	50	5	1
Hot Mustard	1 pkg (1 oz)	60	4	0
Light Mayonnaise	1 pkg (0.4 oz)	40	5	1
McChicken	1 (5.2 oz)	430	23	5
McChicken Hot 'n Spicy	1 (5.1 oz)	450	26	5
Quarter Pounder	1 (6.1 oz)	420	21	8
Quarter Pounder Double w/ Cheese	1 (9.9 oz)	760	48	20
Quarter Pounder w/ Cheese	1 (7 oz)	530	30	13

FOOD	PORTION	CALS	FAT	SAT FAT
Sweet 'N Sour Sauce	1 pkg (1 oz)	50	0	0
SALAD DRESSINGS				
Newman's Own Cobb	1 pkg (2 oz)	120	9	2
Newman's Own Creamy Caesar	1 pkg (2 oz)	190	18	4
Newman's Own Low Fat Balsamic Vinaigrette	1 pkg (1.5 oz)	40	0	0
Newman's Own Ranch	1 pkg (2 oz)	290	30	5
SALADS AND SALAD BARS				
Bacon Ranch w/o Chicken	1 serv (7.1 oz)	140	10	5
Caesar w/o Chicken	1 serv (6.7 oz)	90	4	3
California Cobb w/o Chicken	1 serv (7.6 oz)	160	11	5
Crispy Chicken Bacon Ranch	1 serv (10.4 oz)	370	21	7
Crispy Chicken Caesar	1 serv (10 oz)	310	16	5
Crispy Chicken California Cobb	1 serv (10.9 oz)	380	23	7
Croutons Butter Garlic	1 pkg (0.5 oz)	50	2	0
Grilled Chicken Bacon Ranch	1 serv (10.2 oz)	270	13	5
Grilled Chicken Caesar	1 serv (9.8 oz)	210	7	4
Grilled Chicken California Cobb	1 serv (10.7 oz)	280	14	6
Side Salad	1 (3.1 oz)	15	0	0
MR. HERO				
DESSERTS				
Cheesecake	1 serv	350	27	15
Cheesecake w/ Cherries	1 serv	385	25	15
MAIN MENU SELECTIONS				
Breadsticks w/ Sauce	1 serv	291	9	2
Cheddar Cheese Sauce	1 serv	60	5	1
Onion Rings	1 serv	564	32	14
Potato Wafers	1 serv	334	18	5
Spaghetti Dinner	1 serv	606	8	2
Spaghetti w/ Meatballs	1 serv	846	26	2
SALAD DRESSINGS				
Buttermilk	1 serv (2 oz)	290	29	–
Creamy Italian	1 serv (2 oz)	190	17	–
Fat Free French	1 serv (2 oz)	70	0	0
Fat Free Ranch	1 serv (2 oz)	70	0	–
SALADS AND SALAD BARS				
Croutons	1 serv	59	2	–
Garden Salad	1 serv	36	tr	0
Grilled Chicken	1 serv	225	10	3

FOOD	PORTION	CALS	FAT	SAT FAT
Seafood Crab	1 serv	452	37	7
Side Salad	1 serv	27	tr	0
Tuna	1 serv	745	69	13
SANDWICHES				
Cheesesteaks Grilled Steak Philly	7 inch	450	14	6
Cheesesteaks Hot Buttered Deluxe	7 inch	566	33	18
Cold Subs Classic Italian	7 inch	586	36	9
Cold Subs Tuna & Cheese	7 inch	666	47	9
Cold Subs Turkey & Cheese	7 inch	453	21	5
Cold Subs Ultimate Italian	7 inch	608	33	11
Hot Subs Grilled Chicken Philly	7 inch	438	14	5
Hot Subs Meatball	7 inch	620	32	3
Hot Subs Romanburger	7 inch	717	47	15
Round Bacon Cheeseburger	1	352	23	7
Round Chicken	1	420	23	5
Round Fish	1	412	23	4
Round Tuna	1	302	34	6
MR. PITA				
Cranberry Turkey	1 reg	424	1	tr
Grilled Raspberry Chicken	1 reg	342	3	1
Grilled Chicken & Broccoli	1 reg	373	4	1
Grilled Chicken Caesar	1 reg	353	4	1
Grilled Hawaiian Chicken	1 reg	375	4	1
Ultra Combo	1 reg	354	3	1
Ultra Grilled Chicken	1 reg	367	4	1
Ultra Supreme	1 reg	350	3	1
Ultra Turkey	1 reg	343	1	tr
MRS. FIELDS				
Brownie Double Fudge	1 (3.1 oz)	420	20	11
Brownie Fudge Walnut	1 (3.4 oz)	500	29	10
Brownie Pecan Fudge	1 (2.8 oz)	390	21	9
Brownie Pecan Pie	1 (3 oz)	400	21	7
Cookie Chewy Fudge	1 (1.7 oz)	230	12	7
Cookie Coconut Macadamia	1 (1.7 oz)	250	15	7
Cookie Milk Chocolate Chip	1 (1.7 oz)	240	12	7
Cookie Milk Chocolate Macadamia	1 (1.7 oz)	250	14	7
Cookie Milk Chocolate w/ Walnuts	1 (1.7 oz)	250	13	7
Cookie Oatmeal Raisin	1 (1.7 oz)	220	10	5
Cookie Peanut Butter	1 (1.7 oz)	240	13	6

FOOD	PORTION	CALS	FAT	SAT FAT
Cookie Semi-Sweet Chocolate	1 (1.7 oz)	230	12	7
Cookie Semi-Sweet Chocolate w/ Walnuts	1 (1.8 oz)	240	13	7
Cookie Triple Chocolate	1 (1.7 oz)	230	12	7
Cookie White Chunk Macadamia	1 (1.7 oz)	260	15	7
Muffin Banana Walnut	1 (3.9 oz)	460	24	5
Muffin Blueberry	1 (4 oz)	390	15	6
Muffin Chocolate Chip	1 (4 oz)	450	19	8
Muffin Mandarin Orange	1 (4 oz)	420	17	7
Peanut Butter Dream Bar	1 (5 oz)	750	40	18
Stokabunga Energy Cookie	1 (5 oz)	750	48	—

MY FAVORITE MUFFIN

FOOD	PORTION	CALS	FAT	SAT FAT
Basic Muffin	⅓ muffin	220	10	2
Double Chocolate	⅓ muffin	190	8	2
Fat Free Bavarian	⅓ muffin	100	0	0
Fat Free Bavarian Chocolate	⅓ muffin	130	0	0

NEWPORT CREAMERY

BEVERAGES

FOOD	PORTION	CALS	FAT	SAT FAT
Skim Milk	1 serv (16 oz)	206	5	—

ICE CREAM

FOOD	PORTION	CALS	FAT	SAT FAT
Reduced Fat No Sugar Added Chocolate	½ cup (2.6 oz)	110	3	2
Reduced Fat No Sugar Added Coffee	½ cup (2.6 oz)	100	4	2
Soft Serve Nonfat Frozen Yogurt Cone or Dish	1 reg (5 oz)	125	0	0

SALAD DRESSINGS

FOOD	PORTION	CALS	FAT	SAT FAT
Corn Oil & Vinegar	1 tbsp	45	6	0
Fat Free Ranch	1½ oz	48	0	0
Low-Cal French	1½ oz	48	0	0

SALADS AND SALAD BARS

FOOD	PORTION	CALS	FAT	SAT FAT
Chef's Salad	1 serv	215	8	—
Chicken Fajita	1 serv	295	20	—
Grilled Chicken	1 serv	247	13	—

SANDWICHES

FOOD	PORTION	CALS	FAT	SAT FAT
Lite Chicken Salad	1	379	19	—
Lite Grilled Cheese	1	274	17	—
Lite Grilled Chicken Breast Pocket	1	327	12	—
Lite Sliced Turkey	1	288	12	—
Lite Tuna Salad	1	358	21	—

FOOD	PORTION	CALS	FAT	SAT FAT
Lite Vegetarian Pocket Broccoli Mushrooms Onions Peppers Cheese	1	211	5	—
Lite Vegetarian Pocket Broccoli Cheese	1	214	5	—
Lite Vegetarian Pocket Peppers Onions Mushrooms Cheese	1	230	6	—
Low Fat Cheese	1 slice	73	4	—
Mayonnaise	2 tsp	71	8	—
Smart Sides Broccoli	1 serv	23	tr	—
Smart Sides Cottage Cheese	1 serv	90	4	—
Smart Sides Side Salad	1 serv	30	0	0

OLIVE GARDEN

FOOD	PORTION	CALS	FAT	SAT FAT
Garden Fare Apple Carmellina	1 serv (12.2 oz)	560	2	1
Garden Fare Dinner Capellini Pomodoro	1 serv (21.1 oz)	610	16	3
Garden Fare Dinner Capellini Primavera	1 serv (20.1 oz)	400	7	4
Garden Fare Dinner Capellini Primavera w/ Chicken	1 serv (23.8 oz)	560	10	5
Garden Fare Dinner Chicken Giardino	1 serv (20.6 oz)	550	11	4
Garden Fare Dinner Linguine Alla Marinara	1 serv (16.3 oz)	500	9	2
Garden Fare Dinner Penne Fra Diavolo	1 serv (14.3 oz)	420	7	3
Garden Fare Dinner Shrimp Primavera	1 serv (28.4 oz)	740	15	5
Garden Fare Lunch Capellini Pomodoro	1 serv (11.7 oz)	360	9	2
Garden Fare Lunch Capellini Primavera	1 serv (11.2 oz)	260	5	3
Garden Fare Lunch Capellini Primavera w/ Chicken	1 serv (14.9 oz)	420	8	4
Garden Fare Lunch Chicken Giardino	1 serv (12.8 oz)	360	9	4
Garden Fare Lunch Linguine Alla Marinara	1 serv (10.2 oz)	310	6	1
Garden Fare Lunch Penne Fra Diavolo	1 serv (10.2 oz)	300	5	2
Garden Fare Lunch Shrimp Primavera	1 serv (15.2 oz)	410	8	3
Minestrone Soup	1 serv (6 oz)	80	1	0

P.J. CHANG'S CHINA BISTRO

FOOD	PORTION	CALS	FAT	SAT FAT
Cantonese Scallops	1 serv	305	8	—

FOOD	PORTION	CALS	FAT	SAT FAT
Chicken w/ Black Bean Sauce	1 serv	426	11	—
Plain Rice Noodles	1 serv	270	2	—
Vegetable Chow Fun	1 serv	677	18	—

PANDA EXPRESS

FOOD	PORTION	CALS	FAT	SAT FAT
Beef & Broccoli	1 serv (5 oz)	180	9	2
Black Pepper Chicken	1 serv (5 oz)	210	9	2
Chicken w/ Mushrooms	1 serv (5 oz)	170	3	0
Chicken w/ String Beans	1 serv (5 oz)	180	9	2
Egg Flower Soup	1½ cups	80	0	0
Egg Rolls	2 (3 oz)	190	6	1
Hot & Sour Soup	1½ cups	110	4	1
Lo Mein	1 serv (8 oz)	300	10	2
Mixed Vegetables	1 serv (5 oz)	80	3	—
Orange Chicken	1 serv (5 oz)	310	13	3
Spicy Chicen w/ Peanuts	1 serv (5 oz)	510	29	5
Steamed Rice	1 serv (8 oz)	220	0	0
Sweet & Sour Pork	1 serv (4 oz)	310	20	7
Sweet & Sour Sauce	1 serv (2 oz)	60	0	0
Vegetable Chow Mein	1 serv (8 oz)	300	10	2
Vegetable Fried Rice	1 serv (8 oz)	410	19	3

PANERA BREAD
BAGELS AND SPREADS

FOOD	PORTION	CALS	FAT	SAT FAT
Bagel Asiago Cheese	1	330	5	3
Bagel Blueberry	1	320	2	0
Bagel Cinnamon Crunch	1	490	9	5
Bagel Dutch Apple & Raisin	1	340	3	0
Bagel Everything	1	290	2	0
Bagel French Toast	1	340	5	1
Bagel Mochachip Swirl	1	340	4	2
Bagel Nine Grain	1	290	1	0
Bagel Peanut Butter Crunch	1	400	6	3
Bagel Plain	1	280	1	0
Bagel Sesame	1	310	3	0
Cream Cheese Hazelnut Reduced Fat	1 serv (2 oz)	150	11	7
Cream Cheese Honey Walnut Reduced Fat	1 serv (2 oz)	150	11	7
Cream Cheese Mocha Reduced Fat	1 serv (2 oz)	160	11	30
Cream Cheese Plain	1 serv (2 oz)	190	18	12
Cream Cheese Plain Reduced Fat	1 serv (2 oz)	130	12	8

FOOD	PORTION	CALS	FAT	SAT FAT
Cream Cheese Raspberry Reduced Fat	1 serv (2 oz)	120	10	7
Cream Cheese Smoked Salmon Reduced Fat	1 serv (2 oz)	120	10	6
Cream Cheese Sun Dried Tomato Reduced Fat	1 serv (2 oz)	140	11	7
Cream Cheese Veggie Reduced Fat	1 serv (2 oz)	130	11	7
Hummus Roasted Garlic	1 serv (2 oz)	100	5	1
BEVERAGES				
Caffe Mocha	1 serv (11.5 oz)	360	16	55
Homestyle Lemonade	1 serv (16 oz)	80	0	0
Hot Chocolate	1 serv (11 oz)	350	15	10
IC Cappuccino Chip	1 serv (16 oz)	590	35	26
IC Caramel	1 serv (16 oz)	550	24	15
IC Honeydew Green Tea	1 serv (16 oz)	270	13	0
IC Mocha	1 serv (16 oz)	520	24	15
IC Spice	1 serv (16 oz)	470	22	13
Iced Green Tea	1 serv (16 oz)	60	0	0
Latte Caffe	1 serv (8.5 oz)	120	5	3
Latte Caramel	1 serv (11 oz)	400	16	9
Latte Chai Tea	1 serv (10 oz)	210	5	3
Latte House	1 serv (10.8 oz)	320	13	8
Sierra Turkey	1	950	55	13
BREADS				
Artisan Country	1 slice	120	0	0
Artisan French	1 slice (2 oz)	110	0	0
Artisan Kalamata Olive	1 slice (2 oz)	140	2	0
Artisan Multigrain	1 slice (2 oz)	120	1	0
Artisan Raisin Pecan	1 slice (2 oz)	140	3	0
Artisan Sesame Semolina	1 slice (2 oz)	120	0	0
Artisan Stone Milled Rye	1 slice (2 oz)	110	0	0
Artisan Three Cheese	1 slice (2 oz)	120	2	1
Artisan Three Seed	1 slice	130	2	0
Ciabatta	1 (6 oz)	430	10	2
Cinnamon Raisin	1 slice (2 oz)	160	3	1
Focaccia Asiago Cheese	1 slice (2 oz)	150	6	2
Focaccia Basil Pesto	1 slice (2 oz)	150	6	2
Focaccia Rosemary & Onion	1 slice (2 oz)	140	5	1
French	1 slice (2 oz)	130	1	0
French Roll	1 (2.25 oz)	140	1	0
Holiday	1 slice (2 oz)	150	1	0

FOOD	PORTION	CALS	FAT	SAT FAT
Honey Wheat	1 slice (2 oz)	140	3	1
Nine Grain	1 slice (2 oz)	150	3	1
Rye	1 slice (2 oz)	140	3	1
Sourdough	1 slice (2 oz)	120	0	0
Sourdough Roll	1 (2.5 oz)	160	0	0
Sourdough Soup Bowl	1 serv (8 oz)	500	2	0
Sunflower	1 slice (2 oz)	160	5	1
Tomato Basil	1 slice (2 oz)	130	1	0
DESSERTS				
Bear Claw	1	380	21	11
Brownie Caramel Pecan	1	470	24	5
Brownie Chocolate Raspberry	1	370	18	5
Brownie Very Chocolate	1	460	22	5
Cinnamon Roll	1	560	26	12
Cobblestone	1	560	9	2
Coffee Cake Cherry Cheese	1	190	10	5
Cookie Chocolate Chipper	1	420	22	13
Cookie Chocolate Duet w/ Walnuts	1	410	25	17
Cookie Nutty Chocolate Chipper	1	440	26	12
Cookie Nutty Oatmeal Raisin	1	350	14	7
Cookie Shortbread	1	340	21	13
Croissant Apple	1	260	11	7
Croissant Cheese	1	300	16	10
Croissant Chocolate	1	440	23	13
Croissant French	1	265	15	9
Croissant Raspberry Cheese	1	280	13	8
Danish Apple	1	510	30	15
Danish Cheese	1	590	35	19
Danish Cherry	1	520	26	14
Danish Georgia Peach	1	580	30	15
Danish German Chocolate	1	770	46	24
Macaroon Chocolate Hazelnut	1	270	15	10
Mini Bundt Cake Carrot Walnut	1	430	21	3
Mini Bundt Cake Lemon Poppyseed	1	460	20	4
Mini Bundt Cake Pineapple Upside Down	1	450	20	8
Muffie Banana Nut	1	260	12	2
Muffie Chocolate Chip	1	240	10	3
Muffie Pumpkin	1	270	6	2
Muffin Banana Nut	1	470	20	3

FOOD	PORTION	CALS	FAT	SAT FAT
Muffin Blueberry	1	450	15	3
Muffin Chocolate Chip	1	540	22	8
Muffin Pumpkin	1	510	12	3
Muffin Low Fat Tripleberry	1	300	3	1
Pecan Roll	1	520	31	6
Scone Cinnamon Chip	1	560	27	16
Scone Orange	1	530	25	15
Strudel Apple Raisin	1	390	22	6
Strudel Cherry	1	400	24	6
SALADS				
Asian Sesame Chicken	1 serv	370	19	3
Caesar	1 serv	350	26	7
Caesar Grilled Chicken	1 serv	470	27	7
Classic Cafe	1 serv	380	36	5
Fandango	1 serv	400	28	7
Greek	1 serv	520	48	10
SANDWICHES				
Asiago Roast Beef	1	730	35	16
Bacon Turkey Bravo	1	770	28	9
Chicken Salad On Artisan Sesame Semolina	1	730	26	4
Chicken Salad On Nine Grain	1	640	29	5
Garden Veggie	1	570	23	7
Italian Combo	1	1050	54	18
Panini Coronado Carnitas	1	810	35	11
Panini Portobello & Mozzarella	1	650	29	10
Panini Turkey Artichoke	1	810	38	11
Peanut Butter & Jelly On French	1	450	15	3
Panini Frontega Chicken	1	860	42	12
Smoked Ham On Artisan Stone Milled Rye	1	930	31	10
Smoked Ham On Rye	1	650	34	11
Smoked Turkey Breast On Artisan Country	1	590	16	2
Smoked Turkey On Sourdough	1	440	15	2
Tuna Salad On Artisan Multigrain	1	830	41	5
Tuna Salad On Honey Wheat	1	720	43	6
Turkey Fresco	1	580	17	5
Tuscan Chicken	1	950	56	10

FOOD	PORTION	CALS	FAT	SAT FAT
SOUPS				
Baked Potato	1 serv	260	16	8
Boston Clam Chowder	1 serv	210	11	6
Broccoli Cheddar	1 serv	230	16	9
Cream Of Chicken & Wild Rice	1 serv	200	12	6
Forest Mushroom	1 serv	140	7	4
French Onion	1 serv	220	10	5
Low Fat Chicken Noodle	1 serv	100	2	0
Low Fat Vegetarian Garden Vegetable	1 serv	90	1	0
Low Fat Vegetarian Black Bean	1 serv	100	1	0
Vegetarian Santa Fe Roasted Corn	1 serv	130	4	1
PAPA MURPHY'S				
MAIN MENU SELECTIONS				
Calzone Combo	⅛ pie	450	20	9
Calzone Italian	⅛ pie	480	23	9
Calzone Veggie	⅛ pie	410	17	7
Cheesy Bread	1 serv	180	7	2
PIZZA				
Deeper Dish Traditional	⅛ pie	440	24	10
Gourmet Family Size Chicken Garlic	1/12 pie	320	15	6
Gourmet Family Size Classic Italian	1/12 pie	360	19	8
Gourmet Family Size Veggie	1/12 pie	300	14	6
Papa's Family Size All Meat	1/12 pie	370	19	8
Papa's Family Size Cheese	1/12 pie	270	10	5
Papa's Family Size Cowboy	1/12 pie	370	19	7
Papa's Family Size Favorite	1/12 pie	380	20	8
Papa's Family Size Hawaiian	1/12 pie	290	11	5
Papa's Family Size Murphy's Combo	1/12 pie	480	20	7
Papa's Family Size Pepperoni	1/12 pie	310	15	7
Papa's Family Size Perfect	1/12 pie	300	13	6
Papa's Family Size Rancher	1/12 pie	330	15	7
Papa's Family Size Specialty	1/12 pie	340	17	6
Papa's Family Size Veggie Combo	1/12 pie	300	13	5
Stuffed Big Murphy	⅛ pie	380	17	7
Stuffed Chicago Style	⅛ pie	370	16	7
Stuffed Chicken & Bacon	1/16 pie	370	16	6
SALADS				
Chicken & Bacon w/o Dressing	1 serv	370	23	6
Italian Salad w/o Dressing	1 serv	260	21	8

FOOD	PORTION	CALS	FAT	SAT FAT
Veggie Salad w/o Dressing	1 serv	140	8	5

PERKINS

FOOD	PORTION	CALS	FAT	SAT FAT
Low Fat Brownie	1 (5.4 oz)	260	1	–
Low Fat Muffin Banana	1 (5.8 oz)	330	3	–
Low Fat Muffin Blueberry	1 (5.8 oz)	270	3	–
Low Fat Muffin Honey Bran	1 (5.8 oz)	270	3	–
Low Fat Muffin Plain	1 (5.8 oz)	300	3	–

PICCADILLY CAFETERIA

BAKED SELECTIONS

FOOD	PORTION	CALS	FAT	SAT FAT
Corn Sticks	1 (2 oz)	165	10	–
French Bread	1 slice	132	2	–
Garlic Bread	1 serv (15.8 oz)	1154	24	–
Mexican Corn Bread	1 piece	220	14	–
Roll	1 (2 oz)	130	2	–
Roll Whole Wheat	1 (1.7 oz)	117	1	–
Texas Toast	1 serv (15.5 oz)	1088	17	–

BEVERAGES

FOOD	PORTION	CALS	FAT	SAT FAT
Iced Tea	1 serv (6.5 oz)	2	0	–
Punch	1 serv (9 oz)	133	0	–

DESSERTS

FOOD	PORTION	CALS	FAT	SAT FAT
Apple Pie	1 slice (7.2 oz)	439	19	–
Cantaloupe	1 serv (5.5 oz)	55	tr	–
Cantaloupe	1 serv (9 oz)	89	1	–
Chocolate Cream Pie	1 slice (7.5 oz)	512	25	–
Custard	1 cup (5.4 oz)	183	1	–
Custard Pie	1 slice (6.2 oz)	412	18	–
Dole Whip Topping	1 serv (3 oz)	68	1	–
Fresh Fruit Plate	1 serv (21.1 oz)	389	5	–
Gelatin	1 serv (4.75 oz)	128	4	–
Honeydew Melon	1 serv (9 oz)	89	tr	–
Honeydew Melon	1 serv (5.5 oz)	55	tr	–
Lemon Chiffon Pie	1 slice (6.3 oz)	481	20	–
Pound Cake	1 slice (3.8 oz)	371	17	–
Watermelon	1 serv (11 oz)	100	1	–

MAIN MENU SELECTIONS

FOOD	PORTION	CALS	FAT	SAT FAT
Au Jus	1 serv (3 oz)	5	tr	–
Baby Lima Beans	1 serv (4.5 oz)	151	6	–
Baked Potato	1	218	tr	–
Baked Potato w/ Topping	1	350	15	–

FOOD	PORTION	CALS	FAT	SAT FAT
Beef Chopped Steak Fried	1 serv (4 oz)	311	23	−
Beef Leg Roast	1 serv (4 oz)	311	18	−
Beef Liver Fried	1 serv (4.5 oz)	430	29	−
Beef Tips Braised	1 serv (10 oz)	470	26	−
Black-eyed Peas w/ Pork Jowls	1 serv (4 oz)	108	6	−
Broccoli Buttered	1 serv (4 oz)	77	6	−
Broccoli & Rice Au Gratin	½ cup	184	9	−
Carrots Young Buttered	½ cup	90	6	−
Cauliflower Buttered	1 serv	80	6	−
Chicken Baked w/o Skin	¼ chicken	352	11	−
Chicken Teriyaki	1 serv (4 oz)	445	22	−
Chicken Teriyaki Polynesian	1 serv (4 oz)	537	27	−
Corn	1 serv (4.5 oz)	128	7	−
Cornbread Stuffing	1 serv (4.5 oz)	164	9	−
Crackers	4 (0.4 oz)	51	1	−
Cranberry Sauce	1 serv (1.5 oz)	64	tr	−
Eggplant Escalloped	½ cup	180	10	−
Fish Baked	1 serv (7 oz)	195	10	−
Green Beans	1 serv (4.5 oz)	77	6	−
Ham Baked	1 serv (4 oz)	224	10	−
Macaroni & Cheese	½ cup	317	11	−
Mashed Potatoes	1 serv (4.8 oz)	120	3	−
Meatballs Baked & Spaghetti	1 serv (11.5 oz)	108	5	−
New Potatoes Boiled	½ cup	148	12	−
Okra Smothered	1 serv (4 oz)	121	10	−
Onion Sauce	1 serv (4 oz)	152	7	−
Rice	½ cup	99	tr	−
Rice Polynesian	1 serv (4 oz)	140	6	−
Spaghetti Baked	1 serv (9.5 oz)	256	10	−
Squash Baked Italian	1 serv (4.75 oz)	73	3	−
Squash Mixed Yellow & Zucchini	1 serv (4 oz)	72	5	−
Squash Yellow Baked French Style	⅓ cup	86	5	−
Turkey Breast	1 serv (3 oz)	99	2	−
Vegetables Unseasoned	1 serv (5 oz)	29	tr	−
SALADS AND SALAD BARS				
Broccoli Salad	1 serv (4 oz)	202	20	−
Cabbage Combination Salad	1 serv (4.5 oz)	50	tr	−
Carrot & Raisin Salad	1 serv (4.5 oz)	321	23	−
Cole Slaw w/ Cream	1 serv (4 oz)	182	18	−
Cucumber & Celery Salad	1 serv (4 oz)	82	6	−

FOOD	PORTION	CALS	FAT	SAT FAT
Fruit Salad	1 serv (6 oz)	59	1	—
Neptune Salad	1 serv	361	34	—
Spinach Tossed Salad	1 serv (4 oz)	88	6	—
Spring Salad Bowl	1 serv (4 oz)	22	tr	—
SOUPS				
Gumbo Chicken	1 serv (8 oz)	92	2	—
Gumbo Seafood	1 serv (8 oz)	98	2	—
Vegetable	1 serv (8 oz)	49	tr	—

PIZZA HUT
APPETIZERS

FOOD	PORTION	CALS	FAT	SAT FAT
Breadstick	1	150	6	1
Breadstick Cheese	1	200	10	4
Breadstick Dipping Sauce	1 serv (3 oz)	50	0	0
Hot Wings	2 pieces	110	6	2
Mild Wings	2 pieces	110	7	2
Wing Blue Cheese Dipping Sauce	1 serv (1.5 oz)	230	24	5
Wing Ranch Dipping Sauce	1 serv (1.5 oz)	210	22	4
BEVERAGES				
Diet Pepsi	1 med (14 oz)	0	0	0
Mt. Dew	1 med (14 oz)	190	0	0
Pepsi	1 med (14 oz)	180	0	0
DESSERTS				
Apple Pizza	1 slice	260	4	1
Cherry Pizza	1 slice	240	4	1
Cinnamon Sticks	2	170	5	1
White Icing Dipping Cup	1 serv (2 oz)	170	0	0
PIZZA				
Fit 'N Delicious Diced Chicken Mushroom Jalapeno	1 med slice	170	5	2
Fit 'N Delicious Diced Chicken Red Onion Green Pepper	1 med slice	170	5	2
Fit 'N Delicious Green Pepper Red Onion Diced Red Tomato	1 med slice	150	4	2
Fit 'N Delicious Ham Pineapple Diced Red Tomato	1 med slice	160	4	2
Fit 'N Delicious Ham Red Onion Mushroom	1 med slice	160	5	2
Fit 'N Delicious Tomato Mushroom Jalapeno	1 med slice	150	4	2

FOOD	PORTION	CALS	FAT	SAT FAT
Hand Tossed Cheese	1 med slice	240	8	5
Hand Tossed Chicken Supreme	1 slice	230	6	3
Hand Tossed Ham	1 med slice	220	6	3
Hand Tossed Meat Lover's	1 med slice	300	13	6
Hand Tossed Pepperoni	1 med slice	250	9	5
Hand Tossed Pepperoni Lover's	1 med slice	300	13	7
Hand Tossed Sausage Lover's	1 med slice	280	12	5
Hand Tossed Super Supreme	1 med slice	300	13	6
Hand Tossed Supreme	1 med slice	270	11	5
Hand Tossed Veggie Lover's	1 med slice	220	6	3
Marinara Dipping Sauce	1 serv (3 oz)	45	0	0
Pan Cheese	1 med slice	280	13	5
Pan Chicken Supreme	1 med slice	280	12	4
Pan Ham	1 med slice	260	11	4
Pan Meat Lover's	1 med slice	340	19	2
Pan Pepperoni	1 med slice	290	15	5
Pan Pepperoni Lover's	1 med slice	340	19	7
Pan Sausage Lover's	1 med slice	330	17	6
Pan Super Supreme	1 med slice	340	18	6
Pan Supreme	1 med slice	320	16	6
Pizone Classic	1	1220	42	22
Pizone Pepperoni	1	1220	44	22
Thin'N Crispy Cheese	1 med slice	200	8	5
Thin'N Crispy Chicken Supreme	1 med slice	200	7	4
Thin'N Crispy Ham	1 med slice	180	6	3
Thin'N Crispy Meat Lover's	1 med slice	270	14	6
Thin'N Crispy Pepperoni	1 med slice	170	10	5
Thin'N Crispy Pepperoni Lover's	1 med slice	260	14	7
Thin'N Crispy Super Supreme	1 med slice	260	13	6
Thin'N Crispy Supreme	1 med slice	240	11	5
Thin'N Crispy Veggie Lover's	1 med slice	180	7	3

POPEYE'S

FOOD	PORTION	CALS	FAT	SAT FAT
Apple Pie	1 serv (3.1 oz)	290	16	—
Biscuit	1 serv (2.3 oz)	250	15	—
Breast Mild	1 (3.7 oz)	270	16	—
Breast Spicy	1 (3.7 oz)	270	16	—
Cajun Rice	1 serv (3.9 oz)	150	5	—
Cole Slaw	1 serv (4 oz)	149	11	—
Corn On The Cob	1 serv (5.2 oz)	127	3	—

FOOD	PORTION	CALS	FAT	SAT FAT
French Fries	1 serv (3 oz)	240	12	—
Leg Mild	1 (1.7 oz)	120	7	—
Leg Spicy	1 (1.7 oz)	120	7	—
Nuggets	1 serv (4.2 oz)	410	32	—
Nuggets Mild Tender	1 (1.2 oz)	110	7	—
Nuggets Spicy Tender	1 (1.2 oz)	110	7	—
Onion Rings	1 serv (3.1 oz)	310	19	—
Potatoes & Gravy	1 serv (3.8 oz)	100	6	—
Red Beans & Rice	1 serv (5.9 oz)	270	17	—
Shrimp	1 serv (2.8 oz)	250	16	—
Thigh Mild	1 (3.1 oz)	300	23	—
Thigh Spicy	1 (3.1 oz)	300	23	—
Wing Mild	1 (1.6 oz)	160	11	—
Wing Spicy	1 (1.6 oz)	160	11	—

QUINCY'S

BAKED SELECTIONS

FOOD	PORTION	CALS	FAT	SAT FAT
Banana Nut Bread	1 serv (2 oz)	165	7	1
Biscuit	1 (2.5 oz)	270	15	4
Cornbread	1 serv (2 oz)	140	5	1
Yeast Roll	1 (2 oz)	160	4	tr

BREAKFAST SELECTIONS

FOOD	PORTION	CALS	FAT	SAT FAT
Bacon	1 serv (0.25 oz)	35	3	1
Corned Beef Hash	1 serv (4.5 oz)	210	15	8
Country Ham	1 serv (1.5 oz)	90	6	2
Escalloped Apples	1 serv (3.5 oz)	120	2	0
Oatmeal	1 serv (1 oz)	175	2	0
Pancakes	1 (1.5 oz)	95	3	1
Sausage Gravy	1 serv (4 oz)	70	6	2
Sausage Links	1 (2 oz)	225	22	8
Sausage Patties	1 (2 oz)	230	23	9
Scrambled Eggs	1 serv (2 oz)	95	7	2
Steak Fingers	1 serv (3.5 oz)	360	25	11
Syrup	1 oz	75	0	0

DESSERTS

FOOD	PORTION	CALS	FAT	SAT FAT
Banana Pudding	1 serv (5 oz)	240	12	9
Brownie Pudding Cake	1 serv (4 oz)	310	5	tr
Caramel Topping	1 serv (1 oz)	105	1	tr
Chocolate Chip Cookies	1 (0.5 oz)	60	8	1
Cobbler Apple	1 serv (6 oz)	255	8	2

FOOD	PORTION	CALS	FAT	SAT FAT
Cobbler Cherry	1 serv (6 oz)	410	8	2
Cobbler Peach	1 serv (6 oz)	305	8	2
Frozen Yogurt	1 serv (4 oz)	135	2	1
Fudge Topping	1 serv (1 oz)	105	4	1
Sugar Cookie	1 (0.5 oz)	60	3	1
MAIN MENU SELECTIONS				
⅓ Pound Hamburger	1 serv (8 oz)	565	33	16
BBQ Beans	1 serv (4 oz)	114	1	1
Bacon Cheese Burger	1 (9 oz)	663	41	17
Baked Potato	1 (6 oz)	115	0	0
Broccoli	1 serv (4 oz)	34	0	0
Cheese Sauce	1 serv (1 oz)	58	5	2
Chopped Steak Steak	1 serv (8 oz)	499	42	20
Cinnamon Apples	1 serv (4 oz)	172	5	1
Corn	1 serv (4 oz)	96	1	0
Country Steak w/ Gravy	1 serv (8 oz)	530	25	7
Cowboy Steak	1 serv (14 oz)	580	33	15
Filet w/ Bacon	1 serv (8 oz)	340	17	7
Green Beans	1 serv (4 oz)	61	4	1
Grilled Chicken	1 reg serv (5 oz)	120	2	0
Grilled Chicken Sandwich	1 (9 oz)	324	4	1
Grilled Salmon	1 serv (7 oz)	228	4	1
Homestyle Chicken Fillet	1 serv (3 oz)	217	9	2
Junior Sirloin Steak	1 serv (5.5 oz)	194	10	5
Large Sirloin Steak	1 serv (10 oz)	368	20	9
Mashed Potatoes	1 serv (4 oz)	54	6	1
NY Strip Steak	1 serv (10 oz)	450	26	13
Philly Cheese Steak	1 serv (11 oz)	588	30	11
Porterhouse Steak	1 serv (17 oz)	683	46	23
Regular Sirloin Steak	1 serv (8 oz)	285	16	7
Ribeye Steak	1 serv (10 oz)	452	29	13
Rice Pilaf	1 serv (4 oz)	119	2	0
Roasted BBQ Chicken	1 serv (14 oz)	941	65	17
Roasted Herb Chicken	1 serv (14 oz)	875	65	17
Sirloin Tips w/ Mushroom Gravy	1 serv (6 oz)	196	7	3
Sirloin Tips w/ Peppers & Onions	1 serv (5 oz)	203	8	3
Smothered Steak Sandwich	1 (9 oz)	429	15	6
Smothered Strip Steak	1 serv (10 oz)	622	41	16
Southern Breaded Shrimp	1 serv (7 oz)	546	31	6
Spicy BBQ Chicken Sandwich	1 (10 oz)	368	1	1

FOOD	PORTION	CALS	FAT	SAT FAT
Steak & Shrimp	1 serv (9 oz)	677	39	12
Steak Fries	1 serv (4 oz)	358	19	6
T-Bone Steak	1 serv (13 oz)	521	35	18
SALAD DRESSINGS				
Blue Cheese	1 serv (1 oz)	155	16	3
French	1 serv (1 oz)	125	12	1
Honey Mustard	1 serv (1 oz)	100	6	tr
Italian	1 serv (1 oz)	135	14	2
Light Creamy Italian	1 serv (1 oz)	65	4	0
Light French	1 serv (1 oz)	85	4	0
Light Italian	1 serv (1 oz)	20	2	0
Light Thousand Island	1 serv (1 oz)	65	4	0
Parmesan Peppercorn	1 serv (1 oz)	150	14	0
Ranch	1 serv (1 oz)	110	11	2
SOUPS				
Chili With Beans	1 serv (6 oz)	235	11	2
Clam Chowder	1 serv (6 oz)	180	9	1
Cream Of Broccoli	1 serv (6 oz)	170	10	1
Vegetable Beef	1 serv (6 oz)	90	2	1
QUIZNO'S				
Cookie Oatmeal Chocolate Chip	1	360	17	5
Cookie w/ Reese's Pieces	1	360	17	3
Sub Honey Bourbon Chicken	1 sm	329	6	1
Sub Sierra Turkey w/ Raspberry Chipotle Sauce	1 sm	350	6	0
Sub Turkey Lite	1 sm	334	6	1
Sub Tuscan Chicken Salad	1 sm	326	6	1
RALLY'S				
BEVERAGES				
Coke	1 serv (20 oz)	177	0	—
Coke	1 serv (16 oz)	132	0	—
Coke	1 serv (32 oz)	264	0	—
Coke	1 serv (42 oz)	372	0	—
Diet Coke	1 serv (20 oz)	1	0	—
Diet Coke	1 serv (32 oz)	1	0	—
Diet Coke	1 serv (42 oz)	2	0	—
Fanta Orange	1 serv (42 oz)	424	0	—
Fanta Orange	1 serv (32 oz)	301	0	—
Fanta Orange	1 serv (16 oz)	150	0	—

FOOD	PORTION	CALS	FAT	SAT FAT
Fanta Orange	1 serv (20 oz)	202	0	–
Mr. Pibb	1 serv (42 oz)	334	0	–
Mr. Pibb	1 serv (16 oz)	113	0	–
Mr. Pibb	1 serv (20 oz)	159	0	–
Mr. Pibb	1 serv (32 oz)	237	0	–
Root Beer	1 serv (16 oz)	146	0	–
Root Beer	1 serv (42 oz)	414	0	–
Root Beer	1 serv (32 oz)	294	0	–
Root Beer	1 serv (20 oz)	197	0	–
Shake Banana	1 serv	399	11	–
Shake Chocolate	1 serv	411	12	–
Shake Strawberry	1 serv	399	11	–
Shake Vanilla	1 serv	320	11	–
Sprite	1 serv (16 oz)	132	0	–
Sprite	1 serv (32 oz)	264	0	–
Sprite	1 serv (42 oz)	338	0	–
Sprite	1 serv (20 oz)	161	0	–
MAIN MENU SELECTIONS				
Big Buford	1	743	46	–
Chicken Fillet Sandwich	1	399	15	–
Chili w/ Cheese & Onion	1 serv (7 oz)	360	22	–
Chili w/ Cheese & Onion	1 serv (13 oz)	669	41	–
French Fries	1 extra lg (8 oz)	423	21	–
French Fries	1 lg (6 oz)	317	16	–
French Fries	1 reg (4 oz)	211	11	–
Onion Rings	1 serv	210	2	–
Rallyburger	1	433	22	–
Rallyburger w/ Cheese	1	488	35	–
Spicy Chicken Sandwich	1	437	18	–
Super Barbecue Bacon	1	593	31	–
Super Double Cheeseburger	1	762	48	–

RANCH 1
MAIN MENU SELECTIONS

FOOD	PORTION	CALS	FAT	SAT FAT
Baked Potato w/ Broccoli	1 serv	510	1	0
Baked Potato w/ Cheese	1 serv	790	25	12
Baked Potato w/ Chicken	1 serv	610	4	1
Chicken Tenders	1 serv	370	15	3
Fajita Grilled Chicken	1	330	16	7
Fruit Cup	1 serv	90	1	0

FOOD	PORTION	CALS	FAT	SAT FAT
Hot Pasta Grilled Chicken	1 serv	590	10	2
Platter Grilled Chicken & Vegetables	1 serv	790	7	2
Ranch Fries	1 reg	350	14	5
Ranch Fries	1 lg	420	17	5
Sandwich American Rancher	1	390	10	4
Sandwich Grilled Chicken Philly	1	450	14	5
Sandwich Ranch Classic	1	370	5	1
Sandwich Spicy Grilled Chicken	1	420	11	2
Sandwich Club	1	470	16	6
SALADS				
Gourmet Greens	1 serv	220	7	3
Gourmet Greens w/ Chicken	1 serv	350	11	4
Zesty Caesar	1 serv	180	3	2
Zesty Chicken Caesar	1 serv	290	6	2

RED LOBSTER
CHILDREN'S MENU SELECTIONS

FOOD	PORTION	CALS	FAT	SAT FAT
Cheeseburger	1 serv	1040	56	18
Fried Chicken Fingers	1 serv	680	33	6
Fried Shrimp	1 serv	650	33	6
Grilled Chicken Tenders	1 serv	580	24	4
Hamburger	1 serv	920	47	12
Popcorn Shrimp	1 serv	650	35	6
Popcorn Shrimp & Cheesesticks	1 serv	750	41	9
Spaghetti & Cheesesticks	1 serv	830	39	6
DESSERTS				
Carrot Cake	1 serv (6.5 oz)	730	31	–
Cheesecake	1 serv (5.5 oz)	530	41	–
Fudge Overboard	1 serv	620	23	12
Ice Cream	1 serv (4.5 oz)	140	7	5
Key Lime Pie	1 serv (5 oz)	450	15	–
Raspberry Cobbler	1 serv (3 oz)	530	33	–
Sensational 7	1 serv	790	41	19
MAIN MENU SELECTIONS				
Admiral's Feast	1 serv	1060	52	12
Appetizer Calamari	1 serv	350	22	6
Appetizer Chicken Fingers	1 serv	390	18	4
Appetizer Chilled Shrimp In The Shell	1 serv (6 oz)	110	2	0
Appetizer Crab & Shrimp Cakes	1 serv	480	24	6
Appetizer Crab Add-On	1 serv	60	1	0

FOOD	PORTION	CALS	FAT	SAT FAT
Appetizer Fresh Fried Mushrooms	1 serv	790	51	13
Appetizer Lobster Quesadilla	1 serv	760	47	24
Appetizer Lobster Stuffed Mushroom	1 serv	400	26	13
Appetizer Mozzarella Cheesesticks	1 serv	730	46	20
Appetizer Parmesan Zucchini	1 serv	620	40	11
Appetizer Shrimp Cocktail	1 serv	50	1	0
Appetizer Stuffed Mushrooms	1 serv	420	27	13
Applesauce	1 serv (4 oz)	90	0	0
Atlantic Cod	1 lunch serv (5 oz)	110	1	0
Atlantic Cod	1 serv (8 oz)	200	2	0
Atlantic Salmon	1 lunch serv (5 oz)	200	9	2
Atlantic Salmon	1 serv (8 oz)	340	15	3
Baked Atlantic Cod	1 serv	220	6	1
Baked Atlantic Haddock	1 serv	220	6	1
Baked Flounder	1 lunch serv	190	7	1
Baked Potato	1 (8 oz)	130	0	0
Broccoli	1 serv (3 oz)	25	0	0
Broiled Fisherman's Platter	1 serv	600	23	4
Broiled Rock Lobster Tail	1 tail	190	6	1
Broiled Seafarer's Platter	1 serv	450	19	2
Caesar Salad w/ Dressing	1 serv	240	21	4
Catfish	1 serv (8 oz)	220	3	1
Catfish	1 lunch serv (5 oz)	130	2	0
Catfish Santa Fe	1 serv	340	9	2
Catfish Sante Fe	1 lunch serv	180	6	1
Chicken Fingers	1 lunch serv	390	18	4
Chicken Fresco	1 lunch serv	660	36	17
Chicken Fresco	1 serv	1320	73	33
Clam Strips	1 lunch serv	360	19	5
Clam Strips	1 serv	720	39	9
Cocktail Sauce	1 oz	30	0	0
Cole Slaw	1 serv (4 oz)	190	16	2
Crab Alfredo	1 lunch serv	590	33	17
Crab Alfredo	1 serv	1170	66	35
Fish & Shrimp Combo	1 serv	730	35	9
Fish Nuggets	1 lunch serv	320	14	4

FOOD	PORTION	CALS	FAT	SAT FAT
Fish Seasoning Add On For Blackened Dinner	1 serv	70	5	1
Fish Seasoning Add On For Blackened Lunch	1 serv	50	4	1
Fish Seasoning Add On For Broiled Dinner	1 serv	45	5	1
Fish Seasoning Add On For Broiled Lunch	1 serv	35	4	1
Fish Seasoning Add On For Grilled Dinner	1 serv	35	4	1
Fish Seasoning Add On For Grilled Lunch	1 serv	25	3	1
Fish Seasoning Add On For Lemon Pepper Dinner	1 serv	35	4	1
Fish Seasoning Add On For Lemon Pepper Lunch	1 serv	30	3	1
Fish Seasoning Add On For Sante Fe Style Dinner	1 serv	60	4	1
Fish Seasoning Add On For Sante Fe Style Lunch	1 serv	40	3	1
Flounder	1 lunch serv (5 oz)	130	2	2
Flounder	1 serv (8 oz)	220	3	1
French Fries	1 serv (4 oz)	350	22	3
Fried Flounder	1 lunch serv	230	10	3
Fried Shrimp	12 lg	500	27	7
Fried Shrimp	1 lunch serv	270	15	4
Garden Salad w/o Dressing	1 serv	50	1	0
Garlic Cheese Biscuit	1	140	8	3
Grilled Cheeseburger	1	580	34	15
Grilled Chicken Breasts	1 serv	230	7	2
Grilled Chicken Salad w/o Dressing	1 serv	320	10	2
Grouper	1 serv (8 oz)	220	3	1
Grouper	1 lunch serv (5 oz)	130	2	0
Haddock	1 serv (8 oz)	210	2	0
Haddock	1 lunch serv (5 oz)	120	1	0
Halibut	1 lunch serv (5 oz)	150	4	0

FOOD	PORTION	CALS	FAT	SAT FAT
Halibut	1 serv (8 oz)	260	6	1
King Salmon	1 serv (8 oz)	420	25	6
King Salmon	1 lunch serv (5 oz)	250	15	4
Lake Trout	1 lunch serv (5 oz)	200	9	2
Lake Trout	1 serv (8 oz)	340	16	3
Lemon Pepper Grilled Mahi Mahi	1 serv	240	7	1
Lobster Shrimp & Scallop Scampi	1 lunch serv	430	16	3
Lobster Shrimp & Scallop Scampi	1 serv	870	33	5
Mahi Mahi	1 serv (8 oz)	220	3	1
Mahi Mahi	1 lunch serv (5 oz)	130	2	0
Maine Lobster Steamed	1 serv (1.25 lb)	160	1	0
Maine Lobster Stuffed	1 serv (2 lb)	430	10	2
Marinara Sauce	1 serv	50	4	0
Melted Butter	1 oz	200	22	14
Neptune's Feast	1 serv	1210	62	14
New York Strip Steak	1 serv	560	34	13
Perch	1 serv (8 oz)	220	3	1
Perch	1 lunch serv (5 oz)	130	2	0
Pollack	1 lunch serv (5 oz)	120	2	0
Pollock	1 serv (8 oz)	120	2	0
Popcorn Shrimp	1 serv	580	37	9
Popcorn Shrimp	1 lunch serv	380	24	6
Red Rockfish	1 lunch serv (5 oz)	130	2	1
Red Rockfish	1 serv (8 oz)	230	4	1
Red Snapper	1 lunch serv (5 oz)	140	2	0
Red Snapper	1 serv (8 oz)	240	3	1
Rice Pilaf	1 serv (4 oz)	180	2	0
Roasted Vegetables	1 serv (6 oz)	120	4	1
Roasted Vegetables	1 lunch serv (4 oz)	80	3	1
Sailor's Platter	1 lunch serv	250	12	2
Sandwich Blackened Catfish	1	340	9	2
Sandwich Broiled Fish	1	300	8	2

FOOD	PORTION	CALS	FAT	SAT FAT
Sandwich Cajun Grilled Chicken	1	370	14	3
Sandwich Classic Fish	1	520	23	9
Sandwich Grilled Chicken	1	290	7	2
Sassy Sauce	1 oz	80	6	1
Seafood Broil	1 lunch serv	310	14	2
Shrimp & Chicken	1 serv	340	15	4
Shrimp Caesar Salad w/o Dressing	1 serv	240	11	4
Shrimp Carbonara	1 serv	1290	76	38
Shrimp Carbonara	1 lunch serv	650	38	19
Shrimp Combo	1 serv	380	23	5
Shrimp Feast	1 serv	470	24	5
Shrimp Milano	1 serv	1190	65	35
Shrimp Milano	1 lunch serv	590	33	17
Shrimp Scampi	1 lunch serv	110	7	1
Smothered Chicken	1 serv	530	31	15
Snow Crab Legs	1 serv	110	2	0
Sockeye Salmon	1 lunch serv (5 oz)	240	12	2
Sockeye Salmon	1 serv (8 oz)	410	21	4
Sole	1 serv (8 oz)	220	3	1
Sole	1 lunch serv (5 oz)	130	2	0
Soup Bread Salad w/o Dressing	1 lunch serv	430	18	7
Steak & Fried Shrimp	1 serv	780	46	15
Steak & Rock Lobster Tail	1 serv	570	31	11
Swordfish	1 lunch serv (5 oz)	170	6	2
Swordfish	1 serv (8 oz)	290	10	3
Tartar Sauce	1 oz	160	17	3
Teriyaki Grilled Chicken Breast	1 serv	240	7	2
Twice Baked Potato	1	430	23	14
Walleye	1 lunch serv (5 oz)	120	2	0
Walleye	1 serv (8 oz)	210	3	1
Yellow Lake Perch	1 lunch serv (5 oz)	130	2	0
Yellow Lake Perch	1 serv (8 oz)	220	3	1
SALAD DRESSINGS				
Blue Cheese	1 serv	170	18	3
Buttermilk Ranch	1 serv	110	11	2

FOOD	PORTION	CALS	FAT	SAT FAT
Caesar	1 serv	170	18	3
Dijon Honey Mustard	1 serv	140	13	2
Fat Free Ranch	1 serv	50	0	0
Lite Red Wine Vinaigrette	1 serv	50	3	0
SOUPS				
Bayou Style Gumbo	1 serv (6 oz)	120	4	1
Broccoli Cheese	1 serv	160	9	6
Clam Chowder	1 serv (6 oz)	130	5	3
RUBY TUESDAY'S				
Cajun Chicken Salad w/ Ranch Dressing	1 serv	636	46	–
Peppercorn Mushroom Sirloin	1 serv	947	57	–
SBARRO				
Baked Ziti	1 serv (14 oz)	830	42	21
Meat Lasagna	1 serv (17 oz)	730	38	17
Pizza Cheese	1 serv (6 oz)	450	14	7
Pizza Pepperoni	1 serv (6 oz)	510	21	10
Pizza Sausage	1 serv (10 oz)	640	29	14
Pizza Sausage & Pepperoni Stuffed	1 serv (11 oz)	880	44	19
Pizza Spinach & Broccoli Stuffed	1 serv (11 oz)	710	26	10
Pizza Supreme	1 serv (10 oz)	600	25	12
Pizza Veggie Slice	1 serv (10 oz)	490	12	5
Spaghetti w/ Sauce	1 serv (18 oz)	630	18	3
SCHLOTZSKY'S DELI				
SALADS AND SALAD BARS				
Caesar	1 serv (7 oz)	150	8	4
Chicken Caesar	1 serv (9 oz)	250	10	5
Chinese Chicken	1 serv (9 oz)	150	3	1
Choice Potato Salad	1 serv (5 oz)	250	18	3
Country Style Cole Slaw	1 serv (4 oz)	230	16	3
Garden	1 serv (9 oz)	60	1	0
Greek	1 serv (12 oz)	220	12	8
Smoked Turkey Chef	1 serv (13 oz)	240	10	5
SANDWICHES				
Light & Flavorful Albacore Tuna	1 (13 oz)	530	16	4
Light & Flavorful Chicken Breast	1 (15 oz)	540	10	3
Light & Flavorful Dijon Chicken	1 sm (10 oz)	330	4	1
Light & Flavorful Dijon Chicken	1 (15 oz)	500	6	1

FOOD	PORTION	CALS	FAT	SAT FAT
Light & Flavorful Pesto Chicken	1 (14 oz)	510	9	2
Light & Flavorful Santa Fe Chicken	1 (17 oz)	640	19	9
Light & Flavorful Smoked Turkey Breast	1 (13 oz)	500	7	1
Light & Flavorful The Vegetarian	1 (12 oz)	520	17	7
Original Cheese	1 (14 oz)	850	44	23
Original Ham & Cheese	1 (17 oz)	790	32	12
Original Turkey	1 (17 oz)	1020	51	20
Specialty Deli Albacore Tuna Melt	1 (16 oz)	820	40	16
Specialty Deli BLT	1 (10 oz)	580	24	7
Specialty Deli Chicken Club	1 (16 oz)	690	23	9
Specialty Deli Corned Beef	1 (12 oz)	590	15	3
Specialty Deli Corned Beef Reuben	1 (15 oz)	830	35	13
Specialty Deli Pastrami & Swiss	1 (15 oz)	860	37	17
Specialty Deli Pastrami Reuben	1 (16 oz)	920	43	18
Specialty Deli Roast Beef	1 (14 oz)	620	17	3
Specialty Deli Roast Beef & Cheese	1 (17 oz)	850	34	14
Specialty Deli Texas Schlotzsky	1 (16 oz)	820	37	16
Specialty Deli The Philly	1 (16 oz)	820	32	14
Specialty Deli Turkey & Bacon Club	1 (17 oz)	870	40	15
Specialty Deli Turkey Guacamole	1 (16 oz)	680	24	3
Specialty Deli Turkey Reuben	1 (16 oz)	860	39	16
Specialty Deli Vegetable Club	1 (13 oz)	580	24	7
Specialty Deli Western Vegetarian	1 (12 oz)	650	33	14
The Original	1 (14 oz)	940	50	22

SEE'S CANDIES

FOOD	PORTION	CALS	FAT	SAT FAT
Bridge Mix	14 pieces (1.4 oz)	200	12	6
Dark Chocolate Bordeaux	2 (1.4 oz)	170	27	1
Dark Chocolates	2 (1.2 oz)	160	10	5
Lollypop Butterscotch	1	90	3	2
Lollypop Cafe Latte	1	90	3	2
Lollypop Chocolate	1	90	5	3
Lollypop Peanut Butter	1	90	4	1
Marshmints	3 (1.4 oz)	140	4	3
Milk Chocolate Bordeaux	2 (1.4 oz)	170	8	5
Milk Chocolate Butter	2 (1.4 oz)	190	9	6
Milk Chocolate Buttercreams	2 (1.4 oz)	180	8	5
Milk Chocolate California Brittle	2 (1.3 oz)	220	16	8

FOOD	PORTION	CALS	FAT	SAT FAT
Milk Chocolate Nuts & Chews	3 (1.7 oz)	250	16	7
Milk Chocolate Peanuts	3 (1.5 oz)	230	17	6
Milk Chocolate Soft Centers	2 (1.4 oz)	170	9	5
Milk Chocolates	2 (1.2 oz)	160	9	5
Nuts & Chews	3 (1.6 oz)	240	16	6
P-Nut Crunch	2 (1.4 oz)	220	15	6
Peanut Brittle	1.5 oz	230	16	6
Pecan Buds	3 (1.7 oz)	270	21	6
Red Hot Swamp Goo	3 pieces (1.4 oz)	140	4	3
Soft Centers	2 (1.4 oz)	170	9	5
Truffles Black or Gold	2 (1.4 oz)	180	11	6
Truffles Mint	3 (1.6 oz)	200	11	7
Victoria Toffee	1.5 oz	250	19	7

SIZZLER
DESSERTS

FOOD	PORTION	CALS	FAT	SAT FAT
Chocolate & Vanilla Soft Serve	4 oz	136	4	4
Chocolate Syrup	1 oz	90	0	0
Strawberry Topping	1 oz	70	0	0
Whipped Topping	1 tbsp	12	1	1

HOT BUFFET

FOOD	PORTION	CALS	FAT	SAT FAT
Broccoli Cheese Soup	1 serv (4 oz)	139	9	2
Chicken Noodle Soup	1 serv (4 oz)	31	1	0
Chicken Wings	1 oz	73	4	1
Clam Chowder	1 serv (4 oz)	118	6	0
Fettucine	2 oz	80	1	0
Focaccia Bread	2 pieces	108	7	1
Marinara Sauce	1 oz	13	0	0
Meatballs	4	157	11	5
Minestrone Soup	1 serv (4 oz)	36	0	0
Nacho Cheese Soup	1 serv (4 oz)	120	10	5
Potato Skins	2 oz	160	8	1
Refried Beans	¼ cup	62	1	2
Saltine Crackers	2	25	1	0
Spaghetti	2 oz	80	0	0
Taco Filling	2 oz	103	9	4
Taco Shells	1	50	2	0
Vegetable Sirloin Soup	1 serv (4 oz)	60	2	1

MAIN MENU SELECTIONS

FOOD	PORTION	CALS	FAT	SAT FAT
Buttery Dipping Sauce	1 serv (1.5 oz)	330	37	7

FOOD	PORTION	CALS	FAT	SAT FAT
Cheese Toast	1 piece	273	21	5
Cocktail Sauce	1 serv (1.5 oz)	40	0	0
Dakota Ranch Steak	1 (9.5 oz)	500	32	13
Dakota Ranch Steak	1 (8 oz)	421	27	11
Dakota Ranch Steak	1 (6 oz)	316	20	8
French Fries	1 serv (4 oz)	358	12	6
Hamburger	1	626	33	12
Hibachi Chicken Breast w/ Pineapple	5 oz	193	3	1
Hibachi Sauce	1 serv (1.5 oz)	57	0	0
Lemon Herb Chicken Breast	5 oz	140	3	1
Malibu Chicken Patty	1	310	19	3
Malibu Sauce	1 serv (1.5 oz)	283	31	6
Margarine Whipped	1½ tbsp	105	12	2
Potato Baked Plain	1 (4 oz)	105	0	0
Rice Pilaf	1 serv (6 oz)	256	5	1
Salmon	8 oz	110	12	2
Sante Fe Chicken Breast	5 oz	150	3	1
Shrimp Broiled	5 oz	150	6	1
Shrimp Fried	4 pieces	223	2	0
Shrimp Mini	4 oz	152	1	0
Shrimp Scampi	5 oz	143	3	1
Sour Dressing	2 tbsp	60	6	5
Swordfish	8 oz	315	14	3
Tartar Sauce	1 serv (1.5 oz)	170	17	3
SALAD DRESSINGS				
Blue Cheese	1 oz	111	12	4
Honey Mustard	1 oz	160	16	2
Italian Lite	1 oz	14	0	0
Japanese Rice Vinegar Fat Free	1 oz	10	0	0
Parmesan Italian	1 oz	100	10	2
Ranch	1 oz	120	12	2
Thousand Island	1 oz	143	15	2
SALADS AND SALAD BARS				
Alfafa Sprouts	¼ cup	2	0	0
Avocado	½	153	15	2
Bean Sprouts	¼ cup	8	0	0
Beets	¼ cup	13	0	0
Bell Peppers	2 oz	8	0	0
Broccoli	½ cup	12	0	0
Cabbage Red	¼ cup	5	0	0

FOOD	PORTION	CALS	FAT	SAT FAT
Cantaloupe	½ cup	28	0	0
Carrot & Raisin Salad	2 oz	130	10	2
Carrots	¼ cup	12	0	0
Chinese Chicken Salad	2 oz	54	2	0
Chives	1 oz	62	6	1
Cottage Cheese	2 oz	51	1	1
Cucumber	2 oz	7	0	0
Eggs	1 oz	44	3	1
Garbanzo Beans	¼ cup	63	1	1
Grapes	½ cup	29	0	0
Guacamole	1 oz	42	4	1
Honeydew Melon	½ cup	30	0	0
Iceberg Lettuce	1 cup	7	0	0
Jicama	2 oz	13	0	0
Kidney Beans	¼ cup	52	0	0
Kiwifruit	2 oz	35	0	0
Mediterranean Minted Fruit Salad	2 oz	29	0	0
Mexican Fiesta Salad	2 oz	54	1	0
Mushrooms	¼ cup	4	0	0
Old Fashioned Potato Salad	2 oz	84	5	1
Onions Red	2 tbsp	8	0	0
Peaches	¼ cup	34	0	0
Peas	¼ cup	31	0	0
Pineapple	½ cup	38	0	0
Real Bacon Bits	1 tbsp	27	2	0
Red Herb Potato Salad	2 oz	121	9	1
Romaine Lettuce	1 cup	9	0	0
Salsa	1 oz	7	0	0
Seafood Louis Pasta Salad	2 oz	64	2	0
Seafood Salad	2 oz	56	3	1
Spicy Jicama Salad	2 oz	16	0	0
Spinach	½ cup	6	0	0
Strawberries	½ cup	22	0	0
Teriyaki Beef Salad	2 oz	49	2	1
Tomatoes Cherry	¼ cup	12	0	0
Tuna Pasta Salad	2 oz	133	10	7
Turkey Ham	1 oz	62	5	2
Watermelon	½ cup	26	0	0
Zucchini	¼ cup	5	0	0

FOOD	PORTION	CALS	FAT	SAT FAT
SMOOTHIE KING				
Activator Chocolate	1 (20 oz)	429	1	tr
Activator Strawberry	1 (20 oz)	559	1	tr
Activator Vanilla	1 (20 oz)	429	1	tr
Banana Boat	1 (20 oz)	520	14	8
Coconut Surprise	1 (20 oz)	457	6	2
Coffee Smoothies Hazelnut	1 (20 oz)	118	tr	tr
Coffee Smoothies Amaretto	1 (20 oz)	118	tr	tr
Coffee Smoothies French Roast	1 (20 oz)	164	tr	tr
Coffee Smoothies French Vanilla	1 (20 oz)	118	tr	tr
Coffee Smoothies Irish Creme	1 (20 oz)	118	tr	tr
Coffee Smoothies Mocha	1 (20 oz)	206	1	tr
HeaterZ Banana Nut	1	400	22	–
HeaterZ Blueberry Muffin	1	370	26	–
HeaterZ Chocolate Peanut Butter Cup	1	380	13	–
HeaterZ Cinnamon Oatmeal Raisin	1	420	3	–
HeaterZ Coconut	1	440	13	–
HeaterZ Coffee Amaretto	1 (12 oz)	177	2	1
HeaterZ Coffee French Roast	1 (12 oz)	172	2	1
HeaterZ Coffee French Vanilla	1 (12 oz)	177	2	1
HeaterZ Coffee Hazelnut	1 (12 oz)	177	2	1
HeaterZ Coffee Irish Creme	1 (12 oz)	177	2	1
HeaterZ Coffee Mocha	1 (12 oz)	266	2	1
High Protein Almond Mocha	1 (20 oz)	402	13	2
High Protein Banana	1 (20 oz)	412	14	2
High Protein Chocolate	1 (20 oz)	401	13	2
High Protein Lemon	1 (20 oz)	390	13	2
High Protein Pineapple	1 (20 oz)	380	13	2
Hot Coffee Amaretto	1 (12 oz)	168	tr	tr
Hot Coffee French Roast	1 (12 oz)	164	tr	tr
Hot Coffee French Vanilla	1 (12 oz)	168	tr	tr
Hot Coffee Hazelnut	1 (12 oz)	168	tr	tr
Hot Coffee Irish Creme	1 (12 oz)	168	tr	tr
Hot Coffee Mocha	1 (12 oz)	209	1	tr
Iced Coffee Amaretto	1 (20 oz)	168	tr	tr
Iced Coffee French Roast	1 (20 oz)	164	tr	tr
Iced Coffee French Vanilla	1 (20 oz)	168	tr	tr
Iced Coffee Hazelnut	1 (20 oz)	168	tr	tr
Iced Coffee Irish Creme	1 (20 oz)	168	tr	tr
Iced Coffee Mocha	1 (20 oz)	209	1	tr

FOOD	PORTION	CALS	FAT	SAT FAT
Kid Cup Berry Interesting	1	150	0	0
Kid Cup Choc-A-Laka	1	210	2	0
Kid Cup Gimmi-Grape	1	170	0	0
Kid Cup Smarti Tarti	1	150	0	0
Low Carb All Flavors	1 (20 oz)	225	6	3
Low Fat Angel Food	1 (20 oz)	330	1	tr
Low Fat Blackberry Dream	1 (20 oz)	343	tr	tr
Low Fat Caribbean Way	1 (20 oz)	392	tr	tr
Low Fat Celestial Cherry High	1 (20 oz)	285	tr	tr
Low Fat Cherry Picker	1 (20 oz)	360	1	tr
Low Fat Cranberry Supreme	1 (20 oz)	577	1	tr
Low Fat Cranberry Cooler	1 (20 oz)	538	tr	tr
Low Fat Grape Expectations	1 (20 oz)	399	tr	tr
Low Fat Grape Expectations II	1 (20 oz)	529	tr	tr
Low Fat Hearty Apple	1 (20 oz)	380	2	1
Low Fat Immune Builder	1 (20 oz)	333	1	tr
Low Fat Instant Vigor	1 (20 oz)	359	1	tr
Low Fat Island Treat	1 (20 oz)	334	1	tr
Low Fat Lemon Twist Banana	1 (20 oz)	339	tr	tr
Low Fat Lemon Twist Strawberry	1 (20 oz)	399	tr	tr
Low Fat Light & Fluffy	1 (20 oz)	389	tr	tr
Low Fat Mangofest	1 (20 oz)	320	0	0
Low Fat Muscle Punch	1 (20 oz)	339	1	tr
Low Fat Muscle Punch Plus	1 (20 oz)	340	1	tr
Low Fat Orange Ka-BAM	1 (20 oz)	320	0	0
Low Fat Peach Slice	1 (20 oz)	341	tr	tr
Low Fat Pep Upper	1 (20 oz)	334	1	tr
Low Fat Pineapple Pleasure	1 (20 oz)	331	tr	tr
Low Fat Pineapple Surf	1 (20 oz)	440	1	0
Low Fat Raspberry Sunrise	1 (20 oz)	335	1	tr
Low Fat Strawberry X-Treme	1 (20 oz)	370	0	0
Low Fat Strawberry Kiwi Breeze	1 (20 oz)	300	0	0
Low Fat Youth Fountain	1 (20 oz)	267	tr	tr
Malts	1 (20 oz)	887	41	26
Mo'cuccino	1 (20 oz)	420	12	7
Peanut Power	1 (20 oz)	502	21	4
Peanut Power Plus Grape	1 (20 oz)	703	21	4
Peanut Power Plus Strawberry	1 (20 oz)	632	21	4
Pina Colada Island	1 (20 oz)	550	11	9
Power Punch	1 (20 oz)	430	1	tr

FOOD	PORTION	CALS	FAT	SAT FAT
Power Punch Plus	1 (20 oz)	499	2	tr
Shakes	1 (20 oz)	875	41	25
Slim-N-Trim Chocolate	1 (20 oz)	270	2	1
Slim-N-Trim Orange Vanilla	1 (20 oz)	199	1	0
Slim-N-Trim Strawberry	1 (20 oz)	357	1	tr
Slim-N-Trim Vanilla	1 (20 oz)	227	1	tr
Super Punch	1 (20 oz)	425	tr	tr
Super Punch Plus	1 (20 oz)	516	tr	tr
The Hulk Chocolate	1 (20 oz)	846	29	17
The Hulk Strawberry	1 (20 oz)	953	29	16
The Hulk Vanilla	1 (20 oz)	846	29	16
Yogurt D-Lite	1 (20 oz)	335	4	2

SONIC DRIVE-IN
ADD-ONS

FOOD	PORTION	CALS	FAT	SAT FAT
Bacon	1 serv (0.5 oz)	80	7	3
Cheddar Cheese Shredded	1 serv (1 oz)	104	9	6
Cheese	1 serv (0.7 oz)	70	6	4
Chili	1 serv (1 oz)	52	4	2
Cone Coat Chocolate	1 serv (1 oz)	143	8	7
Green Chilies	1 serv (1 oz)	10	0	0
Hickory Barbecue Sauce	1 serv (1 oz)	41	0	0
Honey Mustard Dressing	1 serv (1.1 oz)	110	9	1
Jalapenos Nachos Sliced	1 serv (1 oz)	5	0	0
Malt	1 serv (1 oz)	104	1	0
Maraschino Cherry	1 serv (8 g)	10	0	0
Marinara Sauce	1 serv (1 oz)	15	0	0
Ranch Dressing	1 serv (1 oz)	147	16	2
Slaw	1 serv (0.9 oz)	45	3	0
Sweet Pickle Relish	1 serv (1.1 oz)	40	0	0
Syrup Blue Coconut	1 serv (1 oz)	65	0	0
Syrup Cherry	1 serv (1 oz)	64	0	0
Syrup Chocolate	1 serv (1 oz)	74	0	0
Syrup Grape	1 serv (1 oz)	61	0	0
Syrup Vanilla	1 serv (1 oz)	61	0	0
Syrup Watermelon	1 serv (1 oz)	71	0	0
Thousand Island Dressing	1 serv (1 oz)	150	15	2
Topping Pineapple	1 serv (1.5 oz)	108	0	0
Topping Strawberry	1 serv (1.2 oz)	38	0	0
Topping Strawberry	1 serv (1 oz)	101	4	3

FOOD	PORTION	CALS	FAT	SAT FAT
BEVERAGES				
Barqs Root Beer	1 sm	160	0	0
Barqs Root Beer	1 lg	333	0	0
Coca-Cola	1 lg	291	0	0
Coca-Cola	1 sm	139	0	0
Diet Coca-Cola	1 sm	1	0	0
Diet Coca-Cola	1 lg	3	0	0
Diet Sprite	1 lg	8	0	0
Diet Sprite	1 sm	4	0	0
Dr Pepper	1 sm	144	0	0
Dr Pepper	1 lg	300	0	0
Float Or Flurry Blue Coconut Slush	1 reg	424	12	12
Limeade	1 sm	143	0	0
Limeade	1 lg	303	0	0
Limeade Cherry	1 sm	169	0	0
Limeade Cherry	1 lg	361	0	0
Limeade Strawberry	1 sm	172	0	0
Limeade Strawberry	1 lg	341	0	0
Slush Blue Coconut	1 lg	521	0	0
Slush Watermelon	1 lg	526	0	0
Sprite	1 sm	138	0	0
Sprite	1 lg	288	0	0
BREAKFAST SELECTIONS				
Breakfast Burrito	1	731	47	22
Fruit Taquitos	1 serv	302	7	1
Sunrise	1 reg	224	0	0
Sunrise	1 lg	368	0	0
Toaster Bacon Egg & Cheese	1	500	20	11
Toaster Ham Egg & Cheese	1	436	19	7
Toaster Sausage Egg & Cheese	1	570	36	14
DESSERTS				
Banana Split	1 serv	467	11	10
Chocolate Covered Shake Banana	1 reg	625	25	23
Chocolate Covered Shake Cherry	1 reg	587	24	23
Chocolate Covered Shake Peanut Butter	1 reg	678	34	25
Chocolate Covered Shake Strawberry	1 reg	608	24	23
Cream Pie Shake Banana	1 reg	775	27	21
Cream Pie Shake Chocolate	1 reg	795	27	21
Cream Pie Shake Coconut	1 reg	721	26	21

FOOD	PORTION	CALS	FAT	SAT FAT
Dish Of Vanilla	1 serv	265	11	11
Float Or Flurry Cherry Slush	1 reg	421	12	12
Float Or Flurry Coca-Cola	1 reg	379	12	12
Float Or Flurry Dr Pepper	1 reg	377	12	12
Float Or Flurry Grape Slush	1 reg	423	12	12
Float Or Flurry Orange Slush	1 reg	422	12	12
Float Or Flurry Rootbeer	1 reg	386	12	12
Float Or Flurry Watermelon Slush	1 reg	427	12	12
Ice Cream Cone	1	285	11	11
Shake Banana	1 reg	508	18	18
Shake Chocolate	1 reg	564	18	18
Shake Pineapple	1 reg	615	18	18
Shake Strawberry	1 reg	510	18	18
Shake Vanilla	1 reg	454	18	18
Sonic Blast Butterfinger	1 reg	636	26	23
Sonic Blast M&M	1 reg	641	27	24
Sonic Blast Oreo	1 reg	638	27	21
Sonic Blast Reese's	1 reg	658	30	23
Sundae Chocolate	1 serv	362	11	11
Sundae Hot Fudge	1 serv	392	15	15
Sundae Pineapple	1 serv	399	11	11
Sundae Strawberry	1 serv	322	11	11
MAIN MENU SELECTIONS				
Ched'R'Peppers	1 serv	256	12	5
Cheese Fries	1 reg	265	17	6
Cheese Fries	1 lg	322	19	6
Cheese Tater Tots	1 reg	329	22	7
Cheese Tots	1 lg	435	27	8
Chicken Strip Dinner	1 serv	749	32	5
Chicken Strip Snack	1 serv	272	13	2
Chicken Strips	2	184	9	1
Chili Cheese Fries	1 reg	299	19	6
Chili Cheese Fries	1 lg	357	22	7
Chili Cheese Tater Tots	1 reg	363	25	7
Chili Cheese Tots	1 lg	547	36	11
Corn Dog	1	262	17	5
Extra Long Coney Plain	1	483	27	10
French Fries	1 lg	252	13	2
French Fries	1 reg	195	11	2
Fritos Chili Pie	1 serv	611	44	13

FOOD	PORTION	CALS	FAT	SAT FAT
Hot Dog Plain	1	262	16	5
Jr. Burger	1	353	21	6
Mozzarella Sticks	1 serv	382	19	11
No.1 Hamburger	1	577	36	7
No.1 Sonic Cheeseburger	1	647	42	11
No.2 Hamburger	1	481	25	5
No.2 Sonic Cheeseburger	1	551	31	9
Onion Rings	1 lg	507	35	7
Onion Rings	1 reg	331	23	5
Regular Coney Cheese	1	366	24	10
Sandwich Breaded Chicken	1	582	23	4
Sandwich Country Fried Steak	1	748	47	12
Sandwich Grilled Chicken	1	343	13	2
Super Sonic No.1	1	929	66	19
Super Sonic No.2	1	839	56	17
SuperSonic Onion Rings	1 serv	706	10	1
SuperSonic Tots	1 serv	485	28	5
SuperSonic Fries	1 serv	358	18	3
Tater Tots	1 lg	365	21	4
Tater Tots	1 reg	259	16	3
Toaster Sandwich BLT	1	581	41	9
Toaster Sandwich Bacon Cheddar Burger	1	675	38	11
Toaster Sandwich Chicken Club	1	675	29	8
Toaster Sandwich Country Fried Steak	1	708	45	11
Toaster Sandwich Grilled Cheese	1	282	12	5
Wrap Chicken Strip	1	574	29	5
Wrap Grilled Chicken	1	539	27	5
Wrap w/o Ranch Chicken Strip	1	428	13	2
Wrap w/o Ranch Grilled Chicken	1	393	12	3

STARBUCKS
BAKED SELECTIONS

Baby Bundt Cake Chocolate	1	330	15	7
Bagel	1	430	1	0
Bagel Cinnamon Raisin	1	440	1	0
Bagel Sesame	1	440	3	0
Bar Caramel Apple	1	310	16	8
Bar Carrot Cake	1	420	25	9
Bar Lemon	1	310	14	8

FOOD	PORTION	CALS	FAT	SAT FAT
Bar Oreo Dream	1	420	30	15
Bar Toffee Crunch	1	430	21	8
Biscotti Chocolate Hazelnut	1	110	5	2
Biscotti Vanilla Almond	1	110	5	2
Brownie Caramel	1	580	36	12
Brownie Enrobed Espresso	1	430	25	16
Brownie Espresso	1	370	21	13
Brownie Milk Chocolate Peanut Butter	1	460	29	9
Bundt Cake Lemon Yogurt	1 serv	350	13	5
Caramel Pecan Sticky Roll	1	730	40	7
Cinnamon Roll	1	620	29	7
Cinnamon Twist	1	320	17	2
Coffee Cake	1 serv	570	28	10
Coffee Cake Apple Walnut	1 serv	320	17	5
Coffee Cake Blueberry Walnut	1 serv	340	18	5
Coffee Cake Cinnamon Walnut	1 serv	360	18	5
Coffee Cake Crumble Berry	1 serv	520	26	10
Coffee Cake Hazelnut	1 serv	630	35	14
Coffee Cake Sour Cream	1 serv	420	25	12
Cookie Black And White	1	430	17	3
Cookie Double Chocolate Chunk	1 serv	430	21	7
Cookie Oatmean Raisin	1	390	15	2
Cookie White Chocolate Macadamia Nut	1	470	27	8
Crisp Cinnamon Twist	1	60	2	1
Croissant Almond	1	330	18	7
Croissant Butter w/ Apricot Glaze	1	320	17	2
Croissant Raspberry & Cream Cheese	1	260	12	7
Crumb Cake	1 serv	670	32	15
Crumb Cake Key Lime	1 serv	550	27	10
Danish Apple w/ Mocha Swirls	1	370	19	2
Danish Cheese w/ Mocha Swirls	1	460	28	7
Danish Raspberry w/ Mocho Swirls	1	370	19	2
Graham Dark Chocolate	1	140	8	5
Graham Milk Chocolate	1	140	8	5
Madeline	1	80	4	2
Muffin Blueberry	1	380	19	4
Muffin Cranberry Orange	1	410	20	4
Muffin Morning Sunrise	1	330	12	5

FOOD	PORTION	CALS	FAT	SAT FAT
Muffin Chocolate Cream Cheese	1	450	24	6
Pound Cake Banana	1 serv	360	18	11
Pound Cake Cranberry Walnut	1 serv	390	21	9
Pound Cake Iced Carrot	1 serv	540	13	3
Pound Cake Iced Lemon	1 serv	500	23	12
Pound Cake Marble	1 serv	400	21	11
Pound Cake Orange Poppy	1 serv	490	27	12
Pound Cake Pumpkin	1 serv	310	12	2
Pound Cake Zucchini	1 serv	370	19	2
Pullman Banana	1 serv	400	17	5
Pullman Chocolate	1	380	17	7
Pullman Cranberry Walnut	1	360	15	4
Pullman Lemon Glazed	1	370	15	9
Pullman Marble Chocolate Chip	1	440	20	12
Pullman Orange Poppy Cheese	1	450	22	13
Pullman Pumpkin	1	370	17	3
Scone Blueberry	1	460	18	4
Scone Butterscotch Pecan	1	520	27	11
Scone Cinnamon Chip w/ Icing	1	510	23	10
Scone Maple Oat w/ Icing	1	490	22	9
Scone Apricot Currant	1	450	17	8
Scone Raspberry	1	440	18	8
Shortbread	1	100	6	3
BEVERAGES				
Apple Juice	1 grande	230	0	0
Blended Coffee Of The Week	1 grande	10	0	0
Caffe Americano	1 grande	150	0	0
Caffe Au Lait Nonfat Milk	1 grande	90	0	0
Caffe Au Lait Soy Milk	1 grande	110	3	0
Caffe Latte Whole Milk	1 grande	260	14	9
Caffe Misto Au Lait Whole Milk	1 grande	140	8	5
Caffe Mocho Whip Whole Milk	1 grande	400	22	13
Caffe Latte Soy Milk	1 grande	210	6	1
Caffe Mocha No Whip Whole Milk	1 grande	300	12	7
Caffe Mocha No Whip Nonfat Milk	1 grande	230	2	0
Caffe Mocha No Whip Soy Milk	1 grande	260	6	1
Caffe Mocha Whip Nonfat Milk	1 grande	330	12	7
Caffe Mocha Whip Soy Milk	1 grande	360	16	7
Caffe Latte Nonfat Milk	1 grande	160	0	0
Cappuccino Nonfat Milk	1 grande	100	0	0

FOOD	PORTION	CALS	FAT	SAT FAT
Cappuccino Soy Milk	1 grande	120	3	0
Caramel Mocha No Whip Soy Milk	1 grande	340	6	1
Caramel Macchiato Nonfat Milk	1 grande	230	2	2
Caramel Macchiato Soy Milk	1 grande	300	8	2
Caramel Macchiato Whole Milk	1 grande	320	14	8
Caramel Mocha Whip Soy Milk	1 grande	440	16	7
Caramel Apple Cider No Whip	1 grande	300	0	0
Caramel Apple Cider Whip	1 grande	410	10	7
Caramel Mocha No Whip Whole Milk	1 grande	370	11	6
Caramel Mocha Whip Nonfat Milk	1 grande	410	12	7
Caramel Mocha Whip Whole Milk	1 grande	470	21	12
Caramel Mocha No Whip Nonfat Milk	1 grande	300	3	0
Chocolate Nonfat Milk	1 grande	240	2	0
Chocolate Whole Milk	1 grande	340	15	8
Cinnamon Spice Mocha No Whip Nonfat Milk	1 grande	250	1	0
Cinnamon Spice Mocha No Whip Whole Milk	1 grande	330	12	7
Cinnamon Spice Mocha Whip Nonfat Milk	1 grande	350	11	6
Cinnamon Spice Mocha Whip Whole Milk	1 grande	430	22	14
Cinnamon Spice No Whip Soy Milk	1 grande	290	6	1
Cinnamon Spice Whip Soy Milk	1 grande	390	15	7
Espresso Decaf Coffee Of The Week	1 grande	10	0	0
Frappuccino Blended Coffee	1 grande	230	3	2
Frappuccino Blended Coffee Mocha Coconut No Whip Whole Milk	1 grande	400	10	7
Frappuccino Caramel Blended Coffee No Whip	1 grande	280	4	2
Frappuccino Caramel Blended Coffee Whip	1 grande	430	16	10
Frappuccino Chocolate Blended Creme Whip	1 grande	530	19	10
Frappuccino Chocolate Blended Creme No Whip	1 grande	400	7	2
Frappuccino Chocolate Brownie Blended Coffee No Whip	1 grande	370	9	6
Frappuccino Chocolate Brownie Blended Coffee Whip	1 grande	510	22	15

FOOD	PORTION	CALS	FAT	SAT FAT
Frappuccino Chocolate Malt Blended Creme Whip	1 grande	610	22	11
Frappuccino Mocha Blended Coffee No Whip	1 grande	290	4	2
Frappuccino Mocha Blended Coffee Whip	1 grande	420	16	10
Frappuccino Mocha Coconut Blended Coffee Whip	1 grande	550	22	16
Frappuccino Mocha Malt Blended Coffee No Whip	1 grande	430	7	4
Frappuccino Mocha Malt Blended Coffee Whip	1 grande	570	20	12
Frappuccino Tazo Chai Creme Blended Tea No Whip	1 grande	370	5	1
Frappuccino Tazo Chai Creme Blended Tea Whip	1 grande	500	17	9
Frappuccino Tazoberry Blended Tea	1 grande	190	0	0
Frappuccino Tazoberry Creme Blended Tea No Whip	1 grande	330	2	0
Frappuccino Tazoberry Creme Blended Tea Whip	1 grande	460	14	9
Frappuccino Vanilla Blended Creme No Whip	1 grande	350	5	1
Frappuccino Vanilla Blended Creme Whip	1 grande	480	17	9
Frappuccino White Chocolate Mocha Blended Coffee No Whip	1 grande	320	5	3
Frappuccino White Chocolate Mocha Blended Coffee Whip	1 grande	450	17	11
Hot Chocolate No Whip Whole Milk	1 grande	340	15	8
Hot Chocolate No Whip Nonfat Milk	1 grande	240	2	0
Hot Chocolate Whip Nonfat Milk	1 grande	340	12	7
Hot Chocolate Whip Whole Milk	1 grande	440	24	15
Iced Caffe Mocha Whip Whole Milk	1 grande	350	20	12
Iced Caffe Latte Whole Milk	1 grande	160	8	5
Iced Caffe Mocha Whip Nonfat Milk	1 grande	310	14	9
Iced Caffe Mocha Whip Soy Milk	1 grande	330	17	9
Iced Caffe Americano	1 grande	20	0	0
Iced Caffe Mocha No Whip Whole Milk	1 grande	220	8	4

FOOD	PORTION	CALS	FAT	SAT FAT
Iced Caffe Latte Nonfat Milk	1 grande	100	0	0
Iced Caffe Latte Soy Milk	1 grande	120	5	0
Iced Caffe Mocha No Whip Nonfat Milk	1 grande	180	2	0
Iced Caffe Mocha No Whip Soy Milk	1 grande	200	5	1
Iced Caramel Macchiato Nonfat Milk	1 grande	100	1	1
Iced Caramel Macchiato Soy Milk	1 grande	230	5	1
Iced Caramel Macchiato Whole Milk	1 grande	270	10	6
Iced Shaken Coffee	1 grande	80	0	0
Iced Tazo Chai Nonfat Milk	1 grande	230	0	0
Iced Tazo Chai Whole Milk	1 grande	270	7	4
Iced White Chocolate Mocha No Whip Soy Milk	1 grande	340	8	5
Iced White Chocolate Mocha No Whip Whole Milk	1 grande	360	11	8
Iced White Chocolate Mocha Whip Nonfat Milk	1 grande	450	18	12
Iced White Chocolate Mocha Whip Soy Milk	1 grande	470	20	13
Iced White Chocolate Mocha Whip Whole Milk	1 grande	490	24	16
Iced White Chocolate No Whip Nonfat Milk	1 grande	320	6	5
Milk Nonfat	1 grande	160	0	0
Steamed Apple Cider	1 grande	230	0	0
Steamed Nonfat Milk	1 grande	160	0	0
Steamed Whole Milk	1 grande	270	15	9
Tazo Chai Whole Milk	1 grande	290	7	5
Tazo Chai Nonfat Milk	1 grande	230	0	0
Tazo Iced Tea	1 grande	80	0	0
Tazo Tea Lemonade	1 grande	120	0	0
Vanilla Creme Whip Nonfat Milk	1 grande	340	9	6
Vanilla Creme Whip Whole Milk	1 grande	440	24	15
Vanilla Creme No Whip Nonfat Milk	1 grande	240	0	0
Vanille Creme No Whip Whole Milk	1 grande	340	14	9
White Chocolate Mocha No Whip Nonfat Milk	1 grande	340	5	4
White Chocolate Mocha No Whip Whole Milk	1 grande	410	15	10

FOOD	PORTION	CALS	FAT	SAT FAT
White Chocolate Mocha Whip Nonfat Milk	1 grande	440	14	10
White Chocolate Mocha Whip Whole Milk	1 grande	510	24	16
White Chocolate No Whip Soy Milk	1 grande	370	14	22
White Chocolate Whip Soy Milk	1 grande	440	15	8
White Hot Chocolate No Whip Nonfat Milk	1 grande	390	6	5
White Hot Chocolate No Whip Whole Milk	1 grande	480	18	12
White Hot Chocolate Whip Nonfat Milk	1 grande	490	15	11
White Hot Chocolate Whip Whole Milk	1 grande	580	28	19
Whole Milk	1 grande	270	15	9

TOPPINGS

FOOD	PORTION	CALS	FAT	SAT FAT
Caramel	1 tbsp	15	1	0
Chocolate	1 tsp	5	0	0
Flavored Sugar Free Syrup	1 pump	0	0	0
Flavored Syrup	1 pump	20	0	0
Mocha Syrup	1 pump	25	1	0
Sprinkles	1 serv	0	0	0

STUFF'N TURKEY

FOOD	PORTION	CALS	FAT	SAT FAT
Chef's Salad	1 serv	288	9	3
Grilled Turkey Breast	1 serv	244	3	1
Homemade Turkey Salad	1 serv	651	29	5
Real Fresh Roasted Turkey Breast	1 serv	384	5	1
Rotisserie Turkey Breast	1 serv	251	3	1
Thanksgiving Dinner On A Sandwich	1 serv	605	16	4
Turkey Barbecue	1 serv	478	6	1
Turkey Powerhouse	1 serv	482	11	5

SUBWAY
BEVERAGES

FOOD	PORTION	CALS	FAT	SAT FAT
Fruizle Smoothie Berry Lishus	1 sm (13 oz)	113	0	0
Fruizle Smoothie Berry Lishus w/ Banana	1 sm (17 oz)	221	1	0
Fruizle Smoothie Peach Pizazz	1 sm (12 oz)	103	0	0
Fruizle Smoothie Pineapple Delight w/ Banana	1 sm (17 oz)	241	1	0

FOOD	PORTION	CALS	FAT	SAT FAT
Fruizle Smoothie Pineapple Delite	1 sm (13 oz)	133	0	0
Fruizle Smoothie Sunrise Refresher	1 sm (12 oz)	119	0	0
COOKIES				
Chocolate Chip	1	215	10	4
Chocolate Chunk	1	217	10	4
Double Chocolate	1	209	10	4
M&M	1	215	10	4
Oatmeal Raisin	1	210	8	3
Peanut Butter	1	221	12	4
Sugar	1	227	12	4
White Macadamia Nut	1	221	11	4
SALAD DRESSINGS				
Fat Free French	1 serv (2 oz)	70	0	0
Fat Free Italian	1 serv (2 oz)	20	0	0
Fat Free Ranch	1 serv (2 oz)	60	0	0
SALADS AND SALAD BARS				
BMT	1 serv	275	19	8
Cold Cut Trio	1 serv	234	15	6
Ham	1 serv	112	3	1
Meatball	1 serv	320	20	9
Roast Beef	1 serv	117	3	1
Roasted Chicken Breast	1 serv	130	3	1
Seafood & Crab	1 serv	197	11	4
Steak & Cheese	1 serv	181	8	4
Subway Club	1 serv	146	4	2
Subway Melt	1 serv	203	10	5
Tuna	1 serv	238	16	2
Turkey Breast	1 serv	105	2	0
Turkey Breast & Ham	1 serv	117	3	1
Veggie Delight	1 serv	50	1	0
SANDWICHES				
6 Inch Steak & Cheese	1	362	13	5
6 Inch Subway Melt	1	384	15	5
6 Inch Sub BMT	1	456	24	9
6 Inch Sub Cold Cut Trio	1	415	20	7
6 Inch Sub Ham	1	261	5	2
6 Inch Sub Meatball	1	501	25	10
6 Inch Sub Roast Beef	1	267	5	2
6 Inch Sub Roasted Chicken Breast	1	291	5	2
6 Inch Sub Seafood & Crab	1	378	16	5

FOOD	PORTION	CALS	FAT	SAT FAT
6 Inch Sub Subway Club	1	296	5	2
6 Inch Sub Tuna	1	419	21	5
6 Inch Sub Turkey Breast	1	254	4	1
6 Inch Sub Turkey Breast & Ham	1	267	5	1
6 Inch Sub Veggie Delight	1	200	3	1
American Cheese Triangles	2	41	4	2
Asiago Caesar Sauce	1.5 tbsp	110	11	2
Bacon Strips	2	45	4	2
Breakfast Bacon & Egg	1	321	16	5
Breakfast Cheese & Egg	1	317	15	5
Breakfast Ham & Egg	1	338	14	4
Breakfast Western Egg	1	300	12	4
Cheddar Triangles	2	59	5	3
Cucumber Slices	3	2	0	0
Deli Ham	1	210	4	2
Deli Roast Beef	1	223	5	2
Deli Tuna	1	325	16	5
Deli Turkey Breast	1	215	4	2
Deli Style Roll	1	165	3	1
Dijon Horseradish	1.5 tbsp	91	10	2
Dijon Horseradish Melt	6 inch	465	22	7
Fat Free Red Wine Vinaigrette	1.5 tbsp	29	0	0
Fat Free Sweet Onion	1.5 tbsp	38	0	0
Green Pepper Strips	3 (0.2 oz)	2	0	0
Hearty Italian Bread	6 inch	207	3	2
Honey Mustard	1.5 tbsp	28	0	0
Honey Mustard Ham	6 inch	311	5	2
Honey Oat Bread	6 inch	249	4	1
Italian Bread	6 inch	178	2	1
Lettuce	1 serv (0.7 oz)	3	0	0
Mayonnaise	1 tbsp	111	12	3
Mayonnaise Light	1 tbsp	46	5	1
Monterey Cheddar Bread	6 inch	235	6	4
Mustard	2 tsp	7	0	0
Olive Oil Blend	1 tsp	45	5	1
Olive Rings	3 (3 g)	3	tr	0
Onions	1 serv (0.5 oz)	5	0	0
Parmesan Oregano Bread	6 inch	211	4	2
Pepperjack Cheese Triangles	2	40	4	2
Pickle Chips	3 pieces (0.3 oz)	1	0	0

FOOD	PORTION	CALS	FAT	SAT FAT
Provolone Circles	2 halves	51	4	2
Red Wine Vinaigrette Club	6 inch	350	6	3
Roasted Garlic Bread	6 inch	225	3	2
Sourdough Bread	6 inch	208	3	1
Southwest Sauce	1.5 tbsp	86	9	2
Southwest Turkey Bacon	6 inch	407	17	5
Sweet Onion Chicken Teriyaki	6 inch	374	5	2
Swiss Triangles	2	53	4	3
Tomato Slices	3 (1.2 oz)	7	0	0
Vinegar	1 tsp	1	0	0
Wheat Sub	6 inch	186	2	0
Wrap Chicken Bacon Ranch w/ Swiss	1	480	27	—
Wrap Turkey Bacon Melt	1	430	25	—
SOUPS				
Black Bean	1 cup	180	5	2
Brown & Wild Rice w/ Chicken	1 cup	190	11	5
Cheese w/ Ham & Bacon	1 cup	230	16	6
Chicken & Dumplings	1 cup	130	5	3
Cream Of Broccoli	1 cup	130	7	2
Cream Of Potato w/ Bacon	1 cup	210	12	4
Golden Broccoli Cheese	1 cup	180	12	4
Hearty Chili Beef	1 cup	250	7	3
Minestrone	1 cup	70	1	0
New England Clam Chowder	1 cup	140	5	1
Potato Cheese Chowder	1 cup	210	10	7
Roasted Chicken Noodle	1 cup	90	4	1
Tomato Bisque	1 cup	90	3	1
Vegetable Beef	1 cup	90	2	1

TACO BELL
BEVERAGES

FOOD	PORTION	CALS	FAT	SAT FAT
2% Lowfat Milk	1 serv (8 oz)	110	5	3
Coffee Black	1 serv (12 oz)	5	0	0
Diet Pepsi	1 serv (16 oz)	0	0	0
Dr. Pepper	1 serv (16 oz)	208	0	0
Lipton Iced Tea Sweetened	1 serv (16 oz)	140	0	0
Lipton Iced Tea Unsweetened	1 serv (16 oz)	0	0	0
Mountain Dew	1 serv (16 oz)	227	0	0
Orange Juice	1 serv (6 oz)	80	0	0
Pepsi Cola	1 serv (16 oz)	200	0	0

FOOD	PORTION	CALS	FAT	SAT FAT
Slice	1 serv (16 oz)	200	0	0
BREAKFAST SELECTIONS				
Breakfast Quesadilla Cheese	1 (5.5 oz)	380	21	9
Breakfast Quesadilla w/ Bacon	1 (6 oz)	450	27	11
Breakfast Quesadilla w/ Sausage	1 (6 oz)	430	25	10
Country Breakfast Burrito	1 (4 oz)	270	14	5
Double Bacon & Egg Burrito	1 (6.25 oz)	480	27	9
Fiesta Breakfast Burrito	1 (3.5 oz)	280	16	6
Grande Breakfast Burrito	1 (6.25 oz)	420	22	7
Hash Brown Nuggets	1 serv (3.5 oz)	280	18	5
MAIN MENU SELECTIONS				
7-Layer Burrito	1 (10 oz)	530	23	7
BLT Soft Taco	1 (4.5 oz)	340	23	8
Bacon Cheeseburger Burrito	1 (8.5 oz)	570	31	12
Bean Burrito	1 (7 oz)	380	12	4
Big Beef Burrito Supreme	1 (10.5 oz)	520	23	10
Big Beef MexiMelt	1 (4.75 oz)	290	15	7
Big Chicken Burrito Supreme	1 (9 oz)	510	24	7
Border Sauce Fire	1 serv (0.3 oz)	0	0	0
Border Sauce Hot	1 serv (0.3 oz)	0	0	0
Border Sauce Mild	1 serv (0.3 oz)	0	0	0
Burger Sauce	1 serv (0.5 oz)	60	5	1
Burrito Supreme	1 (9 oz)	440	19	8
Cheddar Cheese	1 serv (0.25 oz)	30	2	2
Cheese Quesadilla	1 (4.25 oz)	350	18	9
Chicken Fajita Wrap	1 (8 oz)	470	22	6
Chicken Fajita Wrap Supreme	1 (9 oz)	520	25	8
Chicken Quesadilla	1 (6 oz)	410	21	10
Chicken Club Burrito	1 (8 oz)	540	32	10
Chili Cheese Burrito	1 (5 oz)	330	13	6
Choco Taco Ice Cream Dessert	1 serv (4 oz)	310	17	10
Cinnamon Twists	1 serv (1 oz)	140	6	0
Club Sauce	1 serv (0.5 oz)	80	8	1
Double Decker Taco	1 (5.75 oz)	340	15	5
Double Decker Taco Supreme	1 (7 oz)	390	19	8
Fajita Sauce	1 serv (0.5 oz)	70	7	1
Green Sauce	1 serv (1 oz)	5	0	0
Grilled Chicken Burrito	1 (7 oz)	410	15	5
Grilled Chicken Soft Taco	1 (4.5 oz)	240	12	4
Grilled Steak Soft Taco	1 (4.5 oz)	230	10	3

FOOD	PORTION	CALS	FAT	SAT FAT
Grilled Steak Soft Taco Supreme	1 (5.75 oz)	290	14	5
Guacamole	1 serv (0.75 oz)	35	3	0
Mexican Pizza	1 serv (7.75 oz)	570	35	10
Mexican Rice	1 serv (4.75 oz)	190	9	4
Nacho Cheese Sauce	2 serv (2 oz)	120	10	3
Nachos	1 serv (3.5 oz)	320	18	4
Nachos Beef Supreme	1 serv (7 oz)	450	24	8
Nachos Bellgrande	1 serv (11 oz)	770	39	11
Picante Sauce	1 serv (0.3 oz)	0	0	0
Pico De Gallo	1 serv (0.75 oz)	5	0	0
Pintos 'n Cheese	1 serv (4.5 oz)	190	9	4
Red Sauce	1 serv (1 oz)	10	0	0
Soft Taco	1 (3.5 oz)	220	10	5
Soft Taco Supreme	1 (5 oz)	260	14	7
Sour Cream	1 serv (0.75 oz)	40	4	3
Steak Fajita Wrap	1 (8 oz)	470	21	6
Steak Fajita Wrap Supreme	1 (9 oz)	510	25	8
Taco	1 (2.75 oz)	180	10	4
Taco Supreme	1 (4 oz)	220	14	7
Taco Salad w/ Salsa	1 (19 oz)	850	52	15
Taco Salad w/ Salsa w/o Shell	1 (16.5 oz)	420	22	11
Three Cheese Blend	1 serv (0.25 oz)	25	2	1
Tostada	1 (6.25 oz)	300	15	5
Veggie Fajita Wrap	1 (8 oz)	420	19	5
Veggie Fajita Wrap Supreme	1 (9 oz)	470	22	7
TACO CABANA				
Black Beans	1 serv (4 oz)	111	tr	—
Borracho Beans	1 serv (4 oz)	108	3	—
Breakfast Taco Bacon & Egg	1	246	12	—
Breakfast Taco Barbacoa	1	307	15	—
Breakfast Taco Chorizo & Egg	1	248	12	—
Breakfast Taco Potato & Egg	1	234	10	—
Burrito Bean & Cheese	1	710	27	—
Burrito Beef	1	653	24	—
Burrito Black Bean	1	559	11	—
Burrito Chicken	1	665	26	—
Calabacita	1 serv (4 oz)	78	5	—
Chips	1 serv (2 oz)	285	14	—
Elotes	1	220	11	—

FOOD	PORTION	CALS	FAT	SAT FAT
Fajitas Beef	1 serv (4 oz)	245	12	—
Fajitas Chicken Dark	1 serv (4 oz)	236	11	—
Fajitas Chicken White	1 serv (4 oz)	191	6	—
Grilled Chicken Dark	1 serv (4.5 oz)	298	18	—
Grilled Chicken Dark No Skin	1 serv (3.4 oz)	170	7	—
Grilled Chicken White	1 serv (5 oz)	295	14	—
Grilled Chicken White No Skin	1 serv (3.8 oz)	167	3	—
Guacamole	1 serv (1 oz)	48	4	—
Queso	1 serv (3 oz)	184	12	—
Refried Beans	1 serv (4 oz)	171	6	—
Sour Cream	1 serv (1 oz)	57	5	—
Spanish Rice	1 serv (4 oz)	181	5	—
Taco Bean & Cheese	1	292	12	—
Taco Black Bean	1	216	5	—
Taco Carne Guisada	1	202	8	—
Taco Crispy Beef	1	148	7	—
Taco Soft Chicken	1	217	9	—
Tortilla Corn	1 6-inch	70	1	—
Tortilla Flour	1 6-inch	129	3	—
Tortilla Soup	1 lg	371	13	—
Tortilla Soup	1 sm	249	8	—

TACO JOHN'S
CHILDREN'S MENU SELECTIONS

Kid's Meal Crispy Taco	1 serv (8 oz)	579	34	10
Kid's Meal Softshell Taco	1 serv (8.5 oz)	617	33	10

DESSERTS

Choco Taco	1 serv (3.5 oz)	320	17	11
Churro	1 serv (1.5 oz)	147	8	2
Flauta Apple	1 serv (2 oz)	84	1	tr
Flauta Cherry	1 serv (2 oz)	143	4	1
Flauta Cream Cheese	1 serv (2 oz)	181	8	3
Italian Ice	1 serv (4 oz)	80	0	0

MAIN MENU SELECTIONS

Bean Burrito	1 (6.5 oz)	387	11	5
Beans Refried	1 serv (9.5 oz)	357	9	2
Beef Burrito	1 (6.5 oz)	449	20	9
Chicken Fajita Burrito	1 (6.25)	370	12	5
Chicken Fajita Salad w/o Dressing	1 serv (12.25 oz)	557	33	9
Chicken Fajita Softshell	1 (4.5 oz)	200	7	3

FOOD	PORTION	CALS	FAT	SAT FAT
Chili	1 serv (9.25 oz)	350	21	10
Chimichanga Platter	1 serv (18 oz)	979	38	15
Combination Burrito	1 (6.5 oz)	418	16	7
Crispy Tacos	1 serv (3.25 oz)	182	11	4
Double Enchilada Platter	1 serv (18.25 oz)	967	42	16
Meat & Potato Burrito	1 (7.75 oz)	503	24	7
Mexi Rolls w/ Nacho Cheese	1 serv (9.75 oz)	863	48	11
Mexican Rice	1 serv (8 oz)	567	18	5
Nacho Cheese	1 serv (2 oz)	300	10	0
Nachos	1 serv (3.5 oz)	333	21	2
Potato Oles	1 serv (4.63 oz)	363	23	5
Potato Oles	1 lg serv (6.12 oz)	484	30	7
Potato Oles Bravo	1 serv (8.88 oz)	579	38	7
Potato Oles w/ Nacho Cheese	1 serv (6.63 oz)	483	33	5
Ranch Burrito	1 (7 oz)	447	23	8
Sampler Platter	1 serv (25.5 oz)	1406	61	24
Sierra Chicken Fillet Sandwich	1 (8.5 oz)	534	29	8
Smothered Burrito Platter	1 serv (19.5 oz)	1031	40	16
Softshell Tacos	1 serv (4.25 oz)	230	10	4
Sour Cream	1 oz	60	5	–
Super Burrito	1 (8.5 oz)	465	19	9
Super Nachos	1 serv (13 oz)	919	56	13
Taco Bravo	1 serv (6.25 oz)	346	14	5
Taco Burger	1 (5 oz)	280	12	5
Taco Salad w/o Dressing	1 (12.4 oz)	584	38	11

TACOTIME

FOOD	PORTION	CALS	FAT	SAT FAT
Casita Burrito Meat	1 serv (12 oz)	647	31	15
Cheddar Cheese	1 serv (0.75 oz)	86	7	4
Chicken	1 serv (2.5 oz)	109	6	2
Chips	1 serv (2 oz)	266	12	3
Crisp Burrito Bean	1 (5.25 oz)	427	18	5
Crisp Burrito Chicken	1 (4.75 oz)	422	25	8
Crisp Burrito Meat	1 (5.25 oz)	552	30	10
Crisp Taco	1 (4 oz)	295	17	7
Crustos	1 serv (3.5 oz)	373	15	–
Double Soft Bean Burrito	1 (9.5 oz)	506	12	6
Double Soft Combination Burrito	1 (9.5 oz)	617	23	10
Double Soft Meat Burrito	1 serv (6.5 oz)	726	33	14
Empanada Cherry	1 (4 oz)	250	9	–

FOOD	PORTION	CALS	FAT	SAT FAT
Enchilada Sauce	1 serv (1 oz)	12	0	0
Flour Tortilla 10 in	1 (2.75 oz)	213	4	1
Flour Tortilla 7 in	1 (1.75 oz)	88	1	0
Flour Tortilla 8 in	1 (1.25 oz)	107	3	1
Fried Flour Tortilla 10 in	1 (2.75 oz)	318	16	4
Fried Flour Tortilla 8 in	1 (1.35 oz)	205	11	2
Guacamole	1 serv (1 oz)	29	2	0
Hot Sauce	1 serv (1 oz)	10	0	0
Lettuce	1 serv (0.5 oz)	2	0	0
Mexi Fries	1 reg (4 oz)	266	17	—
Mexi Fries	1 lg (8 oz)	532	34	—
Mexican Dressing No Fat	1 serv (2 oz)	20	0	—
Mexican Rice	1 serv (4 oz)	159	2	1
Nachos	1 serv (10.5 oz)	680	38	19
Nachos Deluxe	1 serv (15.25 oz)	1048	57	23
Natural Super Taco Meat	1 (11.25 oz)	627	27	13
Olives	1 serv (0.50 oz)	16	2	0
Quesadilla Cheese	1 serv (3.25 oz)	205	11	6
Ranchero Salsa	1 serv (2 oz)	21	1	0
Refritos	1 serv (7 oz)	326	10	5
Refritos	1 serv (2.5 oz)	97	0	0
Rolled Soft Flour Taco	1 (7 oz)	512	23	10
Shredded Beef	1 serv (2.5 oz)	70	7	—
Soft Taco Chicken	1 (7 oz)	387	16	6
Sour Cream	1 serv (1 oz)	55	5	3
Sour Cream Dressing	1 serv (1.5 oz)	137	14	5
Super Shredded Beef Soft Taco	1 (8 oz)	368	11	6
Taco Cheeseburger	1 (7.5 oz)	633	36	10
Taco Meat	1 serv (2.5 oz)	208	11	4
Taco Salad Chicken w/o Dressing	1 serv (9 oz)	370	21	7
Taco Salad w/o Dressing	1 serv (7.75 oz)	479	28	11
Taco Shell 6 in	1 (1.25 oz)	110	6	1
Thousand Island Dressing	1 serv (1 oz)	160	16	2
Tomato	1 serv (0.5 oz)	3	0	0
Tostada Delight Salad Meat	1 (9.75 oz)	628	33	14
Value Soft Bean Burrito	1 (6.75 oz)	380	10	4
Value Soft Meat Burrito	1 (6.75 oz)	491	21	8
Value Soft Taco	1 (5.25 oz)	316	15	7
Veggie Burrito	1 (11 oz)	491	16	6
Wheat Tortilla 11 in	1 (3.5 oz)	175	3	1

FOOD	PORTION	CALS	FAT	SAT FAT
TCBY				
Hand Dipped All Flavors 96% Fat Free	½ cup (3 oz)	140	3	2
Hand Dipped All Flavors Nonfat	½ cup (2.9 oz)	120	0	0
Lowfat Ice Cream All Flavors No Sugar Added	½ cup (2.6 oz)	110	3	2
Nonfat Ice Cream All Flavors	½ cup (2.9 oz)	120	0	0
Soft Serve All Flavors 96% Fat Free	½ cup (3.4 fl oz)	140	3	2
Soft Serve All Flavors No Sugar Added Nonfat	½ cup (2.8 oz)	80	0	0
Soft Serve All Flavors Nonfat	½ cup (3.4 oz)	110	0	0
Sorbet All Flavors Nonfat & Nondairy	½ cup (3.4 oz)	100	0	0
TGI FRIDAY'S				
Corn Salsa	1 serv	175	3	–
Fresh Vegetable Medley w/ Potato	1 serv	470	8	–
Fresh Vegetable Medley w/ Rice	1 serv	407	8	–
Friday's Gardenburger	1	445	9	–
Garden Dagwood Sandwich	1 serv	375	11	–
Pacific Coast Chicken	1 serv	415	8	–
Pacific Coast Tuna	1 serv	410	8	–
Pea Salsa	1 serv (6.4 oz)	175	3	–
Plum Sauce	1 serv	105	0	0
Salad & Baked Potato	1 serv	250	5	–
Sizzling Chicken & Broccoli	1 serv	700	40	–
Sizzling NY Strip Steak w/ Blue Cheese & Broccoli	1 serv	684	36	–
Turkey Burger	1 (9.8 oz)	410	19	–
TIM HORTONS				
BAGELS AND CREAM CHEESE				
Blueberry	1	200	2	0
Cinnamon Raisin	1	300	2	0
Cream Cheese	1.5 oz	150	12	8
Cream Cheese	1.5 oz	150	12	9
Cream Cheese Light	1.5 oz	90	7	5
Cream Cheese Plain	1.5 oz	140	14	10
Everything	1	300	2	0
Multigrain	1	300	3	0
Onion	1	295	2	0
Plain	1	290	2	0

FOOD	PORTION	CALS	FAT	SAT FAT
Poppy Seed	1	300	3	0
Sesame Seed	1	300	3	0
Whole Wheat & Honey	1	300	2	0
BAKED SELECTIONS				
Biscuit Southern Country Cranberry	1	470	19	5
Biscuit Southern Country Raspberry	1	470	19	5
Cake Black Forest	1 serv	500	21	14
Cake Celebration	1 serv	500	16	8
Cake Chocolate Fantasy	1 serv	420	15	7
Cake Shadow	1 serv	430	19	10
Cookie Chocolate Chip	1	150	7	3
Cookie Macaroon	1	140	8	7
Cookie Oatcakes	1	190	10	4
Cookie Oatmeal Raisin	1	150	6	2
Cookie Peanut Butter	1	170	10	3
Cookie Peanut Butter Chocolate Chunk	1	170	10	4
Croissant Butter	1	210	11	6
Croissant Cheese	1	240	12	5
Danish Cherry Cheese	1	380	23	9
Donut Apple Fritter	1	300	14	5
Donut Chocolate Dip	1	230	10	3
Donut Chocolate Glazed	1	360	22	7
Donut Dutchie	1	280	13	4
Donut Honey Dip	1	230	10	3
Donut Maple Dip	1	250	10	3
Donut Old Fashion Glazed	1	270	12	4
Donut Old Fashion Plain	1	220	12	4
Donut Sour Cream Plain	1	280	18	6
Donut Sugar Twist	1	230	10	3
Donut Walnut Crunch	1	320	18	5
Donut Filled Angel Cream	1	280	13	4
Donut Filled Blueberry	1	220	8	3
Donut Filled Boston Cream	1	230	8	3
Donut Filled Canadian Maple	1	230	8	3
Donut Filled Strawberry	1	220	8	3
Donuts Honey Stick	1	280	15	5
Muffin Blueberry Bran	1	300	9	2
Muffin Carrot Whole Wheat	1	410	22	2
Muffin Chocolate Chip	1	390	15	4

FOOD	PORTION	CALS	FAT	SAT FAT
Muffin Oatbran 'n Apple	1	350	12	3
Muffin Oatbran Carrot 'n Raisin	1	340	11	2
Muffin Oatmeal Raisin	1	430	11	2
Muffin Raisin Bran	1	380	10	2
Muffin Wild Blueberry	1	330	11	2
Muffin Low Fat Carrot	1	260	2	0
Muffin Low Fat Cranberry	1	260	2	0
Muffin Low Fat Honey	1	290	2	0
Pie Apple	1 serv	540	31	6
Pie Banana Cream	1 serv	440	26	13
Pie Cherry	1 serv	570	31	6
Pie Chocolate Cream	1 serv	490	31	16
Tart Fresh Strawberry	1 serv	220	9	2
Tart Raisin Butter	1 serv	330	11	3
Tea Biscuit Plain	1	220	6	2
Tea Biscuit Raisin	1	250	6	2
Timbits Chocolate Glazed	1	70	3	1
Timbits Dutchie	1	60	2	0
Timbits Honey Dip	1	50	1	0
Timbits Old Fashion Plain	1	45	2	0
Timbits Filled Banana Cream	1	45	1	0
Timbits Filled Lemon	1	50	2	0
Timbits Filled Spiced Apple	1	80	1	0
Timbits Filled Strawberry	1	50	1	0
BEVERAGES				
Apple Juice	1 (9 oz)	140	0	0
Cafe Mocha	1 (10 oz)	250	10	4
Cappuccino English Toffee	1 (10 oz)	130	5	4
Cappuccino French Vanilla	1 (10 oz)	130	5	4
Cappuccino Iced	1 (16 oz)	430	23	14
Chocolate Milk	1 (14 oz)	280	5	3
Coffee Decaffeinated + Sugar & Cream	1 (10 oz)	80	4	2
Coffee + Sugar & Cream	1 (10 oz)	80	4	2
Coke	1 (14 oz)	170	0	0
Diet Coke	1 (14 oz)	1	0	0
Fruit Punch	1 (10 oz)	150	0	0
Hot Chocolate	1 (10 oz)	200	6	2
Iced Tea	1 (14 oz)	130	0	0
Milk 2%	1 (14 oz)	210	6	5

FOOD	PORTION	CALS	FAT	SAT FAT
Orange Juice	1 (10 oz)	140	0	0
Sprite	1 (14 oz)	160	0	0
Tea + Sugar & Milk	1 (10 oz)	45	0	0
SANDWICHES				
Albacore Tuna Salad	1 serv	350	8	1
Black Forest Ham & Swiss	1 serv	640	27	9
Chunky Chicken Salad	1 serv	380	10	1
Fireside Roast Beef	1 serv	470	19	3
Garden Vegetable	1 serv	460	24	11
Harvet Turkey Breast	1 serv	470	18	2
SOUPS				
Barley & Wild Rice	1 serv	120	2	0
Chicken Noodle	1 serv	100	3	1
Chili	1 serv	320	9	3
Cream Of Broccoli	1 serv	190	7	2
Cream of Mushroom	1 serv	195	10	3
Hearty Vegetable	1 serv	130	2	0
Minestrone	1 serv	125	2	0
Potato Bacon	1 serv	195	7	2
Vegetable Beef Barley	1 serv	110	2	0

TOGO'S
SALAD DRESSINGS

FOOD	PORTION	CALS	FAT	SAT FAT
1000 Island	1 serv (2.3 oz)	231	22	–
Caesar	1 serv (2.3 oz)	241	23	–
Oriental	1 serv (2.3 oz)	221	14	–
Ranch	1 serv (2.3 oz)	321	33	–
Reduced Calorie Italian	1 serv (2.3 oz)	60	5	–
Reduced Calorie Ranch	1 serv (2.3 oz)	191	16	–
SALADS AND SALAD BARS				
Caesar Salad	1 serv	471	31	–
Garden Salad	1 serv	256	10	–
Oriental Salad	1 serv	499	21	–
Taco Salad	1 serv	943	59	–
SANDWICHES				
Albacore Tuna	1 sm	701	30	–
Avocado & Turkey	1 sm	675	28	–
Avocado Cucumber & Alfalfa Sprouts	1 sm	637	28	–
Bar-B-Q Beef	1 sm	724	22	–
California Roasted Chicken	1 sm	510	15	–

FOOD	PORTION	CALS	FAT	SAT FAT
Cheese Swiss American Provolone	1 sm	859	46	—
Chunky Chicken Salad	1 sm	636	26	—
Egg Salad w/ Cheese	1 sm	728	35	—
Ham & Cheese	1 sm	661	26	—
Hot Pastrami	1 sm	705	26	—
Hummus	1 sm	668	21	—
Italian Salami & Cheese	1 sm	770	33	—
Italian Salami Capicolla Mortadella Cotto & Provolone	1 sm	736	32	—
Meatballs w/ Pizza Sauce & Parmesan	1 sm	707	28	—
Pastrami Reuben	1 sm	875	45	—
Roast Beef Hot & Cold	1 sm	552	11	—
Turkey & Cranberry	1 sm	623	13	—
Turkey & Bacon Club	1 sm	667	26	—
Turkey & Cheese	1 sm	638	23	—
Turkey & Ham w/ Cheese	1 sm	670	25	—

TROPIGRILL

FOOD	PORTION	CALS	FAT	SAT FAT
Banana Tropical	1 serv (7.55 oz)	498	14	—
Black Beans (combo meal portion)	1 serv (4.78 oz)	153	2	—
Black Beans (side)	1 serv (8.39 oz)	269	4	—
Boiled Yuca	1 serv (12 oz)	334	0	—
Boneless Breast	1 serv (3.14 oz)	140	4	—
Cheese Potatoes	1 serv (7.42 oz)	177	6	—
Chicken ¼ Dark Meat	1 serv (4.52 oz)	298	18	—
Chicken ¼ Dark Meat w/o Skin	1 serv (3.42 oz)	170	7	—
Chicken ¼ White Meat	1 serv (5.09 oz)	295	14	—
Chicken ¼ White Meat w/o Skin	1 serv (3.82 oz)	167	3	—
Chicken Caesar Sandwich	1 (6.4 oz)	457	20	—
Chicken Sandwich	1 (7.92 oz)	442	19	—
Congri	1 serv (7.08 oz)	439	13	—
Vegetable Kabob	1 (3.07 oz)	106	1	—
White Rice	1 serv (6.82 oz)	341	6	—
Yellow Rice	1 serv (7 oz)	294	5	—
Yucatan Fries	1 serv (5.3 oz)	440	24	—

VILLAGE INN

FOOD	PORTION	CALS	FAT	SAT FAT
French Toast Cinnamon Raisin	1 serv	809	16	4
Fruit & Nut Pancakes Low Cholesterol	1 serv	936	19	2
Omelette Chicken & Cheese	1 serv	721	19	4
Omelette Fresh Veggie	1 serv	704	18	4

FOOD	PORTION	CALS	FAT	SAT FAT
Omelette Mushroom & Cheese	1 serv	680	18	4
Turkey & Vegetable Scrambled Sensation	1 serv	726	19	4

WENDY'S
BEVERAGES
Cola	11 oz	130	0	0
Diet Cola	11 oz	0	0	0
Frosty Junior	6 oz	170	4	3
Frosty Medium	16 oz	440	11	7
Frosty Small	12 oz	330	8	5
Lemon-Lime Soda	11 oz	130	0	0

CHILDREN'S MENU SELECTIONS
French Fries Kid's Meal	1 serv (3.2 oz)	270	13	2
Kid's Meal Cheeseburger	1 (4.2 oz)	310	12	6
Kid's Meal Hamburger	1 (3.9 oz)	270	9	3
Kids'Meal Chicken Nuggets	4 pieces (2.1 oz)	190	13	3

MAIN MENU SELECTIONS
¼ lb Hamburger Patty	1 (2.6 oz)	200	14	6
2 Oz Hamburger Patty	1 (1.3 oz)	100	7	3
American Cheese	1 slice (0.6 oz)	70	6	4
American Cheese Jr.	1 slice (0.4 oz)	45	4	3
Bacon	1 strip (4 g)	20	2	1
Baked Potato Chili & Cheese	1 (15.4 oz)	630	24	9
Big Bacon Classic	1 (9.9 oz)	580	30	12
Breaded Chicken Fillet	1 (3.5 oz)	230	11	2
Cheddar Cheese Shredded	2 tbsp (0.6 oz)	70	6	4
Cheddar Shredded	2 tbsp (0.6 oz)	70	6	4
Chicken Breast Fillet Sandwich	1 (7.3 oz)	430	16	3
Chicken Club Sandwich	1 (7.6 oz)	470	20	5
Chicken Nuggets	5 pieces (2.6 oz)	230	16	3
Chili	1 sm (8 oz)	210	7	3
Chili	1 lg (12 oz)	310	10	4
Classic Single w/ Everything	1 (7.6 oz)	410	19	7
French Fries	1 Great Biggie (6.7 oz)	570	27	4
French Fries	1 Biggie (5.6 oz)	470	23	4
French Fries	1 med (5 oz)	420	20	3
Grilled Chicken Fillet	1 (2.9 oz)	110	3	1
Grilled Chicken Sandwich	1 (6.6 oz)	300	7	2

FOOD	PORTION	CALS	FAT	SAT FAT
Honey Mustard Reduced Calorie	1 tsp (7 g)	25	2	0
Hot Stuffed Bake Potato Plain	1 (10 oz)	310	0	0
Hot Stuffed Baked Potato Bacon & Cheese	1 (12.6 oz)	530	18	4
Hot Stuffed Baked Potato Broccoli & Cheese	1 (14.4 oz)	470	14	3
Jr. Bacon Cheeseburger	1 (5.8 oz)	380	19	7
Jr. Cheeseburger	1 (4.5 oz)	310	12	6
Jr. Cheeseburger Deluxe	1 (6.3 oz)	360	16	6
Kaiser Bun	1 (2.5 oz)	200	3	1
Ketchup	1 tsp (7 g)	10	0	0
Lettuce	1 leaf (0.5 oz)	0	0	0
Mayonnaise	1½ tsp (9 g)	30	3	0
Mustard	½ tsp (5 g)	5	0	0
Nuggets Sauce Barbeque	1 pkg (1 oz)	45	0	0
Nuggets Sauce Honey Mustard	1 pkg (1 oz)	130	12	2
Nuggets Sauce Sweet & Sour	1 pkg (1 oz)	50	0	0
Onion	4 rings (0.5 oz)	5	0	0
Pickles	4 slices (0.4 oz)	0	0	0
Saltines	2 (0.2 oz)	25	1	0
Sandwich Bun	1 (2 oz)	160	2	0
Spicy Chicken Fillet	1 (3.6 oz)	210	9	2
Spicy Chicken Sandwich	1 (7.5 oz)	410	14	3
Tomatoes	1 slice (0.9 oz)	5	0	0
Whipped Margarine	1 pkg (0.5 oz)	70	7	2
SALAD DRESSINGS				
Blue Cheese	1 pkg (2 oz)	360	36	7
French	1 pkg (2 oz)	250	21	3
Hidden Valley Ranch	1 pkg (2 oz)	200	20	3
Hidden Valley Ranch Reduced Fat Reduced Calorie	1 pkg (2 oz)	120	11	2
Italian Reduced Fat Reduced Calorie	1 pkg (2 oz)	80	7	1
Italian Caesar	1 pkg (1.5 oz)	230	24	4
Thousand Island	1 pkg (2 oz)	260	25	4
SALADS AND SALAD BARS				
Bacon Bits	2 tbsp (0.5 oz)	45	2	1
Caesar Side Salad w/o Dressing	1 (3.2 oz)	110	5	3
Chicken Salad	2 tbsp (1.2 oz)	70	5	1
Deluxe Garden Salad w/o Dressing	1 (9.5 oz)	110	6	1
Grilled Chicken Salad w/o Dressing	1 (11.9 oz)	200	7	2

FOOD	PORTION	CALS	FAT	SAT FAT
Side Salad w/o Dressing	1 (5.4 oz)	60	3	1
Soft Breadstick	1 (1.5 oz)	130	3	1
Taco Chips	15 (1.5 oz)	210	9	2
Taco Salad w/o Dressing	1 (16.4 oz)	380	19	10

WHATABURGER
BAKED SELECTIONS

FOOD	PORTION	CALS	FAT	SAT FAT
Biscuit	1	280	13	—
Blueberry Muffin	1	239	8	—
Cinnamon Roll	1	320	16	—
Cookie Chocolate Chunk	1	247	16	—
Cookie White Chocolate Macadamia Nut	1	269	16	—
Fried Apple Turnover	1	215	11	—

BEVERAGES

FOOD	PORTION	CALS	FAT	SAT FAT
Cherry Coke	1 reg	227	0	0
Coffee	1 sm	5	0	0
Coke Classic	1 reg	211	0	0
Creamer	1 pkg	10	1	—
Diet Coke	1 reg	2	0	0
Dr. Pepper	1 reg	207	1	—
Iced Tea	1 reg	5	0	0
Lemon Juice	1 pkg	1	0	0
Milk 2%	1 serv	113	4	—
Orange Juice	1 serv (10 oz)	140	0	0
Root Beer	1 reg	237	0	0
Shake Chocolate	1 junior	364	9	—
Shake Strawberry	1 junior	352	9	—
Shake Vanilla	1 junior	325	10	—
Sprite	1 reg	211	0	0
Sugar	1 pkg	15	0	0
Sweet And Low	1 pkg	4	0	0

BREAKFAST SELECTIONS

FOOD	PORTION	CALS	FAT	SAT FAT
Biscuit w/ Bacon	1	359	20	—
Biscuit w/ Bacon Egg & Cheese	1	511	33	—
Biscuit w/ Egg & Cheese	1	434	26	—
Biscuit w/ Sausage	1	446	29	—
Biscuit w/ Sausage Egg & Cheese	1	601	42	—
Biscuit w/ Sausage Gravy	1	479	27	—
Breakfast Platter w/ Bacon	1 serv	695	44	—

FOOD	PORTION	CALS	FAT	SAT FAT
Breakfast Platter w/ Sausage	1 serv	785	53	—
Breakfast On A Bun w/ Bacon	1	365	19	—
Breakfast On A Bun w/ Sausage	1	455	28	—
Butter	1 pkg	36	4	—
Egg Omelette Sandwich	1	288	13	—
Grape Jelly	1 pkg	45	0	0
Hashbrowns	1 serv	150	9	—
Honey	1 pkg	25	0	0
Margarine	1 pkg	25	3	—
Pancake Syrup	1 pkg	180	0	0
Pancakes	3	259	6	—
Pancakes w/ Bacon	1 serv	335	12	—
Pancakes w/ Sausage	1 serv	426	21	—
Scrambled Eggs	2	189	15	—
Strawberry Jam	1 pkg	40	0	0
Taquito Bacon & Egg	1	335	16	—
MAIN MENU SELECTIONS				
Bacon	1 slice	38	3	—
Cheese Slice	1 lg	89	7	—
Cheese Slice	1 sm	46	4	—
Chicken Strips	2	120	5	—
Club Crackers	1 pkg	30	2	—
Croutons	1 pkg	30	1	—
Fajita Beef	1	326	12	—
Fajita Grilled Chicken	1	272	7	—
French Fries	1 junior	221	12	—
French Fries	1 lg	442	24	—
French Fries	1 reg	332	18	—
Garden Salad	1	56	1	—
Grilled Chicken Salad	1 serv	150	1	—
Grilled Chicken Sandwich	1	442	14	—
Grilled Chicken Sandwich w/o Bun Oil w/ Mustard	1	300	3	—
Grilled Chicken Sandwich w/o Bun Oil & Dressing	1	358	6	—
Grilled Chicken Sandwich w/o Dressing	1	385	9	—
Jalapeno Pepper	1	3	tr	—
Justaburger	1	276	11	—
Ketchup	1 pkg	30	0	0